HANDBOOK OF SEXUAL DYSFUNCTIONS

Related Titles of Interest

Karen S. Calhoun and Beverly M. Atkeson
Treatment of Rape Victims: Facilitating Psychosocial Adjustment
ISBN: 0-205-14296-6 (paper)
ISBN: 0-205-14297-4 (cloth)

Robert G. Meyer
The Clinician's Handbook, Third Edition
ISBN: 0-205-14230-3

C. Eugene Walker, Barbara L. Bonner, and Keith L. Kaufman
The Physically and Sexually Abused Child: Evaluation and Treatment
ISBN: 0-205-14493-4 (paper)
ISBN: 0-205-14494-2 (cloth)

Mark G. Winiarski
AIDS-Related Psychotherapy
ISBN: 0-205-14511-6

HANDBOOK OF
SEXUAL DYSFUNCTIONS
Assessment and Treatment

Edited by

WILLIAM O'DONOHUE
Northern Illinois University

JAMES H. GEER
Louisiana State University

Allyn and Bacon

Boston   London   Toronto   Sydney   Tokyo   Singapore

Library of Congress Cataloging-in-Publication Data

Handbook of sexual dysfunctions : assessment and treatment / edited by
  William O'Donohue, James H. Geer
     p.   cm.
  Includes bibliographical references and index.
  ISBN 0-205-14787-9
  1. Psychosexual disorders.   2. Sexual disorders.   I. O'Donohue,
William T.   II. Geer, James.
  [DNLM: 1. Psychosexual Disorders—diagnosis.   2. Psychosexual
Disorders—therapy.   3. Sex Disorders—diagnosis.   4. Sex Disorders—
therapy.   WM 611 H2363]
RC556.H36   1993
616.6'9—dc20
DNLM/DCL
for Library of Congress   92-48984
                                          CIP

ISBN 0-205-14787-9
H47871

ABOUT THE EDITORS

William O'Donohue is currently Assistant Professor of Psychology at Northern Illinois University. He received a Ph.D. in clinical psychology from the State University of New York at Stony Brook in 1987. He also pursued graduate study in philosophy and the philosophy of science at Indiana University. He has previously co-edited (with James H. Geer) *Theories of Human Sexuality* (1987; Plenum Press), *The Sexual Abuse of Children: Theory and Research,* and *The Sexual Abuse of Children: Clinical Issues* (both 1992; Lawrence Erlbaum). He has published works on premature ejaculation, the roles of conditioning in sexual arousal, psychophysiological assessment of sexual arousal, and various aspects of child sexual abuse.

James H. Geer received his B.S., M.S., and Ph.D. degrees from the University of Pittsburgh. He has held faculty positions at the State University of New York at Buffalo, the University of Pennsylvania, the State University of New York at Stony Brook, and Louisiana State University, where he is currently Professor in the Department of Psychology. Dr. Geer has had visiting appointments at universities in England and The Netherlands. He is a Fellow of the American Psychological Society and the American Psychological Association. Dr. Geer has published widely in the areas of emotion and psychophysiology. For the past 15 years, he has concentrated on research in human sexuality.

ABOUT THE CONTRIBUTORS

J. Gayle Beck received a Ph.D. in Psychology from the State University of New York at Albany and is currently Associate Professor at the University of Houston. She has published extensively in the areas of sexual dysfunctions, behavior therapy, and adult anxiety disorders. Dr. Beck is the author of *Patterns of Sexual Arousal: Psychophysiological Processes and Clinical Applications* (along with Raymond Rosen, Ph.D.), as well as numerous research articles and chapters.

Joost Dekker, Ph.D., is both a scientist and a practitioner. In his research he has focused on psychophysiological studies on sexual arousal and studies on sex therapy. As a practitioner he is concerned with sexual dysfunctions and sexual paraphilias. His current research is in the field of behavioral medicine.

Walter Everaerd is Professor and Chair of the Department of Clinical Psychology at the University of Amsterdam. He is on the board of the Institute of Emotion and Motivation, also in Amsterdam. His research has moved from behavior therapy to behavioral medicine, with a special interest in psychophysiological symptom perception research and sex research.

Ruth G. Gold received her master's degree in Clinical Psychology in 1980 and her master's in Business Administration in 1990, both from Western Carolina University. Currently she is Assessment Coordinator at Northern Illinois University. Her research interests include sexual abuse and its consequences, as well as treatment of adult sexual dysfunction.

Steven R. Gold received his Ph.D. in Clinical Psychology from Purdue University in 1969. He is currently Professor of Psychology and Director of Clinical Training at Northern Illinois University. His research interests include sexual fantasy, sexual and dating aggression, and consequences of child sexual abuse.

Benjamin Graber, M.D., currently president of the Graber Company, prefers to think of himself as a naturalist. A former Professor of Psychiatry, selected for the International Academy of Sex, Dr. Graber's 1975 publication *Woman's Orgasm* remains in print. His parents were proudest of his two appearances on the Phil Donahue Show in the 1970s.

David Kresin, M.D., practices family medicine in Aurora, Colorado and teaches residents as Assistant Clinical Professor at the University of Colorado School of Medicine, Department of Family Practice.

Elizabeth Letourneau is currently working toward a Ph.D. in Clinical Psychology at Northern Illinois University. She received her M.A. in Clinical Psychology from Northern Illinois University in 1992 and her B.A. from the State University of New York at Buffalo in 1988. Ms. Letourneau has co-authored articles and chapters on a variety of topics, including sexual dysfunctions, physiological assessment of male sexual arousal, and treatment issues in sexual paraphilias. In conjunction with Dr. William O'Donohue, she has developed a sex fantasy questionnaire for male paraphilics.

Todd E. Lininger, M.D., is currently Assistant Clinical Professor of Anesthesiology at Wayne State University School of Medicine and Director of the North Oakland Pain Management Service in Waterford, Michigan. His clinical interests include reflex sympathetic dystrophy, post-herpetic neuralgia, and chronic myofascial pain.

Patricia J. Morokoff is Associate Professor of Psychology at the University of Rhode Island. She received her Ph.D. in Clinical Psychology from the State University of New York at Stony Brook in 1980. Dr. Morokoff has published research and theoretical papers in the psychophysiology of sexual arousal, hormones and

sexual behavior, gender issues in sexuality, and women's health, including prevention of AIDS in women.

Randal P. Quevillon, Ph.D., is currently Professor and Chair of Psychology at the University of South Dakota and is on the faculty of the Clinical Psychology doctoral training program. He has published papers in the areas of depression, self-control, community psychology, sexual dysfunction, disaster response, and rural mental health. Dr. Quevillon can be contacted at the Psychology Department, University of South Dakota, Vermillion, SD 57069-2390.

Richard Reid, M.D., Director of Gynecologic Laser Services at Sinai Hospital and Assistant Professor of Obstetrics and Gynecology at Wayne State University School of Medicine, has focused his professional interest on the study of cervical neoplasia, including the relationship of human papillomavirus to lower genital tract neoplasia. Dr. Reid has authored over 100 international journal articles and has contributed to 12 books on gynecology and oncology. He is also a member of the Committee for Medical Devices of the Federal Drug Administration. Dr. Reid's special area of research recently has been in the treatment of vulvodynia (an illness characterized by intense burning or itching of the vulva). He has pioneered the use of the flash-pumped dye laser in treating this disease. In addition, he has developed an operation utilizing the CO_2 laser for the removal of the Bartholin's glands.

Kathleen Blindt Segraves, Ph.D., is Assistant Professor of Psychiatry at the Case Western Reserve University School of Medicine and Director of the Behavioral Medicine Treatment Unit at MetroHealth Medical Center, both in Cleveland, Ohio. Dr. Segraves has co-authored numerous chapters and scientific articles in the fields of behavioral medicine and sexual disorders. A distinguished authority in the field of sex therapy, she has lectured and consulted widely on the effects of pharmacological agents on female sexuality.

Robert Taylor Segraves, M.D., Ph.D., is Professor of Psychiatry at the Case Western Reserve University School of Medicine and Associate Director of the Department of Psychiatry at MetroHealth Medical Center, both in Cleveland, Ohio. Dr. Segraves has authored and edited several texts in the field of marital therapy and sexual disorders. He is past President of the Society for Sex Therapy and Research and currently Editor of the *Journal of Sex Education and Therapy*.

Wendy Stock, Ph.D., is a clinical psychologist and Assistant Professor at Texas A&M University. Dr. Stock received her doctoral degree from the State University of New York at Stony Brook. She received both clinical and research training at the Sex Therapy Center at Stony Brook.

CONTENTS

PREFACE

Human sexual functioning is an important topic. Satisfactory sexual functioning is a significant element in living a good, full life. It is involved in creating children, in forming a special kind of bond with another, in the pursuit and giving of a special kind of physical pleasure, in adult play, and even in our images of ourselves. Because sex is interpersonal in nature, satisfactory sexual functioning in one individual is also critical to the pursuit of these ends by another.

It is also a subject as difficult as any. Perhaps one of the most salient facts about human sexuality is that accurate information about it is hard to come by. Clinicians and researchers alike know that individuals often refuse to disclose sexual information or give only distorted information. This reticence might have something to do with the power and importance of sex alluded to above, but also there might be something inherently private about it. After all, individuals and couples almost always choose to make the sexual acts themselves private. Moreover, sex-

ual functioning is difficult to study because of the number of factors affecting it in complex ways.

The importance of sex to a healthy life makes it an important area for scientific study. Humans suffer from their sexual problems and those of their partners and seek help to alleviate these problems. This book attempts to bring together the best information available on the diverse sexual problems, as well as describing the research agenda for the future. We have followed the taxonomy of sexual dysfunctions contained in the DSM-III-R, as this seems to be the classification system that is currently the most widely used. We have asked each chapter author to write on the psychopathology, assessment, and treatment of each disorder, and also to outline important questions for future research.

For each group of dysfunctions (desire, arousal, orgasm, and pain disorders), the book also contains a chapter written by a physician on the medical aspects of that group of dysfunctions. A knowledge of medical factors is essential. Sexual functioning has a physiological substrate, which may be disordered and may require medical treatment for its amelioration. Of course, the converse is also true: Psychological and social variables affect sexual functioning and, when disordered, may require direct psychological intervention. It is hoped that these chapters will provide an increased understanding of the interplay of these two domains, so as to bring about better understanding and treatment of the sexual dysfunctions.

We are indebted to many individuals. Our foremost thanks go to the chapter authors for the efforts that culminated in their excellent contributions to this work. Without their countless hours of hard work, this project would not have been possible. We would also like to thank the late Jerry Frank of Pergamon Press; his helpfulness, support, and astute judgment will always be fondly remembered. Our new editor at Allyn and Bacon, Mylan Jaixen, has already demonstrated encouragement, acumen, and patience that we have found most beneficial. We express our great appreciation to Gary Coover, who provided invaluable assistance by reading chapters with a critical eye. Finally, we are also indebted to Cindy Buck, Judy Atherton, and Cheryl Ross for their help with diverse aspects of the manuscript.

Last but far from least, we would like to express our appreciation to our families—Jane, Katherine, Jean, John, and David—for their support and encouragement.

William O'Donohue
James H. Geer

CHAPTER 1

RESEARCH ISSUES IN THE SEXUAL DYSFUNCTIONS

William O'Donohue, Northern Illinois University
James Geer, Louisiana State University

In this chapter we will outline the corpus of knowledge that is required for a comprehensive understanding and effective treatment of the sexual dysfunctions (SDs). It is our goal to identify some of the major questions within the field, so as to provide a perspective on the complexity and interdependence of these problems. The emphasis on complexity is not intended to give rise to undue skepticism or to be overly critical of extant work, but rather to provide a synoptic view of the difficulties and subtleties involved in many of the major problems in the field. Thus, the following clusters of research problems relevant to these goals will be examined: descriptive pathology (including taxonomic, epidemiological, etiological, and pathophysiological issues), assessment problems (including the psychometric adequacy of various assessment strategies relevant to SDs, as well as the multivariate nature of SDs), and intervention issues (including identifying effective interventions, their relative efficacy, and effective preventive programs).

We will support our claim that this information is required for a comprehensive understanding and effective clinical response by citing a few examples of the roles some of this information plays in the spectrum of clinical activities, as follows. (1) Preventive programs require an accurate understanding of the etiology of a SD, because to prevent some effect, one must block a necessary cause and all sufficient causes from actualizing. Thus, to have any effect on the prevention of a sexual dysfunction, the clinician must have some knowledge of etiology of that SD. (2) In the effective treatment of an existing SD, the clinician must accurately assess what problems the individual has and the magnitude of those problems. Moreover, accurate assessment is necessary in order to understand the extent to which the intervention actually is helpful (or harmful). Hence, the clinician must have knowledge of assessment issues. (3) Finally, in order to choose among a plethora of possible interventions, a clinician must know which of these is the best for the particular disorder and client. Therefore, intervention issues become relevant.

By explicating various questions in this area, we hope to facilitate a greater understanding of the structure and complexity of the field. Also, the somewhat unsystematic and informal responses to these problems can thus be exposed to the light of criticism, and this critical feedback can produce a growth of knowledge. Many complex questions arise in any attempt to understand and change human behavior—more so when investigating sexual behavior, given its manifold relationships with interpersonal functioning, values, and physiology.

For each of the chapters that follow, we encourage the reader to examine the degree to which the foregoing questions have been adequately answered for each subtype of sexual disorder. The reader should distinguish between unsupported assertions, partially supported hypotheses, and well-corroborated claims. Knowledge has been defined as justified true belief (Cornman, Lehrer, & Pappas, 1982), and in the empirical sciences, justification is taken to be a function of properly designed experiments. The reader is therefore encouraged to examine critically the methodological characteristics of studies that are cited as evidence in support of any particular conclusion.

DESCRIPTIVE PATHOLOGY

Taxonomic Issues

Attempts at classification in the behavioral sciences have proven controversial, as classification is closely connected with fundamental questions about human nature and methodological controversies concerning the study of humans. Some question whether classification is possible, due to the allegedly essentially idiosyncratic nature of each individual. Others carry on a wide-ranging debate as to what features to pick out, among many possible candidates for the classification scheme.

Taxonomies serve a number of functions. Any classification system provides the basic ontology of the field: It makes basic claims about what is said to exist. Moreover, the science's search for regularities and laws depends on the use of the right categories—ones that "carve nature at its joints." The ancient Greek cosmologist Anaximander attempted to analyze all things into the four basic elements of fire, earth, air, and water. However, this rudimentary chemistry failed because it did not yield accurate predictions and explanations. A successful classification system provides the categories that will serve as the essential constituents in scientific laws. A taxonomy should also provide homogenous groupings in which the classification principles are specified, as well as the criteria that distinguish different kinds of entities. As a result, like things are treated alike, and different things are treated differently by the classification system. More pragmatically, a taxonomy provides the *lingua franca* of the discipline. Supplying the standard vocabulary of the field, it provides a structure for information storage and retrieval. Thus, for economy of expression, a satisfactory classification system should make all necessary distinctions without losing any relevant information, and, for the sake of efficiency, it should make no unnecessary distinctions.

The following are among the many fundamental taxonomic questions in the field of sexual dysfunction. *What constitutes a sexual problem?* Should sexual problems be defined in relation to descriptive information about average sexual behavior in some population? (If so, how is the norm to be determined, and what becomes a clinically significant deviation?) Should problems be defined in relation to an individual's goals? (If so, can the individual's goals themselves be problematic?) Or should they be defined in relation to some set of values regarding what constitutes sexual health? This last possibility gives rise to the following questions. *(1) What constitutes healthy (or "normal," "nondisordered," etc.) sexual functioning? (2) Can a sexual problem be defined entirely in value-free, empirical terms, or are value and ethical judgments inevitably embedded in any definition of a sexual problem?* For example, what constitutes a sexual desire problem? For St. Augustine (Lord, give me continence, but not now!), the presence of sexual desire is problematic (Szasz, 1980), but in current thinking only low desire (not high) is considered problematic (American Psychiatric Association, 1987). Others have found an implicit bias in current sex therapy toward "hypersexuality," especially for women (LoPiccolo & Heiman, 1978). If a sexual problem cannot be completely defined in value-free, empirical terms, how can we determine what value and ethical judgments are correct? Do health professionals have expertise in this area?

A related question is, *Are sexual problems mental disorders?* Or are these problems actually physiological, social, religious, or political problems? Szasz (1980) argues that medical professionals have typically made pronouncements about sexual behavior that are clearly reflections of values, not products of their legitimate expertise in physiology and pathophysiology. For example, in the seventeenth and eighteenth centuries physicians such as Benjamin Rush indicated that masturbation (particularly by females) resulted in harmful physical and psychological effects, including masturbatory insanity. However, today's physicians typically advocate masturbation—sometimes as a cure (e.g., for female anorgasmia) and sometimes as a prevention. Szasz's point is that in both cases physicians have overstepped their bounds of legitimate expertise and couched general cultural biases in pseudomedical claims. Others maintain that the sex therapists' advocacy of masturbation must be understood in the context of Kinsey's (1948) findings that the frequency of masturbation was significantly higher in the upper social classes than in the lower classes. Sex therapists and their clients tend to come from the upper social strata, and modern sex therapy may be an imposition of the values of the upper classes on the lower classes (Robinson, 1976).

As another example of the conflation of the descriptive and the normative, Szasz takes issue with the argument of Masters and Johnson that homosexuality should be accepted as a normal response pattern, based on their findings that the "orgasmic experience" of homosexuals and heterosexuals is indistinguishable:

> For those who regard homosexuality as sinful—for example, because of the Judeo-Christian religious teaching on the subject—Masters and Johnson's physiological argument for equality between heterosexuals and homosexuals must appear sophomoric. Suppose that a gastrointestinal physiologist were to claim (as indeed he might, with veracity) that because the gastric juices secreted in response to beef, pork and human flesh are identical—eating pork is not sinful for Orthodox Jews, and eating human flesh is not sinful for anyone. I am not arguing, of course, that homosexual acts are sinful. I am arguing that their sinfulness or nonsinfulness cannot depend on the physiology of orgasms in homosexuals (Szasz, 1980, pp. 38–39).

Szasz's point is relevant not only for religious judgments (sinfulness) but also for secular judgments as to whether an act is moral or immoral. What seems to be clear is that modern sex therapists have reacted against Victorian influences in Western culture and advocated a very inclusive acceptance of a wide variety of sexual activities. Thus, the problem is no longer that "health professionals" are disseminating Victorian prejudices against sex. Rather, the opposite concern emerges: Are professionals overly permissive in their views of sexuality, to the extent that a dogmatic, hypersexual perspective dominates the field? For example, where is the controlled experimental evidence that masturbation has no negative effects?

Even if we disregard these more fundamental questions and take sexual problems to be mental disorders, another question emerges: Does the current classification system adequately emphasize the possible embeddedness of sexual functioning in relationship, religious, political, and physiological contexts? In the DSM-

III-R these factors are not given an essential role in the diagnostic criteria. However, if it is the case that such factors as quality of relationship, religious beliefs about sex, and a sexually oppressive and violent society do heavily influence sexual functioning, then perhaps these factors need to be given a larger role. It is interesting to note that what are now regarded as sexual dysfunctions became mental disorders only in 1980 with the publication of the DSM-III (American Psychiatric Association, 1980). The first two editions of the diagnostic manual (aside from a vague category, "psychophysiologic genito-urinary disorder," in DSM-II) included only "sexual deviations" such as pedophilia and homosexuality (American Psychiatric Association, 1980, 1968).

After these sorts of questions have been addressed, other questions arise. For example, *What kinds of sexual problems are there?* Does the DSM-III-R provide an exhaustive and properly differentiating categorization? Does this classification system miss any problems? (For example, is there such a thing as excessive sexual desire disorder, or post-traumatic (e.g., rape) sexual dysfunction disorder, or sexual communication disorder?) Does the DSM-III-R ever blend together two distinct problems? Does it make all the necessary distinctions in terms of subtypes (and subtypes of subtypes)? *Are some problems that have sexual aspects better classified as subtypes of other, more general problems?* Is there something similar to a sexual aversion that is best categorized as an anxiety disorder—e.g., a sexual phobia? On the other extreme, is there a "sexual addiction" that is best seen as a species of abuse/dependence disorder? *Should the sexual disorders be primarily classified by a sexual arousal cycle? If so, what is the proper sexual arousal cycle?* The latter question is controversial. For example, Kaplan (1979) has had a significant influence in amending Masters and Johnson's original four-phase cycle by adding a desire phase. Are any other alterations necessary—e.g., a "satisfaction phase" after the refractory phase? *Does the current classification system have any unwanted bi-*

ases (e.g., toward heterosexuality, or genital sex, or a phallocentric perspective)? For example, feminists have argued that sex therapy, because of its emphasis on genital sexual performance, has an implicit male-oriented bias (Stock, 1988).

Currently, the taxonomy generally accepted in the field—that found in the DSM-III-R—rests on at least the following presuppositions. (1) Male and female sexual functioning are essentially alike, since both can be considered in terms of the same sexual response cycle (Robinson, 1976). (2) Problems are confined to one phase—i.e., problems are so phase-specific that they can be captured by reference to a single phase. (3) A certain sexual response cycle exists or at least is adequate as an analytic framework. As noted, a desire phase has recently been added to Masters and Johnson's original four-phase cycle, and Masters and Johnson sometimes appeared to need to make further divisions (e.g., "advanced plateau phase," "high plateau"). (4) There is a high degree of synchrony between subjective and physiological changes during this response cycle. (5) To the extent that physiological variables determine the boundaries of the phases and the dimensions of the cycle, sexual functioning becomes mechanistic and materialistic. This list is not exhaustive; further explication of the presuppositions of the current taxonomy might be useful.

The final taxonomic question to be discussed here has typically been of greatest concern to the individuals constructing the diagnostic criteria used in the various editions of the DSM. *Does the DSM-III-R provide adequate inclusion and exclusion criteria for reliable and valid diagnosis?* For example, the sole diagnostic criterion for premature ejaculation is the following:

> Persistent or recurrent ejaculation with minimal sexual stimulation or before, upon, or shortly after penetration and before the person wishes it. The clinician must take into account factors that affect duration of the excitement phase, such as age, novelty of the sexual partner or situ-

ation, and frequency of sexual activity (American Psychiatric Association, 1987, p. 295).

This leaves the clinician considerable flexibility in determining what exactly counts as "persistent," "recurrent," "minimal," and "shortly after." Individuals' "wishes" may also be quite variable. Finally, what exact factors to take into account, and precisely how they are to be "taken into account," is also open to debate.

Have sexual dysfunctions been characterized sufficiently well to produce reliable and valid diagnoses? Field trials involving 339 subjects of all diagnoses of the DSM-III reported a kappa coefficient of .92 for psychosexual disorders and a kappa of 1.0 for psychosexual dysfunctions—numbers that represent excellent reliability (American Psychiatric Association, 1980). However, there are three problems. First, these are interrater reliabilities for the broad categories only, not the reliabilities of specific diagnoses. Thus, clinicians tended to agree that an individual had some psychosexual disorder or had some SD, but this is not evidence that the clinicians could agree on the specific diagnosis. Second, the sample size for these diagnoses was abysmally small. The kappa for the psychosexual disorder was based on seven cases; for psychosexual dysfunction, only five. Third, in a second phase of the field trials, based on five and four subjects, the kappas were .75 and .86, respectively. Thus, these data should not be taken as empirical evidence for the reliability of specific diagnoses.

INCIDENCE AND PREVALENCE

Given some level of agreement in defining what constitutes sexual problems, there arises a set of questions about the frequency of those problems. The study of the incidence and prevalence of health problems is known as *epidemiology*. The term *incidence* refers to the number of new cases of some problem in a certain population in a given period of time. *Prevalence* is the number of individuals with that problem at any given time. Thus, incidence reflects the rate of increase of a problem. Prevalence is often given in terms of *current* (or *point*) *prevalence* (indicating the number of individuals experiencing the problem at any point in time) or *lifetime prevalence* (which indicates the number of individuals who have had the problem at some time in their lives—not necessarily now). Epidemiologists also often gather other information (e.g., demographics), in order to identify risk factors, and collect therapy utilization information so as to identify barriers to entering therapy (Myers et al., 1984).

Epidemiological information, beyond being of interest in its own right, is regarded as useful for several other reasons. (1) It establishes base rates, which play an important role in prediction and in the evaluation of assessment instruments. (2) Such information helps in making decisions about the allocation of scarce resources, especially in cases of latent needs. (3) The identification of risk factors can aid in focusing prevention programs, as well as being useful in developing and evaluating etiological theories.

What, then, is known about the incidence and prevalence of what are currently taken to be sexual problems? Before we address this question, two preliminary points must be made. First, the quality of this information depends on the existence of good taxonomic categories and definitions of these, as well as reliable and valid measures of the problems. We will review the latter issue below. (Note a further difficulty: The problem is partly reflexive. Base rates and clear constructs are important in the evaluation of assessment instruments, and good assessment instruments are essential in gathering epidemiological information and determining the homogeneity of constructs.) Second, the most extensive and methodologically adequate series of epidemiological studies on mental health—the NIMH Epidemiological Catchment Area Program—unfortunately failed to report any information on sexual disorders (Myers et al., 1984; Regier et al., 1988; Robins et al., 1984).

However, Spector and Carey (1990) provide a useful and methodologically critical review of epidemiological studies of sexual problems. Of the 23 studies reviewed, none reported incidence information. Thus, nothing is known about the rate of development of sexual disorders. Moreover, Spector and Carey conclude, "Stable community estimates with regard to the current prevalence of female sexual arousal disorder, vaginismus and dyspareunia are not available" (p. 389). They also conclude that studies utilizing community samples indicate a current prevalence of 5–10% for inhibited female orgasm, 4–9% for male erectile disorder, 4–10% for inhibited male orgasm, and 36–38% for premature ejaculation.

The existing epidemiological studies of sexual dysfunction suffer from numerous methodological problems. Small sample sizes are common; the range is from 58 to several thousand in the Kinsey studies. Poor sampling technique is also a problem. Only one study—Kinsey, Pomeroy, and Martin (1948)—used a stratified sample, but even this included only white Americans and Canadians; most studies used clinic samples. The definitions of sexual dysfunctions are often poor or unstated. Also, the psychometrics of assessment measures are often unknown (e.g., magazine questionnaires or clinical interviews). Furthermore, no distinction is sometimes made between primary dysfunction (lifelong) and secondary dysfunction (acquired after some period of problem-free functioning) (Spector & Carey, 1990). Unfortunately, the most methodologically sound studies are the original Kinsey studies (Kinsey et al., 1948; Kinsey et al., 1953), and these are obviously quite dated.

Given the paucity of studies, the methodological problems of these, and the possibility that the most methodologically adequate ones may be out of date, only the most tentative claims can be advanced regarding the prevalence of SDs. This is most unfortunate—not only because this is interesting information in its own right. It also hampers efforts at developing sound theories of etiology, in that risk factors have not been identified, and hinders

the development of assessment instruments, since base rate prediction can only be calculated with a considerable margin for error.

THEORIES OF ETIOLOGY

Currently, there is no confirmed or generally accepted theory of either abnormal or normal sexual functioning. A well-supported theory of normal sexual behavior and functioning would be extremely useful, as it could provide the context for understanding abnormal sexual functioning. For example, if we understood what mechanisms control normal sexual functioning, perhaps abnormal functioning could be seen in terms of an abnormal magnitude of some of the parameters of these mechanisms.

There is a tremendously wide variety of theories of human sexuality. Geer and O'Donohue (1987) identified at least 14 different accounts, including theological, feminist, sociobiological, phenomenological, developmental, anthropological, Marxist, behavioral/ conditioning, cognitive, scripting theory, psychoanalytic, and physiological. Money (1973) also upheld the multidisciplinary view of sexology in an appropriately titled article, "Sexology: Behavioral, Cultural, Hormonal, Neurological, Genetic, etc." We would add that emphasis should be placed on the "etc."

How is one to decide among these various accounts? It should be emphasized that these diverse accounts are logically compatible, so a choice under pain of logical consistency is not necessary. That is, the truth of the assertions of one approach does not entail the falsity of the assertions of another approach. To a large extent, this compatibility is due to the fact that the various approaches are investigating different questions and problems. For example, a statement made by a sociologist of sex, "Social class influences sexual response A" is inconsistent with the assertions, "It is not the case that social class influences sexual response A" and "Social class never influences sexual responding." However, it is perfectly consistent with claims such as "Electrical shock contingent upon increased penile tumescence in situation *S* will decrease the probability of future occurences of penile tumenscence in situation *S*,'' or ''In the New Testament, Jesus said that sexual practice *B* is morally wrong.''

Admittedly, there are certain tensions involved in allegiances to one approach over another. Individuals committed to the *Weltanschaung* of a material determinism might have little interest in or credence for a theological (or for that matter perhaps a sociological) approach but would probably have strong affinities toward genetic and physiological accounts of human sexuality. Thus, commitments to, and interests in, a certain approach to the understanding of sexual behavior might be largely influenced by general metaphysical positions and ways of viewing the world. Historically, accounts of human sexuality have paralleled the predominant worldview. When humans sought to understand the world in supernatural terms, sex was viewed in supernatural terms; when humanism and rationalism held sway, sex was understood in these terms; and more recently, when humans were inclined to naturalistic and mechanical views, sexual behavior was explained in like terms (Bullough, 1987). The various present-day approaches to understanding human sexuality, although not necessarily opposed to each other on logical grounds, may have connotations related to metaphysical positions and favored levels of analysis; a theory may win favor or disfavor at these levels rather than on an empirical basis.

However, the multitude of theories does serve to call attention to the multivariate nature of sexual functioning and dysfunction. If the goal of a theory is to provide accurate and complete explanations and predictions of the phenomenon of interest (in more technical terms, to account for all the variance), then it must contain all the variables that affect that phenomenon.

For example, Newton's law of gravitational attraction asserts that only a very few factors are relevant to gravitational attraction. His equation,

$$F_g = \frac{m_1 m_2}{r^2},$$

where F_g is the force of gravitational attraction, m_1 and m_2 are the masses of the two objects, and r is the distance between the two objects, indicates that only three things are involved in the explanation or prediction of gravitational attraction: the masses of the two objects and the distance between them. *Nothing else matters*. By this law, a large number of possibly relevant factors are in fact not relevant. Among these are the color and shape of the object, its elemental makeup, and its cognitive state (if it happens to be human).

What variables, then, cannot possibly be relevant to sexual behavior? What factors (such as color in the case of gravitational attraction) can we exclude without loss of explanatory power or accuracy of prediction? Table 1.1 is an admittedly incomplete list of factors that *are* relevant. If we assume that each of the factors on the list has several values, and if we admit the possibility of interaction among these variables, then we see how daunting a task it will be to provide complete explanations and accurate predictions regarding sexual behavior. The task becomes all the more difficult because we cannot confidently confine the possible variables affecting sexual behavior to those listed in Table 1.1. This list is admittedly incomplete, so it cannot be said that nothing else is relevant.

PATHOPHYSIOLOGY AND PSYCHOPATHOLOGY

Another fundamental question concerns the relationship between psychological and physiological factors in SDs. The DSM-III-R states, ''This diagnosis [sexual dysfunctions] is not made if the Sexual Dysfunction is attributed entirely to organic factors, such as a physical disorder or a medication . . .'' (p. 290). Thus, according to the DSM-III-R, a sexual problem is misclassified as a mental disorder if it turns out that it is entirely due to physiological factors. This volume contains a chapter on the medical aspects of each major subdivision of the SDs (sexual desire disorders, sexual

Table 1.1. Factors Possibly Influencing Sexual Behavior

1. Physiological factors
   a. General health
   b. Age
   c. Hormonal levels and sensitivities
   d. Integrity of sexual anatomy
   e. Genetic factors
2. Cultural factors
   a. Laws relevant to sexual behavior
   b. Power relations having to do with sex/gender (e.g., patriarchy)
   c. Levels of general stress in society
   d. Cultural sexual scripts
   e. Economic variables related to resources relevant to sexual behavior
3. Interpersonal factors
   a. Attractiveness
   b. Social skills
   c. Sex role/gender identity behavior
4. Intrapersonal factors
   a. Social anxiety
   b. Sexual scripts
   c. Ethical beliefs regarding sex
   d. Attitudes toward sex and related issues
      i. Sex guilt
      ii. Acceptance of sex role
      iii. Fear of pregnancy
5. Learning/conditioning factors
   a. Previous traumatic sexual experiences
   b. Early childhood experiences with sex
   c. Modeling of significant others (e.g., mother, father)
6. Practical factors
   a. Opportunities for sexual contact
   b. Sexually transmitted disease rates in society
   c. Access to contraception

arousal disorders, orgasm disorders, and sexual pain disorders). In these chapters the pathophysiological aspects of the disorders are discussed, along with physiological problems that mimic the disorders (e.g., side effects of drugs).

However, no firm conclusions can be made at this time about the relation of physiological and psychological processes in these problems. This is due in part to the relative infancy of research programs in physiological and psychological factors in the SDs. Some proponents of the medical model hypothesize that the problems (or subsets of these) are largely or entirely organically based and thus indeed are misclassified as mental disorders. Much energy is currently devoted to ways of making a valid differential diagnosis between organic and functional sexual dysfunction (e.g., nocturnal penile tumescence).

Moreover, the underlying dichotomy between mind and body presumed in the DSM-III-R has been questioned both on philosophical grounds (Cornman, 1975) and on empirical grounds (Schwartz, 1982). Taylor (1986) advocates what is known as the biopsychosocial model:

> The biopsychosocial model maintains that *health and illness are caused by multiple factors and produce multiple effects.* The model further maintains that the *mind and body cannot be distinguished* in matters of health and illness because both so clearly influence an individual's state of health. The biopsychosocial model *emphasizes both health and illness* rather than regarding illness as a deviation from some steady state (1986, p. 12, emphasis in original).

At this stage several fundamental questions remain. (1) Is some sexual dysfunction in fact entirely due to physiological problems, and therefore misclassified as a mental disorder and mistreated by psychotherapy? (2) Are there two distinct subtypes of certain SDs—e.g., male erectile disorder caused entirely by organic complications and male erectile disorder due to psychological factors? (3) Is the biopsychosocial model correct that all SDs should be viewed from an integrationist point of view, eschewing any distinctions between mental and physical disorders? Clearly, more research and thought are required.

THE ASSESSMENT OF SEXUAL BEHAVIOR

The ability to assess accurately sexual dysfunction and variables related to it is essential to the growth of the scientific study of SDs. If something cannot be accurately measured, several significant barriers emerge against progress. At one level, accurate measurement is needed to detect the presence or absence of the phenomenon of interest. So to what extent can the presence or absence of various SDs be accurately measured? As stated previously, the DSM field trials give us little information to the point. Detecting the presence or absence of something often involves categorical measures, which can be the least complex type of measurement.

At another level, accurate measurement is needed to track different magnitudes of the phenomenon of interest. It may not be enough to detect presence or absence; the phenomenon may be present in varying degrees of magnitude. For example, in the case of female sexual arousal disorder, can the magnitude of the lubrication-swelling response and the subjective sense of sexual excitement be accurately tracked? Table 1.2 lists factors that must

Table 1.2. Factors Requiring Assessment in DSM-III-R Sexual Dysfunction Diagnoses

1. Sexual fantasies (presence and deficiency)
2. Sexual desire (presence and degree)
3. Other Axis I diagnoses (and their constituents)
4. Sexual aversion
5. Sexual avoidance
6. Lubrication-swelling response (presence and degree)
7. Completion of sexual activity
8. Subjective sense of sexual excitement (for male and female)
9. Subjective sense of sexual pleasure (for male and female)
10. Erection (presence and degree)
11. Presence of orgasm (in male and female)
12. Delay in orgasm (in male and female)
13. Presence of normal sexual excitement phase (in male and female)
14. Focus of sexual activity (in male and female)
15. Intensity of sexual activity (in male and female)
16. Duration of sexual activity (in male and female)
17. Degree of sexual stimulation (detection of "minimal")
18. Penetration
19. Desire for timing of orgasm
20. Novelty of sexual partner
21. Frequency of sexual activity
22. Genital pain
23. Involuntary spasm of the musculature of the outer third of the vagina
24. Degree of interference with coitus

be measured for diagnosis of the sexual dysfunctions as defined in the DSM-III-R.

Moreover, in clinical and research endeavors, one must also be able to measure accurately the variables that play a causal role in sexual dysfunction. The clinician is interested in evaluating these in terms of their possible etiological role as well as utilizing them as points of intervention. Ideally, one should be able to measure accurately the presence or absence (and preferably even the magnitude) of each of the variables given in Table 1.2, as at least a subset of these might be highly relevant to a particular case.

Therefore, as a rough estimate, we would need to be able to measure approximately 40 variables in order to understand the dependent measures of interest and the nexus of potentially causal variables. Fortunately, it may also be the case that certain problems will not require all 40 to be considered.

Certain aspects of human sexuality and sexual dysfunction make accurate measurement quite difficult. First, there is reason to believe that sexual functioning is reactive. The problem is that measured sexual behavior may be significantly different from naturally occurring, unmeasured behavior. Second, sexuality is a sensitive topic, so there are significant barriers to accurate disclosure. Individuals may refuse to disclose information about their sexual functioning or may distort the truth so as to increase social desirability or to protect self-esteem. Third, some of the variables of interest are complex and therefore difficult to measure accurately. For example, "subjective sense of sexual excitement" is a variable related to the diagnosis of the arousal disorders, but fundamental questions about it remain unanswered. (1) Is this a one-dimensional or a multidimensional construct? (2) How is subjective sexual excitement best operationalized? (3) How can subjects be trained to be accurate reporters concerning their subjective sense of sexual excitement?

To what extent do we possess the ability to measure the variables described above? Conte (1983) provides a useful review of self-report assessment techniques. Self-report measures should be considered carefully, because they probably constitute the most frequently used assessment strategy. Conte concludes that reliable and valid assessment instruments exist for the measurement of sexual functioning. "They are, however, few in number, and some are psychometrically deficient and/or clinically incomplete assessments of sexual functioning and satisfaction . . ." (p. 573).

Conte recommends that the investigator interested in the extent of an individual's sexual experience use Bentler's (1968a, 1968b) or Zuckerman's (1973) heterosexual experience scales; for measurement of attitudes toward sexual behavior, she recommends the use of the Sexual Interest Questionnaire (Harbison et al., 1974); for female sexual arousability, the Sexual Arousability Index (Hoon et al., 1976) for females; and for males either the Clarke Sex History Questionnaire for Males (Paitich et al., 1977) or a questionnaire developed by Marks and Sartorius (1968). The Sexual Interaction Inventory developed by LoPiccolo and Steger (1974) is recommended as it is the only instrument designed to assess both partners and their interactions. Finally, she states that the Derogatis Sexual Functioning Inventory (1978) is the most comprehensive and potentially useful inventory, and it also has more psychometric data than others.

Although these assessment measures do have some merit, they also have significant psychometric shortcomings. For example, there are data indicating excellent reliability for Bentler's and Zuckerman's scales of heterosexual experience, but Conte states that there is no validity data. As another example, the questionnaire developed by Marks and Sartorius, which Conte recommends for the attitudes toward sexual behavior, has a test-retest reliability coefficient of only .6. This means that its validity is severely limited, as it could account for only 36% of the variance. Thus, Conte appears to be too generous in her evaluations of these instruments; many more psychometric studies need to be conducted.

In recent years, partly to overcome problems with self-reporting and partly to obtain direct real-time measurements of sexual arousal, professionals have turned to the use of the polygraph and direct genital measurement. Rosen and Beck (1988) provide an excellent review of the psychophysiological measurement of sexual dysfunction. Although it is beyond the scope of this chapter to provide a thorough review of this literature, a few uses will be mentioned. Measurement of nocturnal penile tumescence has been used in an attempt to differentiate organic erectile dysfunction from psychogenic dysfunction. The hypothesis is that an inability to produce an erection during REM sleep corroborates a diagnosis of organic impairment. However, investigators reach varying conclusions regarding the reliability and validity of this procedure (Rosen & Beck, 1988). For females, psychophysiological sexual techniques have been used less in diagnosis and more in treatment. Biofeedback has been utilized in the treatment of inhibited sexual desire and arousal and orgasmic dysfunction; vaginal vasocongestive measures have been used in the evaluation of treatment outcomes for more traditional forms of sex therapy (Rosen & Beck, 1988). Again, however, these studies have emerged only recently; more studies of the psychometric properties of this technology with various SDs should be conducted.

Thus, it is not at all clear that the field currently possesses instruments that can accurately measure variables of interest. Since accurate measurement technology is a prerequisite for progress in any science—consider the influence of the telescope on astronomy or the microscope on biology—the development and evaluation of accurate and useful assessment instruments should be a priority in this field. Questions of the relationships among variables must be secondary in importance to the measurement of those variables.

The existence of accurate assessment instruments is important not only for diagnosis (and thereby properly beginning therapy), but also for tracking treatment progress and long-term treatment outcome. Therefore, any problems with the quality of assessment methodologies have a direct impact on the evaluation, and thereby the development, of effective treatments for SDs.

THE TREATMENT OF SEXUAL PROBLEMS

The twentieth century has seen a wide variety of therapeutic approaches to sexual dysfunction. The classical Freudian view is that SDs are manifestations of underlying psychopathology, to be treated indirectly by long-term psychoanalysis. Therapy is to focus on uncovering psychodynamic problems, particularly with id impulses, which were thought to have emanated from childhood disturbances in psychosexual development. The neo-Freudians were quite heterodox, expressing a range of views on the nature and treatment of sexual problems. Even more than Freud, Wilhelm Reich emphasized the importance of sexuality (particularly the orgasm) in the causes and cure of all "neuroses." Reichian therapy emphasized the primacy of the orgasm for understanding human functioning and used orgone energy accumulators and direct sexual exercises to unblock dammed-up libidinal energy, in order to allow the patient to achieve maximum orgasmic potential. On the other hand, the ego analysts and object relation analysts deemphasized the role of sexual issues behind various pathologies (including SDs), so treatment for sexual problems again became more indirect. The behavior therapists, beginning with Wolpe (1958), viewed dysfunction as an outcome of inappropriate learning. They therefore used counterconditioning techniques, such as systematic desensitization, for the treatment of sexual problems. Paralleling these views has been a plethora of proposed medical interventions, ranging from genital surgeries to hormone therapies and from brain surgeries to vitamin therapies.

However, it is the work of Masters and Johnson, beginning in the 1970s, which is most often discussed using terms such as "groundbreaking," "watershed," and "landmark." Masters and Johnson provided intensive therapy (lasting about weeks) that included educative, behavioral, and medical components for various sexual problems. Their work has been extremely influential, sometimes functioning as the foundation for subsequent work. However, a reappraisal of their earlier work has occurred in recent years—especially when subsequent researchers found drastically poorer outcome results. We will briefly review some of the major criticisms of the work of Masters and Johnson.

Zilbergeld and Evans (1980) provided one of the most penetrating methodological critiques of the work of Masters and Johnson. They specify six major problems with *Human Sexual Inadequacy*. (1) There was no clear specification of the criteria for the evaluation of treatment outcome. (2) Masters and Johnson reported only failure rates and thus gave no information on the exact degree of change. Moreover, Masters and Johnson clearly stated that failure rates could not be translated into success rates, thus rendering totally obscure a piece of information that later came to be regarded as relevant (see Table 1.3). (3) There were sampling biases—unidentified, but certainly present. Masters and Johnson failed to specify clearly their screening procedures and their sampling biases, although it appears that their sample was heavily skewed toward urban, intelligent, affluent, well-motivated, relatively healthy, and sexually oriented individuals. (4) There appeared high and possibly differential mortality of subjects in their long-term outcome data. (5) The duration and specifics of treatment were unclear. (6) Information about the harmful effects of treatment was lacking. These obviously significant methodological shortcomings render Masters and Johnson's research difficult, if not impossible, to interpret.

Admittedly, it is difficult to conduct methodologically sound research into sex therapy treatment outcomes. Obtaining a representative sample is a difficult problem that has plagued much sex research, beginning with Kinsey. Without a representative sample, generalization may be unfounded. Warner and Bancroft (1986) state that the predominant

Table 1.3. Results of Sex Therapy at the Masters & Johnson Institute (1959–1977)

	N	FAILURES	SUCCESSES	SUCCESS RATE
Primary impotence	51	17	34	66.7%
Secondary impotence	501	108	393	78.4%
Premature ejaculation	432	17	415	96.1%
Ejaculatory incompetence	75	18	57	76.0%
Male totals	1,059	160	899	84.9%
Primary anorgasmia	399	84	315	79.0%
Situational anorgasmia	331	96	235	71.0%
Vaginismus	83	1	82	98.8%
Female totals	813	181	632	77.7%
Combined totals	1,872	341	1,531	81.8%

From Kolodny, R. C. (1981). Evaluating sex therapy: Process and outcome at the Masters and Johnson Institute. *Journal of Sex Research, 17,* 301–318. Reprinted from *The Journal of Sex Research,* a publication of The Society for the Scientific Study of Sex; P.O. Box 208; Mount Vernon, Iowa 52314 USA.

findings of sex therapy outcome research have been largely negative. Therapies are found not to be superior to waiting list or placebo controls (Bancroft, 1983); no differential superiority of one treatment over another is shown; no difference is evident between treatment by one or by two therapists (Heiman & LoPiccolo, 1983) or between spaced or massed therapy sessions (Arentewicz & Schmidt, 1983). Warner and Bancroft cite a combination of logistical and methodological reasons. First, they suggest that sample sizes may be inadequate, relative to the variance attributable to sources other than the treatment method, to detect clinically important differences. They recommend the use of power analysis in treatment designs. Based on a reinterpretation of their own negative results (Bancroft et al., 1986), they report that if they wanted to show a clinically superior treatment that would improve success rates by 15% (to 45%) and sought greater power (90%), then the calculated required sample sizes would be 200 in each group! Given the logistical problems in obtaining subjects that are relatively homogeneous for a treatment study, Warner and Bancroft suggest that most such studies will report negative results due to inadequate sample sizes.

They also stress the importance of controlling for prognostic factors that make some cases much more difficult to treat than others.

This presents a dilemma: Although we know little about what prognostic factors are relevant, if we do not take prognostic variability into account in the analysis, "it will remain as part of the 'experimental error' (i.e., the unexplained or residual error) serving to inflate it. Since the statistical significance of a treatment effect is measured in relation to this residual error, moderate treatment effects would thus remain undetectable (unless sample size can be increased sufficiently to maintain power, as has been discussed)" (p. 856). Warner and Bancroft recommend further research into commonsense prognostic indicators such as the quality of the couple's relationship and motivation (see Hawton & Catalan, 1986), the development of adequate measurement of the variables and the use of composite prognostic scores (e.g., discriminant function scores), by which subjects can then be blocked into two groups. Warner and Bancroft believe that the homogeneity within blocks will be improved, with a corresponding reduction in residual error.

The most useful question to address in treatment outcome research is "What therapy, delivered by what kind of therapist, for which problem, for which type of client, in which set of circumstances is how effective, and how does this come about?" Table 1.4 translates this question to domains of variables that can

Table 1.4. Domains of Variables in Treatment Outcome Research

1. Clients
   a. Specifics of problem (e.g., subtype, primary vs. secondary, duration)
   b. Relatively stable personal-social characteristics (e.g., degree of other pathology, motivation, previous sexual adjustment)
   c. Physical-social life environment (e.g., quality of previous sexual adjustment)
2. Therapists
   a. Therapeutic techniques (e.g., educational, sensate focus, and various combinations; frequency of sessions, duration of therapy)
   b. Relatively stable personal-social characteristics (e.g., gender, sexual orientation, sexual attitudes, attractiveness)
   c. Physical-social treatment environment (single vs. cotherapists, couple vs. individual treatment)
3. Time (includes initial client contact, termination, and follow-up)
4. Criteria
   a. Treatment effectiveness
   b. Social validation

affect sex therapy and therefore must be considered in therapy design. Of course, these variables should be viewed in the context of factors that influence internal validity, such as the presence of control groups for spontaneous remission (no treatment controls), placebo effects (placebo controls), and experimenter bias (double blind). This sort of research is admittedly difficult to conduct. But it is necessary in order to make the results interpretable and potentially to capture the complex relationships that might be at work.

CONCLUSION

The chapters that follow critically review the state of information regarding sexual dysfunctions, using the taxonomy provided by the DSM-III-R. Each author attempts to address many of the questions outlined in this chapter. We encourage the reader to keep two thoughts in mind. What information, of what quality, is available concerning any one of these questions? Perhaps more important, what future research would be valuable to help address the questions?

REFERENCES

American Psychiatric Association. (1968). *Diagnostic and statistical manual of mental disorders* (2nd ed.). Washington, DC: Author.

American Psychiatric Association. (1980). *Diagnostic and statistical manual of mental disorders* (3rd ed., rev.). Washington, DC: Author.

American Psychiatric Association. (1987). *Diagnostic and statistical manual of mental disorders* (3rd ed., rev.). Washington, DC: Author.

Arentewicz, G. & Schmidt, G. (1983). *The treatment of sexual disorders*. New York: Basic Books.

Bancroft, J. (1983) *Human sexuality and its problems*. Edinburgh, UK: Churchill Livingstone.

Bancroft, J., Dickerson, M., Fairburn, C. G., Gray, J., Greenwood, J., Stevenson, N., & Warner, P. (1986). Sex therapy outcome research: A reappraisal of methodology. *Psychological Medicine, 16,* 851–863.

Bentler, P. M. (1968a). Heterosexual behavior assessment. I. Males. *Behavior Research and Therapy, 6,* 21–25.

Bentler, P. M. (1968b). Heterosexual behavior assessment. II. Females. *Behavior Research and Therapy, 6,* 27–30.

Bullough, V. L. (1987). A historical approach. In J. Geer & W. O'Donohue (Eds.), *Theories of human sexuality*. New York: Plenum.

Conte, H. R. (1983). Development and use of self-report techniques for assessing sexual functioning: A review and critique. *Archives of Sexual Behavior, 12,* 555–576.

Cornman, J. W. (1975). *Perception, common sense and science*. New Haven, CT: Yale University Press.

Cornman, J. W., Lehrer, K., & Pappas, G. S. (1982). *Philosophical problems and arguments: An introduction*. New York: Macmillan.

Derogatis, L. R. (1978). *Derogatis Sexual Functioning Inventory* (rev. ed.). Baltimore, MD: Clinical Psychometrics Research.

Geer, J. H., & O'Donohue, W. (Eds.). (1987). *Theories of human sexuality*. New York: Plenum.

Harbison, J. J. M., Graham, P. J., Quinn, J. T., MacAllister, H., & Woodward, R. (1974). A questionnaire measure of sexual interest. *Archives of Sexual Behavior, 3,* 357–366.

Hawton, K., & Catalan, J. (1986). Prognostic factors in sex therapy. *Behaviour Research and Therapy*.

Heiman, J. R., & LoPiccolo, J. (1983). Clinical outcome of sex therapy. *Archives of General Psychiatry, 40,* 443–449.

Hoon, E. F., Hoon, P. W., and Wincze, J. P. (1976). An inventory for the measurement of female sexual arousability: The SAI. *Archives of Sexual Behavior, 5*, 291–300.

Kaplan, H. S. (1979). *Disorders of sexual desire*. New York: Brunner/Mazel.

Kinsey, A. C., Pomeroy, W. B., & Martin, C. (1948). *Sexual behavior in the human male*. Philadelphia: W. B. Saunders.

Kinsey, A. C., Pomeroy, W. B., Martin, C., & Gebhard, P. (1953). *Sexual behavior in the human female*. Philadelphia: W. B. Saunders.

Kolodny, R. C. (1981). Evaluating sex therapy: Process and outcome at the Masters & Johnson Institute. *Journal of Sex Research, 17*, 301–318.

Leroy, D. H. (1972). The potential criminal liability of human sex clinics and their patients. *St. Louis University Law Journal, 16*, 589–599.

LoPiccolo, J., & Heiman, J. (1978). The role of cultural values in the prevention and treatment of sexual problems. In C. B. Qualls, J. P. Wincze & D. H. Barlow (Eds.), *The prevention of sexual disorders* (pp. 43–74). New York: Plenum.

LoPiccolo, J., & Steger, J. C. The Sexual Interaction Inventory: A new instrument for the assessment of sexual dysfunction. *Archives of Sexual Behavior, 3*, 585–595.

Marks, I. M., & Sartorius, N. H. (1968). A contribution to the measurement of sexual attitude. *Journal of Nervous and Mental Disease, 145*, 441–451.

Money, J. (1973). Sexology: Behavioral, cultural, hormonal, neurological, genetic, etc. *The Journal of Sex Research, 9*, 3–10.

Myers, J. K., Weissman, M. M., Tischler, G. L., Holzer, C. E., Leaf, P. J., Orvaschel, H., Anthony, J. C., Boyd, J. H., Burke, J. D., Kramer, M., & Stoltzman, R. (1984). Six month prevalence of psychiatric disorders in three communities: 1980–1982. *Archives of General Psychiatry, 41*, 959–970.

Paitich, D., Langevin, R., Freeman, R., Mann, K., & Handy, L. (1977). The Clarke SHQ: A clinical sex history questionnaire for males. *Archives of Sexual Behavior, 6*, 421–436.

Regier, D. A., Boyd, J. H., Buke, J. D., Rae, D. S., Myers, J. K., Kramer, M., Robins, L. N., George, L. K., Karno, M., & Locke, B. Z. (1988). One-month prevalence of mental disorders in the United States: Based on five epidemiologic catchment area sites. *Archives of General Psychiatry, 45*, 977–986.

Robins, L. N., Helzer, J. E., Weissman, M. M. Orvaschel, H., Gruenberg, E., Burke, J. D., & Regier, D. A. (1984). Lifetime prevalence of specific psychiatric disorders in three sites. *Archives of General Psychiatry, 41*, 949–958.

Robinson, P. (1976). *The modernization of sex*. New York: Harper & Row.

Rosen, R. C., & Beck, J. G. (1988). *Patterns of sexual arousal: Psychophysiological processes & clinical applications*. New York: Guilford.

Schwartz, G. E. (1982). Testing the biophysical model: The ultimate challenge facing behavioral medicine? *Journal of Consulting and Clinical Psychology, 50*, 1040–1053.

Spector, I. P., & Carey, M. P. (1990). Incidence and prevalence of the sexual dysfunctions: A critical review of the empirical literature. *Archives of Sexual Behavior, 19*, 389–408.

Stock, W. (1988). Propping up the phallocracy: A feminist critique of sex therapy and research. *Women and Therapy, 7*, 23–41.

Szasz, T. (1980). *Sex by prescription*. Garden City, NY: Anchor Press.

Taylor, S. E. (1986). *Health psychology*. New York: Random House.

Warner, P., & Bancroft, J. (1986). Methodological considerations—the importance of prognostic variability. *Psychological Medicine, 16*, 855–863.

Wolpe, J. (1958). *Psychotherapy by reciprocal inhibition*. Stanford, CA: Stanford University Press.

Zilbergeld, B., & Evans, M. (1980). The inadequacy of Masters and Johnson. *Psychology Today, 14*, 29–34.

Zuckerman, M. (1973). Scales for sex experience for males and females. *Journal of Consulting and Clinical Psychology, 41*, 27–29.

CHAPTER 2

MEDICAL ASPECTS OF INHIBITED SEXUAL DESIRE DISORDER

David Kresin,* University of Colorado, School of Medicine

The intent of this chapter is to develop a medical framework in which to conceptualize the origins of inhibited sexual desire in men and women. Human sexual desire has been the object of extensive literary and political debate in one form or another for centuries, but it is only in recent years that inhibited sexual desire has become an object of medical and psychological concern. Lief (1977) and Kaplan (1977) independently first described the inhibited or hypoactive sexual desire (HSD) patient, and in 1980 the DSM-III included the condition in its listing of sexual disorders. Southren (1985) has defined HSD as follows:

> Hypoactive sexual desire (HSD) is a condition characterized by a discrepancy between actual and desired frequencies of sexual activities in intimate partners and a deficit in sexual interest in one partner (p. 55).

The assessment of the prevalence of HSD is limited by several factors. It is mainly the HSD patient who has an unsatisfied partner, or a partner who is able to motivate him or her to seek help, who will receive evaluation or treatment. Also, given the nature of the disorder, not all HSD patients have a sexual partner; of those without a partner, some may attribute their low libido to lack of opportunity for sexual interaction. These limiting factors, along with the patients' and many physicians' general inhibition regarding discussion of sexual matters, all tend to minimize the true incidence of HSD. Schreiner-Engel and Schiavi (1986), in a review of epidemiological studies, found that HSD

* The author wishes to thank Professor David L. Nanney of the University of Illinois, for his guidance and inspiration.

prevalence in the population ranged from 1% to 15% for men and 1% to 35% for women.

Because it has been only in recent years that the subject of desire (and specifically inhibited sexual desire) has been treated as a legitimate field of concern and study, research on the topic is limited relative to other areas of human sexuality. However, a thorough if not exhaustive effort will be made here to represent the findings available on medical etiologies presently known for HSD.

Evaluation of the HSD patient requires a thorough history, physical examination, and laboratory studies specifically tailored to the history and physical examination (H&P). The specific requirements of the medical workup will be delineated, along with an extensive review of the various medical conditions that may contribute to the HSD condition. It is necessary to have an understanding of the dynamic interactions of the central nervous system (CNS) with the sexual organs (gonads—testicles and ovaries). Hormonal and neuropeptide releasing factors will be discussed, and pertinent research will be presented to elucidate their importance in sexual desire.

Also, the effects of several drugs, used both medicinally and recreationally, will be considered, followed by a discussion of several environmental and occupational toxins that may affect levels of sexual desire. Although there is a paucity of research available on the topic of HSD in the homosexual population, brief mention will be made of gay male sexual desire issues. Finally, numerous studies from the past two decades will be presented to support a genetic, neuroanatomic, neurochemical model of human sexuality.

HISTORY OF THE STUDY OF DESIRE

Rosen and Leiblum (1989) provide a synopsis of the onset of research in, and recognition of, the HSD condition. Masters and Johnson (1966, 1970) first outlined a four-stage sexual response cycle, which they used to develop treatment protocols for sexual dysfunction. The sexual dysfunction addressed by this model mainly involved problems of erection and ejaculation in males and arousal, penetration, and orgasm in women. As noted by Rosen and Leiblum (1989), this early assessment of sexual dysfunction did not specifically address the issue of inhibited desire. However, this deficiency was addressed independently seven years later by Harold Leif (1977) and Helen Singer Kaplan (1977). Leif (1977) coined the term *inhibited sexual desire* (ISD) for patients who chronically fail to initiate or respond to sexual stimuli, whereas Kaplan promoted the term *hypoactive sexual desire* (HSD). Kaplan espoused a triphasic approach to sexual response, with desire being the primary component of sexual arousal and the other stages being excitement and orgasm. Zilbergeld and Ellison (1980) developed their own model, with a five-stage sexual response cycle: interest, arousal, physiologic readiness, orgasm, and satisfaction.

The study of HSD took on additional legitimacy in 1980, when the DSM-III (*Diagnostic and Statistical Manual* of the American Psychiatric Association) considered inhibited sexual desire as a new diagnostic category. The DSM-III-R (American Psychiatric Association, 1987) categorizes the sexual response cycle in four phases: appetitive, excitement, orgasm, and resolution. The DSM-III-R defines hypoactive sexual desire disorder as follows:

> a) persistent or recurrent deficiency or absence of sexual fantasies and desire for sexual activity. The judgment of deficiency or absence is made by the clinician, taking into account factors that affect sexual functioning, such as age, sex, and the context of the person's life.
> b) occurence not exclusively during the course of another Axis I disorder (other than sexual dysfunction), such as major depression (p. 293).

CURRENT STATE OF THE SCIENCE OF DESIRE

Normal sexual functioning requires adequate sexual desire, which is brought on by various hormonal/neurochemical/neuropeptides, which in turn are affected by olfactory, visual, and tactile stimulation. This process begins with a complex interplay of the brain and genital organs, commonly interpreted as arousal. Arousal allows genital engorgement/erection, which heightens the sensation of arousal. Interactions between the brain and autonomic nervous system (sympathetic and parasympathetic) allow for the maintenance of adequate genital engorgement, emission, and then ejaculation in the male, followed by a refractory period. In the female there are corresponding changes, with a variable refractory period.

Our understanding of the neuroanatomical/neuropeptide model of sexual desire is fragmentary at best. The following is a basic neuroanatomical description of the vital sexual components of the central nervous system. The main components of the CNS are the brain and spinal cord. The brain may be divided into telencephalon (cerebral hemisphere—cortex), diencephalon (thalamus, hypothalamus, septal area, etc.), mesencephalon, metencephalon, myelencephalon (brainstem—midbrain, pons, cerebellum, and medulla). (See Figure 2.1.) See Nolte (1988) for more detailed neuroanatomy. The cortex processes gross motor/sensory functions as well as intellectual functions. As the brain structures descend (ventral/caudal/inferior) there is more primitive/more automatic/less conscious intervention required to control basic functions (e.g., the reflex networks that control focusing or tracking of the eye).

The hypothalamus is located within the diencephalon. The hypothalamus consists of clusters of nerve bodies and groups of nerve axons. The pituitary gland has an anterior lobe that the hypothalamus accesses via its blood supply (hypophyseal portal system). The posterior pituitary lobe has direct nerve projections from the hypothalamus.

The hypothalamus produces and expresses releasing hormones and many neurotransmitters: gonadotropin releasing hormones (GRH) or luteinizing hormone releasing hormone (LHRH), thyrotropin releasing hormone (TRH), and oxytocin and vasopressin. The pituitary responds to the hypothalamus releasing hormones by secreting its own hormones—e.g., follicle stimulating hormone (FSH), luteinizing hormone (LH), and thyroid stimulating hormone (TSH) to stimulate endocrine gland activity. TSH stimulates the thyroid gland to produce thyroid hormone. LH and FSH stimulate the gonads (ovaries and testicles) to produce sex hormones (testosterone, progesterone, estrogen). The gonadal and thyroid hormones then influence the pituitary and hypothalamus through both direct and indirect actions.

Finally, a brief description of the sexually active limbic system is necessary. The limbic system influences emotions, defense/aggression, eating, and sexuality. It physically and functionally links the telencephalon (cortex) and diencephalon (hypothalamus). The limbic system consists of cingulate and parahippocampal gyri (cortex), the hippocampal formation (a ventral portion of the brain that contains allegedly more primitive cortex—archicortex), the amygdala, the septal area, the hypothalamus portions of the midbrain reticular formation, and the olfactory area.

The hypothalamus has significant impact on sexual desire. Moss et al. (1989), in a review of investigations of the female rat has demonstrated the role of the hypothalamus in sexual desire. DuBois (1974), Naik (1976), and Setalo

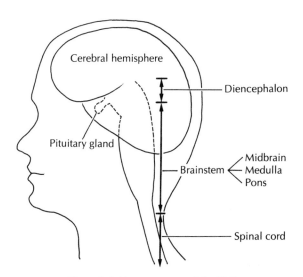

Figure 2.1. Neuroanatomy of the CNS.

et al. (1976) found that the hypothalamus releases neuropeptides; of particular interest is the luteinizing-releasing hormone LHRH. Hormonal fluctuations observed during the estrous cycle in the rat are correlated with LHRH content in specific hypothalamic sites (medial preoptic area, arcuate nucleus, and ventromedial nucleus) as well as in extrahypothalamic (midbrain central gray) sites. Kalra (1976) and Kobayashi et al. (1978) found that estrogen, a steroid hormone critical for the display of sexual receptivity in the female rat, has also been shown to cause changes in the hypothalamic LHRH content.

Moss et al. (1989) cite Blake (1978) and Kalra and Kalra (1983) that the onset of female rat sexual heat and ovulation is precipitated by hypothalamic LHRH stimulating LH release. This LH surge is followed a few hours later by classical receptive female behavior. Endogenous LHRH is critical to the expression of the lordotic behavior. It demonstrates in the rat the physiologic role of the decapeptide LHRH, with its initiation and maintenance of mating behavior.

Moss et al. (1989) cite Dudley and Moss's (1986) study, in which it was found that $LHRH^{1-10}$ may be fractionated and that $Ac-LHRH^{5-10}$ is able to modify membrane responsiveness of single neurons located in the ventromedial nucleus. Moss et al. (1989) cite Krause et al. (1982) and Advis et al. (1982) in discussion of how the naturally occurring physiologic degradation of $LHRH^{1-10}$ into $LHRH^{1-5}$ and $LHRH^{6-10}$ varies throughout the estrous cycle, with a decrease at the onset of the first estrous cycle.

The anterior pituitary gland contributes numerous hormones to the systemic blood supply. One of the major hormones produced by this gland is a 199 amino acid long molecule called prolactin. Cook (1989) cites Segal et al. (1979) to state that human male hyperprolactinemic states are associated with diminished potency and libido (occasionally hypogonadism), which are reversible by lowering the prolactin levels. Cook (1989) cites the finding of Svare et al. (1979) of suppressed rat copulatory behavior (without altering testosterone levels) induced by grafting pituitaries into kidneys. Svare et al.

(1979) suggest that some of the rat's hyperprolactinemic state of diminished libido may be mediated by direct action on the brain. Cook (1989) believes that this is supported by the failure of testosterone administration in hyperprolactinemic males to restore libido.

Blumer and Walker (1975) state that most temporal lobe epileptics have a decrease in sexual interest. They state that seizures originating in the medial temporal region can, however, cause arousal. Remillard et al. (1983) found that this arousal occurs early in the seizure and is more common in women than in men. McGlone and Young (1990) found that lesions in either lobe may cause decreased sexual desire and behavior, and lesions in both lobes may produce Kluver-Bucy syndrome (a state of hypersexuality and increased oral behavior). Taylor (1959) found that up to 72% of patients with temporal lobe seizures have been shown to have decreased sexual drive. Pritchard (1980) states that hyposexuality is not correlated with the site of epileptic focus, drug therapy, or seizure control. He claims that an epileptic focus in the mesobasal area does seem to be related to hyposexuality.

The scientific study of human sexual desire is generally limited by the subjective self-report of desire. Wallen (1990) argues that profound differences exist between female rodents and female primates: Female primates can mate without hormonal input, unlike female rodents. Therefore, female sexual initiation is argued to be the only valid indicator of female sexual motivation. In future human studies of desire sexual initiation, it is to be hoped that a less subjective parameter than self-report of the level of desire will be used.

DEMOGRAPHIC AND HORMONAL ASPECTS OF HSD

The degree or prevalence of HSD has been an illusive number for researchers to agree on. The goal of quantifying HSD in the general population is limited by numerous factors. Nathan (1986) reanalyzed 22 general population surveys to assess the prevalence and distribution of DSM-III-defined psychosexual dysfunction. After accounting for methodological shortcomings in analyzing information obtained for other purposes, inhibited sexual desire was found to range from 1% to 15% for men and from 1% to 35% for women.

Schein et al. (1988), in a study of 212 patients in a family practice center (with a wide representation of age, sex, race, and social class), surveyed sexual identity and function. They found that 16% of individuals reported a deficient libido and 11% reported an absence of motivation for sexual behavior with a partner. Females reported this deficiency at approximately three times the reported male rate ($p<0.05$). This study will later be used to support an innate biological difference in male-female desire levels.

Schreiner-Engel and Schiavi (1986) studied 46 married couples with DSM-III ISD and 36 matched controls. They found that ISD patients had "nearly normal psychological profiles" at assessment time but had significantly increased histories of affective disorders. ISD patients were found to have approximately twice the incidence of major and/or intermittent depression. Interestingly, there appeared to be a temporal link between the onset of ISD and the initial episode of depression. They suggested that a mutual biologic entity may be shared in ISD and depression, or the depression may contribute to the ISD pathology. Similarly, Jupp and McCabe (1989) studied 153 women (mean age 29.5) and found a significant correlation between general arousability and neuroticism ($r = 0.45$, $p < .001$). They also found a curvilinear correlation between general arousability and sexual dysfunction, and a negative relationship between levels of desire and sexual dysfunction.

Stuart et al. (1987) conducted a multipurpose study to identify differences in biopsychosocial criteria between a clinical group of 59 married women with ISD and 39 married women with normal sexual desire. They found no statistical group difference in hormonal (prolactin or testosterone), demographic, or personality variables. The differences in prolactin could have been missed, however, due to acknowledged "limited financial resources." Single hormonal blood studies were procured during the first ten days of the menstrual cycle. Tennekoon and Lenton (1985) state that prolactin levels have diurnal cycles and also vary through the menstrual cycle.

Schreiner-Engel et al. (1989) specifically tailored a study to evaluate more critically the lack of hormonal differences between HSD women and normal controls. Blood samples were drawn from 17 HSD women and 13 controls (between 8:00 A.M. and 10:00 A.M.) every three to four days for one menstrual cycle. The samples were analyzed with radioactive immune assay (RIA) testing for testosterone, sex hormone binding globulin (SHBG—used in calculation to determine biologically available testosterone), estradiol, progesterone, prolactin, and luteinizing hormone. They found no evidence of hormonal fluctuation (testosterone, free testosterone, and prolactin) differences that would support the theory that reproductive hormones are influential in determining sexual desire in eugonadal women.

Schiavi et al. (1988) found mixed results in a study of 17 HSD men and matched controls. Six men had problems of arousal, and eleven had secondary erectile failure. The patients (aged 27–55) were studied for four nights in a sleep laboratory; on the final night, blood was sampled every 20 minutes. They found lower plasma testosterone (measured hourly at night) in the HSD patients compared to the controls. They also found a positive correlation between testosterone and sexual behavior. In free testosterone, prolactin and estradiol, however, they found no differences between control and HSD groups.

Adams et al. (1978) and Matteo and Rissman (1984) found that both heterosexual and lesbian women exhibit a periovulatory increase in female-initiated sexual behavior. Bancroft et al. (1983), Singer and Singer (1972), and Cavanagh (1969) reached a variety of conclusions regarding the timing of peak sexual desire. Stanislaw and Rice (1988) evaluated data for 22,635 menstrual cycles from 1066 subjects from five countries (Canada, Columbia, France, Mauritius, and the United States). They found that an increase in sexual desire occurred a few days prior to ovulation (the fertile time having been detected by measurements of basal body temperature shifts).

The research seems to indicate that there are no significant serum hormonal measurements to explain decreased desire in women. However, Stanislaw et al. (1988), Adams et al. (1978), and Matteo and Rissman (1984) all present strong evidence that some sort of biologically driven desire mechanism has a periovulatory peak of desire. Schiavi et al. (1988) demonstrate a decrease in nocturnal testosterone in HSD men. Again, it appears that there is no clear evidence for a specific serum hormone level to control desire. However, I hypothesize that there are testosterone receptors in specific areas of the limbic system whose receptor affinity varies from male to female and has various higher-cortical influences. (The specifics will be discussed at the end of this chapter.)

MEDICAL CONDITIONS/DISEASES THAT AFFECT DESIRE

While it is reasonable to surmise that most disease states could potentially affect sexual desire, this has been inadequately studied. The inadequacy is in part due to the fact that there has only recently been medical/psychological acknowledgment of the importance of sexual desire. The progress of research is further hampered by the fact that desire is quantifiable in human studies only through self-report, and such measures have unknown psychometric properties. Money and Higham (1989) state that nothing is as yet known about the relationship of gonadal hormones during childhood to sexually dimorphic behavior. They discuss the currently popular and most frequently quoted version of innate hormonal determinism. This pertains to a male hermaphroditic pedigree discovered in the isolated mountain villages of the Dominican Republic. In this pedigree there is a deficiency of an enzyme responsible for converting testosterone to dihydrotestosterone. This deficiency is lifelong and prevents the testosterone from becoming active at sites of primary and secondary sexual development. Unlike other cases of five alpha-reductase deficiencies, feminization does not occur, and the affected individuals develop as moderately virilized males or as eunuchoids.

In cases of total androgen insensitivity or testicular feminizing syndrome (TFS), the individual is externally (somatically) a female with a shortened vagina, small uterus, and intraabdominal testicles. At puberty, female secondary sexual characteristics develop.

Alvarez et al. (1983) viewed ten cases of testicular feminization and found that intellectual achievement was normal and that psychological stability based on the MMPI showed no typical profile of the group. There was a lack of strong maternal drive, however. The personality profile manifested two outstanding traits in the group: dominance and shrewdness, the former being remarkably high for a female sample. They hypothesize a psychological alteration of the possible role of partial androgenization of the central nervous system in these patients.

However, Vague (1983) found that phenotypical males with TFS demonstrate truly feminine conciousness of gender identity, normal extragenital erotogenic sensitivity, suppressed or very reduced clitoral sensitivity and reaction, normal reactions of the labia minora and the vagina (which deepens with the renewal of intercourse), realization of pleasure, climax without clonicotonic orgasm and followed by resolution, and a normal maternal attitude. In short, the above all seem to characterize sexual behavior in a complete or almost complete TFS individual.

Money and Higham (1989) state that Turner's syndrome is present in a female individual who lacks one X chromosome and consequently fails to develop gonads. In childhood these females dream of romance, marriage, and motherhood. As adults they have desire for marriage and motherhood, but their delayed growth and corresponding delayed social maturity frequently lead to confusing and diminished libido or relative romantic and erotic inertia.

Money and Matthews (1982) found that women with progestin-induced hermaphroditism (women who were exposed to progesterone intrautero (prenatally) in an attempt to prevent miscarriages in their mothers) were indistinguishable from their unaffected age mates in both romantic and sexual interest. Money, Schwartz, and Lewis (1984) report that women with congenital adrenal hyperplasia were mostly heterosexual. However, two-fifths reported bisexual or homosexual dreams, fantasies, or practices.

Money and Higham (1989) contend that hyperandrogenism does not appear to exist. However, they state that if an excess of hormone is given, it would be spilled out in the urine, and the remainder would act as a replacement for the natural products of the testes, which would be temporarily deactivated. They also state that hypoandrogenism is associated with "sexual inertia" (HSD) but not with homosexuality or bisexuality. Hyperestrogenism in the male does not produce homosexuality or bisexuality, but rather hypoandrogenism and "sexual inertia."

Parks et al. (1974) found homosexual males to be hormonally the same as heterosexual males. Money and Higham (1989) state the same to be true of transexual and transvestite males. They state that there are no known correlations between paraphilic behavior and hormonal function in either males or females. Money and Higham (1989) articulately summarize:

The phyletic program of sexually dimorphic behavior is initiated by the chromosomes, which dictate gonadal morphology, which in turn, affect the CNS as well as the genital anatomy. Postnatally the effects of social biography are imprinted during the period of gender-identity formation in early life. Prenatal and postnatal effects act conjointly to establish sexually dimorphic patterns of behavior that are highly resistant to change. Prepubertal gender-identity/role differentiation prepares the individual for the sexual dimorphism of puberty and adulthood. At puberty, androgen alters the threshold for erotic arousal in both males and females, but it does not control the imagery of eroticism or the sex of the partner in a pair-bond. Estrogen subserves the reproductive functions in the female. Its role in male reproductive status is unknown. Its cyclic effect on mood, affect, and eroticism in women is incompletely understood. Psychosocial events and hormonal events co-vary, but the mechanism by which this occurs is not known (p. 1858).

A variety of endocrine diseases have varying effects on sexual desire. Randall (1989) states that acromegalic females may show no effect on their libido or menses early in the course of the disease. (Acromegaly is a medical condition in which the pituitary gland has increased secretion of growth hormone to produce giantism.) As the disease progresses, so do the changes in their libido and menses. Randall also states that males in the early stages of the disease have increased libido, which diminishes as time progresses.

Testosterone's influence on male sexual erection and desire has long been recognized. The major source of testosterone in males is the Leydig cells—interstitial cells of the testes. Odell (1989) states that mature Leydig cells are unresponsive to FSH. FSH functions to induce prepubertal Leydig cell LH receptor formation. FSH and/or human chorionic gonadotropin (HCG)—"an LH-like hormone" (p. 2140) are critical during fetal Leydig cell development. LH can then induce Leydig cell testosterone production.

Men were surgically castrated (eunuchs) to be servants for women in ancient courts. Bancroft (1984) states that androgens are necessary for normal levels of sexual appetite in men. In studies of hypogonadal men on androgen replacement therapy (including those castrated for testicular neoplasms), sexual interest and sexual activity declines within two to three weeks after removal of exogenous androgens. In addition, ejaculation and usually the capacity for orgasm also cease. On reintroduction of exogenous androgens, these functions start to return within one to two weeks. In laboratory studies of hypogonadal men, Bancroft (1984) established that erections stimulated by erotic films occur to a normal extent. But their androgen deficiency is demonstrated by their loss of sexual interest and activity. Hypogonadal men experience the usual increase in sexual interest and activity when given hormone replacement but do not show any further improvement in their erectile response to erotic films. He also found that their capacity to respond to fantasy was reduced in the androgen-deficient state and that it increased with exogenous androgens.

O'Carroll and Bancroft (1984) conducted a double-blind crossover comparison study of testosterone and placebo injection with two groups of men with normal testosterone levels, of whom ten experienced a loss of sexual interest and ten experienced erectile failure. Testosterone injections produced a significant increase in sexual interest but had no effect on erectile function. O'Carroll and Bancroft contend that these findings further support the libido-enhancing effect of testosterone in the previously cited hypogonadal male testosterone study, and that they further advance the testosterone enhancing libido effect even in men with normal levels of circulating testosterone.

Buvat et al. (1987) used human chorionic gonadotropin (HCG) to treat 39 patients with non-organic erectile failure and 6 patients with a lack of sexual desire. (HCG stimulates the testicles to produce testosterone.) This treatment was found to be significantly better than placebo (47% vs. 12%, $p<0.5$) in treatment of HSD and improved six of seven sexual parameters, compared to two of seven for placebo. Unfortunately, the sexual parameter desire for sexual activity "was not included because the observations were not reliable" (p. 217).

Prolactin, the hormone secreted by the anterior pituitary gland into the bloodstream, is vital in lactation. Weizman et al. (1983) and Bancroft (1984) report that hyperprolactinemia in males and females can cause sexual impairment. Weizman et al. (1983) studied a group of patients undergoing hemodialysis (a time-consuming treatment for patients who suffer kidney failure due to a variety of medical conditions), all of whom were dependent on dialysis for the duration of their lives. Approximately 50% (38 males and 21 females) reported sexual dysfunction. Patients reporting sexual dysfunction were found to have a significantly higher serum prolactin level than those with normal sexual function. Bromocryptine treatment of five hyperprolactinemic patients (four male, one female) reduced serum prolactin levels to a normal range and improved sexual function. (All experienced increased libido.) However, there was no placebo control group.

Bancroft (1984) anecdotally describes a patient in whom hyperprolactinemia (belatedly discovered) was seen, with loss of sexual interest and erectile failure. The patient initially received placebo and counseling. At a six-month follow-up he reported that there was a substantial improvement in the sexual relationship between himself and his wife. Three years later the patient's initial prolactin level was measured (due to the fortuitous discovery of the initial serum sample), and he was found to have been hyperprolactinemic at the beginning of treatment, but at the six-month follow-up there was no evidence of recurrence of erectile failure, although his level of sexual interest had declined and he was still found to be hyperprolactinemic. (No evidence of a pituitary tumor was found.) Bromocryptine produced a significant improvement in his level of sexual interest, although this change was not great and did not have much impact on his level of sexual activity with his wife. Bancroft concluded that the effects of the hyperprolactinemia were confined to a dimunition of the man's sexual interest and that his partner's psychological reactions to this had a much greater impact on their sexual relationship. Bancroft hypothesizes that the effects of increased prolactin in males are comparable to the effects of diminished testosterone.

Declining sexual activity has long been associated with aging. Women in menopause experience primary ovarian failure, punctuated by the cessation of menses (i.e., menopause) and may often experience a decline in sexual desire and function.

Davidson et al. (1982) cites Kinsey et al.

(1948) and Verwoerdt et al. (1969) to substantiate the statement that there is a progressive decline in sexual desire and functioning as men age. He also cites Vermeulen et al. (1972), Baker et al. (1976), and Stearns et al. (1976) that this decline in male sexual desire and functioning is mirrored by corresponding diminution in plasma testosterone and a reciprocal increase in gonadotropin level. Davidson et al. (1982) state that these studies have been used to substantiate the existence of a male climacteric (a counterpart to female menopause).

Davidson et al. (1982) studied 220 ambulatory men aged 49 to 93, measuring total T, SHBG, LH, FSH, prolactin, and estradiol. They found decreased total T, increased SHBG, subsequent greater decrease in free T (than total T), increased LH and FSH, and static estradiol and prolactin levels. Analysis of the data revealed that significant correlations between hormonal and behavioral (libido or performance) factors are of low order. This suggests a weak hormone/behavior relationship. Hormone variables affect performance parameters more than they affect libido. Total T is not correlated with behavioral parameters.

Davidson et al. noted that these correlations tend to diminish when they are run within decades of life (eliminating most of age influences on hormones). Multiple regression analyses revealed that age accounted for a larger behavioral variance than hormone levels. Dividing the age groups into tertiles of free T or LH (high, medium, or low), Davidson et al. a significant effect of age on libido and performance, but not on free T. LH had no effect on libido but a significant effect on performance ($p < 0.02$).

Davidson et al. (1982) cite Harman and Tsitouras (1980) and Sparrow and Rowe (1980) in stating that no significant diminution in total T or free T were found in older men who were specifically selected for physical and mental health and intellectual/educational level. Davidson et al. (1982) summarize:

Frank hypogonadism may be almost as rare in the aging population as among younger adults, and the aging decrease in androgen is apparently not sufficient to have a major impact on sexuality. It remains possible, however, that sexual decline represents a quite variable change in androgen sensitivity of the behavioural target tissues (wherever they are!), so that the severity of this defect (in receptors?) is not correlated well with the level of free or total T. The fact that there is a somewhat better relationship to LH is consistent with this idea. LH increase signifies the response of hypothalamic-pituitary tissue to lowered androgen and might therefore reflect a shift in CNS androgen receptor sensitivity which is also relevant to behaviour change (pg. 606).

If the reader wishes more information on androgen replacement therapy, see Segraves (1988) and Davidson et al. (1982).

The study of sexual desire in women has been facilitated by natural and artificial hormonal influences in women's lives. These include changes in desire after cessation of endogenous hormonal production (natural menopause) or surgical menopause. This cessation of normal ovarian function is punctuated by subsequent cessation of menstruation. Also interesting to note is the supplementation hormonal therapy in postmenopausal females—estrogen, estrogen-progesterone, estrogen-testosterone. The widespread use of oral contraceptive pills (estrogen and estrogen-progesterone combinations) and the studies of the normal hormonal fluctuations associated with the menstrual cycle have facilitated our understanding of the relationship between hormones and sexual desire.

Menopause can be viewed from numerous perspectives, but in general it is simply the cessation of menses. Menopause has numerous hormonal, biological, and sociocultural effects. The hormonal changes in menopause are simply a diminution of estrogen and progesterone production; these changes are reflected in diminished negative feedback on the pituitary gland, which leads to increased levels of LH and FSH. (Increased FSH and LH are a good marker of menopause.)

It is important to note the abrupt reversal in the use of estrogen replacement therapy (ERT) in menopausal women in the past decade. The risks of estrogen's possible oncogenic effects on breast and uterus have been reappraised, and these risks may be mitigated. Lindsay et al. (1984) found that a minimal dose of estrogen is effective in preventing osteoporosis (a significant causal agent in postmenopausal morbidity and mortality). Matthews et al. (1989) state that natural menopause has an undesirable effect on lipid metabolism, which may lead to a corresponding increase in heart disease. They found that hormone replacement therapy in menopausal women may ameliorate some of the deleterious lipid changes.

Vermeulen (1983) has found that as estrogen levels decrease in the perimenopausal period, testosterone levels may decrease, remain unchanged, or actually increase for a few years. The increased testosterone is secondary to ovarian stromal hyperplasia (due to high LH stimulation of the ovaries). The cessation of ovarian hormonal production causes numerous end organ changes, primarily vasomotor symptoms (e.g., unpleasant hot flushing sensation and sweating, so profuse that a change of clothing is often required). Semmens and Wagner (1982) state that estrogen deficiency impairs vaginal transudation and lubrication and can lead to dyspareunia (discomfort/pain during intercourse). Estrogen tends to thicken or cornify cells of the vaginal lining. Tsai et al. (1987) found that vaginal blood flow and vaginal transport mechanism decrease in the postmenopausal female.

However, Segraves (1988) cites Morrell et al. (1984) and Myers and Morokoff (1985), who used photoplethysmography to measure pre- and postmenopausal women's vaginal response to erotic stimuli. Morrell et al. (1984) found a decreased vasocongestive response in postmenopausal women, but subjective arousal ratings did not vary between pre- and postmenopausal responses. Myers and Morokoff (1985) failed to find a differential vasocongestive response, although postmenopausal women (non-ERT) reported decreased vaginal lubrication.

The psychological impact of the cessation of menses can be as traumatic as that of the onset of menses. The changes that women experience due to menopause are not limited to ovarian failure. Especially in Western, youth-oriented society, advancing age can be associated with perceptions of loss of attractiveness and desirability. Benedek's (1950) pointed use of the term *climacteric* to describe the menopause certainly emphasizes its effect. This orientation of Western society compounds sexual damage in the menopausal woman, since men are more prone to die at an earlier age —leaving their female partners alone, feeling unattractive, in an age group that is predominately female. Hysterectomy also has an impact on the sexuality of Western women. Flint (1975) and Aoz et al. (1977) found that the negative experience of women in Western societies during menopause is further highlighted when compared with non-Western cultures, where women may view menopause in a more positive light and therefore experience fewer menopausal problems.

Diminished sexual function has been noted by numerous researchers following menopause, but the type and degree of diminution has varied. There is even significant debate as to whether this diminution actually exists. Kinsey et al. (1953) reported that 48% of women experiencing menopause felt that their sexual response had decreased, and the incidence of coitus was also observed to decrease. Individual activities of women (masturbation, nocturnal dreams to orgasm) were not observed to decline until the sixth decade of life.

Bachmann (1990) provides a succinct review of menopausal sexual issues. She cites Cutler et al. (1987), who studied 52 perimenopausal females and was unable to demonstrate any correlation of sexual expression (change of sexual desire, response, or satisfaction) with ovarian hormonal profile except at estradiol levels less than 35 mg/pL. (These women reported reduced coital activity.) Bachmann (1990) also cites Channon and Ballinger (1986), whose study of 274 perimenopausal women showed that anxiety was the most significant factor decreasing coital frequency and that depression was correlated with a diminution in libido.

Bachmann et al. (1985) studied sexual desire in 22 postmenopausal women and found no correlation between gonadotropins and loss of sexual desire. About 50% of the women experienced no decline in sexual interest with menopause, and less than 20% reported a significant decrease. The researchers found a positive relationship between sexual desire and a measure of marital adjustment, using the Locke-Wallace marital adjustment test. They did note that coital frequency following menopause decreased from approximately twice a week to once a week, but this was not correlated with a change in desire.

Hällström and Samuelsson (1990) performed general population studies of 677 urban middle-aged women on two occasions, six years apart. Of these women, 197 were married or cohabiting on both occasions. The data indicated that 27% noted a decrease in sexual desire, and 10% noticed an increase in sexual desire between the two interviews. Predictors of decreased desire were age, high sexual desire at first interview, lack of a confiding relationship, insufficient support from spouse, alcoholism in spouse, and major depression. The predictors of increase in sexual desire were weak desire at first interview, negative marital relations before first interview, and mental disorder at first interview. Note that the strongest predictors of change in sexual desire (strength of desire at first interview and weakness of desire at first interview) were strongly correlated with change. This reflects a regression toward the mean. Hällström and Samuelsson (1990) found that sexual desire is characterized by overall moderate temporal stability in middle-aged women. However, a substantial percentage of middle-aged women experience major changes in sexual desire—mostly a decrease. Many women who reported a lack of sexual interest initially regained their desire spontaneously in the six years between interviews. It is interesting to note that there were no subjects who indicated strong sexual desire beyond the age of 50. No clear cohort effects emerged.

Experimentally, it is difficult to make a clear separation between increased libido from ERT

and the symptomatic treatment of somatic complaints/increased sense of well-being (decreased hot flashes, vaginal irritation, or dyspareunia). Bancroft (1984) states, "But as yet no one has demonstrated convincingly, either in a positive or negative direction, that this postmenopausal loss of libido is estrogen dependent" (p. 15). Segraves (1988) notes numerous studies in which there are conflicting opinions about estrogen's effect on the libido. Bancroft (1984) notes that endocrinologists have used progesterone in the treatment of excess sexuality in women.

Human male sexual behavior has long been believed to be influenced by testosterone. Testosterone was first recognized as possibly affecting female sexual behavior when Waxenberg et al. (1959) demonstrated a diminution in sexual desire, activity, and responsivity following adrenalectomy in women who had previously been oophorectomized (in an attempt to treat metastatic breast cancer). Willson et al. (1975) anecdotally note a marked increase in sex drive in women receiving testosterone for treatment of metastatic cancer. Carney, Bancroft, and Matthews (1978) studied a group of women with diminished sexual desire. In the study, one-half of the group was treated with therapy and testosterone, while the other half was treated with therapy and diazepam (an antianxiety drug). At six months the testosterone group showed greater improvement in sexual desire. Later, Bancroft (1984) attempted to replicate the earlier findings, with testosterone and placebo rather than testosterone and diazepam. He found no difference between testosterone and placebo and concluded that the first study had demonstrated a negative effect of diazepam rather than a positive effect of testosterone.

Sherwin et al. (1985) performed a prospective crossover study of 53 surgically menopausal women, who were divided into five study groups. One group consisted of simple hysterectomy without bilateral salpingo-oophorectomy (BSO). The other four groups of women received an intramuscular combination of estrogen and androgen, estrogen alone, androgen alone, or placebo. Analysis (ANOVA) of sexual desire and fantasy scores demonstrated a significant group X time interaction ($p < .001$). Desire and fantasy scores directly rose and fell significantly ($p<0.01$) between testosterone treatment months and the withdrawal month. There was no evidence found that testosterone affected physiologic response or interpersonal aspects of sexual behavior. This result led the authors to conclude that the major impact of androgen on women relates to sexual motivation, not activity.

Sherwin and Gelfand (1987) studied 44 women who had undergone hysterectomy and bilateral salpingo-oophorectomy. One group received estrogen androgen injections monthly since their surgery, the second group received estrogen alone, and the third group received a placebo or was untreated. Testosterone levels were measured at six different days following the monthly injections. Women receiving estrogen and androgen reported higher rates of sexual desire ($p<0.01$), sexual arousal ($p<0.01$), and number of fantasies ($p<0.01$) than those who were given estrogen alone or were untreated. It was also found that these behaviors covaried with plasma testosterone levels, but not with estradiol levels. Higher testosterone levels found during the first two postinjection weeks were associated with higher rates of coitus and orgasm in the estrogen androgen group ($p<0.01$). Sherwin and Gelfand also state that 15–20% of women receiving estrogen and testosterone developed mild facial hirsutism, which is reversible with dosage modification. A deepening of the voice as a result of this treatment is rare and reversible with dosage modification.

Stanislaw and Rice (1988) report a multicountry study of over 1000 subjects and 22,000 menstrual cycles. The timing of sexual desire is positively correlated with the onset of the basal body temperature shift—the ovulation date. The researchers compiled various studies in which arousability and desire are said to increase at various times throughout the menstrual cycle. Stanislaw and Rice (1988) cite Adams et al. (1978) and Matteo and Rissman (1984), who report of a periovulatory peak in female-initiated sexual behavior in both heterosexual and homosexual women. Bancroft et al. (1983) report in-

creased levels of testosterone and androstenedione in the late follicular, early luteal phase of the menstrual cycle. Persky et al. (1978) found that intercourse frequency was related to wives' testosterone levels at their ovulation peaks, confirming the peak Bancroft et al. (1983) had previously demonstrated around periovulatory time. Also noteworthy is a positive relationship between each male's average testosterone level and his wife's or his own sex drive, possibly indicative of testosterone enhancement of sexual desire in both sexes. Persky et al. found that the higher the baseline level of testosterone in the female, the greater the average gratification scores—suggesting a testosterone-dose-related effect.

Disease states are characterized by an absence of health, which frequently is related to diminution of the patient's state of well-being. This can, in turn, be hypothetically linked to a diminution in sexual desire. However, it has been difficult to document this diminution in the medical literature. Thyroid hormonal disturbances have been associated with alterations in sexual desire. Thyroid hormones can be thought of on a simplistic level as controlling the body's thermostat. Thyroid or metabolic rate is controlled by the pituitary gland, which secretes thyroid stimulating hormone (TSH), which acts upon the thyroid gland to secrete thyroid hormone. The pituitary gland, in turn, is controlled by the hypothalamus, which releases thyrotropin releasing hormone (TRH), which controls TSH release. (See Figure 2.2.) Hall et al. (1982) state that in cases of acute failure of the thyroid gland (myxedematous crises), hypersexuality states have been reported. However, myxedematous states are extremely rare and very dramatic. Wortsman et al. (1987) report that hypothyroidism has been associated with a history of impotence and decreased sexual drive. Gold et al. (1981) did a study on 250 consecutive psychiatric patients who were hospitalized for the treatment of depression or anergia. They found that 26% of them had varying degrees of hypothyroidism. Half of the patients' hypothyroidisms were detectable only with TRH testing (the patients had normal T3U, T4, and TSH levels

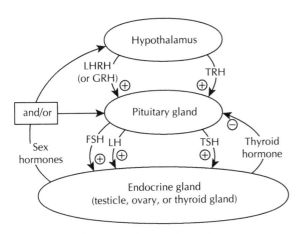

Figure 2.2. Hormone interaction.

but have increased reactions of TSH to administration of TRH). Gold suggests that TRH testing might be helpful in those patients who have atypical depression or are resistant to treatment.

In states of hyperthyroidism McKenzie and Zakarija (1989) found that "libido, in either sex, may be enhanced but is, in our experience more commonly decreased, at times severely" (p. 659). Kidd et al. (1979) found that 71% of patients with thyrotoxicosis (hyperthyroidism) experienced a loss of libido and 56% experienced decreased potency.

Damage to male sexual functioning from advanced diabetes mellitus, well documented in any medical textbook, ranges from neuropathies to advanced atherosclerotic vascular changes that can lead to organic impotence. However, the effects of diabetes mellitus on male sexual desire have not been well documented in the medical literature. Jensen (1981) found that 50% of male diabetics developed erectile failure within six years of the onset of disease. Newman and Bertelson (1986) examined 81 insulin-treated diabetic women 18–50 years of age who had reported coital activity during the previous year, all of whom were not pregnant and had not had a hysterectomy. A diagnosis of sexual dysfunction was made in 47% of the subjects, and 32% of those reported inhibited sexual excitement, 21% inhibited sexual desire, 21% dyspareunia, and 14% inhibited orgasm. Jensen

(1986) performed a longitudinal study, initially of 80 diabetic women and then six years later of 50 insulin-treated Type I diabetic women 26–45 years of age. Initially, 18% had reduced sexual desire, and six years later 20% had reduced sexual desire. He found that peripheral neuropathy, retinopathy, nephrophyhy, autonomic neuropathy and metabolic control were not correlated with sexual dysfunction ($p<.05$). Curiously, six of the fourteen women in the initial study who were sexually dysfunctional recovered normal function (some of them in spite of objective evidence of neuropathy; none of the women had been in psychotherapy for their sexual problems). Overall, marital and social situation was found to be the most important factor in the spontaneous remission rate.

Schreiner-Engel et al. (1987) studied 35 Type I and 23 Type II diabetic women, with matched controls, ranging in age from 20 to 63. No statistical difference was found between Type I diabetics and their matched controls in sexual desire, partner's sexual desire, sexual arousal, lubrication, orgasm frequency, frequency of sexual activity, or sexual satisfaction. However, Type II diabetics statistically differed from their matched controls, with desire ($p<.05$), lubrication ($p<.04$), orgasm frequency ($p<.03$), and sexual satisfaction ($p<.04$). (Of the Type I diabetics, 100% were on insulin, whereas 57% of the Type II diabetics were on insulin and 43% were controlled by diet or oral hypoglycemic agents.)

Lipe et al. (1990) compared 41 married men with Parkinson's disease (a progressive central neurologic disease) to a group of 29 married men with arthritis. He found that total sexual functioning and categories of desire, arousal, orgasm, and satisfaction did not differ significantly between patients with PD and arthritis. He found reduced sexual function associated with both arthritis and PD, severity of illness, and depression. It is of interest that medications used to treat PD have been reported to cause hypersexuality and impotence.

Bach et al. (1989) conducted a study of 150 women aged 26–76 with nonalcoholic liver disease; 33% reported a diminution in sexual desire (of whom 27% were premenopausal and 37% postmenopausal). However, this difference did not reach statistical significance. Bach et al. state that nonalcoholic liver disease does not affect sexual desire, function, or performance, and that women with liver disease may be reassured that they can maintain normal sexual relations.

Grunert et al. (1988) studied a population of 120 patients who had traumatic hand injuries. Six months posttrauma, 49% of the patients experienced sexual dysfunction. At six months posttrauma, 19% continued to experience sexual dysfunction (23 patients: 20 men and 3 women, ranging in age from 21 to 57), of whom 65% reported reduced sexual desire, 35% impotence, and 39% rejection of sexual contact by partner. The four major causes of impaired sexual functioning were: (1) pain, 22%; (2) deformity anxiety, 52%; (3) replant anxiety, 9%; and (4) contagious anxiety, 39%.

Pregnancy and puerperium cause multiple changes in both women and their partners. Reamy and White (1987) have done a superior review of this subject, in which they state that pregnancy tends to have a negative effect on sexual desire, expression, and satisfaction, which increases as pregnancy approaches term. They summarize their review in stating,

> Most research respondents reported gradual return to prepregnancy levels of sexual desire, enjoyment, and coital frequency, with a minority in most cited studies indicating sexual interest and coitus levels below prepregnancy levels up to one year after delivery. The most frequently listed reasons for poor postpartum sexual enjoyment include episiotomy discomfort, fatigue, vaginal bleeding or discharge, dyspareunia, insufficient lubrication, fears of awakening the infant or not hearing him/her, fear of injury, and decreased sense of attractiveness (p. 165).

Blumer and Walker (1975) note that temporal lobe epilepsy is clearly associated with abnormal sexual behavior. In temporal lobe epileptics, they contend, sexual normality is the exception, and global hyposexuality is the pre-

dominant aspect of their sexual behavior. They state that patients who develop temporal lobe epilepsy prior to or at the time of puberty may never or only rarely be sexually aroused. Blumer and Walker list the symptomatology associated with psychomotor ictal (seizure) sexual arousal in three categories: (1) precipitating or triggering mechanisms, (2) primictal, (3) ictal equivalence. Precipitating or triggering mechanisms consist of sexual intercourse or masturbation, erotically charged objects or events, hypnosis or suggestion, and self-stimulation. Primictal symptomology consists of epigastric sensation, chest or anal sensation, abdominal pain, and olfactory sensation. Ictal equivalence consists of fear (prepubertal), paradoxical painful experience, and urinary incontinence. Blumer and Walker cite Mitchell et al. (1954) and Hunter et al. (1963) regarding two cases in which temporal lobe abnormalities were closely related with perversion, which was completely abolished following the cure of a temporal lobe epilepsy by unilateral lobectomy.

In summary, numerous medical conditions have been found to influence sexual desire negatively. Testosterone has been found to increase desire in both hypogonadal and eugonadal HSD males. Hyperprolactinemia has been found to be a treatable/curable cause of HSD. However, in aging males experiencing diminished desire, desire has been correlated to age and minimally to testosterone, leading Davidson et al. (1982) to propose decreased "androgen receptor sensitivity" (p. 606).

Testosterone has not been shown to be effective in enhancing desire in HSD women. Middle-aged women's desire seems to fluctuate temporally as they experience a gradual decrease. Testosterone has been demonstrated to increase desire in surgically menopausal women.

Menstrual cycles have been proposed to have various temporal effects on desire. The most convincing studies link the peak of desire to ovulation. Evolutionarily and physiologically, this link makes sense, since increased desire increases the potential for sexual activity during the fertile period of ovulation, and there is a preovulatory surge of LH and a subsequent peak of testosterone. There is strong medical evidence to link testosterone to both male and female desire. This will be expanded upon in the theory section of this chapter.

Hypothyroidism and hyperthyroidism are associated with HSD. Both medical conditions are easily treated/cured; unfortunately, there is no mention of return to normal levels of desire with corrections of these states.

The severe and organ damage experienced in diabetes mellitus (DM) and the complex (vulnerable) vascular/neuronal interplay required for adequate erection/ejaculation have overshadowed and limited reports on the effects of DM on male desire. (The effects of DM on male desire are unknown). Of interest is the fact that the physically devastating insulin-dependent DM seems to have no effect on desire in women, while the obesity-related DM has been seen to have significant effects on desire.

Women with nonalcoholic liver disease experience no significant effects on sexual desire. Traumatic hand injury patients may experience diminished desire. Pregnancy seems to have a progressive negative effect on desire, which is gradually reversed with partuition. Temporal lobe epilepsy is associated with abnormal sexual behavior, with HSD being the norm.

In brief, testosterone is influential in various disease states, as well as normal physiological changes. Many medical conditions/diseases produce mixed but generally negative effects on sexual desire.

DRUG EFFECTS ON SEXUAL DESIRE

Medicinal and recreational drugs have long been thought to affect sexuality. William Shakespeare's play *MacBeth* is commonly referenced as one of the earlier literary allusions to alcohol's ability to increase desire but effectively impair performance. Folklore, too, contains numerous references to libidinal enhancement by ingestion of various herbs, vegetables, and the like. Buffum (1982) performed an exhaustive survey of pharmacosexology; the following is a partial summary of his excellent review as it pertains to desire. By definition, libido-affecting drugs would act upon the central nervous system. In naming certain drugs that block dopamine receptors, his findings are consistent with the dopaminergic theory of sexual behavior. Gessa and Tagliamonte (1974) believe that cerebral serotonin and dopamine may exert reciprocal control on male sexual behavior, which may biochemically explain the aphrodisiac effect of L-DOPA seen in some rats and Parkinsonian patients. Various androgens have inhibitory effects on endogenous testosterone. Oncologic chemotherapy could cause overall dysphoria.

When patients have elevated blood pressure, their physicians often prescribe antihypertensive medications to decrease blood pressure and subsequently decrease the patient's risk of developing a crippling or lethal stroke or heart attack. It is unfortunate when these medications impinge on the patient's sexual desires. Pillay (1976), Newman and Salerno (1974), and Horowitz et al. (1967) report that the centrally acting hypotensive agent methyldopa (Aldomet®) has decreased libido in 7–14% of patients. Laver (1974), Mroczek, Leibel, and Finnerty (1972), Onesti et al. (1971), Ebringer et al. (1970), and Khan, Camel, and Perry (1970) report that clonidine, another centrally acting hypotensive agent (Catapres®) can cause decreased libido and failure of erection. (It is interesting to note that a common use of Catapres® is to treat withdrawal cravings—e.g., from opiate and nicotine withdrawal).

Reserpine (Serpasil®) is a hypotensive agent that is infrequently used due to its numerous central nervous system and peripheral side effects, which are caused by its catacholamine- and serotonin-depleting actions. Laver (1974) found a 46% incidence of decreased libido or erection failure. Tuchman and Crumpton (1955) found that one of fourteen patients (a 7% incidence) had decreased libido. A commonly used hypotensive agent is propranolol (Inderal®), a nonspecific B_1 and B_2 andrenergic blocking agent. Serlin et al. (1980)); Burnett and Chahine (1979); Gavras et al. (1979); Bathen (1978); Hollifield (1977); Veteran's Administration (1977); Warren and Warren (1977); Hollifield et al. (1976); Knarr (1976); Warren, Brewer, and Orgain (1976); Zacharias (1976); and Prichard and Gillam (1969) all report that propranolol may cause decreased libido and erectile failure. Hollifield et al. (1976), Knarr (1976) and Prichard and Gilliam (1969) report an incidence of 1–4% of diminished libido. Zarren and Black (1975); Greenblatt and Koch-Weser (1973); Brown et al. (1972); and Spark and Melby (1968) report that (S)pironolactone (Aldactone®), a hypotensive diuretic, acts as a competitive aldosterone-antagonist and can cause decreased libido. Buffum (1982) states that diazide diuretics (a common form of hypotensive diuretic) is thought to be associated with sexual dysfunction. However, he states that there is little data in the literature to support this statement.

The adverse effects of antipsychotics on libido may occur by blocking dopamine effects in the central nervous system and by suppressing the hypothalamic-pituitary-gonadal axis, according to Byck (1975). Kotin et al. (1976), Haider (1966), and Freyhan (1961) report isolated cases of diminished libido associated with thioridazine (Mellaril®). Bartholomew (1968) performed a noncontrolled, nonblind study of subjects on the drug fluphenazine (Prolixin®). He found that 65% of the population on Prolixin® have a diminution of sexual drive and interest following one 25mg injection of Prolixin®.

Antidepressants have also been noted to have effects on sexuality. Hollister (1978a) and Beaumont (1977) state that depression is frequently associated with a decrease in sexual desire, which makes the side effects of antidepressants difficult to separate from those caused by the depression itself. Hollister (1978b) describes imiprimine (Tofiranil®) as a tricyclic antidepressant with equal serotonin- and norepinephrone-blocking characteristics and moderate anticholinergic effects. Glass (1981), Petrie (1980), and Simpson, Blair, and Amuso (1965) report that imiprimine can cause decreased libido, inadequate erection, delayed ejaculation, and delayed orgasm. Hollister (1978b) hypothesizes that amitryptyline might be expected to cause more

decreased libido than other tricyclics because of its greater ability to block serotonin reuptake and its sedative properties. Protriptyline (Vivactil®) has been reported to cause dimunition of sexual desire, impotence, and ejaculation dysfunction. Everett (1975) and Simpson, Blair and Amuso (1965) report that amoxapine (Asendin®) causes decreased libido, impotence and painful ejaculatory inhibition. Kulik and Wilbur (1982); Schwarcz (1982); Hekimian, Friedhoff, and Deever (1978); and Hollister (1978b) all state that tranylcpromine (Parnate®) is a monoamine oxidase (MAO) inhibitor antidepressant that pharmacologically resembles amphetamine. Simpson et al. (1965) report a small study in which tranylcypromine was found to cause increased libido and spontaneous erections. Lithium (Eskalith®) has been used in the treatment of bipolar depression. Vinarova et al. (1972) report lithium to cause "impaired sexual function" and "decreased sexual appetence" (p. 107).

Testosterone administration to hypogonadal males has been shown to enhance sexual desire. Frasier (1973) administered norethandrolone (another anabolic steroid) to seven men for 8 to 25 weeks. He reported they all developed decreased libido and potency, diminished testicular size, and azoospermia. The men appeared to recover in the 24th to 26th weeks after discontinuation of norethandrolone, but permanent testicular damage was noted. Freed et al. (1972) administered methandienone (Dianabol®), another anabolic steroid, to five men at 25 mgs a day. One man complained of marked diminution of libido. No complaints were listed from any of the five men on 10 mg a day.

According to Buffum (1982),

> Up until 1974 there were prescription products on the market that contained testosterone, yohimbine, and nuxvomica (strychine), for example, for treatment of impotence associated with the male "climacteric." It is significant that in spite of all of the double blind crossover studies purporting to show efficacy (Sabotks (1969); Miller (1968); Bruhl and Leslie (1963)), they were pulled off the market (p. 17).

However, Chambers and Phoenix (1989) found old, sexually sluggish rhesus monkey (active when younger) unresponsive to various doses of yohimbine.

Various antiandrogens have been brought onto the market. Cyproterone acetate (Andro-cur®) is one of the most potent antiandrogens known. Murad and Gilman (1975) and Laschet and Laschet (1975) state that it has specific action in the diencephalon, which results in its inhibition of libido. Murad and Gilman (1975) also state that Androcur® has progestational, androgenic, and antiestrogenic activities. Its antiandrogen effects have been used in treating criminal sex offenders, in an attempt to reduce libido and prevent the recurrence of sex crimes. Murad and Gilman (1975) state that decreased libido occurs after ten to fourteen days, and libido returns to normal two weeks after cessation of medication. Berlin and Meinecke (1981) report that medroxyprogesterone acetate (a progestin) has also been used in the treatment of sex offenders. Herrmann and Beach (1980) reviewed 13 articles on antiandrogen use in sex offenders and summarized the following effects:

> 1) physiological sexual function was normal or hypo in hyper or normal offenders. This was dependent on the dose and duration of treatment. 2) Overt sexual behavior was unchanged or reduced in abnormal/illegal offenders. This was also dependent on dose and duration of treatment. 3) Sexual fantasy was decreased, increased or normalized. The characteristics of the sexual offenders were not described. 4) Sexual arousal was decreased but did not disappear completely in hyper or normal offenders. 5) Gender identity and sexual preference were unchanged. 6) Aggression was reduced. 7) Temporary reactive depression, mild sedation and reduced activity also occured (p. 194).

Progestins have primarily been used for female contraception and the treatment of ovarian disorders. Meiraz et al. (1977); Palanca and Juco (1977); Paulson and Kane (1975); and Heller et al. (1959) state, however, that progestin has been used in males for the treatment of urinary tract obstruction secondary to benign prostatic hypertrophy. Various forms of estrogen have been used in women for replacement after the climacteric or in female contraception, and in the treatment of breast and prostate carcinoma in males, according to Murad and Gilman (1975). Estrogen's diminution of libido in these males gave researchers and clinicians the idea of using estrogen to treat deviant sexual behavior. Bancroft (1974) and Golla and Hodge (1949) state that estrogen's decreased libido effect has been used with good results in the treatment of male sexual deviance. Buffum (1982) says there is no consensus on the effects of oral contraceptives on desire. There have been reports of positive, neutral, and negative effects on desire.

Parr (1976); Cicero et al. (1975); Mintz et al. (1974); DeLeon and Wexler (1973); and Cushman (1972) state that heroin (diacetylmorphine), a synthetic morphine derivative, has been reported to cause decreased libido, retarded ejaculation, and impotence. According to Cushman (1972), 61% of heroin addicts reported impaired libido, 76% of former heroin addicts reported impaired or absent libido during heroin use, and 92% reported impaired or absent libido when heroin was ingested. However, the subjects' libido normalized after detoxification. Cushman (1972) found plasma LH levels in heroin addicts to be within normal levels. Cicero et al. (1975) found no significant difference between heroin users and controls in testosterone levels. Cushman (1972) hypothesizes that morphine administration causes alteration in serotonin turnover rates and consequently affects libido. However, Mirin et al. (1980) found decreased testosterone and LH in heroin users and speculated that heroin depressed LH and caused a subsequent drop in the plasma testosterone levels. Espejo, Hogben, and Stimmel (1973); Handbury et al. (1977); Kreek (1973); and Cushman (1972) report that methadone (Dolophine®) use results in an incidence of decreased libido of between 6% and 38%.

CNS stimulants have been found both to increase and decrease sexual desire. Smith, Buxton, and Bammann (1979); Angrist and Gershon (1976); Parr (1976); and Bell and Trethowan (1961) report that males have increased libido, impotence and delayed ejaculation from amphetamine use. Smith, Buxton, and Bammann (1979); Angrist and Gershon (1976); and Bell and Trethowan (1961) state that female amphetamine use has been reported to cause increased libido and delayed orgasm. Buffum (1982) states that changes in sexuality secondary to amphetamine use are quite variable within given studies. Cocaine is used medically primarily as a local anaesthetic; CNS stimulation is the desired effect in nonmedical use. Buffum (1982) reports positive and negative effects on sexuality. Gawin (1978), Ellinwood and Rockwell (1975), and Gay et al. (1975) report that many recreational cocaine users believe it to have an aphrodisiac effect. However, Gay et al. (1975) noted that erections decrease at high cocaine doses.

Alcohol (or ethanol) acts as a general depressant. Mendelson, Mello, and Ellingboe (1977) and Gordon et al. (1976) report that testosterone levels have been shown to decrease with alcohol consumption. Buffum (1982) cites Gordon, Southren, and Leiber (1979) and Van Thiel and Lester (1976) to explain the alcoholism-induced condition of hyperestrogenization, in which the impaired liver increasingly converts androgen to estrogen. The increased estrogen then causes feminization, gynecomastia, decreased desire, impotence, and sterility, all of which can be found in alcoholic males.

Methaqualone (Quaalude®), a sedative hypnotic sleeping medication earlier prescribed in this country, has been off the market for the past several years. Kochansky et al. (1975); Gerald and Schwirian (1973); Inaba et al. (1973); Weissberg (1972); and Hughes (1964) report that methaqualone has a street reputation as an aphrodisiac.

Marijuana's active agent is delta-9-tetrahydrocannabinol (THC). Hollister (1975) and Jaffe (1975) state that THC has a mixture of sedative, stimulant, and hallucinogenic properties. Hollister (1975) and Chopra (1969) say that decreased libido and inability to perform has been reported in chronic hashish abusers in India. (Hashish is a concentrated form of marijuana.) Halikas, Weller, and Morse (1982); Gay et al. (1975); and Nowlis (1975) state that sexual

function has been reported to be enhanced at more moderate dosages.

Cimetadine is an H_2 antagonist, used in medicine to suppress gastric acid production. Buffum (1982) cites Gifford et al. (1980); Biron (1979); Peden et al. (1979); and Wolfe (1979), reporting 31 males who experienced progressive loss of desire and/or impotence within 1 to 28 weeks of using 0.6–1.2 grams/day.

Digoxin (Lanoxin®) has been used in the treatment of cardiac patients for congestive heart failure and arrhythmias. Neri et al. (1980) found that five of fourteen males (36%) had decreased libido, five of the fourteen had decreased erections, and six of them (43%) had decreased frequency of sexual relations following long-term digoxin administration.

Carbonic hydrase inhibitors have been used to reduce intraocular pressure in glaucoma patients, and also for prophylaxis in altitude sickness. Wallace et al. (1979) reports 39 cases of decreased libido return to pretreatment levels after cessation of CAI.

Levodopa (Larodopa®) is a medication used in the treatment of Parkinsonism (it functions as a precursor of dopamine). Goodwin (1971) reports hypersexual behavior in 8 of 908 Parkinson's patients treated with levodopa. Brown et al. (1978) report a study in which 50% of a group of Parkinson's patients demonstrated increased sexual interest or activity unrelated to improved locomotor function.

Deprenyl (Eldepryl®) is a selective B-type monoamine oxidase inhibitor that is used to treat the symptoms of Parkinson's disease. Drago et al. (1986) found deprenyl to enhance aged male rat sexual behavior. Dallo, Lekka, and Knoll (1986) found deprenyl superior in enhancing the ejaculatory behavior of sexually sluggish male rats when compared to apomorphine, bromocriptine, or amphetamine. Knoll, Dallo, and Yen (1989) report prolonging the lifetime duration of male rat sexual activity as well as the animals' overall lifetime.

Chambers and Phoenix (1989) found that various doses of apomorphine, deprenyl, and yohimbine fail to increase sexual behavior in old, sluggish male rhesus monkeys. They hypothesize that these differences may result from variations in neurotransmitters or receptors that facilitate sexual behavior or availability of the drug to the target site.

ENVIRONMENTAL TOXIN EFFECTS ON SEXUAL DESIRE

Toxins in the environment can have various effects on sexual function. Exposures can be occupational, but routine environmental exposures also occur—spills, illegal dumping such as the Kepone® episode reported by Guzelian (1982), and general or environmental pollutants. These toxic exposures can come from cutaneous, respiratory, or gastrointestinal ingestion (contaminated air, fluids, foods, etc.). The workplace can be a source of toxins such as heavy metals, metals, estrogenic compounds, insecticides, and herbicides. Other sources are the home (and associated hobbies such as gardening, fishing, shooting of firearms) and water sources contaminated by old lead pipe and/or lead solder, or even lead crystal decanters. The OSHA lead standard reads, "In male workers exposed to lead there can be a decrease in sexual drive, impotence, decreased ability to produce healthy sperm and sterility."

Guzelian (1982) provides a current review of chlordecone (Kepone®), an organochlorine pesticide. In citing Cannon et al. (1978), he reports that chlorodecone intoxication resulted in more than half of 131 factory workers and many residents of the surrounding area in which the factory had practiced poor industrial hygiene and waste disposal. Guzelian (1982) states that there are no reports of human deaths due to chlorodecone exposure. But 10 of 23 cases of chlorodecone-poisoned workers experienced a prominent weight loss (up to 60 pounds in four months), despite a normal appetite. Guzelian (1982) cites Taylor et al. (1978) in reporting that chlorodecone intoxication produces in humans an irregular, nonpurposive waking tremor involving the extremities, head, and trunk. Guzelian (1982) also cites Anderson et al. (1976) in stating that decreased libido in seven patients was the only symptom in the 28 chlorodecone-

poisoned workers (all had normal T, LH, and FSH).

Nigam et al. (1988) evaluated 75 male workers: 19 handlers, 26 nonhandlers, and 20 maintenance workers who were directly or indirectly exposed to the manufacture of the insecticide BHC. They report that four handlers experienced loss of libido. It is unfortunate that the article does not state statistical significance of the loss of libido in the four handlers compared to the control group that had no history of occupational contact with BHC.

Moses et al. (1984) cite the U.S. Environmental Protection Agency's (1978) statement that 2,4,-5 trichlorothenoxyacetic acid (2,4,-5T) was one of the most commonly used herbicides in the United States for over three decades, until its suspension in the late 1970s by the EPA. They cite DeYoung et al. (1978) that 2,4,-5T was one of the two active ingredients in the Vietnam War herbicide Agent Orange. Moses et al. performed a cross-sectional survey at a plant where 2,4,-5T had been manufactured from 1969 to 1978, and found that 52% of the 266 workers had chloracne (refractory follicular hyperkeratosis). The researchers state that chloracne was significantly correlated with increased reports of sexual dysfunction and inhibited desire (adjusting for age).

Barlow and Sullivan's (1982) research of occupational toxin exposures that can affect libido includes studies on chloroprene, manganese, mercury, lead, and vinyl chloride. In their discussion of chloroprene (a chemical used in the production of a synthetic rubber) they cite a NIOSH report of workers experiencing sexual impotency "involving both libido and sexual dynamics (no other details were given in the original report)" (p. 78). In their discussion of manganese (a metal used in the manufacture of steel, rock crushers, railway points and crossings, wagon buffers, metal alloys, points of dry-cell batteries, glass, ink, ceramics, rubber, wood preservatives, welding rods, and paints), they cite the Schuler et al. (1957) study of 15 severely magnesium-poisoned miners in Chile. They report that four experienced a diminution or abolition of libido.

Barlow and Sullivan next discuss the occupational toxin hazards of mercury, which is used in various pressure-measuring devices, temperature-measuring devices, thermostats, the manufacture of dental amalgams, numerous other pharmaceutical and agricultural applications, and even some latex-based paints. They cite McFarland and Reigel's (1978) study of nine men who were potentially exposed to metallic mercury vapors in an industrial accident. Six of them were hospitalized. Six cases were followed up over a number of years, with varied symptoms evident—the most consistent complaints being nervousness, irritability, lack of ambition, and lack of sexual desire.

In Barlow and Sullivan's discussion of lead (as a component for antiknock mixtures for gasoline), they cite Neshkov's (1971) study of 66 males whose sexual dysfunction was felt to be caused by exposure to tetraethyl lead; nine of the 66 reported decreased desire.

Finally, Barlow and Sullivan discuss vinyl chloride, which is used in the plastic industry, in organic synthesis, and as a refrigerant. They cite Walker (1976), who examined 37 men (average age: 40) employed at a polyvinyl chloride manufacturing plant (average length of employment: two years, eight months). Of the 37 cases, 18 presented with symptoms (in decreasing order of frequency): cold hands, aches in bones, dyspnoea—i.e., paraesthesia, cold feet, aches in muscles, impaired grip, and loss of libido.

Finkelstein et al. (1988) present an interesting case: "The Mortician's Mystery: Gynecomastic Reversible Hypogonadotropic Hypogonadism in an Embalmer," in which a mortician presented with signs of overt estrogen effects but had undetectable levels of endogenous estrogens. When the mortician quit applying embalming cream without wearing gloves, his hypogonadic state reversed. Retrospectively, estrogen receptor studies found an organic extract of the embalming cream with increased affinities for estradiol receptors. It was hypothesized that the reversal of the hypogonadic state upon cessation of contact with cutaneous embalming cream was an indication that the organic extract had a bioactive estrogen-like effect.

GAY MALE SEXUAL DESIRE ISSUES

Reece (1988) discusses the special issues of sexual problems among gay men and summarizes Paff (1985) by stating that 25% of gay male sex-therapy clients, by their psychotherapists' recollection, presented with desire disorders. Reece (1981/82) found that

> Only five percent presented with problems of desire, but . . . this difference in desire phase disorders can partially be accounted for by the fact that Paff included in his 25% those men who presented with lack of interest in, discomfort with, or aversion to anal sex, while such clients were not included in Reece's groups (p. 44).

McWhirter and Mattison (1978) found that 9% of their 22 gay couples presented with desire disorders.

Reece (1987) discusses the anxiety associated with past, current, or future AIDS status as another potentially significant factor for gay couples.

MEDICAL HISTORY AND EXAMINATION OF THE HSD PATIENT

Medical evaluation of the hypoactive sexual desire patient requires a thorough, competent history and physical examination (H&P). A history of the present condition should preferably include the following: the time of first onset of sexual desire, the patient's sexual orientation (preference), frequency of sexual activity, history of physical or sexual abuse, type of sexual activities, (e.g., pornographic movies, sexual appliances), and drug and alcohol use/abuse. A thorough investigation of the patient's family medical history, especially with reference to any surgeries, hospitalizations, or debilitating diseases, is vital. The patient's family medical history should also be elicited to uncover any potentially inheritable illnesses that could affect the patient's sexual desire or ability—e.g., peripheral vascular disease, diabetes, or neurological disease.

A social and occupational history is useful in

determining patient's potential exposure to environmental toxins that could produce a hypoactive sexual state. A wide variety of activities can result in exposure to toxins that may affect libido. The physician should therefore question the patient regarding his or her hobbies. Possible hazards include exposure to ceramics, use of firearms (including reloading bullets), making lead sinkers, furniture refinishing, painting, and even gardening. Included in the social history should be patient's consumption of tobacco and alcohol and recreational use of other drugs. To complete the history, there should be a systematic evaluation of the major organ system functions (a review of systems—ROS) and a complete listing of all prescribed and over-the-counter (OTC) medications.

A thorough physical examination should include the following: assessment of the patient's height, weight, visual acuity, and head, ears, eyes, nose, throat (HEENT); and a neurologic evaluation of the central nervous system—i.e., nystagmus (possibly Wernicke's encephalothapy)—and retinal pathology to identify any systemic diseases or CNS tumors. Examination of the oral mucosa could indicate nutritional/vitamin deficiencies or toxin exposures. Examination of nasal mucosa can reveal ischemia or even septal necrosis, which could be indicative of intranasal cocaine use. In examination of the neck, it is important to note the size and consistency of the thyroid gland and perform auscultation of the carotid arteries (listening for bruits—a sign of possible obstruction of blood flow to the brain).

Examination of the thorax is performed to uncover any signs of possible chronic obstructive pulmonary disease. Examination of the heart should determine if the rate and rhythm are normal and if there are sounds indicating congestive heart failure (i.e., gallop) or murmurs (sounds indicating possible valvular disease). Examination of the abdomen can identify signs of organomegaly (spleenomegaly and hepatomegaly), ascities (intraabdominal fluid, which can be a sign of liver disease), or tumors. Examination of the genitourinary system should include assessment of the adequacy of gonad size and consistency, with no major structural anomalies such as hypospadius (duplicated vaginas), epispadius (penis with abnormal urethra), large hymenal remnants, bifed vaginas, or the like.

The neurological evaluation started in the HEENT portion of the exam is then further continued by assessing sensory/motor reflexes and cerebellar testing to rule out major neurological diseases. Extremities should be evaluated for major surgical or systemic joint dysfunctions or major vascular obstructive conditions. Examination of the integument or skin can be helpful, in that many major systemic hormonal or malignant conditions are manifested by changes in the skin.

Laboratory evaluation of the HSD patient can be useful but must be tailored to the findings of the H&P. For example, clinical hypothyroidism might necessitate a full thyroid panel, including a thyroid-stimulating hormone (TSH) test and possibly even a thyroid-releasing hormone (TRH) test. These laboratory tests may be instrumental in the discovery of previously unrecognized medical conditions that could affect libido.

Essential laboratory evaluation requires a complete blood cell count (CBC), a urinalysis (UA), a fasting biochemical profile (SMA 24), reflexive human immunodeficiency virus test (HIV), (TSH), and prolactin (an expensive test, but one that can show a treatable/curable cause of HSD). A CBC is useful in detecting anemias or possible occult malignancies that could produce diffuse malaise and subsequent depression of the libido. A fasting biochemical profile will help evaluate the status of the adrenal glands, parathyroid glands, kidney, liver, and pancreas. The patient's HIV status is vital knowledge for both patient and clinician. The TSH can demonstrate over- or underactive thyroid conditions.

Optional but sometimes helpful laboratory tests include testosterone, estrogen, progesterone; LH, FSH, ESR (erythrocycte sedimentation rate); hemaglobin A,C; red blood cell cholinesterase; serum lead level; mercury level; arterial blood gases; pulse oximetry, stress EKG; magnetic resonance imaging (MRI) or computerized axial tomography (CAT) scan of the head; chest X ray; pap smear; mammogram;

and flexible sigmoidoscopy. If the patient's social/occupational history or hobby exposures indicate potential toxins, a red blood cell cholinesterase will be useful in detection of exposure to organophosphates (insecticides). Blood lead levels should be drawn for patients with obvious histories of lead exposure—e.g., from lead water pipes, casting bullets or sinkers, lead crystal decanters. Chronic exposure to latex-based paint might produce mercury toxic CNS effect; mercury levels should then be tested.

THEORY

Sexual behavior is distinct from other behaviors in that it is solely responsible for propagation of the species. Evolutionarily, there must exist a strong reinforcement for procreation. I propose, as have many others (Freud (1922), Skinner (1969), and Davidson et al. (1982)), that pleasure (orgasm) is the reinforcement for sexual behavior.

But what is pleasure or orgasm from a neuro-anatomic/neuropeptide perspective? Pleasure must be strong and specific enough to distract or modify daily survival behavior for propagation to occur. In most vertebrate species, ritualistic, cooperative behavior is required in both male and female to ensure successful propagation.

Did evolution produce separate male and female anatomic/neuropeptide mechanisms for pleasure? The process of evolution builds on basic structures, generally with initial minimal modifications. Occum's razor, which mandates the simplest explanation of a given phenomenon, shapes theories by minimizing the number of steps or mechanisms while still retaining the capacity to explain a given phenomenon. Male and female pleasure should be produced by a basic structure having the same type of reinforcement for both sexes. Evolutionary factors could tend to influence sexual desire temporally, via hormonal factors, in such a fashion as to optimize propagation.

I hypothesize that hypothalamic neural pathways primarily drive vertebrate sexual behavior. Specific temporal testosterone exposures direct the development and activity of the hypo-thalamic neural networks. (This does not exclude the necessity of adequate estrogen priming in females.) This network reinforces sexual behavior by rewarding the organism with orgasmic intrahypothalamic oxytocin surges, which are facilitated/enhanced by testosterone.

Elbrecht and Smith (1992) demonstrated testosterone's influence in the development of phenotypic male morphology and behavior through genetic experiments on female chicken embryos. The embryos were exposed to chemicals that interrupted the normal biosynthesis of estrogen from testosterone by inactivating the converting enzyme aromatase. This demonstration of a single enzyme inhibition lends support to testosterone's primary role in the potential priming of sexual development and behavior.

Crews (1987) provides unique insight into the understanding of vertebrate sexuality. He describes naturally occurring genetically identical female lizards (clones) that reproduce through parthenogenesis: No male is required for fertilization/reproduction. The lizard's sexual behavior (sexual orientation) is temporally dependent on the hormonal phase of its ovaries. Early in the ovarian cycle, estrogen predominates and drives the ventral medial hypothalamus (VMH) to produce classical female receptive behavior. Later in the ovarian cycle, progesterone predominates and drives another portion of the hypothalamus, the preoptic area (POA), to produce male-like pseudomounting behavior, which enhances fertility rates (as compared to a lone lizard).

This alternation of classical male/female sexual behavior by a female lizard demonstrates the hormonally dependent plasticity of its hypothalamic neural pathways. The apparent lack of testosterone influence would be explained by a hypothetical high level of aromatase activity, which could account for the increased sensitivity of the POA to another androgen, progesterone. This hypothetical high level of aromatase activity could also allow for progesterone or testosterone priming of the VMH. The androgenic influence could come from the previous ovarian cycle or from the androgenic precursors of estrogen.

The POA-induced pseudomale sexual behavior in the lizard is similar to the MPOA-influenced sexual behavior of the male rat. The importance of the hypothalamic MPOA-influenced male rat behavior is noted by Dornan and Malsbury (1989). They cite Caggiula et al. (1973), Malsbury (1971), and Sachs and Meisel (1988) in stating that the medial preoptic anterior hypothalamic area (MPOA-AH) is a vital area for male rate sexual behavior.

There are numerous neurotransmitters (dopaminergic, cholinergic, and GABA) and neuropeptides that affect sexual behavior. Dornan and Malsbury (1989) condensed Palkovits (1988), and Simerly et al. (1986) to list the following neuropeptides found within rat MPOA: gonadotropin releasing hormone (GRH), corticotropin releasing hormone (CRH), thyrotropin releasing hormone (TRH), somatostatin, prolactin, alpha-MSH, adrenocorticotropic hormone (ACTH), oxytocin, vasopressin, beta-endorphin, Met- and Leu-EnKephalin, dynorphin A (1-8), dynorphin B, substance P, neuropeptide Y, vasoactive intestinal peptide, galanin, calcitonin gene-related peptide, and neurotensin. Dornan and Malsbury (1989) also conveniently list neuropeptides that produce male sexual effects (animal and human): GRH, CRF, prolactin, beta-endorphin, ACTH, alpha-MSH, neuropeptide Y, substance P, CCK-8, and oxytocin.

The following is a basic model to explain some of human sexual behavior. The end expression of sexual behavior is orgasm (and occasionally propagation). It has been shown by Murphy et al. (1987), Carmichael et al. (1987), Murphy et al. (1990) and Carmichael et al. (in press) that human male and female orgasms are punctuated by a significant increase in plasma oxytocin levels. Plasma oxytocin surges may be used to document orgasm biochemically. Application of oxytocin to specific hypothalamic sites has been shown to induce various sexual responses.

For example, Argiolas et al. (1991) found that oxytocin stimulation of the paraventricular nucleus (PVN) produces penile erections. The PVN and POA are located within the hypothalamus. Nolte (1988) states that the PVN is immediately rostral/dorsal to the preoptic nucleus (PON or POA). The ventromedial nucleus (VMN or VMH) is immediately rostral/ventral to the PON.

Argiolas et al. (1991) make several relevant points. (1) Penile erection is induced by dopaminergic agonists by releasing oxytocin PVN. This finding expands Gessa and Taglimonte's (1974) dopaminergic sexual theory, in that it not only demonstrates that dopamine may induce male sexual response, but also gives specific neuro-anatomic location to its action. (2) Penile erection is prevented by opiates' inhibition of oxytocin transmission in the PVN. This finding is consistent with Buffum's (1982) proposal that heroin users may use heroin to self-medicate for premature ejaculation. (3) Penile erections are induced by oxytocin acting on uterine-like receptors. (4) Oxytocin's second messenger is calcium. (See Figure 2.3.)

Arletti et al. (1991) found that oxytocin administration—200 ng intraperitoneally per rat by systemic administration—or 1 ng intracerebroventricularly per rat induces male copulatory behavior and enhances female receptivity. Localized administration of oxytocin at its site of action should require less oxytocin then systemic (generalized) administration.

The chemicals that bathe the brain's neurons

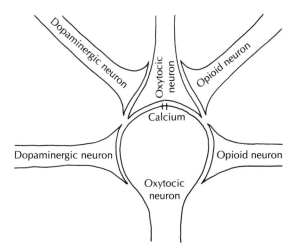

Figure 2.3. Rendering of a diagram presented on a slide during Arletti et al.'s (1991) presentation.

are protected by the blood-brain barrier (BBB). There is no direct access of blood to the tissues of the brain. Oxygen, glucose, drugs, etc. must pass through the blood vessels' walls into the cerebrospinal fluid (CSF), which bathes the brain. The pituitary portal system is a partial exception (discussed earlier in the chapter). However, there are no large corresponding neurovascular structures in the hypothalamus. Generally, the BBB works both ways; it could be assumed that the brain must release a massive amount of oxytocin to allow such a significant pulse of oxytocin in the systemic (plasma) circulation.

What physiological mechanism could account for the massive oxytocin surges seen in human plasma following orgasm? Cutler (1991) states that an epileptic seizure is produced by the excessive discharge of groups of neurons depolarizing in a synchronous manner. I propose that the surge of plasma oxytocin noted with orgasm is the end result of massive recruitment of diencephalic oxytocic neuronal pathways, resulting in localized diencephalic seizure activity, which produces the oxytocin surge. I further propose that arousal behavior is the individual's attempt to bring a localized area of the diencephalon to its seizure threshold, to "tickle the tail of the dragon" (an expression describing the process used in the Manhattan Project, in which increasing amounts of uranium were added in order to determine the critical amount required for the uranium to explode). This neuronal recruitment or tickling and discharge require intact neuronal pathways and adequate hormonal priming.

Taylor (1971) provides an excellent review of the many historical associations between epilepsy and sexual activity. Taylor cites the Roman perspective: "Coitus brevis epileptica est"—orgasm is like a brief seizure. The French refer to orgasm as *la petite mort*—the little death. Taylor draws parallels between sexual activity and epilepsy, which I have modified in Table 2.1.

Heath (1972) reports of human male and female orgasm being facilitated by electrical or chemical stimulation of the septal area of the brain (a diencephalic area with major inputs into the hypothalamus). These orgasms were found

Table 2.1. A Comparison of Seizure Activity and Sexual Activity

SEIZURE ACTIVITY	SEXUAL ACTIVITY
1. Epileptic prodome (period prior to the aura)	1. Sexual prodome (mood of desire)
2. Aura (irreversible awareness of an impending seizure	2. Emission (the sensation immediately prior to ejaculation
3. Ictal—seizure (uncontrolled electrical discharge of brain)	3. Orgasm
4. Postictal (sedated or unconcious state)	4. Postorgasm (desire to rest or sleep)
5. Refractory period (time in which next seizure is unlikely)	5. Refractory period (time in which next orgasm is unlikely

to have localized epileptic-like electroencephalographic (EEG) recordings from deep (diencephalic) electrodes. Heath's surface (scalp) EEG recordings of these orgasms did not demonstrate the seizure activity. Interestingly, Heath felt that Masovich and Tallaferro's (1954) findings of surface EEG in four of six patients demonstrating paroxysmal waves during orgasm might reflect the deeper seizure activity he recorded.

Robinson and Mishkin (1968) mapped numerous areas of the male monkey forebrain in which electrical stimulation could produce erections. Robinson and Mishkin (1966) reported that specific, temporally patterned electrical stimulation to male monkey POA could produce penile erection and ejaculation. No seizure activity was recorded during these orgasms. However, I believe that their pulsed stimulations produced and/or overshadowed any underlining midbrain seizure activity.

If the hypothalamus has the propensity to have massive neuronal recruitment and subsequent seizure activity, it would make physiological sense to have some sort of inhibitory control to prevent biologically unnecessary oxytocin releases that would be potentially dangerous (if sexual behavior became the organism's exclusive behavior).

Lisk (1966) found that electrical lesions from platinum electrodes (to obviate the potential of residual metal deposits producing chronic irrative foci) in the male rat mammillary region markedly increased sexual behavior. Lisk proposed that male rat sexual behavior is an interaction between an activational/integrative (facilitatory) component, probably in the AHPOA, and a regulatory (inhibitory) component in the mammillary bodies.

Dichter (1991) states that hypoxia and ischemia may produce seizures in infants. Human sexual experimentation over the centuries has led some individuals to use hypoxia to facilitate/augment orgasm. Innala and Ernulf (1989) describe asphyxiophilia as a desire for a state of oxygen deficiency (hypoxia), practiced in order to augment sexual excitement and orgasm. Innala and Ernulf (1989) cite Harbitz (1943) that men in Victorian London could receive ''controlled hypoxia'' at a hangmen's club (specialized house of prostitution). Innala and Ernulf (1989) document numerous deaths of practitioners of asphyxiophilia, which may be viewed as an extremely dangerous method of tickling the dragon's tail.

Buffum (1982) cites Sigell et al. (1978) that volatile nitrites (potent vasodilators—''poppers'') are allegedly used prior to orgasm, to prolong orgasm or the perception of orgasm. Buffum (1982) cites Louria (1970) that this effect is mediated by cerebral ischemia (the rapid onset of vasodilation in the body, increasing blood flow to the body and relatively decreasing blood flow to the brain).

Desire is defined as the drive to achieve pleasure/orgasm. Arousal may be viewed as the attempt to stimulate the hypothalamus repetitively in such a manner that pleasure/orgasm is iminent. The cortical/supratentoral influence on sexual activity is hypothesized to occur with the gradual recruitment of oxytocic neuronal pathways. The arousal process functions to excite the diencephalic/hypothalamic area to its seizure threshold. This theory proposes a possible mechanism for observed orgasmically induced oxytocic surges. It would predict that hypothalamic nuclei should demonstrate mating-induced changes in oxytocin levels, synthesis rates, and transport rates.

Jirikowski et al. (1991) present data that *in situ* hybridization findings of oxytocin presence in perikarya (the distal portion of axons) of MPOA neurons are decreased in male and female rats immediately after mating. Radioimmune assays of microdissected forebrain biopsies (hypothalamic—MPOA and surrounding area) revealed increased levels of oxytocin in the male and female rat after mating. However, levels were found to increase in male rats that were allowed to mate repetitively with novel receptive females. The researchers regarded these data as indicating that mating induces MPOA oxytocin axonal transport and secretion.

In late-pregnant and parturient rats, additional oxytocic changes were observed. Jirikowski et al. (1991) believe that oxytocin brain topography is dynamic and influenced by hormonal changes.

A large chasm exists between our understanding of neuronal signals and the behavior they produce. The functional working of many motor/sensory/reflex neuronal pathways is well understood. However, the understanding of how neurons allow or produce perception has been elusive.

Freeman (1991) proposes that perception is a dynamic cooperative interaction of neurons. He proposes a neuronal paradigm using Hebian learning—two simultaneously firing neurons achieving a desired effect that is reinforced with a modulator chemical. Gray et al. (1986) demonstrated that norepinephrine acts as a chemical modulator on learned rabbit behavior, as documented by EEG changes in the olfactory cortex.

Oxytocin may be viewed as a chemical modulator for sexual reinforcement/pleasure. Sexual associations may be viewed as dynamic cooperative interactions of cortical neurons attempting to stimulate specific hypothalamic oxytocic nuclei in the proper way. Sexual associations may have powerful behavioral influences. For example, various smells may produce aversion to arousal/attraction; various kinds of music may induce tranquility or excitement; and various ambient factors (e.g., temperature or lighting) have a variety of influences. Some individuals may develop strong sexual associations that range from benign to unacceptable (e.g., from shoe fetish to pedophilia).

In any dynamic event, proper sequencing is necessary to achieve a desired result. Humans learn from sexual experience the proper way to sequence sensory input for themselves and their mates in order to facilitate sexual activity and orgasm. Optimally, we learn not only to tickle our own dragon's tail, but also our mate's.

Argiolas et al. (1991) state that a baseline level of testosterone is required for oxytocin activity in the male rat. Schumacher et al. (1990) administered progesterone (a hormone with some androgenic properties) to estrogen-primed ovarectomized and adrenalectomized rats. They found a rapid, marked increase in oxytocin receptor affinity in the hypothalamic nuclei, VMH, and surrounding areas. This possible modulation is probably accomplished through a rapid conformational (shape) change in the oxytocin receptor molecule.

I propose that testosterone should have an effect on VMH oxytocin receptor affinity similar to the effect Schumacher et al. (1990) observed with progesterone. Physiologically, the progesterone surge observed in human females occurs after ovulation. There would be no evolutionary/procreative advantage in increasing oxytocin receptor affinity (or desire) after the fertile period (ovulation). Persky et al. (1978), Adams et al. (1978), Bancroft et al. (1983), Bancroft (1984), Matteo and Rissman (1984), Stanislaw and Rice (1988), and Schreiner-Engel et al. (1989) all reported a periovulatory peak in testosterone and/or desire in women. This could potentially result from a gonadotropin message to turn off estrogen production/aromatase activity and allow for a transient, procreatively opportune accumulation of testosterone.

If testosterone is demonstrated to enhance oxytocin receptor affinity, then it may be possible to explain the greater sexual desire in human males, as compared to human females, as being a result of higher perinatal testosterone exposure. This enhancement could be one of the prenatal and postnatal conjoint effects that

produce the recalcitrant sexually dimorphic patterns that Money and Higham (1989) discuss in their summary of sexual behavior.

Symons (1979) summarizes data on late-treated women with adrenogenital syndrome (AGS), a condition in which the individual is constantly exposed to high levels of androgenic hormones from prenatal exposure until adequate treatment. Symons (1979) cites Money and Ehrhardt (1972) and Lev-Ran (1974) to state that late-treated AGS women have dream eroticism similar to that of males. Symons (1979) cites Money (1961, 1965), Ehrhardt et al. (1968), and Lev-Ran (1974) that late-treated AGS women have a high sex drive that may be reversible by cortisone therapy (which would turn off the overproduction of androgenic hormones).

Symons (1979) cites Goy (1968), Goy and Resko (1972), and Phoenix (1974) that pregnant rhesus monkeys injected with testosteone produce normal males but genitally masculinized, "pseudohermaphroditic" females, which exhibit an intermediate level (between male and female) of play initiation, mounting, aggressive play, and threatening behavior.

Symons (1979) reviewed the marked differences between gay men and lesbians and cited Saghir and Robins (1973) to discuss the prevalence of male pornography versus the paucity of female pornography. There seems to be a preponderance of male heterosexual- and homosexual-oriented pornography, a small amount of female-oriented pornography, and a near absence of true lesbian-oriented pornography. Symons (1979) cites the marked increase of sexual partners of homosexual males compared to the number of lesbian sexual partners.

Symons (1979) feels that this and other data suggest that male levels of desire or "tendencies" (p. 291) are dependent on prenatal androgen exposure on the developing brain ("priming the brain"). They are then activated by postpubertal androgen exposure, previously primed at a male level of desire, or "male direction" (p. 291).

The degree of perinatal testosterone priming of oxytocin receptors probably varies among individuals. This variance would most likely produce a Gaussian distribution. Men with the highest oxytocin receptor affinity would be inclined to experience an increased sex drive and might find that most women have such a lesser drive that they would not be adequate sexual partners. Conversely, women with a low oxytocin receptor affinity might find males to have too high a sex drive to be acceptable sexual partners.

It would be unwise to attempt to explain sexual orientation as totally dependent on levels of desire induced by testosterone-mediated variations in oxytocin receptor affinity. Sexual desire is probably heavily influenced by numerous cortical processes (e.g., aversive associations from physical, sexual, and mental abuse could tend to override levels of desire). Not all lesbians have low levels of sexual desire. Some might have major aversions to men, secondary to environmental factors such as incest or rape. Correspondingly, not all gay men have high levels of sexual desire. Again, environmental factors, such as abuse by women, might influence sexual orientation.

Murphy et al. (1990) found that when human males experience orgasm, oxytocin levels rise up to 362% of preorgasmic baseline levels. This surge is not seen when naloxone (Narcan®—an opioid antagonist—is administered intravenously ($p < 0.01$). Murphy et al. also noted a decrease in the level of subjective arousal and pleasure at orgasm. Eight of eight men given naloxone noted lower levels of arousal at full penile erection and sufficient self-perpetuated interest, as well as during masturbation ($p < 0.01$). The reduction of pleasure at orgasm was noted by seven of eight men ($p < 0.05$), but the reduction did not reach the level of absence of pleasure. One subject was noted not to have a rise in plasma oxytocin during orgasm with the placebo infusion. The diminution of pleasure and absence of oxytocin surge during orgasm with naxolone administration constitute further evidence that oxytocin strongly influences human perceptions of pleasure.

The production, release, and receptor affin-

ity of oxytocin is probably dependent on hormones and neurotransmitters. The dynamic interplay of hormones and neurotransmitters ultimately seem to tickle the dragon's oxytocic tail—to drive the organism to seek pleasure (release of oxytocin). I propose that, biochemically, desire is the pursuit of diencephalic/hypothalamic release of oxytocin.

In the future, evaluation of desire disorders may be measured quantitatively from baseline, arousal, or orgasmic oxytocin levels; or some measurement of dynamic oxytocin receptor affinity could replace the patient's subjective response in determining the level of desire.

I also propose that in diencephalic seizures, a cyclic pathway exists within the hypothalamus. The POA or PVN is the probable main input site in the male, and the VMH is the probable main input site in the female.

Freeman (1991) states:

> In short, an active perception is not the copying of an incoming stimulus. It is a step in a trajectory by which brains grow, reorganize themselves, and reach into their own environment to change it to their own advantage.
>
> The poet William Blake wrote, "If the doors of perception were cleansed everything would appear to man as it is, infinite." Such cleansing would not be desirable. Without the protections of the doors of perception—that is, without the self-controlled chaotic activity of the cortex, from which perceptions spring—people and the animals would be overwhelmed by infinity (p. 85).

Perhaps during human orgasm there is a momentary cleansing of the doors of emotional perception. This emotional respite may be briefly experienced as the ultimate reward, or *petite mort*.

In summary I propose that specific hypothalamic areas (POA, PVN, or VMH) drive vertebrate sexual behavior. These areas might have different morphology or chemical sensitivity due to prenatal, pubertal, and adult hormone exposure. Testosterone is the common hormone that prenatally primes the individual's level of desire; at puberty and thereafter, testosterone activates hypothalamic pathways. Testosterone's influence is possibly mediated by conformational (structural) changes in the oxytocin receptor molecule in the hypothalamic neuronal membranes. The sexual behavior is ultimately rewarded by orgasmic seizure-like discharges of hypothalamic oxytocic neurons, which release oxytocin in the brain. The brain then perceives this surge of oxytocin as pleasure.

REFERENCES

Adams, D. B., Gold, A. R., & Burt, A. D. (1978). Rise in female-initiated sexual activity at ovulation and its suppression by oral contraceptives. *New England Journal of Medicine, 299,* 1145–1150.

Advis, J. P., Krause, J. E., & McKelvy, J. F. (1982). Luteinizing hormone-releasing hormone peptidase activities in discrete hypothalamic regions and anterior pituitary of the rat: Apparent regulation during the prepubertal period and first estrous cycle at puberty. *Endocrinology, 110,* 1238–1245.

Alvarez, M. A., Barroso, C. C., & Arce, B. (1983). Psychological characterization of testicular feminization syndrome. *Reproduction, 7*(1–2), 9–15.

American Psychiatric Association. (1987). *Diagnostic and statistical manual of mental disorders* (3rd ed., rev.). Washington, DC: Author.

Anderson, J. H., Jr., Cohn, W. J., Guzelian, P., Taylor, J. R., Griffith, F. D., Blanke, R. V., dos Santos, J. G., & Blackard, W. G. (1976). *Effects of kepone associated toxicity on testicular function.* Presented at Ann. Meet. Endocrine Soc., San Francisco.

Angrist, B., & Gershon, S. (1976). Clinical effects of amphetamine and l-dopa on sexuality and aggression. *Comprehensive Psychiatry, 17,* 715–722.

Aoz, B., Antonovsky, A., Apter, A., et al. (1977). Perception of menopause in five ethnic groups in Israel. *Acta Obstetrica et Gynecologia Scandinavica, 65,* 35–40.

Argiolas, A., Melis, M. R., Stancampiano, R., Gessa, G., & Brodie, B. B. (1991). *Oxytocin stimulation of penile erection: Pharmacology, site and mechanism of action.* Presented at New York Academy of Sciences conference, May 19–22, Cagliari, Italy.

Arletti, R., Benelli, A., & Bertolini, A. 1991. *Oxytocin involvement in male and female sexual behavior.* Presented at New York Academy of Sciences conference, May 19–22, Arlington, VA.

Bach, N., Schaffner, F., & Kapelman, B. (1989). Sexual behavior in women with nonalcoholic liver disease. *Hepatology, 9*(5), 698–703.

Bachmann, G. A. (1990). Sexual issues of menopause. *Annals New York Academy of Sciences, 1*(592), 87–91.

Bachmann, G. A., Lieblum, S. R., Sandler, B., Ainsley, W., Narcessian, R., Sheldon, R., & Nakajima Hymans, H. (1985). Correlates of sexual desire in post-menopausal women. *Maturitas, 7,* 211–216.

Baker, H. W. G., Burger, H. G., deKretser, D. M., Hudson, B., O'Connor, S., Wang, C., Mirovics, A., Court, J., Dunlop, M., & Rennie, G. C. (1976). Changes in the pituitary-testicular system with age. *Clinical Endocrinology, 5,* 349–372.

Bancroft, J. (1984). Hormones and human sexual behavior. *Journal of Sex and Marital Therapy, 10*(1), 3–21.

Bancroft, J., Sanders, D., Davidson, D., & Warner, P. (1983). Mood, sexuality, hormones, and the menstrual cycle. III. Sexuality and the role of androgens. *Psychosomatic Medicine, 45*(6), 509–516.

Bancroft, J., Tennent, G., Loucas, K., & Cass, J. (1974). The control of deviant sexual behavior by drugs: I. Behavioral changes following oestrogens and antiandrogens. *British Journal of Psychiatry, 125,* 310–315.

Barlow, S. M., & Sullivan, F. M. 1982. *Reproductive hazards of industrial chemicals.* New York, Academic Press.

Bartholomew, A. A. (1968). A long-acting phenothiazine as a possible agent to control deviant sexual behavior. *American Journal of Psychiatry, 124,* 77–83.

Bathen, J. (1978). Propranolol erectile dysfunction relieved. *Annals of Internal Medicine, 88,* 716–717.

Beaumont, G. (1977). Sexual side effects of clomipramine (Anafranil). *Journal of International Medical Research, 5*(Suppl.), 37–44.

Bell, D. S., & Trethowan, W. H. (1961). Amphetamine addiction and disturbed sexuality. *Archives of General Psychiatry, 4,* 74–78.

Benedek, T. (1950). Climacterium: Development phase. *Psychoanalytic Quarterly, 19,* 1–27.

Berlin, F., & Meinecke, C. (1981). Treatment of sex offenders with antiandrogenic medication: Conceptualization, review of treatment modalities and preliminary findings. *American Journal of Psychiatry, 138,* 601–607.

Biron, P. (1979). Diminished libido with cimetadine therapy. *California Medical Association Journal, 121,* 404–405.

Blake, C. A. (1978). Neurohumoral control of cyclic pituitary LH and FSH release. *Clinical Obstetrics and Gynecology, 5,* 305–327.

Blumer, D., & Walker, A. E. (1975). The neural basis of sexual behavior. In D. F. Benson (Ed.), *Psychiatric aspects of neurologic disease.* New York: Grune and Stratton.

Brown, E., Brown, G. M., Kofman, O., & Quarrington, B. (1978). Sexual function and affect in parkinsonian men treated with L-dopa. *American Journal of Psychiatry, 135,* 1552–1555.

Brown, J. J., Davies, D., Ferriss, J., Fraser, R., Haywood, E., Lever, A., & Robertson, J. (1972). Comparison of surgery and prolonged spironolactone therapy in patients with hypertension, aldosterone excess, and low plasma renin. *British Medical Journal, 2,* 729–734.

Buffum, J. (1982). Pharmacosexology: The effects of drugs on sexual function. A review. *Journal of Psychoactive Drugs, 14*(1–2), 5–41.

Burnett, W., & Chahine, R. (1979). Sexual dysfunction as a complication of propranolol therapy in men. *Cardiovascular Medicine, 4,* 811–815.

Buvat, J., LeMaire, A., & Buvat-Herbaut, M. (1987). Human chorionic gonadotropin treatment of nonorganic erectile failure and lack of sexual desire: A double-blind study. *Urology, 30*(3), 216–219.

Byck, R. (1975). Drugs and the treatment of psychiatric disorders. In L. Goodman & A. Gilman (Eds.), *The pharmacological basis of therapeutics.* New York: Macmillan.

Caggiula, A. R., Antelman, S. M., & Zigmond, M. J. (1973). Disruption of copulation in male rats after hypothalamic lesions: A behavioral, anatomical, and neurochemical analysis. *Brain Research, 59,* 273–287.

Cannon, S. B., Veazey, J. M., Jr., Jackson, R. S., Burse, V. W., Hayes, C., Straub, W. E., Landrigan, P. J., & Liddle, J. A. (1978). Epidemic Kepone poisoning in chemical workers. *American Journal of Epidemiology, 107,* 529–537.

Carmichael, M. S., Dixen, J., Greenleaf, W., Humbert, R., & Davidson, J. M. (in press). Relationships among cardiovascular, muscular and oxytocin responses during human sexual activity.

Carmichael, M. S., Humbert, R., Dixen, J., Palmi-

sano, G., Greenleaf, W., & Davidson, J. M. (1987). Plasma oxytocin increases in the human sexual response. *Journal of Clinical Endocrinology and Metabolism, 64*(1), 27–31.

Carney, A., Bancroft, J., & Mathews, A. (1978). Combination of hormonal and psychological treatment for female sexual responsiveness: A comparative study. *British Journal of Psychiatry, 133,* 339–346.

Cavanagh, J. R. (1969). Rhythm of sexual desire in women. *Medical Aspects of Human Sexuality, 3*(2), 29–39.

Chambers, K. C., & Phoenix, C. H. (1989). Apomorphine, deprenyl, and yohimbine fail to increase sexual behavior in rhesus males. *Behavioral Neuroscience, 103*(4), 816–823.

Channon, L. D., & Ballinger, S. E. (1986). Some aspects of sexuality and vaginal symptoms during menopause and their relation to anxiety and depression. *British Journal of Medical Psychology, 59,* 173–180.

Chopra, G. S. (1969). Man and marijuana. *International Journal of the Addictions, 4,* 215–247.

Cicero, T. J., Bell, R., Wiest, W., Allison, J., Polakoski, K., & Robins, E. (1975). Function of the male sex organs in heroin and methadone users. *New England Journal of Medicine, 292,* 882–887.

Cook, N. E. (1989). Prolactin. In L. DeGroot (Ed.), *Endocrinology* (2nd ed., pp. 384–407). Philadelphia: W. B. Saunders Co.

Crews, D. (1987). Courtship in unisexual lizards: A model for brain evolution. *Scientific American, 257*(6), 116–121.

Cushman, P. (1972). Sexual behavior in heroin addiction and methadone maintenance. *New York State Journal of Medicine, 72,* 1261–1265.

Cutler, R. W. (1991). Epilepsy. In E. Rubenstein & D. Federman (Eds.), *Scientific American medicine.* New York: Scientific American, Inc.

Cutler, W. B., Garcia, C. R., & McCoy, N. (1987). Perimenopausal sexuality. *Archives of Sexual Behavior, 16,* 225–234.

Dallo, J., Lekka, N., & Knoll, J. (1986). The ejaculatory behavior of sexually sluggish male rats treated with Deprenyl, apomorphine, bromocriptine and amphetamine. *Polish Journal of Pharmacology and Pharmacy, 38*(3), 251–255.

Davidson, J. M., Kwan, M., & Greenleaf, W. J. (1982). Hormonal replacement and sexuality in men. *Clinics in Endocrinology and Metabolism, 11*(3), 599–623.

DeLeon, G., & Wexler, H. L. K. (1973). Heroin addiction: Its relation to sexual behavior and sexual experience. *Journal of Abnormal Psychology, 31,* 36–38.

DeYoung, L. M., Richards, W. L., Bonzelet, W., Tsai, L. L., & Boutwell, R. K. (1978). Localization and significance of γ-glutamyl-transpeptidase in normal and neoplastic mouse skin. *Cancer Research, 38,* 3697–3701.

Dichter, M. (1991). The epilepsies and convulsive disorders. In J. Wilson, E. Braunwald, et al. (Eds.), *Harrison's principles of internal medicine.* New York: McGraw-Hill.

Dornan, W. A., & Malsbury, C. W. (1989). Neuropeptides and male sexual behavior. *Neuroscience and Biobehavioral Reviews, 13,* 1–15.

Drago, F., Continella, G., Spadaro, F., Cavaliere, S., & Scapagninir, U. (1986). Behavioral effects of deprenyl in aged rats. *Functional Neurology, 1*(2), 165–174.

DuBois, B. J. (1974). MP: Immunofluorescence study of the preopticinfundibular LH-RH neurosecretory pathway of the guinea pig during the estrous cycle. *Neuroendocrinology, 15,* 200–208.

Dudley, C. A., & Moss, R. L. (1986). Electrophysiological studies into circuitry involved in the LHRH-mediated sexual behavior. In T. W. Moody (Ed.). *Neural and endocrine peptides and receptors.* New York: Plenum.

Ebringer, A., Doyle, A., Dauborn, J., Johnston, C., & Mashford, M. (1970). The use of clonidine (Catapres) in the treatment of hypertension. *Medical Journal of Australia, 1,* 524–526.

Ehrhardt, A., Evers, K., & Money, J. (1968). Influence of androgen and some aspects of sexually dimorphic behavior in women with late-treated adrenogenital syndrome. *John Hopkins Medical Journal, 123,* 115–122.

Elbrecht, A., & Smith, R. (1992). Aromatase enzyme activity and sex determination in chickens. *Science, 255,* 467–470.

Ellinwood, E. H., & Rockwell, K. (1975). The effect of drug use on sexual behavior. *Medical Aspects of Human Sexuality, 9,* 10–32.

Espejo, R., Hogben, G., & Stimmel, B. (1973). Sexual performance of men on methadone maintenance. *Proceedings of the National Conference of Methadone Treatment,* New York City, *1,* 490–493.

Everett, H. C. (1975). The use of bethanechol chloride with tricyclic antidepressants. *American Journal of Psychiatry, 132,* 1202–1204.

Finkelstein, J. S., McCully, W. F., MacLaughlin, D. T., Godine, J. E., & Crowley, W. F. (1988). The mortician's mystery: Gynecomastia and reversible hypogoadotropic hypogonadism in an embalmer. *New England Journal of Medicine, 318*(5), 961–965.

Flint, M. (1975). The menopause: Reward or punishment? *Psychosomatics, 16,* 161–163.

Frasier, S. D. (1973). Androgens and athletes. *American Journal of Diseases of Children, 125,* 479–480.

Freed, D., Banks, A. J., & Longson, D. (1972). Anabolic steroids in athletics. *British Medical Journal, 3,* 761.

Freeman, W. J. (1991). The physiology of perception. *Scientific American, 264*(2), 78–85.

Freud, S. (1922). *Beyond the pleasure principle.* London: International Psycho-analytical Press.

Freyhan, F. (1961). Loss of ejaculation during Mellaril treatment. *American Journal of Psychiatry, 118,* 171–172.

Gavras, I., Gavras, H., Sullivan, P., Tifft, C., Chobanian, A., & Brunner, H. (1979). A comparative study of the effects of oxyprenolol versus propranolol in essential hypertension. *Journal of Clinical Pharmacology, 19,* 8–14.

Gawin, F. H. (1978). Drugs and eros: Reflection on aphrodisiacs. *Journal of Psychedelic Drugs, 10*(3), 227–236.

Gay, G. R., Newmeyer, J., Elion, R., & Weider, S. (1975). Drug-sex practices in the Haight-Ashbury, or the ''sensitive hippie.'' In M. Sandler & D. L. Gessa (Eds.), *Sexual behavior: Pharmacology and biochemistry.* New York: Raven Press.

Gerald, M. C., & Schwirian, P. M. (1973). Nonmedical use of methaqualone. *Archives of General Psychiatry, 28,* 627–631.

Gessa, G. L., & Tagliamonte, A. (1974). Possible role of brain serotonin and dopamine in controlling male sexual behavior. *Advances In Biochemical Psychopharmacology, 11,* 217–228.

Gifford, L. M., Aeugle, M., Myerson, R., & Tannenbaum, P. (1980). Cimetadine post market outpatient surveillance program—interim report on phase I. *Journal of the American Medical Association, 243,* 1532–1535.

Ginton, A., & Meraril, A. 1976. Long range effects of MPOA lesion on mating behavior in the male rat. *Brain Research, 120,* 158–163.

Glass, R. (1981). Ejaculatory impairment from both phenelzine and imipramine, with tinnitus from phenelzine. *Journal of Clinical Psychopharmacology, 1,* 152–154.

Gold, M. S., Pottash, A. L. C., & Extein, I. (1981). Hypothyroidism and depression. *Journal of the American Medical Association, 245*(19), 1919–1922.

Golla, F. L., & Hodge, R. (1949). Hormone treatment of the sexual offender. *Lancet, 1,* 1006–1007.

Goodwin, F. K. (1971). Behavioral effects of l-dopa in man. *Seminars in Psychiatry, 3,* 477–492.

Gordon, G. G., Altman, K., Southren, L., Rubin, E., & Lieber, C. (1976). The effect of alcohol (ethanol) administration on sex-hormone metabolism in normal men. *New England Journal of Medicine, 295,* 793–797.

Gordon, G. G., Southren, A. L., & Lieber, C. S. (1979). Hypogonadism and feminization in the male: A triple effect of alcohol. *Alcoholism: Clinical and Experimental Research, 3,* 210–211.

Goy, R. W. (1968). Organizing effects of androgen on the behavior of rhesus monkeys. In R. P. Michael (Ed.), *Endocrinology & human behaviour.* London: Oxford University Press.

Goy, R. W., & Resko, J. A. (1972). Gonadal hormones and behavior of normal and pseudohermaphroditic nonhuman female primates. *Recent Progress in Hormone Research, 28,* 707–733.

Gray, C. M., Freeman, W. J., & Skinner, J. E. (1986). Chemical dependencies of learning in the rabbit olfactory bulb: Acquisition of the transient spatial pattern change depends on norepinephrine. *Behavioral Neuroscience, 100*(4), 585–596.

Greenblatt, D. J., & Koch-Weser, J. (1973). Gynecomastia and impotence. Complications of spironolactone therapy. *Journal of the American Medical Association, 223,* 82.

Grunert, B. K., Devine, C. A., Matloub, H. S., Sanger, J. R., & Yousif, N. J. (1988). Sexual dysfunction following traumatic hand injury. *Annals of Plastic Surgery, 21,* 246–48.

Guzelian, P. S. (1982). Comparative toxicology of chlordecone (kepone) in humans and experimental animals. *Annual Review of Pharmacology and Toxicology, 22,* 89–113.

Haider, I. (1966). Thioridazine and sexual dysfunctions. *International Journal of Neuropsychiatry, 2,* 255–257.

Halikas, J., Weller, R., Morse, C. (1982). Effects of marijuana use on sexual performance. *Journal of Psychoactive Drugs, 14*(1–2).

Hall, R., Popkin, M., Devaul, R., et al. (1982). Psychiatric manifestations of Hashimoto's thyroiditis. *Psychosomatics, 23,* 337–342.

Hällström, T., & Samuelsson, S. (1990). Changes in women's sexual desire in middle life: The longitudinal study of women in Gothenburg. *Archives of Sexual Behavior, 19,* 259–268.

Handbury, R., Cohen, M., & Stimmel, B. (1977). Adequacy of sexual performance in men maintained on methadone. *American Journal of Drug and Alcohol Abuse, 4,* 13–20.

Harbitz, F. (1943). *Laerebok: Retsmedicin* (textbook on forensic medicine). Oslo, Norway: Brøggers Boktrykkeris Forlag.

Harman, S. M., & Tsitouras, P. D. (1980). Reproductive hormones in aging men. I. Measurement of sex steroids, basal luteinizing hormone, and leydig cell response to human chorionic gonadotropin. *Journal of Clinical Endocrinology and Metabolism, 51,* 35–40.

Heath, R. C. (1972). Pleasure and brain activity in man: Deep and surface electroencephalograms during orgasm. *Journal of Nervous and Mental Disease, 154*(1), 3–18.

Hekimian, L., Friedhoff, A., & Deever, E. (1978). A comparison of the onset of action and therapeutic efficacy of amoxapine and amitriptyline. *Journal of Clinical Psychiatry, 39,* 633–637.

Heller, C. G., Moore, D. J., Paulsen, G. A., Nelson, W. O., & Laidlaw, W. M. (1959). Effects of progesterone and synthetic progestins on the reproductive physiology of normal men. *Federation Proceedings, 18,* 1057–1065.

Herrmann, W. M., & Beach, R. C. (1980). Pharmacotherapy for sexual offenders: Review of the action of antiandrogens with special reference to their psychic effects. *Modern Problems in Pharmacopsychiatry, 15,* 182–194.

Hollifield, J. W. (1977). Personal communication with J. Buffum.

Hollifield, J. W., Sherman, K., Vander Zwagg, R., & Shand, D. (1976). Proposed mechanisms of propranolol's antihypertensive effect in essential hypertension. *New England Journal of Medicine, 295,* 68–73.

Hollister, L. E. (1975). The mystique of social drugs and sex. In M. Sandler & D. L. Gessa (Eds.), *Sexual behavior: Pharmacology and biochemistry.* New York: Raven Press.

Hollister, L. E. (1978a). Treatment of depression with drugs. *Annals of Internal Medicine, 89,* 78–84.

Hollister, L. E. (1978b). Tricyclic antidepressants. *New England Journal of Medicine, 299,* 1106–1109, 1168–1172.

Horowitz, D., Pettinger, W., Orvis, H., Thomas, R., & Sjoerdsma, A. (1967). Effects of methyldopa in 50 hypertensive patients. *Clinical Pharmacology and Therapeutics, 8,* 224–234.

Hughes, J. M. (1964). Failure to ejaculate with chlordiazepoxide. *American Journal of Psychiatry, 121,* 610–611.

Hunter, R., Logue, V., & McMenemy, W. H. (1963). Temporal lobe epilepsy supervening on longstanding transvestism and fetishism. *Epilepsia, 4,* 60–65.

Inaba, D. S., Gay, G., Newmeyer, J., & Whitehead, C. (1973). Methaqualone abuse—"luding out." *Journal of the American Medical Association, 224,* 1505–1509.

Innala, S. M., & Ernulf, K. E. (1989). Asphyxophilia in Scandinavia. *Archives of Sexual Behavior, 18*(3), 181–189.

Jaffe, J. H. (1975). Drug addiction and alcohol abuse. In L. Goodman & A. Gilman (Eds.), *The pharmacological basis of therapeutics.* New York: Macmillan.

Jensen, S. B. (1981). Diabetic sexual dysfunction: A comparative study of 160 insulin treated diabetic men and women and an age-matched control group. *Archives of Sexual Behavior, 10,* 493–504.

Jensen, S. B. (1986). The natural history of sexual dysfunction in diabetic women: A six year follow up study. *Acta Medica Scandinavica, 219,* 73–78.

Jirikowski, G. F., Caldwell, J. D., & Pederson, C. A. (1991). *Oxytocin immunoreactivity during mating, pregnancy, parturition and lactation.* Presented at conference of the New York Academy of Sciences, May 19–22.

Jupp, J. J., & McCabe, M. (1989). Sexual desire, general arousability, and sexual dysfunction. *Archives of Sexual Behavior, 18*(6), 509–516.

Kalra, S. P. (1976). Tissue levels of luteinizing hormone-releasing hormone in the preoptic area and hypothalamus and serum concentrations of gonadotropins following anterior hypothalamic deafferentation and estrogen treatment of the female rat. *Endocrinology, 99,* 101–107.

Kalra, S. P., & Kalra, P. S. (1983). Neural regulation of luteinizing hormone secretion in the rat. *Endocrine Reviews, 4,* 311–351.

Kaplan, H. S. (1977). Hypoactive sexual desire. *Journal of Sex and Marital Therapy, 3,* 3–9.

Khan, A., Camel, G., & Perry, M. (1970). Clonidine (Catapres): A new hypertensive agent. *Current Therapeutic Research, 12,* 10–18.

Kidd, G. S., Glass, A. R., & Vigersky, R. A. (1979). The hypothalamic-pituitary-testicular axis in thyrotoxicosis. *Journal of Clinical Endocrinology and Metabolism, 48*(5), 798–801.

Kinsey, A. C., Pomeroy, W. B., & Martin, C. E. (1948). *Sexual behavior in the human male.* Philadelphia: Saunders.

Kinsey, A. C., Pomeroy, W. B., Martin, C. E., &
Gebhard, P. H. (1953). *Sexual behavior in the human female.* Philadelphia: Saunders.

Knarr, J. W. (1976). Impotence from propranolol? *Annals of Internal Medicine, 85,* 259.

Knoll, J., Dallo, J., & Yen, T. T. (1989). Striatal dopamine, sexual activity and lifespan. Longevity of rats treated with (−)Deprenyl. *Life Sciences, 45,* 525–531.

Kobayashi, R. M., Lu, K. H., Moore, R. Y., & Yen, S. S. C. (1978). Regional distribution of hypothalamic luteinizing hormone-releasing hormone in proestrous rats: Effects of ovariectomy and estrogen replacement. *Endocrinology, 102,* 98–105.

Kochansky, G. E., Hemenway, T., Salzman, C., & Shader, R. (1975). Methaqualone abusers: A preliminary survey of college students. *Diseases of the Nervous System, 36,* 348–351.

Kotin, J., Wilbert, D., Verburg, D., & Soldinger, S. (1976). Thioridazine and sexual dysfunction. *American Journal of Psychiatry, 133,* 82–85.

Krause, K. E., Advis, J. P., & McKelvy, J. F. (1982). Characterization of the site of cleavage of luteinizing hormone-releasing hormone under conditions of measurement in which LHRH degradation undergoes physiologically related change. *Biochemical and Biophysical Research Communications, 108,* 1475–1481.

Kreek, M. J. (1973). Medical safety and side effects of methadone in tolerant individuals. *Journal of the American Medical Association, 223,* 665–668.

Kulik, F., & Wilbur, R. (1982). Case report of painful ejaculation as a side effect of amoxapine. *American Journal of Psychiatry, 139,* 234–235.

Laschet, U., & Laschet, L. (1975). Anti-androgens in the treatment of sexual deviations in men. *Journal of Steroid Biochemistry, 6,* 821–826.

Laver, M. C. (1974). Sexual behavior patterns in male hypertensives. *Australia-New Zealand Journal of Medicine, 4,* 29–31.

Leif, H. I. (1977). Inhibited sexual desire. *Medical Aspects of Human Sexuality, 7,* 94–95.

Lev-Ran, A. (1974). Sexuality and education levels of women with late treated adrenogenital syndrome. *Archives of Sexual Behavior, 3,* 27–32.

Lindsay, R., Hart, D. M., & Clark, D. M. (1984). The minimum effective dose of estrogen for prevention of postmenopausal bone loss. *Obstetrics and Gynecology, 63*(6), 759–763.

Lipe, H., Longstreth Jr., W. T., Bird, T. D., & Linde, M. (1990). Sexual function in married men with Parkinson's disease compared to married men with arthritis. *Neurology, 40,* 1347–1349.

Lisk, R. D. (1966). Increased sexual behavior in the male rat following lesions in the mammillary region. *Journal of Experimental Zoology, 161*(1), 129–136.

Louria, D. B. (1970). Sexual use of amylnitrite. *Medical Aspects of Human Sexuality, 4,* 89.

Malsbury, C. W. (1971). Facilitation of male rat copulatory behavior by electrical stimulation of the medial preoptic area. *Physiology and Behavior, 7,* 797–805.

Masovich, A., & Tallaferro, A. (1954). Studies on EEG and sex function orgasm. *Diseases of the Nervous System, 15,* 218–220.

Masters, W. H. & Johnson, V. E. (1966). *Human sexual response.* Boston: Little, Brown.

Masters, W. J., & Johnson, V. E. (1970). *Human sexual inadequacy.* Boston: Little, Brown.

Matteo, S., & Rissman, E. F. (1984). Increased sexual activity during the midcycle portion of the human menstrual cycle. *Hormones and Behavior, 18,* 249–255.

Matthews, K. A., Meilahn, E., Kuller, L. H., Kelsey, S. F., Caggiula, A. W., & Wing, R. R. (1989). Menopause and risk factors for coronary heart disease. *New England Journal of Medicine, 321*(10), 641–646.

McFarland, R. V., & Reigel, H. (1978). Chronic mercury poisoning from a single brief exposure. *Journal of Occupational Medicine, 20*(8), 532–534.

McGlone, J., & Young, B. (1990). Cerebral localization. In R. Joynt (Ed.), *Clinical neurology* (Vol. I., pp. 50–51). Philadelphia: J. B. Lippincott.

McKenzie, J. M., & Zakarija, M. (1989). Hyperthyroidism. In L. J. DeGroot (Ed.), *Endocrinology.* Philadelphia: W. B. Saunders.

McWhirter, D. P., & Mattison, A. M. (1978). The treatment of sexual dysfunction in gay male couples. *Journal of Sex and Marital Therapy, 4,* 213–218.

Meiraz, D., Margolin, Y., Lev-Ran, A., & Lazebnik, J. (1977). Treatment of benign prostatic hyperplasia with hydroxyprogesterone-caproate: Placebo controlled study. *Urology, 9,* 144–148.

Mendelson, J. H., Mello, N. K., & Ellingboe, J. (1977). Effects of acute alcohol intake on pituitary-gonadal hormones in normal males. *Journal of Pharmacology and Experimental Therapeutics, 202*(3), 676–682.

Mintz, J., O'Hare, K., O'Brien, C. P., & Goldschmidt, J. (1974). Sexual problems of heroin addicts. *Archives of General Psychiatry, 31,* 700–703.

Mirin, S. M., Meyer, R. E., Mendelson, J. H., & Ellingboe, J. (1980). Opiate use and sexual function. *American Journal of Psychiatry, 137*(8), 909–915.

Mitchell, W., Falconer, M. A., & Hill, D. (1954). Epilepsy with fetishism relieved by temporal lobectomy. *Lancet, 2,* 626–630.

Money, J. (1961). Sex hormones and other variables in human eroticism. In W. C. Young & G. W. Corner (Eds.), *Sex and internal secretions* (Vol. II). Baltimore: Williams and Wilkins.

Money, J. (1965). Influences of hormones on sexual behavior. *Annual Review of Medicine, 16,* 67–82.

Money, J., & Ehrhardt, A. A. (1972). *Man & woman, boy & girl.* Baltimore: John Hopkins University Press.

Money, J., & Higham, E. (1989). Sexual behavior and endocrinology (normal and abnormal). In L. J. DeGroot (Ed.), *Endocrinology,* Philadelphia: W. B. Saunders.

Money, J., & Matthews, D. (1982). Prenatal exposure to virilizing progestins: An adult follow-up study of twelve women. *Archives of Sexual Behavior, 11,* 73–83.

Money, J., Schwartz, M., & Lewis, V. G. (1984). Adult herotosexual status and fetal hormonal masculinization and demasculinization: 46, XX congenital virilizing adrenal hyperplasia (CVAH) and 46 XY androgen-insensitivity syndrome (AIS) compared. *Psychoneuroendocrinology, 9,* 405–414.

Morrell, M. J., Dixen, J. M., Carter, S. C., & Davidson, J. M. (1984). The influence of age and cycling status on sexual arousability in women. *American Journal of Obstetrics and Gynecology, 148,* 66–71.

Moses, M., Lilis, R., Crow, K. D., Thornton, J., Fischbein, A., Anderson, H. A., & Selikoff, I. J. (1984). Health status of workers with past exposure to 2,3,7,8-tetrachlorodibenzo-p-dioxin in the manufacture of 2,4,5-trichlorophenozacetic acid: Comparison of findings with and without chloracne. *American Journal of Industrial Medicine, 5,* 161–182.

Moss, R. L., Dudley, C. A., Gosnell, B. A. (1989). Behavior and the hypothalamus. In L. J. DeGroot (Ed.), *Endocrinology.* Philadelphia: W. B. Saunders.

Mroczek, W. J., Leibel, B. A., & Finnerty, F. A. (1972). Comparison of clonidine and methyldopa in hypertensive patients receiving a diuretic—

double blind cross over study. *American Journal of Cardiology, 29,* 712–717.

Murad, F., & Gilman, A. G. (1975). Androgens and anabolic steroids. In L. Goodman & A. Gilman (Eds.), *The pharmacological basis of therapeutics.* New York: Macmillan.

Murphy, M., Checkley, S., Seckl, J., & Lightman, S. (1990). Naloxone inhibits oxytocin release at orgasm in man. *Journal of Clinical Endocrinology and Metabolism, 71*(4), 1056–1058.

Murphy, M. R., Seckl, J. R., Burton, S., Checkley, S. A., & Lightman, S. L. (1987). Changes in oxytocin and vasopressin secretion during sexual activity in men. *Journal of Clinical Endocrinology and Metabolism, 65*(4), 738–741.

Myers, L., & Morokoff, P. (1985). Physiological and subjective sexual arousal in pre and postmenopausal women. Poster presented at the meeting of the American Psychological Association, Los Angeles.

Naik, D. V. (1976). Immunohistochemical localization of LH-RH during different phases of estrous cycle of rat, with reference to the preoptic and arcuate neurons, and the ependymal cells. *Cell Tissue Research, 173,* 143–166.

Nathan, S. G. (1986). The epidemiology of the DSM-III psychosexual dysfunctions. *Journal of Sex and Marital Therapy, 12*(4), 267–281.

Neri, A., Aygen, M., Zuckerman, Z., & Bahary, C. (1980). Subjective assessment of sexual dysfunction of patients on long-term administration of digoxin. *Archives of Sexual Behavior, 9,* 343–347.

Neshkov, N. C. 1971. The influence of chronic intoxication of ethylated benzene on the spermatogenesis and sexual function of man. *Gigiena Truva: Professional'nye Zaboleveaniya, 13*(2), 45–46.

Newman, A. S., & Bertelson, A. D. (1986). Sexual dysfunction in diabetic women. *Journal of Behavioral Medicine, 9*(3), 261–270.

Newman, R. J., Salerno, H. R. 1974. Sexual dysfunction due to methyldopa. *British Medical Journal,* 4, 106.

Nigam, S. K., Karnik, A. B., Lakkad, B. C., Thakore, K. N., & Joshi, B. H. (1988). Experimental and human surveillance on BHC and DDT insecticides commonly used in India. *Annals of the New York Academy of Sciences, 534,* 694–705.

Nolte, J. (1988). *The human brain.* St. Louis: Mosby.

Nowlis, V. (1975). Categories of interest in the scientific search for relationships (i.e. interactions, associations, comparisons) in human sexual behavior and drug use. In M. Sandler & D. L. Gessa

(Eds.), *Sexual behavior: Pharmacology and biochemistry.* New York: Raven Press.

O'Carroll, R., & Bancroft, J. (1984). Testosterone therapy for low sexual interest and erectile dysfunction in men: A controlled study. *British Journal of Psychiatry, 145,* 146–151.

Occupational Safety and Health Administration (OSHA). (1978). Reproductive toxicity. *OSHA Lead Standard,* 29CFR, 1910.1025. Appendix C.

Odell, W. D. (1989). The leydig cell. In L. DeGroot (Ed.), *Endocrinology.* Philadelphia: W. B. Saunders.

Onesti, G., Bock, K., Heimsoth, V., Kim, K., & Merguet, P. (1971). Clonidine: A new antihypertensive agent. *American Journal of Cardiology, 28,* 74–83.

Paff, B. A. (1985). Sexual dysfunction in gay men requesting treatment. *Journal of Sex and Marital Therapy, 11,* 3–18.

Palanca, E., & Juco, W. (1977). Conservative treatment of benign prostatic hyperplasia. *Current Medical Research and Opinion, 4,* 513–520.

Palkovits, M. (1988). Neuropeptides in the brain. In L. Martini & W. F. Ganong (Eds.), *Frontiers in neuroendocrinology.* New York: Raven Press.

Parks, G. A., Korth-Schutz, S., Penny, R., et al. (1974). Variation in pituitary gonadal function in adolescent male homosexuals and heterosexuals. *Journal of Clinical Endocrinology and Metabolism, 39,* 796–801.

Parr, D. (1976). Sexual aspects of drug abuse in narcotics addicts. *British Journal of Addiction, 71,* 261–268.

Paulson, D. F., & Kane, R. D. (1975). Medrogestone: A prospective study in the pharmaceutical management of benign prostatic hyperplasia. *Journal of Urology, 113,* 815.

Peden, N. R., Cargill, J. M., Browning, M., Saunders, J., & Wormsley, K. (1979). Male sexual dysfunction during treatment with cimetadine. *British Medical Journal, 1,* 659.

Persky, H., Charney, N., Leif, HLIL, O'Brien, C. P., Miller, W. R., & Strauss, D. (1978). The relationship of plasma estradiol level to sexual behavior in young women. *Psychosomatic Medicine, 40,* 523–535.

Persky, H., Leif, H. I., Strauss, D., Miller, W. R., & O'Brien, C. P. (1978). Plasma testosterone level and sexual behavior of couples. *Archives of Sexual Behavior, 7*(3), 157–173.

Petrie, W. M. (1980). Sexual effects of antidepressants and psychomotor stimulant drugs. *Modern Problems in Pharmacopsychiatry, 15,* 77–90.

Phoenix, C. H. 1974. Prenatal testosterone in the nonhuman primate and its consequences for behavior. In R. C. Friedman, R. M. Richart, & R. L. Vande Wiele (Eds.), *Sex differences in behavior.* New York: Wiley.

Pillay, V. K. G. (1976). Some side effects of alphamethyldopa. *South African Medical Journal, 50,* 625–626.

Prichard, B. N. C., & Gillam, P. M. S. (1969). Treatment of hypertension with propranolol. *British Medical Journal, 1,* 7–16.

Pritchard, P. B. (1980). Hyposexuality: A complication of complex partial epilepsy. *Transactions of the American Neurological Association, 105,* 193.

Randall, R. V. (1989). Acromegaly and giantism. In L. J. DeGroot (Ed.), *Endocrinology.* Philadelphia: W. B. Saunders.

Reamy, K. J., & White, S. E. (1987). Sexuality in the puerperium: A review. *Archives of Sexual Behavior, 16*(2), 165–186.

Reece, R. (1981/82). Group treatment of sexual dysfunction in gay men. *Journal of Homosexuality, 7*(2/3), 113–129.

Reece, R. 1987. Causes and treatments of sexual desire discrepancies in male couples. *Journal of Homosexuality, 14*(1/2), 157–172.

Reece, R. (1988). Special issues in the etiologies and treatments of sexual problems among gay men. *Journal of Homosexuality, 15,* 43–57.

Remillard, G. M., Anderman, S., Testa, G., et al. (1983). Sexual ictal manifestations predominant in women with temporal lobe epilepsy. A finding suggesting sexual dimorphism in the human brain. *Neurology, 33,* 323.

Robinson, B. W., & Mishkin, M. (1966). Ejaculation evoked by stimulation of the preoptic area in monkey. *Physiology and Behavior, 1,* 269–272.

Robinson, B. W., & Mishkin, M. (1968). Penile erection evoked from forebrain structures in Macaca mulatta. *Archives of Neurology, 19,* 184–198.

Rosen, R. C., & Leiblum, S. R. (1989). Assessment and treatment of desire disorders. In R. C. Rosen & S. R. Leiblum (Eds.), *Principles and practice of sex theory.* New York: Guilford.

Sachs, B. D., & Meisel, R. L. (1988). The physiology of male sexual behavior. In E. Knobil & J. Neill (Eds.), *The physiology of reproduction.* New York: Raven Press.

Saghir, M. T., & Robins, E. (1973). *Male and female homosexuality.* Baltimore: Williams and Wilkins.

Schein, M., Zyzanski, S. J., Levine, S., Medalie, J. H., Dickman, R. L., & Alemagno, S. A. (1988). The frequency of sexual problems among family practice patients. *Family Practice Research Journal, 7*(3), 122–134.

Schiavi, R. C., Schreiner-Engel, P., White, D., & Mandeli, J. (1988). Pituitary-gonadal function during sleep in men with hypoactive sexual desire and in normal controls. *Psychosomatic Medicine, 50,* 304–318.

Schreiner-Engel, P., & Schiavi, R. (1986). Lifetime psychopathology in individuals with low sexual desire. *Journal of Nervous and Mental Disease, 174*(11), 646–651.

Schreiner-Engel, P., Schiavi, R. C., Vietorisz, D., & Smith, H. (1987). The differential impact of diabetes type on female sexuality. *Journal of Psychosomatic Research, 31*(1), 23–33.

Schreiner-Engel, P., Schiavi, R. C., White, D., & Ghizzani, A. (1989). Low sexual desire in women: The role of reproductive hormones. *Hormones and Behavior, 23,* 221–234.

Schuler, P., Oyanguren, H., Maturana, B., Valenzuela, A., Cruz, E., Plaza, B., Schmidp, E., & Haddad, R. (1957). Manganese poisoning. Environmental and medical study in a Chilean mine. *Industrial Medicine and Surgery, 26,* 167.

Schumacher, M., Coirini, H., Pfaff, D., & McEwen, B. S. (1990). Behavioral effects of progesterone associated with rapid modulation of oxytocin receptors. *Science, 250,* 691–694.

Schwarcz, G. (1982). Case report of inhibition of ejaculation and retrograde ejaculation as side effects of amoxapine. *American Journal of Psychiatry, 139,* 233–234.

Segal, S., Yaffe, H., Lanfer, N., & Ben-David, M. (1979). Male hyperprolactinemia: Effects on fertility. *Fertility and Sterility, 32,* 556–561.

Segraves, R. T. (1988). Hormones and libido. In S. Leiblum (Ed.), *Sexual desire disorders.* New York: Guilford.

Semmens, J. P., Wagner, G. 1982. Estrogen deprivation and vaginal function in postmenopausal women. *Journal of the American Medical Association, 248,* 445–448.

Serlin, M. S., Orme, M., Baber, N., Sibeon, R., Laws, B., & Breckenridge, A. (1980). Propranolol in the control of blood pressure: A dose-response study. *Clinical Pharmacology and Therapeutics, 27,* 586–592.

Setalo, G., Vigh, S., Schally, A. V., et al. (1976). Changing immunoreactivity of the LHRH-containing nerve terminals in the organum vasculosum of the lamina terminalis. *Acta Biologica Hungarica, 27*, 75–77.

Sherwin, B. B., & Gelfand, M. M. (1987). The role of androgen in the maintenance of sexual functioning in oophorectomized women. *Psychosomatic Medicine, 49*, 397–409.

Sherwin, B. B., Gelfand, M. M., Brender, W. (1985). Androgen enhances sexual motivation in females: A prospective, crossover study of sex steroid administration in the surgical menopause. *Psychosomatic Medicine, 47*(4), 339–351.

Sigell, L. T., Kapp, F. T., Fusaro, G. A., Nelson, E. D., & Falck, R. S. (1978). Popping and snorting volatile nitrites: A current fad for getting high. *American Journal of Psychiatry, 135*(10), 1216–1218.

Simerly, R. B., Gorski, R. A., & Swanson, L. W. (1986). Neurotransmitter specificity of cells and fibers in the medial preoptic nucleus: An immunohistochemical study. *Journal of Comparative Neurology, 246*, 343–363.

Simpson, G. M., Blair, J. H., & Amuso, D. (1965). Effects of antidepressants on genito-urinary function. *Diseases of the Nervous System, 26*, 787–789.

Singer, I., & Singer, J. (1972). Periodicity of sexual desire in relation [sic] time of ovulation in women. *Journal of Biosocial Science, 4*, 471–481.

Skinner, B. F. (1969). *Contingencies of reinforcement.* New York: Appleton-Century-Crofts.

Smith, D. E., Buxton, M. E., & Bammann, G. (1979). Amphetamine abuse and sexual dysfunction: Clinical and research considerations. In D. E. Smith (Ed.), *Amphetamine use, misuse and abuse.* Cambridge: G. K. Hall.

Southren, S. (1985). Hypoactive sexual desire: A cognitive model. *Journal of Sex Education and Therapy, 11*(2), 55–60.

Spark, R. F., & Melby, J. C. (1968). Aldosteronism in hypertension—the spironolactone response test. *Annals of Internal Medicine, 69*, 685–691.

Sparrow, D., Bosse, R., & Rowe, J. W. (1980). The influence of age, alcohol consumption, and body build on gonadal function in men. *Journal of Clinical Endocrinology and Metabolism, 51*, 508–512.

Stanislaw, H., & Rice, F. J. (1988). Correlation between sexual desire and menstrual cycle characteristics. *Archives of Sexual Behavior, 17*(6), 499–508.

Stearns, E. L., MacDonnell, J. A., Kaufman, B. J., Lucman, T. S., Winter, J. S., & Faiman, C. (1976).

Declining testicular function with age. *American Journal of Medicine, 57*, 761–766.

Stuart, F. M., Hammond, D. C., & Pett, M. A. (1987). Inhibited sexual desire in women. *Archives of Sexual Behavior, 16*(2), 91–107.

Svare, B., Bartke, A., Doherty, P., et al. (1979). Hyperprolactinemia suppresses copulatory behavior in male rats and mice. *Biology of Reproduction, 21*, 529–535.

Symons, D. (1979). *The evolution of human sexuality.* New York: Oxford University Press.

Taylor, D. C. (1959). Aggression in epilepsy. *Journal of Psychiatric Research, 13*, 29.

Taylor, D. C. (1971). Appetitive inadequacy in the sex behavior of temporal lobe epileptics. *Journal of Neuro-Visceral Relations*, Suppl. X, 486–490.

Taylor, J. R., Selhorst, J. B., Houff, S. A., & Martinez, A. J. (1978). Chlordecone intoxication in man. I. Clinical observations. *Neurology, 28*, 626–630.

Tennekoon, K. H., & Lenton, E. A. (1985). Early evening prolactin rise in women with regular cycles. *Journal of Reproduction and Fertility, 73*, 523–527.

Tsai, C. C., Semmens, J. P., Semmons, E. C., Lam, C. F., & Lee, F. S. (1987). Vaginal physiology in post menopausal women: pH value, transvaginal electropotential difference and estimated blood flow. *Southern Medical Journal, 80*, 987–990.

Tuchman, H., & Crumpton, C. (1955). A comparison of *Rauwolfia serpentina* compounds, crude root, alseroxylon derivative, and single alkaloid in the treatment of hypertension. *American Heart Journal, 49*, 742–750.

U.S. Environmental Protection Agency. 1978. Rebuttable presumption against registration and continued registration of pesticide products containing 2,4,5-T. *Federal Register, 43*(78), 56–57.

Vague, J. (1983). Testicular feminization syndrome. An experimental model for the study of hormone action on sexual behavior. *Hormone Research, 18*(1–3), 62–68.

Van Thiel, D. H., & Lester, R. 1976. Sex and alcohol: A second peek. *New England Journal of Medicine, 15*, 835–836.

Vermeulen, A. (1983). Androgen secretion by adrenals and gonads. In V. B. Mahesh & R. B. Greenblatt (Eds.), *Hirsuitism and virilism.* Boston: John Wright.

Vermeulen, A., Rubens, R., & Verdonck, L. (1972). Testosterone secretion and metabolism in male senescence. *Journal of Clinical Endocrinology and Metabolism, 34,* 730–735.

Verwoerdt, A., Pfeiffer, E., & Wang, H. S. (1969). Sexual behavior in senescence—changes in sexual activity and interest of aging men and women. *Journal of Geriatric Psychiatry, 2,* 163–180.

Veteran's Administration Cooperative Study Group on Antihypertensive Agents. (1977). Propranolol in the treatment of essential hypertension. *Journal of the American Medical Association, 237,* 2303–2310.

Vinarova, E., Uhlir, V., Stika, L. K., & Vinar, O. (1972). Side effects of lithium administration. *Activitas Nervosa Superior, 14,* 105–107.

Walker, A. E. (1976). Clinical aspects of vinyl chloride disease: Skin. *Proceedings of the Royal Society of Medicine, 69,* 286–289.

Wallace, T., Fraunfelder, F., Petursson, G., & Epstein, D. (1979). Decreased libido—a side effect of carbonic anhydrase inhibitor. *Annals of Opthalmology, 11,* 1563–1566.

Wallen, K. (1990). Desire and ability: Hormones and the regulation of female sexual behavior. *Neuroscience & Biobehavioral Reviews, 14,* 233–241.

Warren, S. C., & Warren, S. G. (1977). Propranolol and sexual impotence. *Annals of Internal Medicine, 86,* 112.

Warren, S. G., Brewer, D. L., & Orgain, E. S. (1976). Long-term propranolol therapy for angina pectoris. *American Journal of Cardiology, 37,* 420–426.

Waxenberg, S. E., Drellich, M. G., & Sutherland, A. M. (1959). Changes in female sexuality after adrenalectomy. *Journal of Clinical Endocrinology and Metabolism, 19,* 193–202.

Weissberg, K. (1972). Sopors are a bummer. *Berkeley Barb,* 1–7, 13.

Weizman, R., Weizman, A., Levi, J., Gura, V., Zevin, D., Maoz, B., Wijsenbeek, H., & Ben-David, M. (1983). Sexual dysfunction associated with hyperprolactinemia in males and females undergoing hemodialysis. *Psychosomatic Medicine, 45*(3), 259–269.

Willson, R. J., Beecham, C. T., & Carrington, E. R. (1975). *Obstetrics and gynecology.* St. Louis: Mosby.

Wolfe, M. M. (1979). Impotence on cimetidine treatment. *New England Journal of Medicine, 300,* 94.

Wortsman, J., Rosner, W., & Dufaw, M. L. (1987). Abnormal testicular function in men with primary hypothyroidism. *American Journal of Medicine, 82,* 207–212.

Zacharias, F. J. (1976). Patient acceptability of propranolol and the occurrence of side effects. *Postgraduate Medical Journal, 52*(Suppl. 4), 87–89.

Zarren, H. S., & Black, P. L. (1975). Unilateral gynecomastia and impotence during low-dose spironolactone administration in men. *Military Medicine, 140,* 417–419.

Zilbergeld, B., & Ellison, C. R. (1980). Desire discrepancies and arousal problems in sex therapy. In S. R. Leiblum & L. Pervin (Eds.), *Principles and practice of sex therapy* (pp. 65–104). New York: Guilford.

CHAPTER 3

SEXUAL DESIRE DISORDERS

Elizabeth Letourneau, Northern Illinois University
William O'Donohue, Northern Illinois University

DEFINITION AND DESCRIPTION

Lief (1977) and Kaplan (1977; 1979) are typically credited with suggesting that low sexual desire be classified as a sexual dysfunction. Although Lief (1977) attributes to Freud (1926; 1936) and Rado (1949) the earliest recognition of the importance of desire in sexuality, Lief (1977) coined the term *inhibited sexual desire disorder* (ISD), and he and Kaplan (1977) were instrumental in convincing the mental health community of the importance of sexual desire in sexual functioning. Their influence lay in their independent construction of two models of human sexual functioning, both of which include sexual desire as a basic component of the human sexual response cycle. Prior to these two models, the primary model of sexual functioning was the four-stage model—arousal, plateau, orgasm, and refractory stages—of Masters and Johnson (1970), which did not include

the concept of desire as a basic aspect of sexual functioning.

In his model of human sexual functioning, Lief (1977) added desire to the stages of excitement, plateau, orgasm, and resolution. Kaplan (1977) initially developed a biphasic model that did not include desire, but she went on to add desire, creating a triphasic model of human sexual functioning (Kaplan, 1979) that includes sexual excitement, orgasm, and desire.

Changes to the Masters and Johnson human sexual functioning model were spurred by clinical observations of a subset of sex therapy clients who were particularly resistant to standard sex therapy techniques (Kaplan, 1979; Lief, 1977). These clients differed from other sexual dysfunction clients in that they seemed to engage in sexual activities less frequently, complain of disinterest in sex, have more significant relationship problems, and experience more anxiety about sex (Kaplan, 1979; Lief,

1977). In adding the concept of sexual desire to sexual functioning, Lief and Kaplan were able to offer explanations for the treatment difficulty experienced with these clients—explanations that had treatment implications.

Lief's (1977) and Kaplan's (1979) theories regarding low sexual desire became widely accepted, as evidenced by the changes in the sexual dysfunctions category of the third edition of the *Diagnostic and Statistical Manual* (DSM-III) (American Psychiatric Association, 1980). Although no reference to sexual desire disorder was made in the DSM-II, it was included in the DSM-III, with the following criteria for ISD:

> 302.71 Psychosexual Dysfunctions with Inhibited Sexual Desire
> A. Persistent and pervasive inhibition of sexual desire. The basis for the judgment of inhibition is made by the clinician taking into account age, sex, occupation, the individual's subjective statement as to intensity and frequency of sexual desire, a knowledge of norms of sexual behavior, and the context of the individual's life. In actual practice, this diagnosis will rarely be used unless the lack of desire is a source of distress either to the individual or to his or her partner. Frequently this category will be used in conjunction with one or more of the other dysfunction categories.
> B. The disturbance is not caused exclusively by organic factors and is not symptomatic of another clinical psychiatric syndrome (p. 278).

The most recent DSM, DSM-III-R (American Psychiatric Association, 1987) includes a distinction between clients who have low desire but engage in sexual activity without extreme aversion versus those who exhibit extreme aversion towards sexual activity and/or genitalia (APA, 1987). The latter dysfunction is labeled *sexual aversion* (see Chapter 4 of this book).

The DSM-III also included frequency of sexual fantasies as a diagnostic criterion. Kaplan (1979) and others made the clinical observation that individuals with low sexual desire rarely

fantasized about things sexual. This observation was subsequently supported by research findings suggesting that clients diagnosed with ISD engage in sexual fantasizing less frequently than nondysfunctional individuals (Nutter & Condron, 1983; 1985).

A seemingly minor change made in the sexual dysfunctions category of the DSM-III involved the ISD label. The nomenclature was changed from "inhibited sexual desire dysfunction" to "hypoactive sexual desire dysfunction." This change occurred because the task force making diagnostic recommendations felt that the term *inhibited* implied a psychodynamic causality that was unwarranted for this diagnosis (Lief, 1977). However, issue may also be taken with the value judgment involved in labeling a frequency of activity as "hypoactive" and the one-sided designation of lower rates of sexual activity as psychopathological but not higher rates of sexual activity. This issue will be developed more fully below. The change from one diagnostic label to another would also appear to underline a lack of clarity regarding what actually constitutes clinically low sexual desire—another point to be discussed later in this chapter.

Currently, the criteria for hypoactive sexual desire (HSD) are as follows:

> 302.71 Hypoactive Sexual Desire Disorder
> A. Persistently or recurrently deficient or absent sexual fantasies and desire for sexual activity. The judgment of deficiency or absence is made by the clinician, taking into account factors that affect sexual functioning, such as age, sex, and the context of the person's life.
> B. Occurrence not exclusively during the course of another Axis I disorder (other than a Sexual Dysfunction), such as Major Depression (APA, 1987, p. 293).

An obvious problem with this definition of low sexual desire is its subjective nature. This subjectivity results from two more basic problems: (1) the difficulty of operationally defining *desire* and (2) the lack of valid population norms regarding the experience of sexual desire (Hawton, 1985; Leiblum & Rosen, 1988; O'Donohue & Geer, Chapter 1 of this book). Despite the inherent difficulty of the task, several authors have developed definitions of sexual desire. For example, Lief (1977) defined sexual desire as "a readiness for sexual activity, a mental set, a psychic state" and ISD as "a significant problem in feeling enough desire to initiate or to respond to sexual cues" (p. 94). Leiblum and Rosen (1988), after delineating some of the difficulties in defining sexual desire, also offer a definition: "A subjective feeling state that may be triggered by both internal and external cues, and that may or may not result in overt sexual behavior" (p. 5). Levine (1988) employs a more technical definition of desire, as involving "the psychobiological energy that precedes and accompanies sexual arousal and tends to produce sexual behavior" (p. 33). Levine further states that desire is the product of an interaction between specific neuroendocrine, cognitive, and motivational processes. Levine provides extensive definitions of his terms. However, the accuracy of his definition of sexual desire is difficult to determine, given that knowledge in the areas of psychobiological energy; neuroendocrine, cognitive, and motivational processes; and their relationship to sexual desire is currently incomplete.

Unfortunately, the definitions of desire given above frequently employ rather vague terminology (e.g., "psychic state"). Also, in the case of Leiblum and Rosen (1988), the definition does not seem to be uniquely definitive of sexual desire. The ambiguous nature of these definitions and of diagnostic criteria for low sexual desire may be related to a lack of population norms. For example, if valid population norms were known regarding the occurrence of sexual desire, then clinicians would be able to designate people who experience desire a certain number of standard deviations below the population mean as having significantly lower desire than average. Because this is not the case, diagnostic criteria must rely on less spe-

cific terms such as "low," "hypoactive," or "inhibited," all of which are subjective, vague, and rest upon the views of the clinician making the diagnosis (Leiblum & Rosen, 1988). For some, this is not a particularly troublesome problem, as they believe that judgment of normal or abnormal levels of sexual desire may be validly accomplished even without knowledge of population norms (Kaplan, 1979; Lazarus, 1988; LoPiccolo & Friedman, 1988). For example, Kaplan (1979) argues that "there is enough of a sense of what the normal range of sexual interest is for practical purposes, and while there is confusion in borderline situations, professional consensus is adequate to define the extreme and clearly pathological deviations from the norm" (p. 59). This sentiment is reflected in the DSM-III-R, which calls for the clinician to make "the judgment of deficiency or absence" of desire, although it does not provide any guiding criteria to do so (p. 293). There is, however, reason to be concerned with this reliance on clinical intuition, as this could leave diagnoses open to the cultural, social, and personal biases of clinicians. Moreover, there is no evidence of the interrater reliability of this diagnosis.

By reducing the necessity for vague terminology, epidemiological data regarding base rates of sexual functioning are useful in the process of defining sexual dysfunctions, thus increasing the reliability of these definitions (Nathan, 1986). This type of data may also help to increase the validity of diagnostic criteria. For example, although there are no widely accepted population estimates of the frequency of experiencing desire, there are data suggesting that sexually nondysfunctional women generally experience sexual desire and sexual fantasies less frequently than do nondysfunctional men (Kinsey, Pomeroy, Martin, & Gebhard, 1953; Leiblum & Rosen, 1988). Yet the definitions offered for low sexual desire are generally applied to all individuals without regard to age, gender, or other factors that may be related to differences in desire. If there are true differences in rates of sexual desire between different populations, then clinicians who use only a single "sexual desire continuum," with clinically low desire on one end and high desire on the other (e.g., Lazarus, 1988), will place women at greater risk for receiving a diagnosis of clinically low sexual desire than men, even though these women may be experiencing "normal" levels of desire. This would not only lead to invalid diagnoses, but might also cause detrimental effects to the women whose level of sexual desire has been incorrectly pathologized. By the same token, men would hypothetically be at greater risk for the diagnosis of some sort of "hyperactive sexual desire disorder." However, there is no reference to hyperactive sexual desire in the DSM-III-R. Epidemiological data would help to determine whether different populations required different definitions for "normal" sexual desire levels.

Recognizing the diagnostic and definitional problems with this dysfunction, some authors advocate the use of a "desire discrepancy" as the diagnostic criterion in cases where clients experience sexual desire at a level that causes distress in their sexual relationships (Rosen & Leiblum, 1988). This lets clients, rather than clinicians, determine when low sexual desire is a problem and also allows for the possibility that too much sexual desire may be a problem. However, despite the more neutral terminology, at least part of the treatment focus of those who use this criterion nonetheless appears to be on increasing the sex drive of one of the partners. In addition, it may be that desire discrepancies are "normal" for couples. For example, there is evidence suggesting that men and women experience their "peak" sexual drives at different points in their development (Kinsey, Pomeroy, & Martin, 1948; Kinsey et al., 1953). Thus, when desire discrepancies are treated as pathological, there is still the risk of psychopathologizing normal sexual functioning. Furthermore, although some clients may experience sexual difficulties within the context of a particular relationship, others experience more global lack of desire, which may also be lifelong. Thus, eliminating the individual diagnosis may not be the most

appropriate answer to this dilemma (Friedman & Hogan, 1985; Kaplan, 1983).

The Politics of Desire

Hypoactive, inhibited, and *low* are adjectives that imply a comparison to some standard. What standard, then, ought to be used? What are the values, if any, involved in the use of the standard? We claim that the use of any standards for sexual desire involves value judgments. There are many possible candidates for standards—including reference to some population average or to some notion of "health"—and many ways of defining a clinically significant deviation from the standard—e.g., 1 or 2 standard deviations, or the point at which one partner's complaints are of such and such magnitude. Clearly, choosing among these alternatives reflects values. Moreover, the standards themselves and the very definitions of deviations involve values. Reference to a population average implicitly involves the claim that the population average ought to be approximated, and a "health" standard must rest on some regulative notion of proper functioning: How much desire is healthy? The claim that one partner has hypoactive desire is a judgment, which also implies that the other partner does not have hyperactive desire. Criteria for determining a clinically significant deviation involve values: Complaints of a certain magnitude are abnormal; behavior of a given sort is found only in $x\%$ of the population and therefore is sufficiently rare to be considered abnormal; individuals ought not to have complaints of this magnitude, etc.

So what values are involved in our standards and in our definitions of deviation? Two kinds of values, both potentially problematic, must be carefully considered. The first is a male bias; the second, which is related, is a hypersexual bias.

Desire has proven difficult to measure precisely, and there is controversy as to whether there are gender differences in sexual desire. Those who believe differences do exist have claimed that it is males who are more sexually desirous (Symons, 1987). But is this simply a way in which females are pathologized when they do not conform to male sexual interests? Another related question concerns the object of desire. Desire is not amorphous; it is a desire for something. Patriarchal biases can come into play if males are the ones who have a dominant influence in determining the nature and content of the sexual interaction. A husband may have a disproportionate say in choosing the occasion for the sexual interaction and how it unfolds—little foreplay or romance and few activities pleasing to the wife. In such a case, the female may simply have no desire for such interaction. Since socialization messages place great importance on monogamy (especially for females), this disinterest may become generalized to a disinterest in all sex. A female might reasonably expect that other males would behave in a similar manner. It has been said that the reason women fake orgasm is that men fake foreplay.

The second bias possibly involved in the definition of hypoactive sexual desire is a bias toward hypersexuality. It is revealing that there is no category for hypersexuality in the DSM-III-R. Could this be due to a belief that hypersexuality cannot be a problem? Part of the message of the sexual revolution in the 1960s and '70s was that sex is good—therefore, the more sex, the better. Robinson (1976) has suggested that the major sexologists of the twentieth century (Ellis, Kinsey, and Masters and Johnson) show bias in favor of increasing sexual activity. The point goes beyond contemporary warnings about promiscuous sexuality and its health risks. The point is that human sexual interaction may have a proper role or roles and that its frequency can only be understood in this context. When taken out of context, sexuality can be excessive. For example, according to natural law theorists, sex has a procreative and affiliative function, but it can be misused for other illicit ends. The ends become illicit partly because a thing is being used contrary to its nature, but also because of interference with the pursuit of other ends. St. Augustine, for example, sees sexual desire as potentially interfering with more important spiritual and intellectual pursuits.

We do not wish to suggest that individuals and couples who complain of low sexual desire are not really experiencing a problem. Clearly, the belief that one has abnormally low sexual desire, or that one's sexual relationship is frustrating because of desire discrepancies, may cause serious problems for a person or couple. The rest of this chapter is devoted to a review of what is known about clients who complain of low sexual desire and the treatment of such clients. However, acknowledgment that some individuals are dissatisfied with their level of sexual desire does not prove that the problem is either abnormal or psychological; it may be indicative of sociological phenomena or something altogether different. More must be learned about this aspect of sexual functioning. Meanwhile, in attempting to increase the sexual desire of an individual (usually a woman), we must take care not to propagate a socially biased, male-identified point of view that regards low sexual desire as a problem per se (Apfelbaum, 1988, p. 82).

PSYCHOPATHOLOGY

Incidence and Prevalence

As noted by Nathan (1986) and O'Donohue and Geer (Chapter 1 of this book), information garnered from epidemiological data is useful in determining base rates of the experience of sexual desire. However, several factors generally limit the conclusions that can be drawn from epidemiological data (Hawton, 1985; Nathan, 1986; O'Donohue & Geer, Chapter 1). First, the lack of an adequate definition of the diagnosis is a limiting factor, as is the lack of reliable and valid assessment techniques for making the diagnosis. Nathan notes that surveys of sexual dysfunctions (1) frequently assess skewed samples—better educated, younger, and from higher socioeconomic backgrounds than the normal population. (2) Such surveys often fail to address specific DSM criteria, thus making it difficult to assess actual norms for the specific dysfunctions. For example, data regarding frequency of sexual activity are often used to gauge sexual desire, but this may be unwarranted—for example, people may engage in sexual activities to please their partners rather than as a result of desire. (3) The surveys often do not gather the data necessary for ruling out other, related diagnoses. (4) The data are usually presented in a yes-no format, which leads to a high number of false negatives and false positives. (5) Many surveys do not set a specific time frame, so incidence information is confused with prevalence information. (6) Finally, specific diagnostic criteria may not be addressed because key terms have not been adequately understood or because the use of "clinical judgment" is necessary for making the diagnosis but cannot be accommodated by the survey (p. 265). Hawton (1985) further notes that individuals may be less inclined to reveal sensitive information regarding their sexual functioning, or they may be more open to social biases when responding about sexual functioning than with other topics, thus further limiting the validity of the data. Hawton also points out that nonresponders may differ significantly from those individuals who answer surveys, thus limiting the generalizability of the data.

Obviously, this long list of difficulties will not be overcome completely, and we cannot wait for the "perfect" survey before attempting to understand the epidemiology of clinical disorders (or what are now considered to be disorders). Nonetheless, the results of the existing epidemiological studies must be viewed with caution, as only preliminary estimates of the true prevalence and incidence of low sexual desire (Nathan, 1986).

Since the inclusion of the sexual desire diagnostic category in the DSM-III, low sexual desire has become one of the diagnoses most widely employed by clinicians in the United States (Kaplan, 1979; Knopf & Seiler, 1990; Lief, 1985; Schreiner-Engel & Schiavi, 1986). Surveys of sex therapists indicate that 28–55%

of all sex therapy clients are considered to have desire discrepancies or low sexual desire as the primary therapeutic concern (Bagarozzi, 1987; Hawton, 1985; LoPiccolo & Friedman, 1988; Schover & LoPiccolo, 1982). This trend appears to be increasing over time (LoPiccolo & Friedman, 1988; Rosen & Leiblum, 1989; Schover & LoPiccolo, 1982), although it is difficult to differentiate between possibly increased incidence and the effects of increased public and professional recognition of this diagnostic category. For example, in a reevaluation of over 1000 sex therapy cases covering a span of eight years, LoPiccolo and Friedman reported increasing incidence of sexual desire disorders at their sex therapy clinic. Low sexual desire was determined to be the primary diagnosis in 32% of the couples seen in 1974 and 55% of the couples seen in 1982. However, it is possible that clinicians gathered the type of information that allows for such a diagnosis only in the later period.

Nathan (1986) reviewed the results from 22 surveys of nondysfunctional samples. Regarding low sexual desire, Nathan's findings suggested that unmarried women were most likely to indicate an absence of sexual desire. Specifically, 15–20% of unmarried female respondents indicated a lack of sexual desire, compared with only 1–3% of men and married women. When less strict definitions of low sexual desire were employed (e.g., "disinterested in sex" versus "never felt sexual desire"), the percentage of men and women who indicated that low sexual desire was a problem increased dramatically.

Survey data of sex therapists and the general population indicate a substantial difference between the numbers of men and women who complain of low sexual desire. However, LoPiccolo and Friedman (1988) reported an increase over time in the number of males receiving the diagnosis of low sexual desire. Specifically, in 1974–1976 the gender ratio for low sexual desire at their clinic was approximately 70-30 female. In 1982–1983, the ratio was 45-55, indicating that more men than women received this diagnosis. However, the latter finding appears to be a unique. Most reports indicate that women are far more likely to receive the diagnosis of low sexual desire, even though the incidence rates for males receiving this diagnosis do appear to have increased (Hawton, 1985; LoPiccolo & Friedman, 1988). There are several hypotheses regarding the gender differences found in rates of low sexual desire, including the effect of differential sexual socialization of males and females (Rosen & Leiblum, 1988). Also, women may simply have a lower "base rate" of desire than males. Another explanation involves the higher rates of female children and adults who experience sexual assault (Hawton, 1985). There are some data suggesting a link between sexual assault and sexual dysfunctions, especially sexual desire dysfunctions (Becker, Skinner, Abel, & Treacy, 1982). Finally, sexual desire may be qualitatively different between men and women, with the general and clinical understanding of desire representing a point of view biased toward "male" desire. The popular conception of women as craving more romance and men craving more sex may be indicative of such a difference, though this is highly speculative at present.

Associated Features

The DSM-III-R lists several possible predisposing factors for sexual dysfunction, such as "anxiety," "unusual sensitivity to real or imagined rejection by a sexual partner," and "negative attitude toward sexuality" (p. 292). Other researchers have indicated that these problems may be effects, as well as antecedents, of sexual dysfunction (Hawton, 1985; Kaplan, 1979). Additional emotional reactions which have been cited as accompanying low sexual desire include feelings of anger, fear, depression, and guilt (Hawton, 1985; Kaplan, 1979; Knopf & Seiler, 1990).

Although not all of these associations have been subjected to empirical study, there is some support for the idea that depression and

anxiety are both associated with low desire. Studies presented by Murphy and Sullivan (1981) and Schreiner-Engel and Schiavi (1986) suggest that anxiety and depression are more common in individuals diagnosed with ISD than in nondysfunctional controls.

Low sexual desire obviously can interfere with the sexual functioning of another individual—the sexual partner of the individual who has low desire. Behaviors whose frequency is measurably higher in low-desire women (and which may affect interpersonal relationships) include increased refusal of spouses' sexual overtures by married women with ISD (relative to married women without ISD) and increased likelihood that ISD women would report having engaged in sex to avoid hurting their spouses and to fulfill a marital obligation (Stuart, Hammond, & Pett, 1987). Stuart et al. suggest that these behaviors would appear to lead to a third finding, that spouses of ISD women make fewer sexual overtures (Stuart et al., 1987). These findings are significant; ISD may lead to more general relationship difficulties and consequent risk of divorce or intact but unhappy marriage (APA, 1987; Hawton, 1985; Schwartz & Masters, 1988).

Differential Diagnosis

The DSM-III-R criteria for sexual dysfunctions stipulate that these diagnoses may not be employed if another Axis I mental disorder is determined to be the primary cause of the dysfunction (APA, 1987). As mentioned above, there is evidence linking the affective disorders (especially major depression disorder) with low sexual desire (Schreiner-Engel & Schiavi, 1986). Thus, clinicians must attempt to assess for the presence of depression as well as to determine the temporal order of the different disorders before assigning a diagnosis. Unfortunately, it is not an easy task to determine a cause-and-effect relationship between sexual dysfunction and other disorders (Hawton, 1985), and the DSM-III-R does not specify what course of action to take when it is unclear which disorder occurred first. In cases where a personality disorder is determined to coexist with a sexual dysfunction, both disorders should be diagnosed (APA, 1987). Similarly, when a physical disorder or a V Code condition (e.g., marital discord) is partially responsible for reduction or absence of desire, both diagnoses should be given.

There appears to be substantial comorbidity between various sexual dysfunctions, especially between low desire and sexual arousal dysfunction (APA, 1987; Becker et al., 1982; Schwartz & Masters, 1988; LoPiccolo & Stock, 1986). Thus, attention must be given to whether the low desire is "pure" or whether it coexists with another sexual dysfunction. Additionally, low desire must be distinguished from sexual aversion (APA, 1987; Gold & Gold, Chapter 4 of this book). When another sexual dysfunction is determined to be the primary cause of low desire, both diagnoses should be given (APA, 1987).

Clinicians should be careful to differentiate between couples who need sex therapy and those who need more general relationship or marital therapy (Hawton, 1985). This differentiation is supported by studies indicating that couples with severe relationship difficulties are more resistant to sex therapy than couples whose relationship difficulties are less significant (Hawton & Catalan, 1986).

Course and Subtypes

Within the diagnostic framework of the DSM-III-R, the course of low sexual desire may vary on two dimensions (APA, 1987). The first dimension is time of onset. Low sexual desire may be either lifelong or acquired. When lifelong, the low level or lack of desire has been evident since early adolescence. When acquired, the low level or lack of desire has decreased from a premorbid level.

The second dimension used to differentiate clients with low sexual desire is degree of generalization (APA, 1987). Low desire may be either generalized or situational. Generalized low desire characterizes the person's response to all sexual or potentially sexual situations and cues. In acquired low sexual desire, desire is felt in some but not all sexual situations and cues. Thus, four different courses for low desire are possible: (1) lifelong generalized; (2) lifelong situational; (3) acquired generalized; and (4) acquired situational. Based on clinical observation, it appears that lifelong generalized low desire is the most severe and least common course, and acquired situational low desire is the least severe and most common course (Kaplan, 1979).

Another distinction is that between low desire caused by physical and by psychological factors (APA, 1987; Kaplan, 1979). Kaplan labels physiologically generated low desire as "hypoactive sexual desire" and psychologically caused low desire as "inhibited sexual desire." Sexual desire is not generated in clients who suffer from a relevant physiological cause. In clients with psychological etiology, desire is present but is inhibited by underlying anxiety or anger (Kaplan, 1979). It is unknown to what extent this differentiation is useful, although physiological factors should be taken into consideration if they are a possible cause for the disorder that is being assessed. Unfortunately, there is little data on how physiological disorders affect desire (see Chapter 2 of this book).

On a practical level, it may be useful to distinguish between clients who present themselves to sex therapists because they are concerned with their low levels of desire and clients who present at the request of a partner. It seems intuitive that treatment could differ depending on the motivations of the client (e.g., to appease a partner as against wishing to change desire level for personal reasons).

There may also be a subtype of low-desire individuals who never feel spontaneous sexual desire but who experience desire once their partners have initiated sexual activity (Lazarus, 1988). Again, this is based on clinical speculation. More research is needed to determine whether there are clinically useful subtypes within the diagnostic category of low sexual desire.

THEORIES OF ETIOLOGY

As noted in Chapter 1, a virtually limitless number of possible etiological factors and combinations of factors are involved in the sexual dysfunctions. Even for the relatively new category of desire disorders, etiological theories may be found in several disciplines. (1) Physiology is one causal area: For example, changes in the levels of various hormones affect desire (see Chapter 2). (2) There are sociobiological aspects: For instance, due to selective advantages associated with different reproductive strategies, the male sex drive is more readily activated than the female sex drive (Symons, 1987). (3) Sociological factors play a role—e.g., because of the increased frequency and explicitness of television portrayals of exceptional lovemaking, hypersexual standards have arisen, which may heighten performance anxiety and thus decrease desire (Pietropinto, 1986). (4) Feminist psychology is significant: The women's movement has fostered cultural acceptance of women's sexuality to such an extent that women now feel comfortable asserting their sexual rights, this may cause low-desire spouses to become involved in sex therapy (LoPiccolo & Heiman, 1977).

It is beyond the scope of this chapter to provide detailed descriptions of all the etiological theories that have been proposed regarding low sexual desire. The present focus will instead be on the better-known psychological theories. It should be noted that these theories are based primarily on clinical observation (Barlow, 1986; Hawton, 1985; Schreiner-Engel & Schiavi, 1986; Stuart et al., 1986). Clinical observation and conjecture play an role in the initial formation of hypotheses (Paul, 1969). However, research at more stringent methodological levels must be conducted in order to test these conjectures. Some such research has been done on a few of the theories; this will be reviewed later in the chapter. The etiological theories discussed below should not be regarded as mutually exclusive, as all the theories emphasize the interaction of various etiological factors rather than exclusive reliance upon any one factor.

Underlying Psychopathology

Anxiety

Anxiety is the single most frequently cited factor in the development of low sexual desire. Kaplan (1979) hypothesizes that suppression of sexual desire occurs when severe anxiety is experienced during the desire phase of sexual activity. Numerous subconscious and involuntary variables cause the activation of this anxiety. These include mild sources of anxiety, such as performance anxiety; "mid-level sources of anxiety," such as fear of success and fear of pleasure; and "deep sources of anxiety," such as fears of castration or injury (pp. 87–88). According to Kaplan, although any source of anxiety may cause suppression of desire, the deep sources of anxiety are the most prevalent etiological factors in this dysfunction—which explains the relatively poor success rate in treating desire disorder patients as compared with patients having other sexual dysfunctions.

LoPiccolo and Friedman list several anxiety-provoking fears as causing low desire, such as fear of losing control over sexual urges, fear of becoming pregnant, and fear of becoming too close (and therefore vulnerable) to one's sexual partner (LoPiccolo & Friedman, 1988).

In keeping with Masters and Johnson's original conceptualization of sexual dysfunctions, Schwartz and Masters (1988) indicate that performance anxiety is largely responsible for decreased sexual desire. These authors state that ISD is often secondary to an initial sexual dysfunction rather than being the initial problem. Once a sufficient number of failure experiences have occurred, "feelings of anxiety or even fear of performance will develop in anticipation of, or during further sexual encounters," which leads to the development of low sexual desire (p. 233). Fears of poor sexual performance may also linger in response to childhood trauma (Schwartz & Masters, 1988).

Based on the results of several lines of research, Barlow (1986) suggests a model of psychogenic sexual dysfunction in which cognitive interference interacts with anxiety to cause dysfunction. Although he addresses erectile dysfunction specifically, Barlow suggests that this model may be useful for understanding the causes of other sexual dysfunctions. Barlow's model of dysfunctional individuals progresses from (1) an implicit or explicit demand for sexual performance, which leads to (2) negative affect and other cognitions, which lead to (3) an attentional focus on nonerotic issues, which leads to (4) increased autonomic arousal, which leads to (5) increased attention on nonerotic issues, which results in (6) dysfunctional performance and (7) avoidance of sexual situations (Barlow, 1986).

When discussing the etiological role of anxiety in sexual dysfunctions, authors typically refer to performance anxiety, or fears surrounding pressure to perform sexually (e.g., Barlow, 1986; Kaplan, 1979; Masters and Johnson, 1970). However, Apfelbaum (1988) focuses on a different type of anxiety when explaining the cause of low sexual desire. In a society that pressures individuals to respond positively towards sex (Vandereyeken, 1987), those who respond with negative feelings may experience anxiety, which Apfelbaum labels "response anxiety." Individuals experiencing response anxiety will subsequently repress their negative reactions towards sex and therefore remain unaware that they have these negative responses. These people (typically women) then assume that the problem is something intrinsic to themselves—for example, that they have low levels of sexual desire. Apfelbaum believes that withdrawal and self-blame are essentially the only avenues open to the person experiencing negative feelings about sex. Women are especially subject to the "performance pressure" to experience positive re-

actions to sex, as it is a woman's "role" to be supportive of and grateful for her partner's sexual acts. According to Apfelbaum, therapists perpetuate both the belief that sex must always be desired and that women must support their partners, when they attempt to "uninhibit" women in order to bring about higher levels of sexual desire.

As stated previously, there is some research on the relationship between anxiety and sexual dysfunction. For example, Barlow and colleagues (Barlow, Sakheim, & Beck, 1983; Beck, Barlow, Sakheim, & Abrahmson, 1984) have conducted research involving this relationship. They report that anxiety produced by the threat of noncontingent shock increased the level of sexual arousal in sexually nondysfunctional male subjects. However, the threat of both noncontingent and contingent shock decreased the arousal of sexually dysfunctional males (Beck et al., 1984). Thus, Barlow (1986) concludes that anxiety inhibits arousal in sexually dysfunctional males but facilitates arousal in functional males. Unfortunately, neither Barlow's model nor the research he cites indicate what factors initially cause an individual to become sexually dysfunctional. Anxiety seems to play a maintaining rather than a causal role, according to Barlow's theory.

Limited support for the theory that anxiety is a causative factor in low-desire disorders is suggested by Murphy and Sullivan (1981). These researchers report results from a comparison of "sexual aversion" subjects ($N = 20$) and normal controls ($N = 35$), all of whom were married, middle-class white women. Sexual aversion, in this case, was defined such that it described individuals with low desire. The assessment measures utilized in this study were the State-Trait Anxiety Inventory, the Social-Sexual History Questionnaire, and the Sexual Response Questionnaire. Comparison of results on these measures suggested that the low-desire women were significantly more anxious than the control subjects, both with regard to sexual functioning and in several other areas. In addition, the low-desire women had difficulty with identity and self-acceptance, experienced consistent pressure to perform sexually, and felt that communication with their partners was inadequate. Again, these results do not suggest that cause of the anxiety in the low-desire subjects. Also, as in the research of Barlow (1986), these results do not indicate whether anxiety preceded or followed the onset of low sexual desire.

Depression

Kaplan (1979) describes depression as a common cause of low desire, hypothesizing that during episodes of depression, activity diminishes in the "centers and circuits" that control sexual functioning (p. 80). Kaplan recommends that psychopharmacological therapy or psychotherapy be used to address the depression first—treating the desire disorder (if it still exists) only afterwards. This approach is reflected in the DSM-III-R and by LoPiccolo and Friedman (1988), who indicate that even mild to moderate levels of depression make treatment of low sexual desire difficult.

There is some empirical support for a relationship between depression and low desire (Mathew & Weinman, 1982; Schreiner-Engel & Schiavi, 1986). For example, Mathew and Weinman found that the incidence of desire dysfunctions was significantly greater for depressed subjects than for a control group of nondepressed subjects. However, this finding does not indicate the direction of cause and effect in this relationship. Of greater relevance to the current review is the work of Schreiner-Engel and Schiavi (1986), who examined the differences in lifetime psychopathology of low-desire subjects as compared with normal subjects. Criteria for inclusion in the ISD group ($N = 46$ couples) were reported frequency of sexual activity of less than three times per month for at least the previous six months and a corresponding absence of desire for any sexual activity. Inclusionary criteria for control subjects ($N = 36$ couples) involved a minimum reported frequency of sexual activity averaging once per week (if between the ages of 40 and 55) or twice per week (if between the ages of 25 and 40). In addition, all subjects were screened for currently active major psychopathology other than ISD and for evidence of medical disorders, drug intake, or substance abuse. Lifetime psychopathology was assessed with the Schedule for Affective Disorders and Schizophrenia, Lifetime Version (SADS-L; Endicott & Spitzer, 1978). Current psychological symptom status was assessed with the SCL-90-R (Derogatis, 1977). Past and current psychosexual functioning and premenstrual syndrome (PMS) were assessed via the Personal History Questionnaire (PHQ-C) (abstracted from the PHQ-A, Heiman, 1980). Regarding the "clinical characteristics" of the low-desire subjects, 35% of the men ($N = 22$) and 52% of the women ($N = 49$) reported that they did not masturbate at all, and 45% and 39% of the men and women (respectively) masturbated once per month or less. Most men (85%) had attempted intercourse less than twice per month during the preceding six months, whereas only 37% of the women had intercouse this infrequently. The authors reported that "most" low-desire subjects rarely fantasized, but no percentages were given. The mean length of decreased desire was 5.1 years for men (range = 1–30 years). For women, 42% reported lifelong low desire. The mean length of decreased desire for the remaining female subjects was 3.6 years (range = 2–14 years). Lastly, at least one member in all of the low-desire couples expressed concern regarding the lack of sexual desire in themselves or in their partners. In what must be considered a major defect of this study, information on the "clinical characteristics" of the control group couples was not presented, thus making comparison between groups impossible.

Regarding the SADS-L results, no subject (either dysfunctional or control) met the criteria for a current anxiety, affective, or psychotic disorder. However, significantly more ISD subjects met the criteria for lifetime history of affective disorders (71% and 73% for females and males, respectively) than did control subjects (27% and 32% for females and males, respectively). Approximately half of the male and female ISD subjects experienced episodes of intermittent and/or major depression, compared with approximately one-third of the controls. No significant differences were found between lifetime rates of personality or anxiety disorders for these two groups.

Of the acquired-ISD subjects with histories of affective disorders, loss of interest in sexual activity coincided with or followed the initial depressive episode (Schreiner-Engel & Schiavi, 1986). For those subjects who were diagnosed with lifelong ISD, mood disturbances were reported to have begun sometime during adolescence.

The SCL-90-R did not generally differentiate between the two groups, although the male ISD and control subjects differed significantly on the "depressed affect" subscale. However, the concerns of the male ISD subjects revolved around their sexual dysfunction. Lastly, the female ISD and control groups differed significantly in reported rates of PMS, with 71% of the ISD subjects reporting servere PMS, contrasted with only 20% of the non-LSD subjects.

The authors concluded that ISD individuals have an elevated lifetime prevalence of psychopathology. However, male ISD subjects did not differ significantly from male controls in overall rates of diagnoses based on the SADS-L. Only the female ISD subjects evidenced significantly "elevated" lifetime prevalence of psychopathology, and this group contained the only subjects with lifetime ISD, suggesting that it may have been skewed in the direction of more severe ISD. In fact, as noted by the authors, the stringent inclusionary criteria for the ISD subjects may have resulted in samples representing the extremes of this diagnoses. It is nonetheless interesting that ISD subjects evidenced greater lifetime rates of affective disorders. Although this does not prove that depression causes low desire (e.g., a third variable may influence both problems), it does suggest a need for continued research on this relationship.

Personality Disorders

The DSM-III-R states that personality disorders often occur along with, and possibly play an etiological role in the occurrence of, sexual dysfunctions (APA, 1987). However, in their exploratory study of the biopsychosocial characteristics of low-desire women, Stuart et al. (1987) reported results that did not support a link between low sexual desire and underlying personality variables. The subjects were married women recruited from a sex and marital therapy clinic. Case records were reviewed independently by two investigators, who achieved agreement on 90 of 92 cases. The following criteria were used, three of which had to be present for a diagnosis of ISD: lifelong history of asexuality; phobic avoidance of sex; low level of initiation or sexual receptivity; low frequency of sexual activity; consistent negative reaction to sexual activity; verbal expression of lack of interest in sex; significant decrease in libido from a past norm; engaging in sex for reasons other than desire; and partner complaint. A total of 59 women were assigned to the ISD group, 27 of whom also received additional sexual dysfunction diagnoses. Of the 59 ISD subjects, 11 were judged as having lifelong, global ISD, whereas the wother women had developed ISD sometime during their marriages. In the non-ISD group, 21 received no diagnosis, 7 received a diagnosis of orgasmic dysfunction, and 3 were diagnosed as having vaginismus. The two groups were compared on the results of radioimmunoassay blood samples; the Minnesota Multiphasic Personality Inventory (MMPI; Hathaway & McKinley, 1943); the Dyadic Adjustment Scale (DAS; Spanier, 1976); and a research questionnaire regarding history, current sexual interaction, and relationship interactions (Stuart et al., 1986). Results indicated that testosterone and prolactin levels (as measured by radioimmunoassay) and personality variables (as measured by the MMPI) were not significantly different between groups. The MMPI profiles were classified as subclinical, with most scales within the normal limits, although Scale 2 (D) and Scale 4 (PD) of the MMPI were slightly elevated for both groups. The two groups were significantly different with regard to several relationship variables. For example, on the Dyadic Adjustment Scale (Spanier, 1976), the ISD subjects scored significantly lower on all subscales—indicating lower marital consensus, satisfaction, cohesion, and affection relative to the marriages of the non-ISD subjects. Subjective ratings of relationship interactions further indicated that ISD subjects were less satisfied with conflict resolution and the quality of their spouses' listening ability, and that they felt less emotional closeness, love, and romantic feelings towards their spouses (Stuart et al., 1987). Also, the non-ISD subjects' ratings of their parents' affection and attitudes towards sex were more positive than those of ISD subjects. There were several differences in sexual functioning between these groups. (1) ISD subjects more frequently refused sexual overtures. (2) More of the ISD spouses had stopped making sexual overtures. (3) ISD women reported less subjective arousal during foreplay and intercourse. (4) ISD subjects reported less interest, enjoyment, and emotional satisfaction with sexual experiences. The most prevalent reasons for engaging in intercourse for the non-ISD group were to experience closeness and enjoyment. For the ISD group, the two most common reasons were to avoid hurting their spouses and to fulfill a sense of marital obligation.

A stepwise discriminant analysis was conducted involving all variables not used as criteria for initial group assignment (e.g., psychological characteristics of the women and demographic information). Data from 19 ISD and 12 non-ISD women were excluded due to missing information. The two variables found to be the best predictors of group membership were the extent of feelings of romantic love towards one's spouse and respondents' appraisal of their own ability to listen to their spouses. Women in the ISD group had less feelings of romantic love and were more critical of their own listening ability than the non-ISD women (Wilks lambda for both variables = 0.620, $p < 0.001$). A discriminant function was then derived utilizing canonical correlation, with results indicating a strong correlation between the two variables and group membership (canonical correlation = 0.617). The significance of the discriminating ability of the function was χ_2 (2, $N = 59$) = 26.81, $p < 0.001$. The two variables used together accurately predicted 81% and 81% of the ISD and non-ISD groups, respectively.

The authors concluded that "the majority of disorders of sexual desire bear some relationship to the quality of the marriage" and that "it may be useful to conceptualize sexual desire in interactional terms" (p. 10). These results do not support the assumption that low sexual desire is a result of underlying personality factors (Stuart et al., 1987).

Other sexual dysfunctions may also be relevant in the etiology of low sexual desire (APA, 1987; LoPiccolo & Friedman, 1988). Indirect support for this hypothesis is suggested by findings of relatively high incidence of multiple dysfunctions in low-desire subjects. For example, Stuart and colleagues (1986) reported that 45 percent of ISD subjects received additional sexual dysfunction diagnoses, although the temporal ordering of initial presentation (which came first) is unknown. Multiple diagnoses have also been reported in women who experienced previous sexual assault (Becker et al., 1982). In these cases, it is unknown which dysfunctions appeared first and whether desire disorders would have occurred in response to the trauma regardless of the presence of other dysfunctions.

Sexual Dysfunction and Assault

Sexual assault has also been hypothesized as a cause of decrease in or loss of sexual desire in women (Becker, Skinner, Abel, & Chicon, 1986; Becker et al., 1982; LoPiccolo & Friedman, 1988). In a survey of 83 women who had been either sexually molested by a relative as children or raped as adults, over half were determined to suffer from a sexual dysfunction (Becker et al., 1982). Most of these women (71%) reported that the sexual dysfunction occurred after the sexual assault. Sexual desire dysfunction was indicated in 53% of the cases. In a more extensive survey of 372 female survivors of rape and incest, Becker and colleagues (1986) found similar results. Specifically, 59% of the survivors were determined to suffer from sexual dysfunctions. In a control group of women who had not been assaulted ($N = 99$), only 17% reported experiencing sexual dysfunctions. Of the subjects who experienced assault-related sexual dysfunctions, 66% were diagnosed as having more than one dysfunction.

Interpersonal and Systems Factors

Scharff (1988) employs object relations theory to describe how early family experiences and later adult relationships may influence sexual desire. According to Scharff, children start out with undifferentiated egos, into which all experiences with primary caretakers are internalized. With developing awareness, negative aspects of experiences are separated and repressed. Experiences in which a desire or need is unmet are internalized into the libidinal, or need-exciting, ego and object system. Experiences in which rejection is perceived are internalized into the antilibidinal, or rejecting, ego and object system. When initial relationships with primary caretakers become sexualized during childhood, these experiences are internalized into the libidinal system (as they cannot be fulfilled), and this represents the initial development of sexual desire. Problems may occur if the initial desired object (e.g., the mother) is also perceived as rejecting. In these cases, the antilibidinal system acts to repress the need-exciting system as a defense against the painful feelings of rejection that have been associated with the initial feelings of desire. This is an interesting hypothesis, but empirical support is lacking and would be difficult to obtain due to the theory's focus on the individual's initial experiences and the use of constructs not amenable to measurement (libidinal and antilibidinal ego and object systems).

Bagarozzi (1987) proposes a systems-based theory regarding the development of low sexual desire in one partner of a couple. He begins by presenting Lewis's (1972; cited in Bagarozzi, 1987) development model of processes through which premarital dyads progress. These include the processes of (1) perceiving similarities; (2) achieving pair rapport; (3) inducing mutual self-disclosure; (4) role taking; (5) achieving interpersonal role fit; and (6) achieving dyadic crystallization.

Based on his clinical experience, Bagarozzi believes that couples in which one member has low sexual desire have often married without resolving one or more of the last three stages. For example, if the fourth stage (role taking) is not resolved, and one partner is dissatisfied because there are discrepancies between his or her ideal spouse and the actual spouse, that partner may use punishment in an attempt to make his or her spouse more "ideal." The spouse receiving the punishers may feel resentment and retaliate, which may lead the dissatisfied spouse to experience a decrease in sexual desire for the retaliating spouse. Or, regarding the fifth stage, Bagarozzi states that changes in sexual behavior may occur after marriage if the couple did not previously establish mutual roles. Bagarozzi gives an example in which premarital sexual exchanges are used by one individual (Bagarozzi implies that this would be the woman) to "win over" the other. Subsequent to marriage, the manipulative spouse no longer needs to pretend more sexual desire than she naturally experiences (p. 282), and her spouse perceives what he takes to be a decrease in her desire. Lastly, if dyadic crystallization (the sixth stage) has not been achieved prior to marriage, lack of true intimacy may cause sexual activities to be perceived as "hollow" after a period of time, which may cause a decrease in desire (p. 282). Bagarozzi indicates that the effects on sexual desire of the meanings and rules governing the expression of sexual acts may be unconscious and have "symbolic significance." Although these are interesting conjectures, there is a no empirical research with which to evaluate Bagarozzi's hypotheses, and the concepts lack clarity.

Verhulst & Heiman (1988) present a systemic model for explaining low sexual desire, focusing on the "sexual rhythms" of two partners (p. 244). Each individual is believed to have a sexual rhythm that reflects the interaction of his or her physiological arousal, emotional desire, and cognitive sexual scripts. To the extent that one or more of these factors is out of synchrony with the others, an individual may perceive an absence of sexual feelings. For example, if an individual's cognitive sexual script says that he or she should feel desire more often than is physiologically perceived, then that person may complain of low sexual desire.

For couples to maintain sexual rhythm, they must coordinate their individual rhythms along the levels of "symbolic interactions," "affect-regulated interactions," and "sensate exchanges." Low desire may result when an "interactional fit" does not occur at one or more of these levels. For example, the term *symbolic interactions* refers to views and beliefs regarding how the world operates. To the extent that partners' heritage, language, or background differ, sexual views and beliefs may also differ, leading to perceived discrepancies in desire.

Affect regulation refers to the concept that emotional states govern interactional patterns. For example, desire expressed by one partner may evoke desire in the other partner, but if nonsexual emotions are evoked by a display of desire, then desire discrepancies may occur. Nonsexual emotions highlighted by Verhulst and Heiman include attachment, exploratory, territorial, and ranking-order interactions. When discrepancies occur between partners' perceptions of territorial or ranking-order interactions, a decrease in desire may be used by one partner to make that interaction more acceptable. For example, a lower-ranked partner may use low desire as a way to gain power in the relationship. Thus, low desire may be used to maintain or reestablish boundaries in these interactions.

Sensate exchange refers to the physiological responses and reflexes elicited by partners. Low desire may occur when these are not synchronized (e.g., when intercourse causes pain for one member and pleasure for the other) or when responses occur in the same pattern but at different times for each partner (e.g., when one partner requires a longer period of stimulation than the other). Generally, however, mere sensate disequilibrium does not account for perceptions of significant low desire. Rather, low sexual desire results from a combination of poor interactional fit at various levels.

Cognitive Factors

Rosen and Leiblum (1988) describe sexual scripts as "the cognitive framework that guides the planning, coordination, and expression of

social conduct generally, including sexual behavior" (p. 169). Sexual scripts develop over time, with childhood scripts involving primary sexual information (e.g., expectations regarding sex-role conduct, intimacy, dependency, etc.). These scripts are modified with the acquisition of knowledge and, eventually, adult themes. However, even at the adult level, scripts are frequently modified, as when a couple goes from living in an unmarried to a married state. When individuals are able to accommodate necessary modifications adequately, sexual desire may not be significantly disrupted. However, when couples or individuals find it difficult to accommodate modifications, desire may be lost. Couples who lack adequate communication skills may find script modification too frustrating to be worthwhile. Or individuals with severe medical disorders may lack appropriate models to help them develop new scripts, so sex may be forgone and desire lost.

In addition to providing theories about the etiology of low sexual desire, sexual scripting theory also accounts for differences in levels of sexual desire between women and men (Rosen & Leiblum, 1988). Socially, women's sexual scripts are powerfully influenced by the themes of monogamy and passivity, whereas men's scripts are influenced by expectations of high desire and initiation of sexual acts. There seems little doubt that sociocultural influences influence the expression of sexual desire. Thus, the script approach possesses face validity, although more formal research has not been conducted on Rosen and Leiblum's hypotheses.

Conditioning Factors

There are several conditioning mechanisms that may account for a decrease in sexual desire. First, an individual's sexual arousal may habituate to his or her partner, with a resultant decrease in sexual desire. There is laboratory evidence that sexual arousal habituates to repeated presentations of the same stimulus in males (O'Donohue & Geer, 1985) and in females (Meuwissen & Over, 1990). Moreover, O'Donohue and Plaud (1991) presented data with males indicating that habituation may have long-term effects. In habituation trials held once a week for three weeks, subjects over time began to show less spontaneous remission and began to habituate more quickly. This appears to be the human equivalent of the oft-cited "Coolidge effect," where desire does not decrease in response to a variety of individuals but may decrease with respect to a single individual. Thus, habituation may be a mechanism in the etiology of hypoactive sexual desire, especially in cases of a situational disorder, where the stimulus situation (by definition) is relatively constant. O'Donohue and Plaud cite a possible example of this. In his journal, Richard Burton initially described Elizabeth Taylor as "a wildly exciting lover-mistress. . . . She is beautiful beyond the dreams of pornography. . . . She is an eternal one-night stand." However, a much later journal entry called her "as exiting as a flounder. . . . E.T. beginning to bore, which I would not have thought possible all those years ago."

Another possible mechanism in the etiology of hypoactive sexual desire is operant conditioning, where sexual responding is an operant whose low frequency is due to earlier punishment or extinction experiences. Extinction may occur when the partner's stimulus characteristics become less reinforcing—perhaps due to progressively poorer grooming, weight gain, or aging. Such changes in the attractiveness of individuals are frequently cited by dissatisfied partners as factors causing loss of desire (Kaplan, 1979; LoPiccolo & Friedman, 1988). Note that sexual reinforcement is probably on a continuous schedule, which would seem to be particularly susceptible to extinction. Moreover, extinction may occur when the proprioceptive stimulation from sexual interaction becomes less reinforcing, due perhaps to being out of shape. Finally, previous problems with sexual functioning (such as incidences of arousal problems) may function as punishment trials and therefore function to decrease sexual interest.

The association of certain unsavory stimuli (e.g., poor hygiene) with one's sexual partner may lead through classical conditioning to the experience of lower desire for that partner. Classical conditioning has been found to be a mechanism for changing the strength of desire, although the goals have usually been to increase adult heterosexual desire while decreasing paraphilic desire (Rachman, 1966).

Thus, conditioning processes may provide mechanisms that can produce inhibited sexual desire. However, it should be noted that there is no direct empirical research showing such an etiological pathway. Moreover, these mechanisms seem to be much more useful in accounting for situational desire problems, although large generalization gradients could account for less circumscribed problems.

In summary, it appears that several factors contribute to the etiology of low sexual desire. These factors may operate individually or in combination with other factors. As noted by Friedman and Hogan (1985), different patterns of low desire will emerge, depending on the complex interaction of etiological variables. Assessment of sexual desire must address several areas of functioning if treatment is to address all the variables that may be maintaining the low desire (Friedman & Hogan, 1985). Thus, most authors advocate some form of multistage protocol for the assessment of sexual desire (Friedman & Hogan, 1985; Kaplan, 1983; Lazarus, 1988).

ASSESSMENT

Currently, there is no standard protocol for assessing sexual desire. Differences in definitions of low desire, in the decision whether to focus on individuals or couples, and in the clinician's theoretical paradigm all make the development of a standard assessment protocol difficult. Nonetheless, there is considerable overlap of elements in each of the published protocols reviewed below. There is also overlap in the instruments used by different clinicians and researchers to gather specific assessment data; the properties of several of these instruments are also reviewed. Neither the review of protocols nor the review of assessment devices is exhaustive. Rather, the goal of the following two sections is to impart a general understanding of current assessment practices in the area of sexual desire.

Review of Assessment Protocols

Kaplan (1983) describes the use of semistructured clinical interviewing as the primary method for gathering information regarding sexual dysfunctions. Her determination of the type of material to request, and how to gather it in a sensitive yet thorough manner, was based on 12 years of experience as a sex therapist (Kaplan, 1983). Kaplan's protocol has seven primary components: (1) assessment of the chief complaint, (2) a sexual status exam, (3) assessment of medical status, (4) assessment of psychiatric status, (5) family and psychosexual history, (6) evaluation of the current relationship, (7) summation and recommendations.

In the assessment of the chief complaint, the goal is to elicit a detailed description of the relevant symptoms, onset, and progress of the sexual dysfunction. The sexual status exam is then used to verify and/or correct the diagnostic impression formed from the investigation of the chief complaint. Kaplan compares this portion of the assessment to the functional analysis of behavioral psychologists, but she maintains that it goes beyond an analysis of behavior to include information related to subconscious emotional conflict and other areas not usually assessed by the behaviorist. Regarding the assessment of medical status, Kaplan indicates that some clients may not need a full evaluation. When assessing clients with clearly situational disorders, such as ISD, a brief review of their health history may be all that is necessary to rule out organic etiology. However, clients who appear to have global low desire should be given a thorough medical examination, including analysis of serum testosterone for males and serum prolactin and other hormones for females. Similarly, assessment of a clients' psychiatric status may be relatively brief, depending on the therapist's impression of the client after having conducted the first parts of the clinical interview. A family history and psychosexual history are conducted in order to gather information about deeper psychological causes and their origins. Evaluation of the current relationship aims to determine whether deeper difficulties exist and what part these may play in the maintenance and etiology of the sexual problem. The last phase of assessment takes the form of a meeting between the therapist and the couple. At this meeting, a summary of the therapist's diagnostic impressions is given, along with recommendations regarding treatment. The therapist also explains to the couple what will happen during sex therapy.

Hawton (1985) describes a general assessment procedure for the sexual dysfunctions, the goals of which are to identify the problem, develop hypotheses regarding etiology, and initiate the therapeutic alliance. Hawton focuses on couples, who are initially assessed in terms of their suitability for sex therapy. For clients for whom sex therapy has been determined to be appropriate, couple and individual clinical interviews are held. The following questions are addressed—specific to the assessment of impaired sexual interest. (1) Is the loss of interest complete or more sporadic? (2) Is it only partner-related, or is loss of interest total? (3) Are there other symptoms? (4) Has the problem accompanied other relationship changes? Other areas of inquiry include family background and early childhood; early sexual development and experiences; sexual information and assessment of sexual knowledge; quality of the current relationship; sexual and general relationships; schooling and occupation, interests, religious beliefs; medical, drug, and psychiatric histories; appearance and mood; and goals and motivation.

Rosen & Leiblum (1988) suggest an approach focusing on interpersonal and systemic factors and assessing biological, cognitive, and motivational aspects of sexual desire. They recommend routine assessment of the following areas: (1) the reaction of the nondysfunctional partner to the low desire, (2) the psychiatric history of the low-desire partner, (3) any past sexual abuse, trauma, or physical disorder, and (4) any conflict in sexual or gender orientation. In addition, distinctions should be made between global and situational low desire and low desire secondary to sexual performance problems. In their script approach, Rosen and Leiblum (1989) indicate that it is important to assess what a person's ideal script would be and to check for discrepancies between overt and covert scripts. Both types of scripts should be analyzed in terms of complexity, rigidity, and conventionality. The individuals' satisfaction and comfort level with their covert and overt scripts should be determined. The covert scripts of both partners should be compared. According to these authors, the advantages of using a scripting approach are that it (1) gets away from merely looking at sexual frequency, (2) focuses on discrepancies between partners, thus lessening any blame or the tendency to pathologize the partner who has lower desire, and (3) highlights the importance of understanding the interpersonal context of sexual choices and conduct and reduces any tendency to make value judgments regarding what is "normal" or expected sexual desire.

LoPiccolo and Friedman (1988) recommend beginning a sexual dysfunction assessment with a series of standardized self-report inventories. These help in determining the couple's suitability for sex therapy and provide an avenue for prospective clients to address sensitive issues which is less intense than face-to-face interviewing and which may decrease the influence of social pressures to report that desire is not a problem. LoPiccolo and Friedman use the following devices:

1. The Sex History Form (Nowinski & LoPiccolo, 1979)
2. The Locke-Wallace Marriage Inventory (Kimmel & van der Veen, 1974)
3. The Sexual Interaction Inventory (LoPiccolo & Steger, 1974)
4. The Brief Symptom Inventory (Derogatis, Lipman, & Covi, 1973)
5. The Zung Depression Scale (Zung, 1973)

In addition, medical and health histories are assessed, and a statement of goals for treatment is requested from all clients.

The second phase of LoPiccolo and Friedman's assessment is the initial intake interview. During the first hour the couple is interviewed together, and data are gathered from both individuals regarding development with the family of origin and the current sexual relationship, including nonsexual stressors. The clinician then interviews each partner separately for 15–20 minutes and asks more general, open-ended questions about the current sexual relationship, specific sexual functioning, fantasizing, erotic activities, and the clients' perceptions of their spouses. Each individual is also asked what he or she believes is causing the low sexual desire.

During the last 30 minutes of the intake session, the couple is brought back together and presented with an initial formulation of the problem, the issues that may be explored in treatment, and the question of whether or not sex therapy is the treatment of choice. Sex therapy is deferred if any of the following are present: depression or other severe psychopathology, alcohol or drug abuse, spouse abuse, active extramarital affairs, or severe marital distress with imminent separation or divorce. Presumably, these factors would interfere either with the development of desire or with the motivation to work on sexual issues with the partner (although there is very little data which supports this hypothesis). If the couple is accepted for sex therapy, the low-desire patient is required to undergo a medical evaluation.

The final stage of assessment consists of taking a detailed sex history from each member during individual interviews. The goal of these interviews is to gather information about the onset and history of the desire problems, any situational factors that affect the maintenance of the problem, and possible ways in which the emotional relationship between the couple interacts with their desire problem.

Review of Assessment Devices

Currently, there are few assessment devices that specifically measure sexual desire. Several measures do assess various aspects of sexual functioning, but even those that aspire to be "omnibus" tests of sexual functioning (Derogatis, 1980, p. 117) fail to address desire adequately. For example, the Derogatis Sexual Functioning Inventory (DSFI; Derogatis & Melisaratos, 1979) assesses ten domains related to sexual functioning. Sexual drive (or "libidinal erotic impulses") is one of these domains the one that appears to represent sexual desire (p. 119). However, sexual drive is measured by frequency of explicit sexual behaviors, which is a poor indicant of actual desire, for many reasons. For example, at least one study failed to find significant differences in frequency of sexual intercourse for married women who did or did not have a diagnosis of ISD (Stuart et al., 1987). Thus, the DSFI provides a less than thorough assessment of sexual desire.

The Golombok Rust Inventory of Sexual Satisfaction (GRISS; Rust & Golombok, 1986) was developed to be a short measure of sexual dysfunction in heterosexual couples or individuals currently in a heterosexual relationship. The GRISS contains 56 items (28 for women and 28 for men). It provides an overall measure on quality of sexual functioning for individuals of either sex, as well as 12 other subscale scores. Two subscales—male and female nonsensuality—appear to correspond with drive. However, these scales were not specifically designated as measures of sexual desire, and both test-retest and internal consistency reliability scores were low for both scales ($r = 0.57$ and $r = 0.61$ for test-retest). In addition, the male nonsensuality scale did not differentiate between clinical ($N = 15$) and nonclinical ($N = 29$) samples in a validation study. The female nonsensuality scale differentiated between a clinical sample ($N = 26$) and a nonclinical sample ($N = 30$) at an 0.005 level of significance. As neither scale was shown to have adequate reliability, validity findings must be viewed with caution.

The last measure to be reviewed is the Sexual Interaction Inventory (SII; LoPiccolo & Steger, 1974), which was developed to remedy the lack of measures of actual sexual functioning and satisfaction. It involves a series of 17 sexual activities, arranged from kissing, to manual and oral genital stimulation, to intercourse. The client is asked six questions regarding each of the activities as it pertains to the current relationship. (1) How often does the activity occur in the current relationship, and how often would the respondent like it to occur? (2) How pleasant does the repondent find the activity, and how pleasant does he or she believe the spouse finds it? (3) How pleasant *would* the respondent like to find the activity, and how pleasant would he or she like the spouse to find it? The client uses a six-point rating scale to answer each question (1 = never or extremely unpleasant; 6 = always or extremely pleasant). Several scales are then derived by summing the responses to subsets of the 17 activities. Scales are labeled "frequency satisfaction—male," "self-acceptance—male," "pleasure mean—male," "perceptual accuracy—male of female," "mate acceptance—male of female," plus similar scales for females, and a "total disagreement" scale.

As with the other measures reviewed, the SII does not specifically target sexual desire. However, the authors indicate that low sexual desire may be indicated by a number of response patterns. For example, low desire in an individual's partner may be indicated by high frequency satisfaction and mate acceptance scores, whereas high pleasure scores may indicate loss of sexual interest in the respondent (Nowinski & LoPiccolo, 1979). Specific data on the relationship between response patterns and low sexual desire were based on clinical judgment. Thus, it is not known to what extent the SII may be validly employed to gather information on sexual desire. The SII does appear to have adequate test-retest reliability, with Pearson product-moment correlations for each scale significant to at least the 0.05 level, based on a sample size of 15 married, nondysfunctional couples. Absolute correlations ranged from 0.533 to 0.902. Internal consistency, based on 78 married couples' scores, resulted in coefficients from 0.795 to 0.933. Convergent validity was measured by comparing each scale score with self-reports of sexual satisfaction from 15 couples. All correlations were in the predicted direction, with 9 of 11 correlations significant at the 0.05 level or better, although absolute magnitudes of most correlations were quite low (the range was 0.004 to 0.350). The latter finding indicated that the single "sexual satisfaction score" obtained for couples bore little relationship to the more specific scale scores of the SII (LoPiccolo & Steger, 1974). Discriminant validity was assessed by comparing a sexually dysfunctional group's scores ($N = 28$) with the scores of 63 nondysfunctional couples. Nine of the eleven scales discriminated between the two groups. Those that did not were "mate acceptance—male of female" and "perceptual accuracy—female." Lastly, reactivity to treatment was assessed by comparing the posttherapy results of the dysfunctional couples who completed the 15-session sex therapy program ($N = 16$) with their pretherapy scores. All 11 scales were significantly different across time at the 0.05 level.

Criticisms of these results, noted by the authors, include bias in and small sizes of the samples and the fact that there is some item overlap between scales, which may have inflated the statistical results (LoPiccolo & Steger, 1982). Furthermore, the authors do not address the poor convergent validity results. The SII appears relatively easy to administer and score, although it measures a rather circumscribed set of sexual activities. What's more, these activities are addressed only for opposite-sexed partners, and sexual desire is not directly addressed.

Additional Research

Research on specific prognostic factors regarding treatment outcomes for low-desire individuals and couples may shed light on what factors should be assessed prior to treatment. For example, it has been reported that low-desire individuals fantasize less than do normal individuals and individuals with other sexual dysfunctions (Nutter & Condron, 1983; 1985). Thus, assessment of sexual fantasies may be relevant in diagnostic formulations. Hawton and Catalan (1986) reviewed several possible prognostic factors in sex therapy. Their study included 154

couples who presented at a sex therapy clinic. The mean age for these subjects was 33 years (sd = .94). In 57 couples, the female partner was determined to suffer primarily from "impaired sexual interest," and this occurred only twice with the male partners. Several different therapists ($N = 62$) conducted the assessments and provided treatment based on that described by Masters and Johnson (1970). After the initial interviews, therapists completed a standard form addressing several topics (e.g., demographic factors, presenting sexual problem, sex history, and general relationship with partner). After the third treatment session, therapists were to rate on a five-point scale each couple's progress, as determined by completion of homework assignments. Therapists also rated change in presenting problem for each couple at termination. This rating was a simple five-point scale, ranging from 1 (resolved) to 5 (worse).

All subjects completed two questionnaires twice: after the initial intake and at the end of treatment. These were a relationship questionnaire (Mathews, Whitehead, & Kellet, 1983) and the Pleasant and Unpleasant Feelings Questionnaire (Carney, Bancroft, & Mathews, 1978).

Results indicated that failure to complete therapy (27% of the couples dropped out) was associated with lower social class, lower motivation of the male partner, poorer general relationships (as rated by the therapist), and poorer progress by the third session (as determined by noncompliance with homework assignments). In addition, positive treatment outcome was associated with the following factors: higher ratings of couples' overall sexual and general relationships (both based on a five-point scale), higher ratings by females of the general relationship, therapists' pretreatment assessment of adequate motivation (especially specially the males' motivation), and adequate early progress in treatment (as assessed by homework compliance by the third session).

Although the results were generally not broken down by type of dysfunction, the authors did comment that a thorough assessment of a couple's overall relationship is particularly relevant for couples where the female appears to have impaired sexual interest. Therapists' ratings of the general relationship of these couples were lower than ratings for other couples ($F(1,152) = 9.32$; $P < 0.01$), and this group achieved only moderate success in therapy as compared with groups of subjects who had other dysfunctions. Interestingly, factors that did not affect treatment outcome (although they are often assumed to) included an orthodox religious background, history of incest, presence of psychiatric symptoms or a history of psychiatric illness, and history of an extramarital affair (Hawton & Catalan, 1986).

The assessment protocols reviewed above have many similarities, although different authors rely on different assessment procedures. For example, Kaplan (1983) relies almost exclusively on clinical interviewing and medical examination, whereas LoPiccolo and Friedman (1988) recommend the use of various questionnaires in addition to the clinical interview. Areas that are common to most protocols include assessment of medical and psychiatric history, current relationship, sexual development, and a focus on client couples rather than individual clients. Given our incomplete understanding of human sexual desire, it seems advisable to collect information in each of these areas. Questionnaires and inventories may be useful for initial screening of clients and for gathering responses to standard questions. Medical and psychiatric assessment may be limited to brief reviews of clients' histories, with particular attention to factors associated with changes in sexual desire. Clinical interviews with both members of the couple may facilitate cooperation and the development of a positive therapeutic alliance, as well as allowing the therapist to pursue areas of relevance in more detail than is feasible with questionnaires. Regarding future research, it is recommended that efforts be expended toward the development of a questionnaire that specifically targets sexual desire.

TREATMENT

Treatment protocols for low desire are as numerous and varied as the etiological theories that have been offered for this disorder. Thus, Kaplan's (1979) treatment focuses on underly-

ing sources of anxiety; Rosen and Leiblum's (1989) focuses on script discrepancies; and LoPiccolo and Friedman (1988) propose a more eclectic, "broad-based" therapy package (1988). As was the case with the assessment protocols, common elements run throughout most therapies for low desire or desire discrepancy. In particular, nearly all treatment protocols include the traditional sensate-focus techniques originally described by Masters and Johnson (1970) and Semans (1956). In the following section a brief review of some published therapy protocols is given, followed by a review of relevant outcome literature.

Review of Treatment Protocols

In explaining her treatment protocol, Kaplan (1979) states that both traditional insight therapy and brief sex therapy have proved disappointing for low-desire dysfunction. The insight therapies often overlook the immediate antecedents, whereas brief sex therapy often overlooks deeper conflicts (Kaplan, 1979). Thus, Kaplan recommends a combination of features from both types of therapy in order to "modify the patient's tendency to inhibit his erotic impulses, and to allow these feelings to emerge naturally and without effort as they will in the healthy, conflict-free person" (p. 103). Initially, patients and their partners are usually assigned sensate focus or pleasuring exercises (patterned after Masters & Johnson, 1970). Some patients require only this amount of intervention. However, it is more likely that "resistances" will arise, usually during the first and second sensate-focusing sessions. Resistance at any point provides a therapeutic crisis and the condition for confronting the patient with the existence of his or her sexual block—the involuntary suppression of erotic feelings—and his or her tendency to focus on angry or frightening thoughts during sexual interactions. Ideally, the patient comes to recognize that desire is not lost, but that he or she has chosen not to feel desire. As a result of this mini-crisis and subsequent insight, some patients will respond favorably by "choosing" to not be sexually inhibited any longer. Again, however, further insight is frequently required. This may be fostered by confronting the patient with the consequences of his or her inhibition (e.g., the possibility of divorce). If this does not work, extra treatment sessions may be necessary.

If the underlying conflicts are at "mid-level" consciousness (e.g., fear of success), about 20–30 sessions will allow enough time to foster the necessary insight to overcome inhibitions. If they are on a deeper level, additional therapy is needed. Kaplan emphasizes that therapy must remain flexible so that relevant intrapsychic conflicts of either the patient or the partner can be explored. Flexibility must also be allowed within the experiential aspects of therapy. For example, self-stimulation may be encouraged when a patient cannot respond to a partner, or external erotic stimuli may be employed if the pleasuring techniques do not evoke desire.

Knopf and Seiler (1990) published a self-help book for couples in which one partner has ISD. They present a general overview of ISD and then discuss a home-based treatment plan for couples, which appears to be based primarily on Kaplan's (1979) theories of ISD. Treatment is a combination of marital therapy, cognitive therapy, sexual enhancement exercises (both individual and for couples), and sexual assertiveness activities. The authors suggest that couples seek professional counseling if they do not see improvement within two months.

Knopf and Seiler have presented a novel approach to the treatment of low sexual desire and desire discrepancies. However, their book is relatively long and seems to be geared for college graduates. Furthermore, several of the exercises are complex; it would require a good deal of motivation to follow through with these. For example, in one exercise each partner makes three lists of sexual activities—indicating what he or she would like to try soon, later, and never. These lists are then exchanged, and the partners negotiate over which activities belong on which list. During "sexual caring days" one partner makes a request from his or her lists and the other either agrees to this sexual activity or chooses a different one from the same list. Then each partner discusses how much effort each is

willing to put into this activity, on a scale of 1 to 10. If the combined score is greater than or equal to 10, the activity is carried out; if not, renegotiation occurs. Obviously, a great deal of planning must go into this particular part of the program, and it seems unlikely that many couples would be able to get through it without some formal guidance.

Hawton (1985) recommends that the therapist begin with a formulation of the problem, including a problem description and an account of factors that may have caused the problem. This is to provide clients with further understanding of their difficulties, encourage a sense of optimism, provide a rational basis for treatment, and allow the therapist to check the information obtained from the assessment. These formulations should also include the positive aspects of the relationship. The second part of treatment involves teaching clients the behavioral components of sensate-focus techniques derived from Masters and Johnson (1970) and Kaplan (1979). The purposes of these homework assignments are to provide a structured approach that allows the couple to rebuild their sexual relationship gradually, to help a couple and their therapist identify the specific factors that are maintaining the sexual dysfunctions, and to provide the couple with specific techniques to deal with particular sexual problems. Hawton recommends that a review session be held around the third treatment session, in order to monitor treatment compliance.

Hawton notes that sexual problems, especially low desire, are often related to general relationship problems, which become apparent during treatment. For low-desire couples, Hawton suggests that therapy focus primarily on reestablishing a satisfactory sexual relationship via the sensate focus program and resolving general relationship issues. Regarding the latter goal, Hawton makes the following suggestions:

1. A simple rationale for exploring relationship issues should be given once it becomes apparent that this is necessary.
2. Assessment must be completed to determine whether the relationship problems can be

treated quickly, while the couple continues their sex therapy, or whether they require more intensive marital therapy.

In particular, the therapist should get answers the following questions:

1. What are their complaints?
2. What behaviors does each want the other to change?
3. Under what circumstances does this need to occur?
4. What will be the consequences of such changes for each partner?

Once target behaviors and goals are identified, Hawton recommends using various well-known strategies to ensure that changes actually occur, such as detailed monitoring of progress, specific suggestions when difficulties are encountered, and contracting.

Rosen and Leiblum (1989) recommend that therapy focus on helping the couple to develop compatible sexual scripts. However, they also concur with Kaplan (1979) and others that more in-depth individual treatment may be required to explore early childhood experiences and memories. These authors also endorse the approaches recommended by several other professionals (LoPiccolo & Friedman, Schwartz & Masters, and Verhulst & Heiman) as being occasionally useful. In defense of their therapeutic flexibility, Rosen and Leiblum state that "the line between sex therapy and psychotherapy has become increasingly arbitrary and potentially irrelevant" (p. 30). Unfortunately, the lack of standardization of their treatment protocol would appear to make process and outcome research difficult to conduct, although these authors recognize the necessity of such studies.

Friedman and Hogan (1985) and LoPiccolo and Friedman (1988) discuss the treatment protocol developed at a sex therapy and research clinic at the State University of New York at Stony Brook. Friedman and colleagues note that direct behavioral techniques such as those based on the initial work of Wolpe (1958) and Semans (1956) and popularized by Masters and

Johnson (1970) have not achieved good success in clients who present with sexual desire dysfunction (Friedman & Hogan, 1985). They concur with Kaplan (1979) that desire problems often stem from profound sexual and marital conflict. Thus, therapy in each case must be tailored to the individual's or couple's needs. The treatment of these clients, according to Friedman and Hogan, requires highly trained therapists who have an "eclectic mental set." Additional assumptions include the following. (1) Clients are frequently unaware of the affective responses to sexual stimuli. (2) It is useful for clients to have an understanding of why they experience low desire. (3) There is as yet no evidence that ISD and aversion to sex are qualitatively different, so the treatment concept remains the same for both. (4) Both partners should be involved in treatment. (5) Masters and Johnson's graded series of sexual tasks remains a useful treatment component.

These authors recommend a "broad-spectrum approach" that combines aspects of several different theoretical paradigms (e.g., Gestaltism, behaviorism) (Friedman & Hogan, 1985; LoPiccolo & Friedman, 1988). Four overlapping elements are combined into a brief 15–25-week treatment plan, with emphasis on generalization and maintenance of treatment gains. The four elements are experiential/sensory awareness, insight, cognitive restructuring, and behavior therapy. Sensory awareness is used to help patients become aware of their unacknowledged affective responses to sexual stimuli. Body awareness exercises are used, with the goal that patients recognize early feelings associated with bodily responses and identify and label those feelings.

Insight training may begin concurrently with sensory awareness, or—if the patient resists the experiential exercises—insight may be introduced first. Here, the therapist helps the patient to learn and understand what is causing and maintaining low desire. This helps patients understand and take responsibility for their own behavior and recognize that change is possible.

Cognitive restructuring is used to identify and alter irrational thoughts that inhibit desire. Patients are taught that these self-statements may cause emotional reactions that are unconducive to sexual functioning. The client and therapist then create coping statements that allow the patient to deal actively with negative emotions surrounding sexual situations, as opposed to avoiding these emotional reactions and situations. To help the patient understand how emotions can control cognitions and behaviors, a "modified transactional analysis framework" is introduced. The client imagines having two tapes, a child tape (frightened child on side A of the tape and a playful child on side B) and a parent tape (with judgmental and nurturing sides). It is hypothesized that adults process input from the environment and from all four sides of the tapes to produce rational decisions. The patient is taught to label feelings, thoughts, and behaviors as coming from one of the four imaginary characters; ideally, this increases awareness of negative responses. "Permission" is then given for "the playful child" to be active in sexual situations, in order to reduce further the anxiety felt by the patient in these situations.

Behavioral assignments are used throughout therapy, including the procedures of Masters and Johnson (1970) and other sexual and nonsexual procedures. Behavioral elements are used to enhance the other three components. Behavioral assignments are used to evoke feelings during experiential exercises and to help patients change nonsexual behaviors that may cause or maintain the sexual dysfunction. Assertiveness training, communication training, and skill training in negotiation are some of the techniques used for these purposes. Skill training is used to prepare patients for sexual situations in which they may have had recent practice.

Schwartz and Masters (1988) discuss the "short-term, rapid-treatment approach" of sex therapy as it relates to desire disorders. As this treatment protocol is well known, only those aspects relating specifically to the treatment of low sexual desire will be reviewed here (see Masters and Johnson, 1970 for a complete account of their therapy). According to these authors, even the more complex issues that are

thought to lead to desire disorders may be addressed within the traditional short-term treatment developed by Masters and Johnson. Schwartz and Masters state that isolating a couple for 14 days and conducting daily therapy sessions will usually provide enough opportunities for the manifestation of deep-seated roadblocks of sexual desire in the lower-desire partner. The daily sessions presumably motivate the couple, since they are able to see rapid changes in their sexual functioning, so that a "positive spiral" is initiated. That is, increased self-efficacy leads to more affectionate feelings, which in turn lead to motivation for further positive behavioral change. In addition, low-level affection and alternatives to intercourse are introduced as ways in which spouses can modify their desire discrepancies.

Therapists must also help the partner accept the adjustment in the desire of his or her spouse and must facilitate the exchange of affection between the two partners. If the couple's exchanges are counterproductive to desire, the therapist redirects them to their goals by (1) confronting the transaction, (2) pointing out the potentially destructive consequences, (3) offering skills to improve the couple's interactions, and (4) offering suggestions on ways and means to practice new skills (p. 239). Also, spouses are taught to recognize negative emotional states and to use these as signals for creative action to support the relationship outside of therapy. Thus, each partner is taught to take some responsibility for the relationship, which refocuses them from blaming each other. It is the concept of taking responsibility for happiness that is most relevant to increasing desire, according to Schwartz and Masters. Clients are shown that sexual functioning is under the voluntary control of the individuals.

Review of Therapy Outcome Research

Paul (1969) discusses the importance of therapy outcome research and presents suggestions for conducting adequate outcome studies. The goal of this type of research is to answer the following "ultimate question" (p. 44): "What treatment, by whom, is most effective for this individual with this specific problem, under which set of circumstances, and how does it come about?" Of course, it would be difficult if not impossible for a single study to answer each part of this question. According to Paul, the independent variable most important in the early stages of research is the treatment variable. There is also need for research that systematically varies therapists and client characteristics (LoPiccolo & Stock, 1986; Paul, 1969), but foremost is the establishment of effective treatment techniques for low sexual desire. Fortunately, there is a relatively strong research emphasis within the field of sexual dysfunctions, and research has been conducted in an attempt to determine the cause-and-effect relationship between treatment and change in sexual desire.

Hawton and Catalan (1986) reported on the outcome of 154 couples treated by 62 therapists with traditional methods of sex therapy (i..e., derived from Masters and Johnson, 1970). Couples were seen by a single therapist on a weekly basis for an average of 14 sessions (with a range of 5–37 sessions). At the end of treatment, therapists rated each couple's sexual dysfunction as "resolved," "largely resolved," "some improvement but problems largely unresolved," "no change," or "worse" (p. 380). Based on these ratings, therapy outcome for 56% of the female subjects with impaired sexual interest ($N = 57$) was considered at least reasonably successful. A further 19% of these clients experienced some improvement, while 25% were determined to have experienced no change in sexual desire. Of the two males with impaired sexual interest, one experienced some improvement, and the other was rated as having experienced no change. Relative to the treatment outcome for couples with other sexual dysfunctions, these results represented only a moderate rate of success (Hawton & Catalan, 1986). In determining the outcome for the various groups of clients, the authors included all clients, including those who ended therapy prematurely. Thus, their results may reflect a lower rate of positive outcome than would be the case if only

those couples who completed treatment were included in the results. On the other hand, Hawton and Catalan's estimates may reflect reality better than if they had concentrated only on the "good" clients. This study had several positive methodological features: there were numerous therapists, all of whom were trained in the same clinic, and a substantial number of subjects. However, as with most other studies, the reliability of the outcome measure is unknown, and there was no control group with which to compare rates of spontaneous improvement or the impact of placebo effects. Furthermore, there is no follow-up reported, so the maintenance of treatment effects is not known.

De Amicis, Goldberg, LoPiccolo, Friedman, and Davies (1985) conducted a three-year follow-up study of couples treated at a sex therapy clinic. Of these couples, nine had one partner with a primary problem of low sexual desire (six men and three women). Initial acceptance for sex therapy depended on presence of sexual dysfunction, absence of psychosis or severe depressive symptoms, and absence of impending separation or divorce. Couples were treated by cotherapists ($N = 28$) or an individual therapist ($N = 9$); in one case the therapist data could not be located at follow-up. The treatment protocol used was similar to that of Friedman and colleagues (Friedman & Hogan, 1985; LoPiccolo & Friedman, 1988). The specific content of therapy differed according to the therapists' orientation and the presumed needs of clients, although several components were consistent among all therapists (e.g., home assignments, a focus on sexual interactions, and time-limited therapy of 15 to 20 sessions).

Outcome was assessed by asking individuals whether their dysfunction was worse, the same, or better after therapy. Results at three-year follow-up indicated that clients with desire dysfunction were evenly divided among the three response categories. In all other diagnostic categories, clients rated themselves as better more often than worse or the same. Questionnaire data indicated that although frequency of desire for sexual contact and frequency of sexual contact were improved at termination, both had regressed to worse than pretreatment levels at three-year follow-up for the clients with desire dysfunction.

Schover and LoPiccolo (1982) conducted an earlier review of the treatment outcome for 152 couples with sexual desire disorders who were treated at the same sex clinic as those in De Amicis et al.'s (1985) report. Schover and LoPiccolo reported that treatment gains for these client couples were significant: increases in ratings of overall relationship satisfaction, frequency of sexual activity, positive responses to spouses' sexual advances, and frequency of masturbation. Some of these gains were not maintained at three-month follow-up, such as females' frequency of sexual activity.

Because of the discrepancy between the findings of these two studies, De Amicis et al. (1985) recommended that researchers acknowledge the necessity of long-term follow-up in order to avoid relying on early, possibly inflated outcome statistics. This is no doubt advisable, but De Amicis et al. based their conclusions on the results of a very small number of ISD client couples. The nine couples who were available for three-year follow-up might not be representative of that population in general.

McCarthy (1984) combined written exercises, bibliotherapy, and traditional sex therapy techniques in treating ISD. Protocols were developed for use with males without partners ($N = 10$) and with couples ($N = 20$) diagnosed with ISD. For individual male clients, written exercises were designed to assist in identifying and overcoming blocks to desire. The following four topics were covered: (1) sexual self-concept, (2) body image and attractiveness, (3) sexual fantasies, and (4) development of a positive sexual scenario. Bibliotherapy was employed if the client was determined to hold a poor self-concept. At one-year follow-up, subjects were asked to rate their improvement on a seven-point scale, from "worse" to "resolved." Five of the clients rated improvement at 6 or 7, three rated improvement at 4 or 5, one indicated no improvement, and one indicated a slight worsening of the problem. The two factors most commonly cited as responsible for positive change

were increased involvement in the sexual interaction and increased compatibility of the partners (McCarthy, 1984).

Regarding couples therapy, the focus was on increasing acceptance of the present level of desire in order to decrease "response anxiety"—the anxiety that accompanies negative feelings towards sexual overtures (cf. Apfelbaum, 1988). Concepts emphasized in the four written assignments for couples were (1) increasing intimacy (this included sensate focus exercises), (2) increasing the attraction of partners for one another, (3) increasing trust in the relationship, and (4) developing sexual scenarios (one per partner). At one-year follow-up, at least one partner in 15 of the couples rated improvement at 6 or 7. Three couples rated change as 3 or less. Two couples had separated and were not included in the follow-up.

Based on the results of the couples and individual treatment, McCarthy (1984) concluded that cognitive-behavioral sex therapy appears to hold promise for treatment of low sexual desire in both individuals and couples. This study is clearly preliminary—a small number of clients' results were reviewed—and there were weaknesses in the methodology of both the study and the report. For example, length of treatment was not reported; outcome was based entirely upon self-report; and results immediately after treatment were not reported.) However, McCarthy offers an interesting treatment format, which appears worthy of further investigation, especially as regards the treatment of male ISD clients without partners.

The results from the studies reviewed above do not lend themselves to the formation of general conclusions regarding the treatment of sexual desire dysfunction. Differences in outcome results may be due to differences in determination of outcome (e.g., reliance on clients' versus therapists' judgment) and the varying treatment components employed in these studies. Furthermore, there is currently little consensus as to what constitutes clinically improved sexual desire. Researchers have employed rather vague definitions of treatment success and have made use of outcome assessment methods whose reliability is unknown (e.g., client self-report or therapists' clinical judgment). The importance of explicitly defining outcome criteria with which to assess treatment success has been noted regarding outcome research (Paul, 1969). Another impediment to generalization of the findings is that different treatment components were involved in the various studies, although each incorporated traditional sex therapy techniques. However, there does appear to be some treatment success with a significant proportion of ISD clients and client couples, which may be maintained in at least the first year after therapy. Clearly, there is a need for further research in this area, with the use of more sophisticated outcome assessment.

CONCLUSION

Approximately 20 years ago, the concept of sexual desire was incorporated into models of human sexual functioning and readily accepted by most professionals as a necessary component. It was hypothesized that clients with inhibited sexual desire were more severely distressed than those with other sexual dysfunctions and that this accounted for their lack of response to traditional brief sex therapy. A diagnosis was developed and included in the DSM-III and revised for the DSM-III-R. Inhibited sexual desire dysfunction quickly become one of the most commonly diagnosed sexual dysfunctions. In short, in the 1970s and 1980s, both research and clinical activity reached high levels in this area. Unfortunately, this activity suffered from limitations that are perhaps intrinsic to the diagnosis of low sexual desire. These limitations result from the discrepancies that exist among clinicians and researchers regarding the conceptualization and treatment of low sexual desire. For example, should the focus of assessment and treatment be on the individual, or should desire discrepancies within the couple be addressed? Even more basic questions are also important. What is sexual desire? Is it the same thing for men and women, young and old? How can desire be measured?

The lack of clarity and consensus engendered

by these questions within the area of sexual desire dysfunctions may explain the absence of adequate assessment devices and the discrepancies in research results regarding treatment outcome and maintenance. Clearly, low sexual desire leads to significant problems for individuals and couples, and these problems are at least partially amenable to therapeutic intervention. However, determining the most effective methods for addressing the problems will require clarification of the basic questions discussed above.

REFERENCES

American Psychiatric Association (APA). (1980). *Diagnostic and statistical manual of mental disorders* (3rd ed.). Washington, DC: Author.

American Psychiatric Association (APA). (1987). *Diagnostic and statistical manual of mental disorders* (3rd ed., rev.). Washington, DC: Author.

Apfelbaum, B. (1988). An ego-analytic perspective on desire disorders. In S. R. Leiblum & R. C. Rosen (Eds.), *Sexual desire disorders*. New York: Guilford Press.

Bagarozzi, D. A. (1987). Marital/family developmental theory as a context for understanding and treating inhibited sexual desire. *Journal of Sex and Marital Therapy, 13*(4), 276–285.

Barlow, D. H. (1986). Causes of sexual dysfunction: The role of anxiety and cognitive interference. *Journal of Consulting and Clinical Psychology, 54*(2), 140–148.

Barlow, D. H., Sakheim, D. K., & Beck, J. G. (1983). Anxiety increases sexual arousal. *Journal of Abnormal Psychology, 92*, 49–54.

Beck, J. G., Barlow, D. H., Sakheim, D. K., & Abrahmson, D. J. (1984). Shock threat and sexual arousal: The role of selective attention, thought content and affective states. *Psychophysiology, 24*, 165–172.

Becker, J. V., Skinner, L. J., Abel, G. G., & Cichon, J. (1986). Level of postassault sexual functioning in rape and incest victims. *Archives of Sexual Behavior, 15*(1), 37–49.

Becker, J. V., Skinner, L. J., Abel, G. G., & Treacy, E. C. (1982). Incidence and types of sexual dysfunctions in rape and incest victims. *Journal of Sex and Marital Therapy, 8*(1), 65–74.

Carney, A., Bancroft, J., & Mathews, A. (1978). Combination of hormonal and psychological treatment for female sexual unresponsiveness: A comparative study. *British Journal of Psychiatry, 132,* 339–346.

De Amicis, L. A., Goldberg, D. C., LoPiccolo, J., Friedman, J., & Davies, L. (1985). Clinical follow-up of couples treated for sexual dysfunction. *Archives of Sexual Behavior, 14*(6), 467–489.

Derogatis, L. R. (1977). *The SCL-90-R manual I: Scoring administration and procedures for the SCL-90-R.* Baltimore, MD: Clinical Psychometrics.

Derogatis, L. R. (1980). Psychological assessment of psychosexual functioning. *Psychiatric Clinics of North America,3*(1), 113–131.

Derogatis, L. R., Lipman, R., & Covi, L. (1973). SCL-90: An outpatient psychiatric rating scale. *Psychopharmacology Bulletin, 9*(1), 13–28.

Derogatis, L. R., & Melisaratos, N. (1979). The DSFI: A multidimensional measure of sexual functioning. *Journal of Sex and Marital Therapy, 5*(3), 244–281.

Endicott, J., & Spitzer, R. L. (1978). A diagnostic interview: The Schedule for Affective Disorders and Schizophrenia. *Archives of General Psychiatry, 35,* 837–844.

Freud, S. (1936). *The problem of anxiety.* New York: W. W. Norton. (Original work published in 1926).

Friedman, J. M., & Hogan, D. R. (1985). Sexual dysfunction: Low sexual desire. In D. H. Barlow (Ed.), *Clinical handbook of psychological disorders.* New York: Guilford Press.

Hathaway, S. R., & McKinley, J. C. (1943). *Minnesota Multiphasic Personality Inventory.* Minneapolis: University of Minnesota Press.

Hawton, K. (1985). *Sex therapy: A practical guide.* Oxford, UK: Oxford University Press.

Hawton, K., & Catalan, J. (1986). Prognostic factors in sex therapy. *Behaviour Research and Therapy, 24*(4), 377–385.

Heiman, J. R. (1980). *Personal History Questionnaire.* Unpublished manuscript. University of Washington School of Medicine, Department of Psychiatry and Behavioral Sciences.

Kaplan, H. S. (1977). Hypoactive sexual desire. *Journal of Sex and Marital Therapy, 3,* 3–9.

Kaplan, H. S. (1979). *Disorders of sexual desire.* New York: Brunner/Mazel.

Kaplan, H. S. (1983). *The evaluation of sexual disorders.* New York: Brunner/Mazel.

Kimmel, D. K., & von der Veen, F. (1974). Factors of marital adjustment in Locke's marital adjustment test. *Journal of Marital and Family Living, 29,* 57–63.

Kinsey, A. C., Pomeroy, W. B., & Martin, C. E. (1948). *Sexual behavior in the human male.* Philadelphia: W. B. Saunders.

Kinsey, A. C., Pomeroy, W. B., Martin, C. E., & Gebhard C. E. (1953). *Sexual behavior in the human female.* Philadelphia: W. B. Saunders.

Knopf, J., & Seiler, M. (1990). *Inhibited sexual desire.* New York: William Morrow.

Lazarus, A. A. (1988). A multimodal perspective on problems of sexual desire. In S. R. Leiblum & R. C. Rosen (Eds.), *Sexual desire disorders.* New York: Guilford Press.

Leiblum, S. R., & Rosen, R. C. (1988). Introduction: Changing perspectives on sexual desire. In S. R. Leiblum & R. C. Rosen (Eds.), *Sexual desire disorders.* New York: Guilford Press.

Levine, S. B. (1988). Intrapsychic and individual aspects of sexual desire. In S. R. Leiblum & R. C. Rosen (Eds.), *Sexual desire disorders.* New York: Guilford.

Lewis, R. (1972). A developmental framework for the analysis for premarital dyadic formation. *Family Process, 11,* 17–48.

Lief, H. I. (1977). Inhibited sexual desire. *Medical Aspects of Human Sexuality, 7,* 94–95.

Lief, H. I. (1985). Evaluation of inhibited sexual desire disorders: Relationship aspects. In H. S. Kaplan (Ed.), *Comprehensive evaluation of disorders of sexual desire* (pp. 61–76). Washington, DC: American Psychiatric Press.

LoPiccolo, J., & Friedman, J. (1988). Broad-spectrum treatment of low sexual desire: Integration of cognitive, behavioral, and systemic therapy. In S. R. Leiblum & R. C. Rosen (Eds.), *Sexual desire disorders.* New York: Guilford Press.

LoPiccolo, J., & Heiman, J. (1977). Cultural values and the therapeutic definition of sexual function and dysfunction. *Journal of Social Issues, 33*(2), 166–183.

LoPiccolo, J. & Steger, J. (1974). The sexual interaction inventory: A new instrument for the assessment of sexual dysfunction. *Archives of Sexual Behavior, 3,* 585–595.

LoPiccolo, J. & Stock, W. (1986). Treatment of sexual dysfunction. *Journal of Consulting and Clinical Psychology, 54*(2), 158–167.

Masters, W., & Johnson, V. (1970). *Human sexual inadequacy.* Boston: Little, Brown.

Mathew, R. J., & Weinman (1982). Sexual dysfunctions in depression. *Archives of Sexual Behavior, 11,* 323–328.

Mathews, A., Whitehead, A., & Kellett, J. M. (1983). Psychological and hormonal factors in the treatment of female sexual dysfunction. *Psychological Medicine, 13*(1), 83–92.

McCarthy, B. W. (1984). Strategies and techniques for the treatment of inhibited sexual desire. *Journal of Sex and Marital Therapy, 10*(2), 97–106.

Meuwissen, I., & Over, R. (1990). Habituation and dishabituation of female sexual arousal. *Behavioural Research and Therapy, 28*(3), 217–226.

Murphy, C., & Sullivan, M. (1981). Anxiety and self-concept correlates of sexually aversive women. *Sexuality and Disability, 4*(1), 15–26.

Nathan, S. G. (1986). The epidemiology of the DSM-III psychosexual dysfunctions. *Journal of Sex and Marital Therapy, 12*(4), 267–281.

Nowinski, J., & LoPiccolo, J. (1979). Assessing sexual behavior in couples. *Journal of Sex and Marital Therapy, 5*(3), 225–243.

Nutter, D. E., & Condron, M. K. (1983). Sexual fantasy and activity patterns of females with inhibited sexual desire versus normal controls. *Journal of Sex and Marital Therapy, 9*(4), 276–282.

Nutter, D. E., & Condron, M. K. (1985). Sexual fantasy and activity patterns of males with inhibited sexual desire and males with erectile dysfunction versus normal controls. *Journal of Sex and Marital Therapy, 11*(2), 91–108.

O'Donohue, W. T., & Geer, J. H. (1985). The habituation of sexual arousal. *Archives of Sexual Behavior, 14*(3), 233–246.

O'Donohue, W., & Plaud, J. (1991). The long-term habituation of sexual arousal in the human male. *Journal of Behavior Therapy and Experimental Psychology, 22*(2), 87–96.

Paul, G. (1969). Behavior modification reseach: Design and tactics. In C. M Franks (Ed.), *Behavior therapy: Appraisal and status.* New York: McGraw-Hill.

Pietropinto, A. (1986). Survey analysis. *Medical Aspects of Human Sexuality, 1,* 48–59.

Rachman, S. (1966). Sexual fetishism: An experimental analogue. *Psychological Record, 16,* 293–296.

Rado, S. (1949). An adaptational view of sexual behavior. In *Psychosexual development in health and disease* (pp. 159–189). New York: Grune and Stratton.

Robinson, P. (1976). The modernization of sex. New York: Harper & Row.

Rosen, R. C., & Leiblum, S. R. (1988). A sexual scripting approach to problems of desire. In S. R. Leiblum & R. C. Rosen (Eds.), *Sexual desire disorders.* New York: Guilford Press.

Rosen, R. C., & Leiblum, S. R. (1989). Desire disorders. In S. R. Leiblum & R. C. Rosen (Eds.),

Principles and practices of sex therapy: Update for the 1990s. New York: Guilford Press.

Rust, J., & Golombok, S. (1986). The GRISS: A psychometric instrument for the assessment of sexual dysfunction. *Archives of Sexual Behavior, 15*(2), 157–165.

Scharff, D. E. (1988). An object relations approach to inhibited sexual desire. In S. R. Leiblum & R. C. Rosen (Eds.), *Sexual desire disorders.* New York: Guilford Press.

Schover, L. R., & LoPiccolo, J. (1982). Treatment effectiveness for dysfunctions of sexual desire. *Journal of Sex and Marital Therapy, 8*(3), 179–197.

Schreiner-Engle, P., & Schiavi, R. C. (1986). Lifetime psychopathology in individuals with low sexual desire. *Journal of Nervous and Mental Disease, 174*(11), 646–651.

Schwartz, M. F., & Masters, W. H. (1988). Inhibited sexual desire: The Masters and Johnson Institute treatment. In S. R. Leiblum & R. C. Rosen (Eds.), *Sexual desire disorders.* New York: Guilford Press.

Semans, J. H. (1956). Premature ejaculation: A new approach. *Southern Medical Journal, 49,* 353–357.

Spanier, G. B. (1976). Measuring dyadic adjustment: New scales for assessing the quality of marriage and similar dyads. *Journal of Marriage and the Family, 38*(1), 15–28.

Stuart, F. M., Hammond, D. C., & Pett, M. A. (1986). Psychological characteristics of women with inhibited sexual desire. *Journal of Sex and Marital Therapy, 12*(2), 108–115.

Stuart, F. M., Hammond, D. C., & Pett, M. A. (1987). Inhibited sexual desire in women. *Archives of Sexual Behavior 16*(2), 91–105.

Symons, D. (1987). An evolutionary approach: Can Darwin's view of life shed light on human sexuality? In J. H. Geer & W. T. O'Donohue (Eds.), *Theories of human sexuality.* New York: Plenum.

Vandereyeken, W. (1987). On desire, excitement, and impotence in modern sex therapy. *Psychotherapy and Psychosomatics, 47,* 175–180.

Verhulst, J., & Heiman, J. R. (1988). A systems perspective on sexual desire. In S. R. Leiblum & R. C. Rosen (Eds.), *Sexual desire disorders.* New York: Guilford Press.

Wolpe, J. (1958). *Psychotherapy by reciprocal inhibition.* Stanford, CA: Stanford University Press.

Zung, W. (1973). From art to science: The diagnosis and treatment of depression. *Archives of General Psychiatry, 29,* 325–337.

CHAPTER 4

SEXUAL AVERSIONS: A HIDDEN DISORDER

Steven R. Gold, Northern Illinois University
Ruth G. Gold, Northern Illinois University

Sexual aversion disorder is a new diagnosis, introduced in the DSM-III-R (American Psychiatric Association, 1987). The prior version—the DSM-III (American Psychiatric Association, 1980)—explicitly excluded sexual phobias from the category of phobias, and sexual aversions were not specifically mentioned as a sexual disorder. Therefore, sexual aversion disorders did not fit into any category except "psychosexual disorders not elsewhere classified" until the latest revision. The addition of sexual aversion disorder to the DSM-III-R might suggest that there has been growing interest and research validation for the diagnosis. Unfortunately, although some authors have noted the frequency of sexual aversion disorder in clinical practice (Kaplan, 1987), limited research in the area makes it difficult to draw conclusions or write at length on sexual aversion disorder.

The aims of this chapter are to review the extant literature that describes and differentiates sexual aversion or sexual phobia from similar disorders; discuss its incidence and prevalence; review theories about its etiology; propose separate etiological models for males and females; and, lastly, discuss the assessment and treatment of sexual aversion disorder.

DEFINITION AND CONCEPTUAL ISSUES

The DSM-III-R includes sexual aversion under the heading of sexual desire disorders and defines it as "persistent or recurrent extreme aversion to, and avoidance of, all or almost all, genital sexual contact with a sexual partner" (p. 293). This is similar to the definition of phobias in the DSM-III-R—including the two critical features of (1) having an adverse reaction when faced with circumscribed situations and (2) avoiding such situations. Despite the interchangeable use of the terms *sexual aversion* and *sexual phobia* in the literature, there is an affective and behavioral difference. *Aversion* implies an intense dislike, disgust, or abhorrence, whereas *phobia* refers to an excessive fear but does not contain the element of disgust (Simon & Schuster, 1979). For most people, the thought or image of eating a plate of mud would provoke disgust, yet mud is unlikely to be avoided or to provoke excess fear. Conversely, although we personally are not phobic about the dark, it would stimulate a high level of fear for us to stroll through Central Park at 3:00 A.M. Context seems critical in determining whether a stimulus results in an aversion or a phobia—or is in fact an appropriate, prudent response. Because the literature does not currently differentiate between sexual aversion and sexual phobia, the terms will be used interchangeably in this chapter.

Sexual aversions or sexual phobias can be very general or highly specific (Kaplan, 1987). For example, a person could have an aversion to any sexual stimulus or to even thinking about sexual contact or situations in which sex might be possible. Aversion may be specific to a particular sexual act, such as oral sex, or to a specific aspect of sexuality, such as the texture of sexual secretions. Under the heading of sexual phobias, Kaplan (1987) lists such commonly seen interpersonal fears as fear of "commitment to one partner," of "intimacy and closeness," and of "falling in love and being loved" (p. 13).

Sexual aversions may be primary or secondary—that is, lifelong or developed after having had pleasurable sexual experiences in the past. A primary aversion is one that has theoretically always existed but may or may not become manifest until the individual becomes involved in a relationship. Primary aversion has been regarded as more difficult to treat and is more often found in men, whereas secondary aversion is more frequently found in women and has been suggested to have a better prognosis (Kaplan, 1987). For example, an older male may realize that he feels uncomfortable around women and therefore may avoid close relationships. The sexual aversion becomes apparent only when he finally has a girlfriend and is forced to recognize that he does not want to have sex.

An example of a secondary aversion might be a woman married for a number of years who, over time, has developed a dislike, then an aversion toward intercourse with her husband. As her husband pushes her to have sex, she feels more and more anxious and out of control, so she begins having panic attacks whenever she experiences or even thinks about sex. This reinforces the fear, and she avoids sex even more.

Sexual aversions differ from some other phobias, such as a fear of heights, in the impact the fear has on the individual's lifestyle. With some alterations in their lifestyle, many persons with nonsexual phobias can live full lives and avoid the object or situation they fear. However, it is impossible, short of being alone on a deserted island, for a person with sexual phobia to avoid all sexual stimuli. Individuals with a primary aversion to sex may live without the close interpersonal relationships commonly regarded as essential for good mental and physical health. Although an individual can have an intimate asexual relationship by choice, the primary sex phobic may lack the ability to approach other individuals without being overcome by fear; such a person may not be able to develop close relationships of any kind. Along with sex, the potential for having a family and children is sacrificed. Individuals suffering a secondary or acquired sexual aversion disorder also have problems in close relationships that have the potential for becoming sexual. Although secondary aversion is associated with less psychopathology (Crenshaw, 1985; Kaplan, 1987), it can disrupt marriages, lead to other sexual dysfunctions, and confuse and distress the afflicted individual and the partner.

The rationale for the classification of sexual aversion disorder is unclear. Sexual aversion is categorized as a sexual disorder primarily because the object of the aversion or disgust is sexual. Other characteristics of sexual aversion are similar to anxiety disorders. Just as the term *social phobia* refers to a fear and avoidance of social situations where scrutiny by others is likely, sexual aversion can be a fear and avoidance of sexual situations where some type of evaluative response by a partner is anticipated. For sexual aversion to be unambiguously a sexual disorder, perhaps an additional criterion should be that there is a sexual performance problem concomitant with the aversion. If an individual can perform in an adequate manner when not fearful, the primary problem is anxiety—not a sexual limitation.

Crenshaw (1985) and Kaplan (1987) state that sexual aversion is characterized by an unwillingness to participate in a sexual activity rather than any particular response pattern during the sexual experience. Perhaps outcome research could help clarify this definitional issue. If some clients can be successfully treated by a therapy focusing directly on the anxiety, then these clients should be conceptualized as having an anxiety disorder, not a sexual dysfunction. If other clients require sexual therapy after their anxiety is reduced, it would suggest anxiety and sexual disorder as a dual diagnosis for those clients. If research reveals that sometimes one type and sometimes two types of intervention are necessary, it would support the hypothesis of distinct disorders: (1) anxiety and (2) anxiety with sexual dysfunction.

For example, a male might develop a secondary sexual aversion after experiencing a failure to achieve an erection. Upset by his lack of "manliness," he subsequently avoids all sexual contact for fear of another failure. Systematic desensitization may reduce his fear of trying to perform sexually but still leaves him unable to achieve an erection. After sensate focus exercises with his partner, he overcomes his erectile disorder. In this example, it seems appropriate to diagnose the man's problem as an anxiety disorder with an additional sexual dysfunction. On the other hand, a woman who enjoys intercourse but has never been able to approach touching her partner's penis without intense anxiety or revulsion overcomes her phobia with systematic desensitization and requires no additional sex therapy. Her diagnosis is most appropriately an anxiety disorder. The proposed diagnostic considerations are cumbersome because it is difficult to assess these hidden disorders early in the therapy process, but the benefit is that the establishment of a framework that guides clinicians in their assessment and therapy.

A second issue raised by the DSM-III-R classification of sexual aversion is whether it should be included under the general category of sexual desire disorders. Schover, Friedman, Weiler, Heiman, and LoPiccolo (1982), in their multiaxial approach to the diagnosis of sexual disorders, suggest that sexual desire disorders and sexual aversion disorders represent a behavioral continuum, with avoidance of sex as the unifying aspect. Sexual aversions represent a more extreme avoidance than low sexual desire. Schover et al. (1982) argue that to classify the two disorders separately would imply different etiologies, an assumption that is not based on any data. However, separate classification need not imply unique etiology, as the DSM-III-R system classifies without etiological assumptions. LoPiccolo and Friedman (1988) also posit a close relationship between aversion and desire disorders. They suggest that low-desire men usually have some degree of aversion to female genitalia, and many other clients reporting low desire may have an aversion they are not cognizant of harboring. There are no data reported to substantiate the suggested association between low desire and aversion.

An opposing view is espoused by Kaplan (1987), who argues that sexual aversions should be separate from sexual desire problems because those with sexual aversions can often experience desire, enjoy sexual fantasies, and masturbate to orgasm. On the other hand, those with low sexual desire can engage in sexual activities without anxiety even if they do not experience pleasure. Based on the difference in the subjective experiences of clients with low desire and with aversion, Kaplan conceptualizes these as related but different syndromes. Kaplan further supports the dichotomy with the finding that 25% of the clients seen at her sexual treatment center who found sexual activity aversive also met the criteria for panic disorder, but only 2% of those with low desire also had a panic disorder. Kaplan provided no descriptive data for her sample, which therefore may or may not be representative of sexual aversion clients.

If sexual aversions are to be classified as a sexual disorder, the current DSM-III-R placement with desire disorders seems appropriate. More reliable and valid diagnoses can be made by isolating the underlying behavioral pattern (in this case, avoidance) than by depending primarily on subjective experiences, as proposed by Kaplan. An integrated approach could include the ideas of Schover et al. (1982) and Kaplan's (1987) description of sexual panic. The sexual avoidance continuum can then be described as ranging from a low desire for sexual activity with no experience of anxiety to a panic reaction when faced with a feared sexual situation. Measures of behavior are more easily rated by the client and are less subject to the clinician's interpretation than self-reported internal states. People vary in their ability to identify and label feelings (perhaps especially sexual feelings) but can more easily report what they did and did not do.

A final issue raised by the current definition of sexual aversion is the emphasis on "genital sexual contact." This implies that someone who could achieve sexual intercourse but found touching and kissing aversive would not be diagnosed. The problem with the genital focus is that it supports a widely held stereotype that "real sex" is genital and all the rest just preliminary. It also omits the cognitive aspects of sexuality. Someone who can perform but receives no pleasure or excitement from sex is not diagnosed as having an aversion, although Kaplan lists the absence of pleasure or erotic feelings as a common phobia—a fear of pleasure. The genital emphasis seems to imply a perhaps unintended value judgment about sexuality that sex therapists and sex educators have worked to dispel.

PSYCHOPATHOLOGY

Incidence and Prevalence

The introduction to the DSM-III-R states that in adding new diagnostic categories, primary importance was given to the research support for the diagnosis. In the case of sexual aversion disorder, the research base is absent. The inclusion of the category was based on clinical experience and a theoretical model of the sexual response cycle rather than a research base. The most compelling argument for inclusion was that victims of rape or child sexual abuse often suffer sexual problems that may include an aversion to future sexual interactions. Because it seems inappropriate to classify trauma victims as having low desire, the category of sexual aversions was added to the list of diagnoses despite the absence of a research base (J. LoPiccolo, personal communication, July 10, 1990).

The incidence and prevalence of sexual aversion are unknown. Crenshaw (1985) described it as "a widespread, poorly recognized syndrome" (p. 285), and Kaplan (1987) noted that "despite their high prevalence, sexual panic states have received surprisingly little professional attention" (p. 3). A recent study of the incidence and prevalence rates of sexual dysfunctions does not even mention sexual aversions (Spector & Carey, 1990). It is unclear why a disorder some clinicians report as widespread has received so little research attention. More research is obviously called for, but definitional and comorbidity problems may make it difficult to tease out accurate rates for sexual aversion.

According to LoPiccolo and Friedman (1988), sexual aversions often occur along with another sexual disorder; they may be masked by the other disorder and therefore not be diagnosed. For example, sexual aversions may contribute to inhibited sexual desire, or be a consequence of inhibited desire, but not be recognized by the client or therapist. Also, a panic disorder may be simply a part of the clinical picture but be the sole diagnosis (Kaplan, 1987). The problem of comorbidity or dual diagnosis may be especially cogent for sexual aversions, because clinicians are less familiar with the disorder than other sexual or anxiety disorders. Also, clients may be more comfortable presenting a "traditional" problem and therefore deny or be unaware of an aversion. Because some of the phobias are specific, a clinician may miss the diagnosis by failing to ask about a wide variety of sexual stimuli. Some clinicians might find this exhaustive questioning too intrusive for the client unless the client first brings up the topic. For example, a client with a phobic response to vaginal odors might never divulge this specific symptom to the therapist, thus increasing the difficulty in understanding and treating the client's behavioral manifestation of inhibited desire. Because some individuals with sexual phobias become anxious when they think about sex or anticipate a situation where sex is even remotely possible, they may learn to distract themselves or avoid any sexual thoughts or fantasies and potential sexual stituations. When this defensive pattern succeeds, the phobics have no insight into the source of their sexual avoidance pattern but develop elaborate rationalizations to explain their lack of sexual interest (Kaplan, 1987). It might take a frustrated lover to bring the sex phobic to therapy, but the focus would then be on low desire or another problem. The sexual aversion would not be uncovered unless the therapist probed for its existence. The hidden nature of many aversions may be the reason some therapists do not report treating more of them; it may also be a major block to research investigations.

If, as suggested by LoPiccolo and Friedman (1988), sexual aversions often coexist with inhibited sexual desire, there is indirect evidence that sexual aversions may be more prevalent now than in the past. This conclusion is based on the report that low sexual desire is the most common presenting complaint brought to sex therapists (Knopf & Seiler, 1990) and that the number of complaints of low sexual desire have increased since the 1970s (Spector & Carey, 1990). Spector and Carey reviewed 23 studies that measured the incidence and/or prevalence rates of sexual dysfunction over the past 50 years. They reported that inhibited sexual desire represented 37% of the presenting problems brought to sex clinics in the early 1970s, increasing to 46% by the end of the 1970s and to 55% in the early 1980s. Parallel to this increase has been a shift from the problem being primarily a female presenting complaint in the 1970s to 60% of the presenting partners being male in the 1980s.

Etiology

To investigate the etiology of sexual aversion, we must cast a wide net. Sexual aversion has been linked to anxiety disorders such as phobias, can coexist with panic states, and can lead to or be a consequence of other sexual dysfunctions. Therefore, theories addressing the etiology of anxiety, panic states, and other sexual disorders (especially inhibited sexual desire) are highly relevant. Current theories of anxiety and sexual dysfunctions emphasize an integration of biological, cognitive, behavioral, interpersonal, and psychodynamic approaches (Ballenger, 1989; Jones & Barlow, 1990; Kaplan, 1987). Because sexual aversions occur in both genders and the sexual socialization of men and women is so different, a comprehensive model of etiology needs to address possible gender differences. It is beyond the scope of this chapter to review thoroughly each of the different areas of research, but we will make attempt to highlight key concepts from each domain.

Sexual aversion disorders are unlikely to be due to a single cause. A number of factors have been associated with the development of sexual disorders, all of which may play a role in the formation of sexual phobias. The focus if this chapter will be on etiological factors that are unique or most relevant to sexual aversions. Nonetheless, one must be aware that other factors may play an important role: for example, stress, alcohol and drug use, fear of pregnancy, depression, sexual orientation concerns, relationship problems, paraphilias, hormone levels, and physical health. This section will first review current models of the etiology of sexual aversion and then suggest additional considerations not included in present approaches.

Kaplan and her coworkers have described a model of the etiology of sexual aversions (Kaplan, 1987, 1988; Kaplan, Fyer, & Novick, 1982). The core concept in Kaplan's (1987) model of the etiology of anxiety and panic disorders is a constitutional, biological defect in the central nervous system that results in a low threshold for activation of the alarm response. People born with this biological vulnerability are hyperaroused and more prone to develop anxiety disorders, either in the face of trauma or in the course of normal living. The alarm reaction is a valuable internal stimulus that motivates the individual to take immediate action, such as fight or flight (Jones & Barlow, 1990). The alarm response is similar to a smoke detector. In anxiety states, the alarm is oversensitive. It is set off by false alarms, overreacting to minor dangers as if they were life-threatening or responding when no objective danger is present. It is like a malfunctioning smoke detector that may go off when there is no smoke in the room or fire in the house. The CNS response to danger can be described as either mobilizing the body for action (with increased sympathetic nervous system responses such as heart racing, increased blood pressure, or rapid breathing) or, in contrast, demobilization to shut down the system (with parasympathetic reactions leading to freezing or fainting) (A. T. Beck & G. Emery, 1985). When the alarm response occurs, it takes precedence over all other activities, and eating, playing, or making love are interrupted in order to stay alive.

It should be pointed out that a biological predisposition and the experience of panic attacks are not necessary or sufficient conditions for the development of a sexual aversion. Kaplan (1987) noted that only 25% of those with sexual aversions had diagnosable panic attacks. However, she added that an additional 38% of the patients she treated, who did not recall panic attacks, had some features of a panic disorder. For these 38%, the alarm response did not spontaneously lead to a full panic attack, but these patients were still hyperaroused and sensitive to separation, rejection, and criticism. Perhaps they were sensitive to anxiety cues and avoided the feared situation before the panic response had the opportunity to develop. There is some research to support the concept of subclinical panic disorder. The Anxiety Sensitivity Index (ASI) is a measure of the fear of fear. High

scorers on the ASI believe that symptoms associated with anxiety have harmful effects, and when they experience these symptoms they tend to panic. Donnell and McNally (1990) report that two-thirds of those with high ASI scores had never experienced a panic attack, suggesting that the fear of anxiety can develop through pathways other than direct experience with panic. High ASI scores do seem to be related to panic, as significantly more high scorers seek treatment for anxiety problems and more often have first-degree relatives with a history of panic than those who score low on the ASI (Donnell & McNally, 1990).

Kaplan (1987) also incorporates Klein's theory that panic "represents an abnormal continuation into adult life of the protest phase of the separation response" (p. 44). The protest response is a vulnerable infant's instinctual reaction to scream when separated from the mother, in order to convince her to return. Individuals with panic disorders frequently have a history of difficulty with separations. With a low threshold for alarm responses and the experience of maternal separation, the anxiety-prone individual develops an anticipatory dread of further separations. A vicious cycle is created, with anticipatory anxiety leading to a heightened state of arousal, making the feared event of the next anxiety attack more likely. It is the sense of events being unpredictable and uncontrollable that makes people most vulnerable to anxiety (Jones & Barlow 1990). Kaplan agrees that people with sexual aversions and panic attacks are not actually afraid of sex, but fear panicking and losing control. The trigger is not the fear of sex but rather the fear of fear itself. Her position is consistent with some cognitive models of anxiety, such as those of Beck (A. T. Beck & G. Emery, 1985) and Barlow (Jones & Barlow, 1990), that emphasize the misinterpretation of somatic signals and support viewing sexual aversion as an anxiety response.

Kaplan (1987) identifies two patterns of parenting that undermine children's management of their separation anxiety. In the first maladaptive pattern, a cold, rejecting parent belittles the child's fears. The child then doubts his or her own instinctual ability to react appropriately to fearful stimuli and learns negative self-attributes, such as self-hatred and guilt. In the second maladaptive pattern of parenting, an overprotective parent does not allow the child to develop coping skills and takes the responsibility for dealing with the anxiety away from the child. Such a child grows into an adult who expects to be cared for and who lacks confidence to deal with his or her own anxiety.

Kaplan's model is strongly influenced by psychoanalytic thinking. She offers an integration of biological vulnerability, separation anxiety, and psychosexual development. The anxious child is hypothesized to have a particularly difficult time resolving the Oedipal conflict. Fearful of competing for the love of the opposite-sex parent because of excessive abandonment concerns, the child adopts passive and self-defeating strategies that impair later adult relationships. These speculations are clinically interesting, but no research is cited in support.

Kaplan (1988) has described adults with a biological predisposition to be vulnerable to anxiety as displaying a triad of destructive personality traits: separation anxiety, rejection sensitivity, and overreaction to criticism from significant others such as parents and lovers. These personality characteristics often result in distressed interpersonal relationships. Partners may not always play a central role in the development of aversion disorders, but they often contribute to the maintanance of the problem, especially in secondary aversion disorders. Unrecognized ambivalence toward the partner often characterizes the attitude of those with an aversion disorder. Due to their sensitivity to rejection, they are prone to hide their anger and resentment, with avoidance of sex being the behavioral manifestation of this anger. The ambivalence can be due to any of the issues with which spouses struggle, but power and intimacy conflicts are considered central. The issues with the spouse are further compounded by the projection of the parental figure onto the spouse. Because these vulnerable adults have not re-solved their separation anxiety and are especially attuned to rejection by the parent, the relationship with the spouse can be colored by the projection, and the spouse can become the rejecting parent.

Two patterns of behavior are seen in individuals with intimacy problems: Some express their need for closeness by developing overly intense and dependent attachments, and others defend themselves from pain by avoiding love and commitment. In the first pattern, the individual is so fearful of rejection that he or she demands constant reassurance and declarations of love. The need for closeness is so intense that there is no option for the partner to be distant or apart when desired. Sex becomes not a mutually enjoyable experience but a complicated, symbolic way for the needy partner to achieve closeness. The atmosphere of pressure can be so overburdening for both partners that the afflicted partner or couple begins to avoid sex. In the second pattern, sex can be enjoyed only when there is no emotional involvement, as any hint of intimacy or closeness raises the anxiety to intolerable levels, so the individual pulls back or begins to avoid sex, for self-protection. Both patterns can be described as having a very narrow sexual comfort zone; when the zone is breached, sexual interest is lost.

Problems in interpersonal relationships are not the only pathway to the development of sexual aversions in Kaplan's model. She sees the negative sexual messages given to children about sex (particularly masturbation) as influencing many people to associate sexuality with sin, shame, and guilt. Children with a low panic threshold and excessive separation anxiety may be particularly sensitive to parental messages and highly concerned about not doing anything to incur parental censure. Engaging in sexual activity may be too risky for the anxious, rejection-sensitive child. These early messages are ingrained and overlearned, so rejection-sensitive adults often behave sexually as if their parents were watching. It is then easier to avoid sex than to risk the feared consequences.

The fictitious case of Frieda illustrates how the biological, environmental, cognitive, and emotional aspects of sexual aversion are manifest in one person. Frieda was a fearful, anxious, only child who was reared by overprotective parents. Her mother had frequent panic attacks and worried whenever Frieda was out of her sight. Frieda was totally dependent on her mother and became upset when her mother had a panic attack, so she learned at an early age that the best way to keep her mother calm was to go along with her and try to please her. Frieda was attracted to and married a man who was also shy but caring and protective of her. The big surprise for her came when she attempted to have intercourse with her new husband. When she began to react sexually, her heart rate elevated, and she felt flushed—the same somatic feelings she experienced whenever she was fearful of being abandoned. For her, sexual arousal and anxiety over loss became linked. During sex these feelings frightened Frieda, and the only way she could contain the anxiety was to demand repeated reassurance from her husband that he loved her and would not leave her. Frieda's anxiety distracted her from any sexual enjoyment, and she unconsciously grew to resent her husband for not taking better care of her. Whenever she was in a sexual situation with her husband, Frieda felt conflicted: Emotionally, she wanted to please him, but her somatic response signaled a fear of abandonment. With repeated encounters, Frieda's anxiety mounted to an intolerable level, and she began having panic attacks when approached by her husband.

Kaplan's model, illustrated by the case of Frieda, describes one approach to the development of sexual aversions. Kaplan provides an integrated and clinically heuristic model of sexual aversion. The model has not been corroborated by research support as yet. It is important to be cautious in evaluating Kaplan's model (as well as others to follow), due to the limited database. All the present models could be stamped: "Caution: Conclusions are tentative."

Female Model of Etiology: Sexual Abuse

Clinical experience and recent research point to females' experiences of sexual trauma such as childhood sexual abuse or adult rape as a significant contributor to sexual problems, particularly problems such as sexual aversion that interfere with desire or arousal. This review will focus on childhood sexual experiences, but very similar effects are found for victims of adult sexual traumas (Koss & Burkhart, 1989). Childhood sexual experiences are emphasized here because childhood sexual abuse increases the risk for later sexual abuse and can have long-term personality consequences (Browne & Finkelhor, 1986). An emphasis on childhood trauma as an important etiological factor is not inconsistent with Kaplan's model but rather provides a broader explanation for the development of a pervasive sense of anxiety, in addition to a biological predisposition. The focus on childhood sexual abuse is also consistent with the DSM-III-R, where sexual aversions were added, in part, to account for the sexual responses of women who had been abused as children.

Two models have been proposed to explain the effects of sexual abuse on later adjustment: post-traumatic stress disorder (PTSD) (e.g., Lindberg & Distad, 1985; Wolfe, Gentile, & Wolfe, 1989) and the traumagenic dynamics model of child sexual abuse (TDM) (Finkelhor & Browne, 1985). A brief review of the two models will help clarify the relationship between childhood sexual abuse and subsequent sexual fears.

The PTSD diagnosis is often appropriate for victims of childhood abuse, because the abuse experience fits the definition of a trauma and survivors often have symptoms that are consistent with the description in the DSM-III-R. The diagnostic characteristics of PTSD include intrusive thoughts, avoidance of trauma-related stimuli, numbing of responsivity, and hyperarousal (as shown by sleep disturbances, difficulty concentrating, and heightened irritability).

The TDM explanation of child sexual abuse proposes four dynamics as a consequence of sexual abuse: traumatic sexualization, betrayal, powerlessness, and stigmatization. *Traumatic sexualization* means that "children who have been traumatically sexualized emerge from their experiences with inappropriate repertories of sexual behavior, with confusions and misconceptions about their sexual self-concepts, and with unusual emotional associations to sexual activities" (Finkelhor & Browne, 1985, p. 531). The second dynamic, betrayal, involves the loss of trust and security in the abuser, who is often a significant person in the child's life. This early betrayal can lead to fearfulness and mistrust in close adult relationships, which makes it difficult to engage in intimate partnerships. Powerlessness, the third dynamic, refers to the child's feeling of helplessness in the abusive situation, the feeling that her body is not her own. In adulthood, this can interfere with sexual responsiveness: Sex involves some pleasurable sensation of loss of control, and the abused woman would equate this feeling with earlier powerlessness and fear. It can also develop into the feeling that the woman is unable to act on her own environment and that she is powerless in relationships. This, along with the fourth dynamic, stigmatization, undermines the victim's self-esteem and contributes further to the long-term consequences of her childhood sexual abuse. These TDM dynamics are consistent with Kaplan's model of the development of aversion disorders.

To synthesize both the PTSD and TDM models, it is expected that some victims of childhood sexual abuse will emerge with cognitive, emotional, and interpersonal problems that leave them anxious, fearful of others, and suffering from an impaired sense of self-efficacy and a distorted view of sexuality. It is therefore not surprising that clinicians have noted an association between sexual abuse and sexual aversions.

Crenshaw (1985), based on her clinical experience, listed incest or child molestation as an etiological factor in the development of primary sexual aversions. LoPiccolo and Friedman (1988), also based on clinical experience, noted that women who were sexually molested as children sometimes have sexual aversions that are specific to their experience during the assault and that may result in flashbacks when they attempt to engage in sex. Bass and Davis (1988) have written an excellent book aimed at helping women survivors of sexual abuse heal themselves. Based on their clinical work, they describe the close connection between sexual arousal and fear in survivors and report that many women avoid making love because it evokes too many painful and terrifying feelings. In behavioral terms, the old panic, which was appropriate for the original stimulus of a sexual attack, becomes generalized to all sexual encounters: It becomes the conditioned response to those encounters. Thus, sexual aversions or sex phobias may be highly specific or may apply to all sexual activities. Bass and Davis (1988) also describe the difficulty survivors have in letting anyone get close to them, for fear of being suffocated or overwhelmed or losing control.

Descriptions of sexual abuse survivors derived from clinicians are supported by recent research on the effects of sexual abuse. A wide range of short- and long-term deleterious consequences of sexual abuse have been reported (see Browne & Finkelhor, 1986, for a review of empirical studies on the effects of childhood sexual abuse).

Several recent studies have examined the effects of childhood sexual abuse on the person's subsequent functioning. Generally, the studies reveal two patterns of sexual behavior as a result of child sexual abuse: sexual acting out and sexual avoidance. Kolko, Moser, and Weldy (1988) compared the behavioral and emotional problems of children who suffered sexual or physical abuse in a sample of 103 hospitalized psychiatric patients. The children ranged in age from 5 to 14. Sexually abused children showed more sexual behavior and more fear and mistrust, both at home and in the hospital, than nonabused children. There were no such differences between children who were physically abused and those who were not abused. Deblinger, McLeer, Atkins, Ralphe, and Foa (1989) compared sexually abused, physically abused, and nonabused psychiatrically hospitalized children matched for age, sex, and socioeconomic status. Sexually abused children exhibited significantly higher rates of inappropriate sexual behavior and sexually abusive behavior. Goldston, Turnquist, and Knutson (1989) also reported that sexually abused girls, as compared to other girls referred for mental health problems, more often engaged in a constellation of sexually inappropriate behaviors, including public and private masturbation, sexual precocity, sexual experimentation with younger children, and seductive behaviors toward men. In a study of 71 sexually abused girls and their mothers, Wolfe et al. (1989) reported that the girls had significantly more sex-associated fears and more intrusive and ruminative thoughts about the abuse (which interfered with sleep and led to nightmares) than the general population on which the scales were normed.

The results of the studies of children who were sexually abused are consistent with both the PTSD and TDM models. The female victims who were introduced to sexual experiences at an inappropriate age continue to behave in a sexual manner toward other children and adults. The sexual behavior is thought to be driven by the intrusive recurrence of thoughts and images about their sexually abusive experience. Some of the girls have learned that sex is a means of gaining affection and attention, and they may have a distorted sense of what is socially appropriate because of poor role models. Others may be attempting to gain control over the trauma by reenacting it—but with themselves in charge.

Research has also examined the long-term effects of child sexual abuse by studying the adult adjustment of survivors. Becker, Skinner, Abel, and Cichon (1986) studied 372 sexual assault survivors and 99 women with no history of sexual assault to determine the incidence and type of sexual dysfunctions suffered. The types of assaults experienced included rape, attempted rape, incest, and child molestation, so not all of the women were child victims. Unfortunately, the groups were not divided by age of victimization. Of the assault survivors, 58.6% were experiencing a sexual dysfunction, as opposed to 17.2% of the nonassaulted women. The sexual dysfunctions were divided into four types: early response cycle inhibiting problems (fear of sex, arousal dysfunction, or desire dysfunction), orgasmic problems, intromission problems, and other sexual problems. The vast majority of the dysfunctions (88.2%) occurred in the first category, with over 50% of the survivors reporting each of the three types of early response cycle problems. The sexual assault survivors reported other sexual problems, the predominant one being the experience of flashbacks during sexual activity. The consequences of the assault had lasted as long as 40 years for some victims. A comprehensive theory would need to explain why approximately 40% of the survivors reported no sexual dysfunctions whereas others had sexual dysfunctions that lasted four decades.

Jackson, Calhoun, Amick, Maddever, and Habif (1990) found results similar to Becker et al. in a sample of young adults who had been incest victims before the age of 18. Of the 22 incest survivors, 65% met the criteria for one or more sexual dysfunctions, with 50% of those reporting inhibited desire. The sexual abuse group reported becoming interested in sex at an earlier age than the matched comparison subjects.

Briere (1988) and Briere and Runtz (1989) reported on the symptoms of 195 women who presented at a crisis clinic, 133 of whom had a history of sexual abuse. Briere found that more severe adult problems were associated with extended abuse, involving bizarre sexual acts, with multiple perpetrators and concomitant physical abuse. Briere and Runtz compared the symptoms of the women with and without a history of sexual abuse and found that the sexually abused women reported significantly more sexual problems, fear of men, nightmares, anxiety attacks, and drug and alcohol use.

S. R. Gold (in press) compared the sexual

fantasies of women with and without a history of childhood sexual abuse. Women with a history of abuse had more force in their sexual fantasies, had more sexually explicit fantasies, reported beginning to have sexual fantasies at an earlier age, and had more fantasies with the theme of being under someone's control. Women with a history of physical abuse did not differ in their sexual fantasies from women who had no history of physical abuse, so the fantasy results appear to be specific to sexual abuse. Briere and Runtz (1990) also reported that there are unique effects associated with different types of abuse. They compared women with a history of sexual, physical and psychological abuse and found that sexual abuse was uniquely related to maladaptive sexual behavior.

Evident in the research are two patterns of sexual response as a consequence of child sexual abuse. One pattern is to avoid further sexual behavior, and the second pattern is excessive sexual preoccupation or sexual acting out. The variables mediating these two patterns are unknown at this time, but diverse styles of coping with adult sexual traumas such as rape have also been reported (Burt & Katz, 1987). Some people respond to sexual trauma by trying to minimize the risk of further traumatization through avoidance, while others cope by using increased sexual behavior in an attempt to gain a sense of intimacy, a feeling of being loved, and attention. (Bass & Davis, 1988). It is clear that not all victims develop aversions. Research is needed to determine the factors that influence survivors to adopt different sexual lifestyles.

A key question, not addressed by the PTSD or the TDM model, is who will and will not suffer lasting consequences from childhood sexual abuse. Both the PTSD and TDM approaches are more descriptive than theoretical and therefore do not provide any direction for answering the question. The concept of self-focused attention may be the key to the mediation of the effects of childhood sexual abuse. Excessive self-focus is defined as overattention to self-referent and internally generated thoughts, images, and affect (Ingram, 1990).

When a person focuses on the self, the result is a self-evaluative process, in which individuals tend to compare themselves to certain standards. If they see themselves as falling short and are unable to reduce the discrepancy between the self and the standards, negative affect results. When the discrepancy involves something of central importance, such as a loss that can not be denied, it is difficult to stop thinking about it. Excessive self-focus by the victim is hypothesized to be directly related to the intensity of long-term negative effects. It is hypothesized that women who have been sexually abused as children and engage in excessive self-focus are more likely to experience long-term negative consequences than abused women who do not focus on the self excessively.

Excessive self-focus makes the person more attentive to the self as a cause of the abuse, resulting in a self-blaming attributional style that intensifies negative affect (Pyszczynski & Greenberg, 1987). Self-focus results in a relative lack of attention to externally generated information, making it less likely that social support can help the individual cope with the loss. A negative cycle may be established, with greater self-focus leading to more internal attribution, more attention to somatic symptoms, greater loss of self-esteem, a more chronic sense of helplessness, and more distance from others. Self-focus began as an adaptive attempt to work through problems, but when it is rigid and excessive, more problems are created than are resolved.

Applying the concept of excessive self-focus to childhood sexual abuse suggests that abused females will often dwell on their abusive experiences. When thinking about the abusive experience leads to an acceptance of self and a resolution of angry and hurtful feelings, it is a positive step toward recovery (Bass & Davis, 1988). Self-focus becomes excessive when the victim compares herself to "undamaged" females and cannot stop thinking about herself in negative terms. Focusing on her negative qualities increases the tendency to blame herself for the abuse ("I'm a bad person, so it must be my fault"), and the internal focus does not allow her to attend to and incorporate external contradictory information that she is valued and not to blame for the abuse. An internal attributional style for negative events is associated with poorer adjustment for sexual abuse victims (E. R. Gold, 1986; Wolfe et al., 1989). Dwelling on negative experiences also increases the likelihood that these events will intrude on one's stream of consciousness in images, fantasies, and dreams, as in the reexperiencing aspect of the PTSD syndrome. Excessive self-focus leads to negative affect such as anxiety and guilt, which heightens the negative emotions the abused female already feels about her contribution to the abuse. Guilt feelings only serve to increase intrusive preoccupation (Niler & Beck, 1989) and decrease self-esteem. Preoccupied with internal events, the woman has less time and interest in developing positive relationships. Also, the self-focus makes the female more sensitive to internal events, like somatic responses signaling anxiety, that act as reminders of emotional states experienced during the sexual abuse. Thus, when self-focus continues beyond the time when it helps healing, it adds to the problem by creating more negative emotions, intrusive thoughts, somatic preoccupation, and less involvement with external events.

Excessive self-focus is hypothesized to be a mediating variable between childhood sexual abuse and the severity of the consequences of the abuse, although there is no research support at present. Further research should assess the role of self-focus with female survivors to determine which, if any, symptoms are exacerbated by excessive self-focus and whether the consequences are expressed cognitively, emotionally, behaviorally, or somatically.

Male Model of Etiology: Performance Anxiety

Males may develop sexual aversions as a result of the influence of the etiological factors already discussed. Since boys are sexually abused as children at a much lower rate than females (Finkelhor, 1984), childhood sexual

abuse is less likely to be a cause of sexual aversions in men. The sexual socialization of males in our society, with the emphasis on "real men" being successful, aggressive, and not like women (Doyle, 1983), is considered a primary contributor to the development of sexual aversions.

Applying the "real men" definition to male sexuality results in pressure on men to believe that they must always want sex, orchestrate the whole event, make sure their partners are turned on and satisfied, and make it look natural and spontaneous (Zilbergeld, 1978). Anxiety about the ability to perform has been described as the common pathway to male sexual dysfunctions (Masters & Johnson, 1970). Barlow (1986) has developed a model, emphasizing cognitive interference interacting with anxiety, to explain the development of sexual dysfunctions. Barlow's model, plus the concept of heightened self-focus, will be used to describe a model of the etiology of male sexual aversion, particularly secondary aversion.

Barlow and his colleagues conducted a series of studies to assess how anxiety affects sexual arousal and how sexually functional and sexually dysfunctional men differ in the way they cope with anxiety (Abrahamson, Barlow, Sakheim, Beck, & Athanasiou, 1985; Barlow, Sakheim, & Beck, 1983; J. G. Beck & D. H. Barlow, 1986a, 1986b; J. G. Beck, D. H. Barlow, & D. K. Sakheim, 1983; Sakheim, Barlow, Beck, & Abrahamson, 1984). In contrast to the view of Masters and Johnson and Kaplan (1981), that anxiety is central to the development of sexual dysfunction and treatment must reduce the anxiety, Barlow et al. (1983) reported data that anxiety can facilitate sexual arousal. Male subjects threatened with electric shock if they did not show a penile response to an erotic film, produced greater arousal to the film than subjects not threatened with the shock. The threat of shock lead to different consequences when applied to men who were sexually functional and those who were dysfunctional (having erectile disorders). Anxiety (operationally defined as the threat of shock) increased arousal in sexually functional males but decreased arousal in dysfunctional males (Barlow, 1986). When a film showed a highly aroused and sexually demanding female partner, sexually functional males showed increased arousal, but the dysfunctional males showed lowered arousal (J. G. Beck et al., 1983).

Abrahamson et al. (1985) tested whether the suppression of arousal in sexually dysfunctional males was due to some form of distraction. During an erotic film, subjects heard a nonsexual audiotaped distractor simultaneously with the film. Sexually functional males showed significant detumescence during the distraction, but dysfunctional males were not affected by distracting sounds.

Integrating the research findings, Barlow (1986) suggested that the key to understanding the role of anxiety in sexual arousal is the cognitive interpretation of the anxiety. Sexually functional males' sexual arousal was decreased by tasks that compete with the processing of erotic stimuli but was enhanced by cognitive states related to sexual performance. When watching an aroused and sexually demanding female, the functional males focused on the erotic cues; when threatened with shock, they focused on the somatic elements (e.g., increased heartrate) that are common to sexual arousal. Dysfunctional males responded to implicit or explicit demands for sexual performance with decreased arousal; their cognitive focus was on thoughts of failure and partner frustration. When the distracting stimuli were not related to sexual performance, there was no effect on sexual arousal, because the distraction took the dysfunctional males' attention away from the self-focus on performance anxiety. Dysfunctional men focused on the self at the cost of distracting themselves from erotic thoughts and fantasies and from possible emotional involvement with the partner (J. G. Beck & D. H. Barlow, 1986b).

The development of secondary sexual aversion disorders in males can be understood in terms of Barlow's (1986) cognitive model and the concept of self-focus. With cultural and self-imposed pressure to be "sexual super-men," many men feel anxiety about their sexual performance. If performance anxiety is superimposed on a male who is biologically predisposed to hyperactivity and sensitive to criticism and rejection, the groundwork for an aversion disorder might be present. Concerned about his performance and the risks involved in sexual failure, the aversion-prone male dwells on his performance, which distracts from the erotic experience. In addition, he tends to compare himself to an idealized, highly successful sexual standard and feels inadequate. The inability to reduce the discrepancy between the standard and his view of his own performance results in excessive self-focus and negative affect. The negative affect stimulated by self-focus, coupled with the low threshold for a panic or anxiety response and the tendency to misinterpret somatic changes as a sign of impending disaster, results in high levels of anticipatory anxiety about approaching new sexual situations. Avoidance of all sexual situations, and perhaps panic when confronted with sex, ensues, and an aversion disorder develops.

The development of a primary sexual aversion disorder is expected to follow a divergent pattern. The psychosexual history of primary aversion disorders is characterized by strict moral or religious upbringing, negative messages from parents about sexuality, and an absence of sexual exploration during childhood and adolescence (Crenshaw, 1985; Kaplan, 1987). Males with a primary sexual aversion disorder are likely to have other sexual dysfunctions, such as low sexual desire or erectile disorders, because they have never been comfortable enough with their sexuality to develop sexual confidence or sexual skills.

Barlow's model has been helpful in explaining male sexual dysfunctions, particularly erectile disorders, by expanding our understanding of the role of anxiety. Applying Barlow's model and the concept of excessive self-focus to sexual aversion disorders may similarly add to the knowledge base and suggest more effective treatment strategies for males.

ASSESSMENT OF SEXUAL AVERSION DISORDERS

It is important for clinicians to assess clients for the presence of a sexual aversion, because the aversion must be treated before other sexual dysfunctions can be successfully addressed. To teach ejaculatory control to a premature ejaculator who panics at the thought of any sexual contact with a partner is to work on the wrong end of the problem.

Assessment of sexual aversion disorders is difficult, because many clients are not aware of their aversion or prefer to deny it, and because there are no standard methods of assessment. The key to successful assessment is identifying the stimulus for the anxiety response. There are two relevant self-report measures that may be helpful in the assessment process: the Sex Anxiety Inventory (SAI) (Janda & O'Grady, 1980) and the Sexual Aversion Scale (SAS) (Katz, Gipson, Kearl, & Kriskovich, 1989). The SAI has test-retest reliability of .84 for females and .85 for males with a 10 to 14 day time interval and .86 internal consistency using the Kuder-Richardson formula (Janda & O'Grady, 1980). The SAS has a coefficient alpha of .85 (Katz et al., 1989). Although both scales appear to be psychometrically sound, neither is sufficient for the diagnosis of sexual aversions at present, because their efficacy has yet to be tested with a clinical population.

The SAI measures anxiety and worry about a range of sexual situations such as masturbation, making sexual advances, and telling dirty jokes. It does not assess the intense phobic response and avoidance associated with sexual aversions. The SAS was designed to measure the DSM-III-R category of sexual aversions. Examination of the item content suggests that the SAS taps some fears that are often entirely appropriate to the situation, such as fear of catching AIDS or fear of becoming pregnant. It does however, ask about avoiding sexual situations and the need for help with a sexual problem. Therefore, it is suggested that the SAS be used as a preliminary screening device to help pinpoint the specific fear underlying the aversion and to identify clients who need a more thorough evaluation for sexual aversion disorder.

The more thorough evaluation should include interviews to obtain a complete sex history. Certainly, this is true for all sexual dysfunctions, but to diagnose a sexual aversion, the factors unique to or frequently associated with the disorder (discussed in the section on etiology) must be assessed. This includes a history of childhood sexual abuse, separation anxiety, heightened sensitivity to criticism and rejection, panic attacks, panic disorder in the family, a strong need for control, a tendency to dwell on problems, and self-blame and excessive concerns about sexual performance. The relationship issues to be most sensitive to are a need for unusual levels of closeness or distance in order to be sexual, intense anger or lack of attraction for the partner, a desire to end all sexual encounters as quickly as possible, and a very narrow sexual comfort zone (as evidenced by a preference for sameness in all sexual encounters, with an unwillingness to try new experiences).

Phobias should be distinguished from other reasons people may have for avoiding sex, such as inhibited sexual desire in cases where there is no interest or pleasure from sex but not the fear present with a phobia. Similarly, relationship problems and performance worries can lead to avoidance that does not constitute a sexual aversion disorder. Sexual encounters that result in physical pain or discomfort are likely to be avoided even by people who have no aversion to sex.

TREATMENT APPROACHES TO SEXUAL AVERSION

To treat sexual aversion disorders adequately, we recommend an integrated approach using biological, cognitive, behavioral, and interpersonal approaches, because anxiety, the common core of sexual aversions, is expressed in all modalities (Barlow, 1986). For individual clients, the mix and priority of presentation of these approaches will vary and should be tailored to the etiology of the client's disorder.

Biological

The client should be evaluated for the use of antidepressants to decrease anxiety. According to Kaplan (1987), there is evidence for a biological predisposition to anxiety, and Ballenger (1989) implicates the noradrenergic system, especially the locus ceruleus (LC), as being hyperactive. Medications, including tricyclic antidepressants, MAO inhibitors, and benzodiazepines, reduce the firing rate of the LC and are often helpful in suppressing the panic response. Kaplan et al. (1982) recommend that for simple phobias, benzodiazapines should be reserved for treatment of refractory patients. In any case, medication should not be introduced unless it is determined that the phobic response is so strong that it interferes with the client's ability to respond to other psychological treatment. For example, in utilizing systematic desensitization to help a client with a fear of being nude with her partner, if the client begins to hyperventilate when she takes the first step, such as imagining looking at her own body while alone, the therapist should then collaborate with the client to find a less threatening stimulus. If there is no imagined stimulus within the fear hierarchy that the client can tolerate, medication might help to reduce the somatic symptoms temporarily, until she begins to have some success with the therapy.

Cognitive

Characteristically, the thinking of persons with panic disorder is one of catastrophe—that the bodily sensations they experience portend a situation that could destroy them or drive them insane. Whatever triggers the response, the reaction is the same: a desire to flee. Often these clients are not aware of the cognitive trigger. If so, a first step in therapy is to help them make a connection (LoPiccolo & Friedman, 1988).

Once they learn that the current panic is connected to an old stimulus, they can begin breaking the connection.

In a recent study, Alford, Beck, Freeman, and Wright (1990) evaluated brief, focused cognitive therapy in the treatment of panic disorder. The subject was taught to identify the physiological symptoms leading to panic attacks and to identify the automatic negative thoughts that were attached to the feelings. Once the feelings and thoughts were identified, the client could begin to reinterpret the situation rationally. The client also learned that it was possible to induce panic-like symptoms even when the environment was safe, further clarifying the difference between the somatic responses and her misinterpretation of the consequences. Alford et al. concluded that cognitive therapy was successful in treating panic disorder. However, results of this type of short-term focused therapy with sexual phobias have not been reported.

Sexual aversion disorders or sexual phobias are more complex than simple phobias, so treatment may be much more involved. For example, following the female model of the etiology of sexual aversion disorder, a common contributing factor is sexual abuse, and Bass and Davis (1988) list 14 separate stages that survivors must complete in order to overcome the abusive trauma. The cognitive aspects of these stages include the recognition of the effects of sexual abuse, the belief that one's memories are valid, the alleviation of guilt, the processing of grief, and resolution of the situation. These stages will be experienced and dealt with differently by victims depending on the impact of the trauma, but clearly these stages are too complex to be completed in short-term cognitive restructuring. However, the first steps (identifying and reinterpreting the cognitive triggers) can be dealt with in short-term therapy, provided there is sufficient support for the client, who may then be free to experience the more severe symptoms that had been repressed prior to therapy. The combined PTSD and TDM model of childhood, sexual abuse suggests that anxiety, fear of others, an impaired sense of self-efficacy, and a distorted view of sexuality are issues to be addressed by cognitive therapeutic approaches.

Finally, following the female model of etiology, the issue of excessive self-focus should be addressed. Cognitive restructuring should be aimed at reevaluating the negative thoughts about the self, eliminating the discrepancy between the self and excessively high standards, and reducing the preoccupation with somatic responses. The client should also learn to incorporate externally generated information that can help her break the negative attributional style.

The male model of etiology is based primarily on performance anxiety. In this model, cognitive therapy can be beneficial in helping the client reevaluate his standards for what "real men" should accomplish sexually and in helping him reinterpret the negative statements that he attributes to his partner. Cognitive therapy can assist him in rephrasing some of his thoughts, such as "I have to perform . . ." into "It would be nice to do this, but it is not a disaster if it doesn't happen." As with the female model, cognitive therapy can also produce a reinterpretation of the anxiety symptoms and the catastrophic thinking about what those somatic symptoms might portend. In a more psychodynamic direction, cognitive therapy can help the male deal with his hypersensitivity to criticism and rejection, by looking at the familial antecedents of his reactivity.

Behavioral

Behavioral techniques are among those most commonly used in the treatment of phobias and sexual disorders. There is evidence that behavioral strategies, such as exposure-based therapies, may be superior to psychodynamic treatment in providing stable, long-lasting relief from symptoms because the behavioral techniques provide mastery skills (Hoffart & Martinsen, 1990). Many of the behavioral techniques are no longer used alone but are recommended in conjunction with other therapeutic interventions. Barlow, Craske, Cerny, and Klosko (1989) found that behavioral treatment can be effective in treating panic attacks instead of prescribing

drugs. Barlow et al. (1989) had four treatment conditions: a waiting list (no treatment) condition; progressive muscle relaxation; exposure and cognitive restructuring; and a combination of the relaxation and cognitive restructuring techniques. They found that the exposure/cognitive and combined techniques groups had the highest rate of reduction in panic attacks following treatment.

Wells (1990) found that the use of relaxation training was counterproductive to the treatment of certain panic disorders when the focus of the relaxation was internal. In fact, he found that because relaxation procedures often increase the client's self-focus, this focus can lead to subsequent greater preoccupation with somatic symptoms and may cause relaxation-induced anxiety (RIA). However, when patients were trained to attend to external stimuli (such as specific sounds) in the room, anxiety was reduced. Therefore, clients with sexual aversions may be prone to RIA when relaxation-based treatments increase self-focus by using internal directions. Careful monitoring of clients with sexual aversions is needed to ensure that RIA does not occur.

Interpersonal

When the underlying fear has an interpersonal component, couples therapy will often be necessary (assuming there is a partner). For example, in the case of Frieda, her dependency needs and fear of abandonment are central to her sexual problems. Frieda could benefit from behavioral and cognitive approaches to decrease her anxiety level and somatic preoccupation, but her unrealistic demands on her husband and the anger generated by his failure to meet them requires a conjoint approach. Understanding the basis of the fear will help Frieda separate her past and present feelings and help her husband be more empathic when he recognizes the basis of Frieda's fears in biological factors and her family of origin.

Kaplan (1987) states that the involvement of the partner is necessary in treating sexual dysfunctions. The partner often needs to have an understanding of the rationale for sexual home-work assignments if he or she is to be support-ive. Because the identified client may suffer from separation anxiety, the partner must be careful not to imply rejection during sexual en-counters. Also, the partner may feel threatened when the client changes their sexual behavior, so partner involvement in therapy could allay these fears.

Finally, it is important to recognize that, al-though one partner may display the sexual aver-sion disorder, both partners have some respon-sibility for its maintenance. Couples develop patterns of interactions that are difficult to alter; there is a tendency to maintain a familiar pattern even if dysfunctional. For this reason, the "healthy" partner may unwittingly contribute to the continuation of the sexual phobia, because the pattern is less threatening than change. When the client begins to try new behaviors, the partner may make an effort to change back—to behave in the old, familiar way. For therapy to be successful, both partners must learn to recog-nize their dance of intimacy and be guided to learn new healthy steps (Lerner, 1989).

Integrated Models of Therapy

The last step in the discussion of treatment ap-proaches is to describe two integrated models, which deal with the phobic aspects of the disor-der as well as the sexual dysfunction. LoPiccolo and Friedman (1988) offer an integrated model for therapy of sexual dysfunctions, consisting of four elements: experiential/sensory awareness, insight, cognitive restructuring, and behavioral interventions. It is their hypothesis that patients need to be able not only to identify their negative feelings but also to recognize the early stages and progressive nature of the feelings. There-fore, patients should be taught to attend to bo-dily cues, to recognize stages of responses, and to label the accompanying feelings. Techniques recommended include exercises from Gestalt, sensate focus, fantasy training, and guided fan-tasy. In addition, patients should be encouraged to understand and take responsibility for their behavior and to recognize that change is possi-ble. At this stage of treatment the partner is an important part of the process, in that the couple is learning how both of them are responsible for the maintenance of the dysfunctional behaviors. Cognitive restructuring is also recommended, to alter irrational beliefs and to reinterpret the earlier misinterpretations of somatic responses. Finally, LoPiccolo and Friedman (1988) re-commend behavioral interventions. These tech-niques may include *in vivo* desensitization, as-sertiveness training, communication training, skill training in negotiation, body massage, bib-liotherapy, desire checklist or desire diary, and educational films.

Ballenger's (1989) integrated model of treat-ment is similar. However, it incorporates the psychodynamic model, and his intervention is conceptualized as calming a multimodal hyper-sensitivity. Medication calms the central ner-vous system; cognitive restructuring calms the catastrophic thinking; behavior therapy leads to desensitization of the overactive system; and dynamic therapy introjects and internal object that has a calming, self-regulatory effect.

Outcome Studies

It would be nice to conclude this chapter with a review of outcome studies on the treatment of sexual aversion, but only one outcome study mentioning sexual aversions could be found in the literature. Schover and LoPiccolo (1982), using archival data but no control groups, re-ported on 747 couples treated for sexual desire dysfunctions between 1974 and 1981. Sex ther-apy resulted in significant gains, which were maintained at follow-up, and treatment was equally successful for low-desire and sexual aversion disorders. One exception to the equal effectiveness outcome was that when the pre-senting complaint was female aversion to sex, a temporary worsening of symptoms at three-month follow-up was noted, which was not true for couples with low sexual desire.

The effectiveness of treatment for sexual aversion disorders is open to speculation. It is expected to be very successful for sexual av-ersions with no concomitant sexual dysfunctions (80–85%) and relatively less successful when coexisting with other sexual problems (60–70%). These estimates are based on the success of treatment for phobias and panic disorders (relatively discrete problems), and there is likely to be a dropoff in effectiveness as problems become more complex.

Before estimates about treatment outcome can be tested, more clinicians must develop an awareness of the hidden nature of sexual aversions and become skilled at probing clients who have sexual dysfunctions for the presence of a sexual phobia. We hope this chapter will be a step in that process.

REFERENCES

Abrahamson, D. J., Barlow, D. H., Sakheim, D. K., Beck, J. G., & Athanasiou, R. (1985). Effects of distraction on sexual responding in functional and dysfunctional men. *Behavior Therapy, 16,* 503–515.

Alford, B. A., Beck, A. T., Freeman, A., & Wright, F. D. (1990). Brief focused cognitive therapy of panic disorder. *Psychotherapy, 27,* 230–234.

American Psychiatric Association. (1980). *Diagnostic and statistical manual of mental disorders* (3rd ed.). Wasington, DC: Author.

American Psychiatric Association. (1987). *Diagnostic and statistical manual of mental disorders* (3rd ed., rev.). Washington, DC: Author.

Ballenger, J. C. (1989). Toward an integrated model of panic disorder. *American Journal of Orthopsychiatry, 59,* 284–293.

Barlow, D. H. (1986). Causes of sexual dysfunction: The role of anxiety and cognitive interference. *Journal of Consulting and Clinical Psychology, 54,* 140–148.

Barlow, D. H., Craske, M. G., Cerny, J. A., & Klosko, J. S. (1989). Behavioral treatment of panic disorder. *Behavior Therapy, 20,* 261–282.

Barlow, D. H., Sakheim, D. K., & Beck, J. G. (1983). Anxiety increases sexual arousal. *Journal of Abnormal Psychology, 92,* 49–54.

Bass, E., & Davis, L. (1988). *The courage to heal.* New York: Harper & Row.

Beck, A. T., Emery, G. (1985). *Anxiety disorders and phobias.* New York: Basic Books.

Beck, J. G., & Barlow, D. H. (1986a). The effects of anxiety and attentional focus on sexual responding. I. Physiological patterns in erectile dysfunction. *Behaviour Research and Therapy, 24,* 9–17.

Beck, J. G., & Barlow, D. H. (1986b). The effects of anxiety and attentional focus on sexual responding. II. Cognitive and affective patterns in erectile dysfunctions. *Behaviour Research and Therapy, 24,* 19–26.

Beck, J. G., Barlow, D. H., & Sakheim, D. K. (1983). The effects of attentional focus and partner arousal on sexual responding in functional and dysfunctional men. *Behaviour Research and Therapy, 21,* 1–8.

Becker, J. V., Skinner, L. J., Abel, G. G., & Cichon, J. (1986). Level of postassault sexual functioning in rape and incest victims. *Archives of Sexual Behavior, 15,* 37–49.

Briere, J. (1988). The long-term clinical correlates of childhood sexual victimization. In R. A. Prentky & V. L. Quinsey (Eds.), *Human sexual aggression* (pp. 327–334). New York: New York Academy of Sciences.

Briere, J., & Runtz, M. (1989). The Trauma Symptom Checklist (TSC-33): Early data on a new scale. *Journal of Interpersonal Violence, 4,* 151–163.

Briere, J., & Runtz, M. (1990). Differential adult symptomatology associated with three types of child abuse history. *Child Abuse & Neglect, 14,* 357–364.

Browne, A., & Finkelhor, D. (1986). Impact of child sexual abuse: A review of the research. *Psychological Bulletin, 99,* 66–77.

Burt, M. R., & Katz, B. L. (1987). Dimensions of recovery from rape: Focus on growth outcomes. *Journal of Interpersonal Violence, 2,* 57–81.

Crenshaw, T. L. (1985). The sexual aversion syndrome. *Journal of Sex & Marital Therapy, 11,* 285–292.

Deblinger, E., McLeer, S. V., Atkins, M. S., Ralphe, D., & Foa, E. (1989). Post-traumatic stress in sexually abused, physically abused, and nonabused children. *Child Abuse & Neglect, 13,* 403–408.

Donnell, C. D., & McNally, R. J. (1990). Anxiety sensitivity and panic attacks in a nonclinical population. *Behaviour Research and Therapy, 28,* 83–85.

Doyle, J. A. (1983). *The male experience.* Dubuque, IA: William C. Brown.

Finkelhor, D. (1984). *Child sexual abuse: New theory and research.* New York: Free Press.

Finkelhor, D., & Browne, A. (1985). The traumatic impact of child sexual abuse: A conceptualization. *American Journal of Orthopsychiatry, 55,* 530–541.

Gold, E. R. (1986). The effects of sexual victimization in childhood: An attributional approach. *Journal of Consulting and Clinical Psychology, 54,* 471–475.

Gold, S. R. (In press). History of child sexual abuse and adult sexual fantasies. *Violence and Victims.*

Goldston, D. B., Turnquist, D. C., & Knutson, J. F. (1989). Presenting problems of sexually abused girls receiving psychiatric services. *Journal of Abnormal Psychology, 98,* 314–317.

Hoffart, A., & Martinsen, E. W. (1990). Exposure-based integrated vs. pure psychodynamic treatment of agoraphobic patients. *Psychotherapy, 27,* 210–218.

Ingram, R. E. (1990). Self-focused attention in clinical disorders: Review and a conceptual model. *Psychological Bulletin, 107,* 156–176.

Jackson, J. L., Calhoun, K. S., Amick, A. A., Maddever, H. M., & Habif, V. L. (1990). Young adult women who report childhood intrafamilial sexual abuse: Subsequent adjustment. *Archives of Sexual Behavior, 19,* 211–221.

Janda, L. H., & O'Grady, K. E. (1980). Development of a sex anxiety inventory. *Journal of Consulting and Clinical Psychology, 48,* 169–175.

Jones, J. C., & Barlow, D. H. (1990). The etiology of posttraumatic stress disorder. *Clinical Psychology Review, 10,* 299–328.

Kaplan, H. S. (1981). *The new sex therapy: Active treatment of sexual dysfunctions.* New York: Brunner/Mazel.

Kaplan, H. S. (Ed.). (1987). *Sexual aversion, sexual phobias, and panic disorder.* New York: Brunner/Mazel.

Kaplan, H. S. (1988). Intimacy disorders and sexual panic states. *Journal of Sex & Marital Therapy, 14,* 3–12.

Kaplan, H. S., Fyer, A. J., & Novick, A. (1982). The treatment of sexual phobias: The combined use of antipanic medication and sex therapy. *Journal of Sex & Marital Therapy, 8,* 3–28.

Katz, R. C., Gipson, M. T., Kearl, A., & Kriskovich, M. (1989). Assessing sexual aversion in college students: The Sexual Aversion Scale. *Journal of Sex & Marital Therapy, 15,* 135–140.

Klein, D. F. (1964). Delineation of two drug-responsive anxiety syndromes. *Psychopharmotherapy, 5,* 397–408.

Knopf, J., & Seiler, M. (1990). *Inhibited sexual desire.* New York: Morrow.

Kolko, D. J., Moser, J. T., & Weldy, S. R. (1988). Behavioral/emotional indicators of sexual abuse in child psychiatric inpatients: A controlled comparison with physical abuse. *Child Abuse & Neglect, 12,* 529–541.

Koss, M. P., & Burkhart, B. R. (1989). A conceptual analysis of rape victimization: Long-term effects and implications for treatment. *Psychology of Women Quarterly, 13,* 27–40.

Lerner, H. G. (1989). *The dance of intimacy.* New York: Harper & Row.

Lindberg, F. H., & Distad, L. J. (1985). Post-traumatic stress disorders in women who experienced childhood incest. *Child Abuse & Neglect, 9,* 329–334.

LoPiccolo, J., & Friedman, J. M. (1988). Broad spectrum treatment of low sexual desire: Integration of cognitive, behavioral, and systematic therapy. In S. R. Leiblum & R. C. Rosen (Eds.), *Sexual desire disorders* (pp. 107–144). New York: Guilford.

Masters, W. H., & Johnson, V. (1970). *Human sexual inadequacy.* Boston: Little, Brown.

Niler, E. R., & Beck, S. J. (1989). The relationship among guilt, dysphoria, anxiety and obsessions in a normal population. *Behaviour Research and Therapy, 27,* 213–220.

Pyszczynski, T., & Greenberg, J. (1987). Self-regulatory perseveration and the depressive self-focusing style: A self-awareness theory of reactive depression. *Psychological Bulletin, 102,* 122–138.

Sakheim, D. K., Barlow, D. H., Beck, J. G., & Abrahamson, D. J. (1984). The effect of an increased awareness of erectile cues on sexual arousal. *Behaviour Research and Therapy, 22,* 151–158.

Schover, L. R., Friedman, J. M., Weiler, S. J., Heiman, J. R., & LoPiccolo, J. (1982). Multiaxial problem-oriented system for sexual dysfunctions. *Archives of General Psychiatry, 39,* 614–619.

Schover, L. R., & LoPiccolo, J. (1982). Treatment effectiveness for dysfunctions of sexual desire. *Journal of Sex & Marital Therapy, 8,* 179–197.

Simon & Schuster (Ed.). (1979). *Webster's new twentieth century dictionary.* New York: Author.

Spector, I. P., & Carey, M. P. (1990). Incidence and prevalence of the sexual dysfunctions: A critical review of the empirical literature. *Archives of Sexual Behavior, 19,* 389–408.

Wells, A. (1990). Panic disorder in association with relaxation induced anxiety: An attentional training approach to treatment. *Behavior Therapy, 21,* 273–280.

Wolfe, V. V., Gentile, C., & Wolfe, D. A. (1989). The impact of sexual abuse on children: A PTSD formulation. *Behavior Therapy, 20,* 215–228.

Zilbergeld, B. (1978). *Male Sexuality.* New York: Bantam.

CHAPTER 5

MEDICAL ASPECTS OF SEXUAL AROUSAL DISORDERS

Benjamin Graber, Omaha, Nebraska

This area of sexual dysfunction is not a particularly easy one for taxonimists. In the DSM-III-R (American Psychiatric Association, 1987), sexual arousal disorders (SADs) are included as a subclassification of sexual disorders, labeled sexual dysfunction disorders. The sexual dysfunction disorders are directly linked to Masters and Johnson's (1966) description of human sexual response and are thus described as an "inhibition in the appetitive or psychophysiological changes that characterize the complete sexual response cycle" (APA, 1987, p. 290). The sex response cycle as modified by Kaplan (1983) includes four phases (appetitive, excitement, orgasm, and resolution); the SADs are dysfunctions in the excitement phase. There are two SAD entities: male erectile disorder (MED) and female sexual arousal disorder (FSAD).

MED involves problems in the process of tumescence/erection; it is commonly called *impotence*. For FSAD, the criteria refer to the "lubrication-swelling response" of the female sexual excitement phase. As I have pointed out in the past, the diagnostic criteria for MED lack specificity (Graber & Kline-Graber, 1981). Even in the context of screening tests in a vascular laboratory, Kempczinski (1979) reported that "the distinction between potency and impotence was not always clear" (p. 278). He noted that 38% of patients classified as potent had experienced decreased erectile function with aging or had had intermittent bouts of impotence, and 18% of the "impotent" patients "were occasionally" capable of both achieving and maintaining erections.

FSAD has not often been specified in the literature as a sexual dysfunction. With women, more attention has been directed toward the desire disorders and the orgasm disorders.

ANATOMY AND PHYSIOLOGY

Male

In the male, the genital site of tumescence is the penis. The penis is divided into an attached portion labeled the *radix* or root, which lies in the perineum, and a free pendulous portion called the *corpus* or body. The internal structure of the penis consists of three cylinders. There are two paired bodies known as the *corpora cavernosa* (CCP). They constitute the dorsal and lateral parts of the penis. On the ventral surface of the penis is the unpaired corpus spongiosum (CSP), which is traversed by the urethra. At the distal end of the penis, the CSP expands into the glans penis. The glans is covered by the prepuce in the uncircumcised male. At the tip of the glans is the external urethral orifice. The glans fits like a hood over the paired corpora cavernosa. The bulb of the penis is the conical enlargement of the proximal 4 or 5 cm of the CSP, which is attached in the perineum to the urogenital diaphragm. It is enclosed by the fibers of the bulbocavernosus muscle. The CCP separate into two crura attached to the pubic arch and covered by the ischiocavernosus muscles (Gray, 1985; Williams & Warwick, 1980).

Blood Supply

The internal iliac (hypogastric) arteries (see Figure 5.1) supply the internal pudendal artery, through which the perineal artery supplies the superficial structures of the urogenital dia-

phragm and the ischiocavernosus and bulbocavernosus muscles. In the male the internal pudendal artery continues as the artery of the penis, giving off two branches—the bulbar artery (BAP) and the urethral artery (UAP). The BAP supplies the bulb of the penis, the posterior one-third of the CSP, the urethral mucosa, and the bulbourethral glands. The UAP supplies CSP. The artery then divides into the cavernous artery and the dorsal artery of the penis. The cavernous arteries of the penis enter the crura of the penis bilaterally and travel in the center of the CCP. The dorsal artery of the penis runs on the dorsum of the penis and supplies the glans and the skin of the penis (Lierse, 1982; Lue et al., 1986; Lue & Tanagho, 1988b; Williams & Warwick, 1980).

The deep dorsal veins (DDVP) (Figure 5.2), which can be seen either as a single vessel or an anastomosing net, receive blood from the convoluted veins of the glans by the circumflex veins of the corpora spongiosa and via the venae emissariae of the corpus cavernosum (Figure 5.3). These consist of thin-walled passages through the tunica albuginea that collect blood from the peripheral parts of the erectile tissue. Communication to the superficial dorsal vein (SDVP) also exists. The superficial dorsal vein

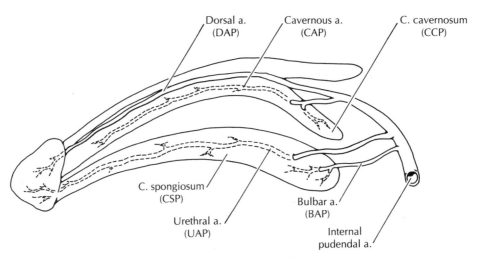

Figure 5.1. Penile arterial supply (modified from Lue & Tanagho, 1988b, Figure 2.1).

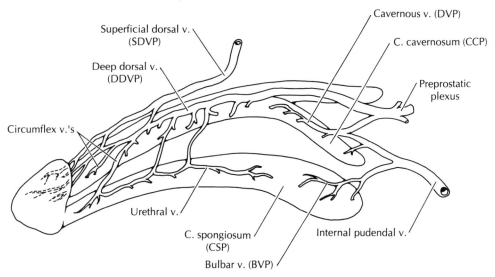

Figure 5.2. Penile venous return (modified from Lue & Tanagho, 1988b, Figure 2.2).

receives branches from the prepuce and penile skin and empties into the saphenous and femoral veins. The deep dorsal vein (DDVP) empties into the lower prostatic venous plexus (IEVP). Blood from the central area of the CCP is drained into the deep (or profunda) vein through short postcavernous veins, which collect blood from the intracavernous spaces and from the capillaries in the cavernous tissue and drain to the prostatic venous plexus. The CSP similarly drains into the bulbar vein (Conti, 1952; Lierse,

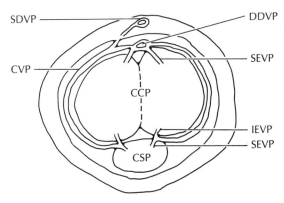

Figure 5.3. Penile intravenous circulation (modified from Newman, 1983, Figure 1).

1982; Lue et al., 1986; Lue & Tanagho, 1988b; Wagner, 1981a).

CCP/CSP Structure and Function

The CCP (Figure 5.4) is described as a sponge-like mesh of endothelium-lined sinusoids and a fibromuscular interstitium, all surrounded by a dense, nonstretchable fibrous tunica albuginea that fluctuates in thickness from 2–3 mm in the flaccid state to 0.5 mm in the erect state (Conti, 1952). The CCP are separated in the pendulous portion of the penis by an incomplete porous and fibrous septum that permits free communication between the two corpora, allowing the CCP to function as one unit. In the flaccid penis, the CCP are empty and collapsed. During erection the CCP increases in diameter or thickness more than in length (Gray, 1985; Lierse, 1982). The tunica albuginea of the CSP is thinner (0.2mm) than in the CCP and contains more elastic fibers. The trabeculae are more delicate, and the cavernous spaces are smaller than in the CCP (Conti, 1952; Gray, 1985; Lierse, 1982). In the flaccid penis the inner spaces of the CSP are always somewhat filled; during erection, the CSP increases in bulk only in the region of the

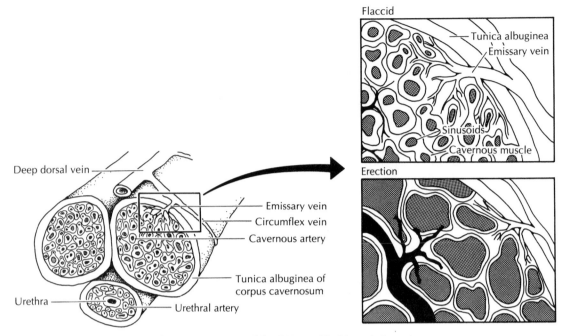

Figure 5.4. Structure of the CCP (modified from deGroat & Steers, 1988, Figure 7-11).

bulb. The increase in the CSP is greater in length than in thickness. The glans has almost no tunica albuginea and little fibrous tissue between the sinusoids, and the epidermis and the overlying skin is thinner and more firmly adherent. While always remaining "soft and yielding," the glans enlarges in all directions during erection (Dickinson, 1949).

Conti's (1952) theories of tumescence and erection, based on his study and interpretation of penile angioarchitecture, have been the subject of much discussion. As recently as 1988, Benson (1988) rejected Conti's major contentions, while Conti (Conti & Virag, 1989) not only defended his position but provided what he reported to be additional anatomical evidence. Two major areas of controversy surround the existence and function of various arterial blockage devices and shunting mechanisms, including arteriovenous anastomoses—direct arterial-venous connections (Lue & Tanagho, 1988a; Newman, 1983; Siroky & Krane, 1983; Wagner, 1981). Various intracavernous anastomoses and shunts have been described (Conti,

1952; Conti & Virag, 1989; Wagner, 1985), including the helicine arteries, which empty directly into the cavernous cavities and are different from the nutritive arterial branches in the CCP, which are found in the trabeculae. The mechanism for restriction of venous outflow required to obtain and maintain an erection also continues to provoke discussion. The juxtaposition of the veins and their passage through the fascial planes (Figure 5.4) most likely play an important role in the hemodynamics of erection (Delcour & Struyven, 1988; Lue & Tanagho, 1988b; Lue & Tanagho, 1988a; Sidi, Koleilat, & Fraley, 1988).

An important step in the understanding of hemodynamics was the induction of the "artificial erection" by Newman, Northup, and Devlin (1964). They used a peristaltic pump to perfuse one corpus of the CCP and measured flow rate through a separate line to the other corpus. At rates of less than 20ml/min, they induced only slight to moderate tumescence. Perfusion of 20–50 ml/min induced an erection, which could be maintained by a rate of 12 ml/min. The perfusion technique has been used to examine the relationship between actual cavernous pressure and penile circumference. This relationship changes during filling due to the relative distensibility of the CCP. The design of the CCP allows for some increase in circumference as pressure increases, but its finite distensibility, due to the lower number of elastic fibers in its composition, is the key factor causing the intracavernous pressure to increase dramatically after the maximum penile circumference is attained. Once the CCP is completely stretched and rigidity occurs, tumescence has proceeded to erection. Wespes and Schulman (1984) have explained a potentially confusing result of the perfusion technique: the lower flow rates neces-

sary to maintain an erection than are necessary to induce it initially. The sinusoids or cavernous spaces of the CCP are elliptical in the flaccid penis and become more circular as tumescence leads to erection. An ellipse has a smaller surface area than a circle of the same perimeter. Thus, a circle with the same perimeter as an ellipse and identical pressure gradients will have 41% less flow.

Innervation

The penis is innervated by both somatic and autonomic nerves (Figure 5.5). The receptors of the glans penis have been extensively studied in

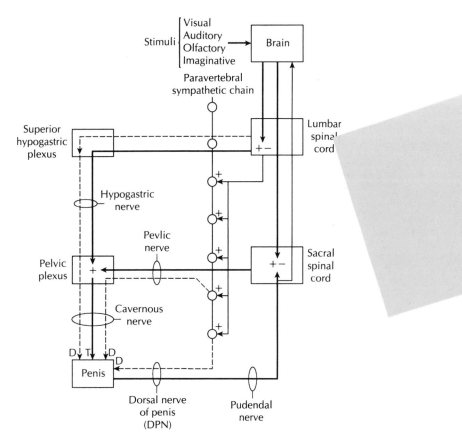

Figure 5.5. Innervation of the penis (modified from deGroat & Steers, 1988, Figure 1.2). D, penile detumescence; T, penile tumescence; synaptic excitatory and inhibitory mechanisms are represented by + and −, respectively.

an attempt to discover any uniqueness as compared to other cutaneous regions (Calaresu & Mitchell, 1969; Campbell, Good, & Kitchell, 1954; Cottrell, Iggo, & Kitchell, 1978; Johnson, Kitchell, & Gilanpour, 1986; Lavoisier, 1982). The somatic innervation is through the pudendal nerve, which arises from the S2 through S4 segment of the spinal cord and is a mixed sensory and motor nerve. The dorsal penile nerve (DPN) carries sensation from the penile skin, prepuce, and glans through the sensory branch of the pudendal. Lesions to the DPN have been shown not to impair erections in cats (Aronson & Cooper, 1967; 1968) or monkeys (Herbert, 1973), but they may do so in rats (Larsson & Sodersten, 1973) and humans (Goldstein, 1988). The efferent fibers of the pudendal nerve innervate the striated musculature of the perineum and pelvis and originate in Onuf's nucleus in the sacral cord in close proximity to autonomic nuclei involved in sexual functioning (Chung, McVary, & McKenna, 1988; deGroat & Booth, 1980; McKenna & Nadelhaft, 1985, 1986) (see Figure 5.6). The autonomic innervation of the

penis includes both sympathetic and parasympathetic fibers. Some sympathetic fibers from T10–L2 segments of the spinal cord form the hypogastric nerve, which joins with the pelvic plexus lateral to the rectum. Other sympathetic preganglionic fibers to the penis arise in the intermediolateral grey of the thoracolumbar cord (Learmonth, 1931; Mitchell, 1953) and synapse in the paravertebral chain ganglia (Booth, Roppolo, & deGroat, 1986). These sympathetic postganglionic axons travel in the pelvic, pudendal, and cavernous nerves (Hulsebosch & Coggeshall, 1982; Kuo, Hisamitsu & deGroat, 1984; Langley & Anderson, 1895). The pelvic plexus lateral to the rectum also contains the parasympathetic nerves arising from S2–S4. The sacral preganglionic fibers to the pelvic plexus are called the *pelvic nerves* or *nervi erigentes* (deGroat & Steers, 1988). The pelvic plexus is a relay point and integration center containing sympathetic and parasympathetic components (Brindley, 1988; Dail, Hamill, & Minorsky, 1986; Hulsebosch & Coggeshall, 1982; Siroky & Krane, 1983a). The autonomic nerve fibers that

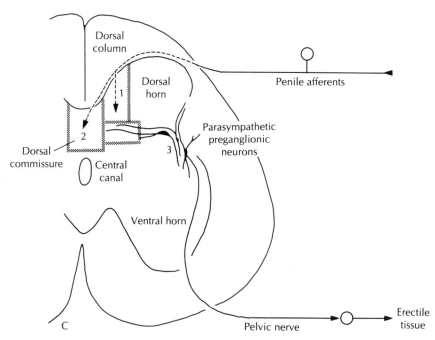

Figure 5.6. Autonomic innervation of the penis (modified from deGroat & Steers, 1988, Figure 1.4).

project to the penis from the pelvic plexus are called the *cavernous nerves*. They travel between the prostatic capsule and the endopelvic fascia and then the lateral surface of the membranous urethra (deGroat & Steers, 1988). One of the most intriguing modern neuroanatomical findings is that the DPN and penile motor neurons originate in the same spinal segments and project to the same laminae in the cord, suggesting a neurobiological structure for somatovisceral integration (see Nunez, Gross, & Sachs, 1986, and Figure 5.6).

Neurophysiological studies have been done on the neurotransmitters involved in these neural pathways. The cholinergic fibers in the sacral parasympathetic pathways were at first the mechanism routinely cited as responsible for erections (Langley & Anderson, 1896), but the role of acetylcholine at neuroeffector junctions in the penis has since come under considerable scrutiny, with conflicting results (Benson, 1988; Newman, 1983; Newman, Northup & Devlin, 1964; Semans & Langworthy, 1938; Sjostrand & Klinge, 1979). Cholinergic (acetylcholinesterase stain positive) neurons have been found in the trabeculae of the CCP, but their density is not clear (Benson, 1988; McConnell, Benson, & Wood, 1979), and atropine does not block pelvic nerve-induced erections (Dorr & Brody, 1967; Henderson & Roepke, 1933). Many studies have been done concerning adrenergic innervation of erection. Adrenergic nerves have been studied by histochemical techniques; they are found in the smooth muscle of the corpora, in the trabeculae of the CCP, in the walls of the blood vessels within the CCP, and less densely in the CSP (McConnell, Benson, & Wood, 1979; Siroky & Krane, 1983). In the rat, this penile innervation has been found to occur through post ganglionic short adrenergic fibers rather than the traditional long fibers (Dail & Evan, 1974; Siroky & Krane, 1983). A number of neuropeptides (see Table 5.1) have been looked at with regard to a role in the vasodilator pathways of the penis, including vasoactive intestinal peptide (VIP), neuropeptide Y (NPY), substance P, and others (Alm, Alumets, Hakanson, Owman, Sjoberg, Sundler, & Walles, 1980; Carvalho, Hodson, Blank, Watson, Mulderry, Bishop, Gu, Bloom,

& Polak, 1986; deGroat & Steers, 1988; Gu, Lazardes, Pryor, Blank, Polak, Morgan, Marangos, & Bloom, 1984; Hedlund & Andersson, 1985).

The role of neurotransmitters (Table 5.1) has been studied by the use of exogenous pharmacologic agents that have been shown to alter penile hemodynamics. Drugs that "promote" smooth muscle relaxation induce erection (Forleo & Pasini, 1980; Lue & Tanagho, 1987; Virag, 1984; Virag, 1985), and drugs that constrict smooth muscles lead to detumescence. Prostaglandin E1, papaverine, and phentolamine (Forleo & Pasini, 1980; Juenemann, Lue, Luo, Jadallah, Nunes, & Tanagho, 1987; Lue & Tanagho, 1987) are examples of drugs used to induce erection; these will also be discussed in the later sections of this chapter relating to the assessment and treatment of MED.

Many interesting supraspinal neuroanatomical and neurochemical mechanisms have been studied for their role in the erectile mechanism, but because most of these experiments use lesioning and electrical or chemical stimulation techniques, they have mostly been done in nonhuman species (Bertolini, Gessa, Vergoni, & Ferrari, 1968; Blumer, 1970; Caggiula, Antelman, & Zigmond, 1973; Clark, 1975; Dua & Maclean, 1964; Eibergen & Caggiula, 1973; Johnston & Davidson, 1972; Kling, 1972; Kluver, 1958; Kluver & Bucy, 1939; Lisk, 1967; Maclean, 1966, 1989; Maclean & Delgado, 1953; Maclean, Denniston, & Dua, 1963; Maclean, Denniston, Dua, & Ploog, 1962; Maclean, Dua, & Denniston, 1961; Maclean & Ploog, 1962; Meisel, Lumia, & Sachs, 1980; Robinson & Mishkin, 1966; Schwartz & Kling, 1961; Slimp, Hart, & Goy, 1978). For a thorough recent summary, see Sachs and Meisel (1988). From these studies it appears that it is the subcortical-rhinencephalic circuitry, rather than that of the neocortex, that is important in the regulation of male sexual behavior. Heath (Heath, 1954; Heath, John, & Fontana, 1968; Heath & Mickle, 1960; Wagner & Green, 1981), during his controversial depth electrode studies, reported that in mentally ill human patients, stimulation of the septal region or the medial forebrain bundle produced pleasurable sensations and sometimes pe-

Table 5.1. Potential Neurotransmitters in the Penis*

SUBSTANCE	DISTRIBUTION	PHARMACOLOGIC EFFECTS IN VITRO	PHARMACOLOGIC EFFECTS IN VIVO	RELEASE FROM PENILE TISSUE
NE	BV (H,M,D,Rb,Rt) CC (H,M,D,C,Rb,Rt) CS (H,M,C,Rt) RP (B,D,C,Rt)	BV + (H,B,D) CC + (H,M,D,C,GP,Rb) CS + (H,M,D,C,GP,Rb,Rt) RP + (B,D,C) BV − (H)	Art. flow O(H,C,Rb) Ven. flow ↓ (B) Pen. vol. O(D,C) ↓ (H,Rb)	↑ (D)
ACH	BV (H,M) CC (H,M,D,C,Rb,Rt) CS (H) RP (B,D,Rb,Rt)	BV + (B) CC + (H,M,D,C,Rb) − (H,Rb) CS + (M,D,C) RP + (B,D,C,Rt)	Art. flow ↑ (D,Rb) Pen. vol. O(D,C)	↑ (H)
VIP	BV (H,M,D,C,GP,Rb,Rt) CC (H,M,D,C,GP,Rb,Rt) CS (H,M) GP (H,M,C)	BV − (H,B,D) CC − (H,M,D,C,GP,Rb) CS − (C,GP,Rb) RP − (B,D,C)	Art. flow ↑ (D) Ven. flow ↓ (D) Pen. vol. ↑ (H,M,D) ↓ (M)	↑ (H,D)
SP	GP (H)	BV O (H) CC ± (H) CS ± (H,Rb) RP + (B,D)	Art. flow O(D) Ven. flow O(D) Pen. vol. ↑ (D)	↑ (D)
NPY	CC (H) CS (H)	BV O (H) CC O (H) CS O (H)	Pen. vol. ↑ (D)	

*Adapted from deGroat & Steers, 1988, Table 1.1.
Abbreviations: NE, norepinephrine; ACH, acetylcholine; VIP, vasoactive intestinal polypeptide; SP, substance P; NPY, neuropeptide Y, BV, blood vessel; CC, corpus cavernosum; GP, glans penis; CS, corpus spongiosum (or cavernosum urethrae); RP, retractor penis; +, contraction; −, relaxation; O, no effect; ↑, increases; ↓, decreases, Art flow, arterial flow; Ven flow, venous flow; Pen. Vol., penile volume, H, human; B, bull; M, monkey; D, dog; C, cat; GP, guinea pig; Rb, rabbit; Rt, rat.

nile erection. However, Sem-Jacobsen, in more extensive stereotaxic stimulation studies (Heath & Mickle, 1960; Sem-Jacobsen, 1968), elicited sexual sensations in two subjects but not erection. The cerebral cortex in the human does receive input from the afferent pathways of the penis (Woolsey, Marshall, & Bard, 1942), which has led to a number of somatosensory evoked potential studies (Goldstein, 1983; Haldeman, Bradley, & Bhatia, 1982; Haldeman, Bradley, Bhatia, & Johnson, 1982, 1983), which will be discussed later in relation to the assessment techniques for MED.

Summary

From the knowledge currently available it is possible to outline, at least broadly, the underlying processes involved in male erectile function. In the flaccid penis, the smooth muscle of the CCP and the helical arteries are contracted in response to baseline adrenergic tone maintained by the sympathetic nervous system. This results in contracted sinusoidal spaces and a slow arterial flow rate of approximately 10 ml/min into the CCP, resulting in a low intracavernous pressure of only 6–8 mm of Hg. In the flaccid penis, there is unobstructed venous outflow through the emissary and deep dorsal veins. Exteroceptive stimuli (visual, olfactory), resulting in higher CNS activation or viscero-somatic reflex activation of the pelvic nerve, result in neurotransmitter release (acetylcholine, vasoactive intestinal peptide, and possibly others) within the CCP. The neurotransmitters induce smooth muscle relaxation, resulting in sinusoidal and arteriolar dilation, decreasing resistance to arterial blood flow, and thereby increasing blood flow to 50–70 ml/min. The enlarged sinusoidal spaces compress the emissary veins, trapping blood in the CCP and resulting in an intracavernous pressure of 90–100 mm of Hg during full erection. Smooth muscle contraction in the walls and valves of veins may also help trap blood. Erection is probably maintained by repetitive release of neurotransmitters. Detumescence occurs when a baseline level of adrenergic neurotransmitters is reestablished (Jamison & Gebhard, 1988; Jevitch, Khawand, & Vidic, 1990; Lewis, 1988; Lue & Tanagho, 1988a; Reiss, Newman, & Zorgniotte, 1982; Sidi, Koleilat, & Fraley, 1988).

Not covered thus far in this section are the hormonal aspects of male erectile function. This is because although it is clear that androgens are essential for the development of male primary and secondary sexual characteristics and the maintenance of male sexual drive, their specific role in erectile mechanics is less clear (deGroat & Steers, 1988; Hart & Haugen, 1968; Johnston & Davidson, 1972; Sachs & Meisel, 1988; Sar & Stumpf, 1973; Schiavi & White, 1976). Because

the role of androgens has been discussed in this book in the section on the medical aspects of sexual desire disorders (see Chapter 2), they are not elaborated here. They will be discussed briefly in the sections below, covering the assessment and treatment of MED.

Female

In the female, the homologous erectile tissues are distributed in the clitoris and circumvaginally (Figures 5.7 and 5.8). The clitoris lies in the anterior labial commissure formed by the labia majora in the vulva and is partially hidden by the anterior ends of the labia minora, which divide around the clitoris, creating the prepuce above and the frenulum below the clitoris. The cleft between the labia minora and behind the clitoris is the vestibule of the vagina, which contains the external urethral orifice and the vaginal orifice.

The body of the clitoris, like the homologous dorsal penis, consists of two small erectile cav-

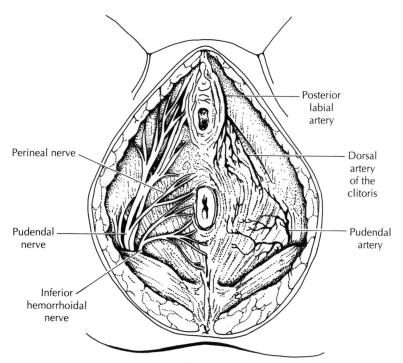

Figure 5.7. Physiological anatomy of the female genitals (modified from Krantz, 1982, Figure 2-12).

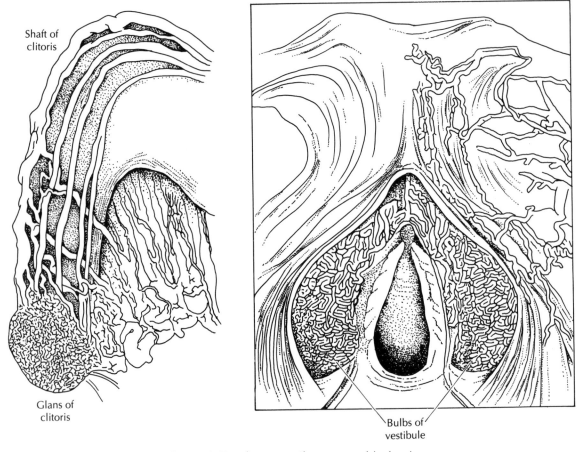

Figure 5.8. Homologous erectile structures of the female
(modified from Dickinson, 1949, Figure 75).

ernous bodies, the crura clitoridis (cf. the CCP of the penis) (Krantz, 1982; Sherfey, 1972). The homologue of the CSP is more diffuse and includes the glans clitorides, the pars intermedia, the vestibular bulbs, and the venous plexi in the walls of the penis. In fact, Kobelt (Lowry, 1978) specifically identifies the vestibular bulbs as the homologue of the bulb of the penis and identifies the widespread venous plexi as the true CSP of the female.

Blood Supply

The blood supply of the vagina (see Figure 5.7) originates superiorly with the uterine artery, which gives off the cervicovaginal artery. On the lateral aspect of the vagina, the vaginal ar-

teries branch to send rami to both the anterior and posterior surfaces. Branches of the internal iliacs, known as the arteriovaginalis, also may supply this region, and when this occurs, the inferior vesical arteries supply the middle half of the vagina. The lower half of the vagina is supplied by the ascending branches of the middle hemorrhoidal arteries which meet to form the azygos artery of the vagina. Also, the urethral branch of the dorsal artery of the clitoris, which originates from the internal pudendal artery, anastomizes with the vaginal branches of the middle hemorrhoidal vessels (Krantz, 1959).

The blood supply of the clitoris is from the dorsal artery of the clitoris, a terminal branch of the internal pudendal artery, itself the terminal division of the posterior portion of the internal iliac. When the dorsal artery enters the clitoris, it divides into the deep and dorsal arteries (and gives off a small branch just before entering the clitoris), which pass posteriorly to supply the external urethral meatus. The venous drainage of the clitoris begins around the corona of the glans and runs along the anterior surface of the clitoris. There it joins the deep vein and continues together with veins from the labia minora, labia majora, and perineum to form the pudendal plexus.

The vagina is drained by a series of venous plexi. In the lower portion of the vagina, the drainage is along the urethra into the dorsal vein of the clitoris, as well as the middle hemorrhoidal venous plexus. The major drainage is through the internal pudendal plexus, terminating in the internal pudendal vein. This vein communicates directly with the hypogastric veins on either side. The upper vaginal venous plexus joins the uterine and cervical veins draining into the hypogastric veins (Krantz, 1959).

Innervation

The innervation of the vagina (Figure 5.7) originates mostly in the plexus uterovaginalis. This plexus is connected to the pelvic plexus. The preganglionic sympathetic nerves of the vagina originate in the thoracolumbar cord and run through the inferior mesenteric through the superior hypogastric ganglion to reach the pelvic plexus. The preganglionic parasympathetic fibers originate in the second through fourth sacral segments (the first is rarely involved, and the fifth more often is). The sensory supply from the vestibule is carried in the pudendal nerve, which also enters the sacral cord through the second through fourth segments. The nerves from the uterovaginal plexus approach the vagina with the arteries of the vagina and send branches to the tunica muscularis and the lamina propria mucosa. The tunica adventitia contains numerous ganglion cells, and the epithelial layer of the vagina contains few, if any, sensory corpuscular terminal organs (Platzer, Poisel, & Hafez, 1978).

The innervation of the female external genitalia originates with the iliohypogastric nerves originating from T12–L1. These divide into the anterior hypogastric nerve, which passes over the symphysis to supply the superior portion of the labia majora and mons pubis, and the second branch, the posterior iliac, which supplies the gluteal area. The ilioinguinal nerve originating from L1, which anastomoses with the iliohypogastric, branches into many small fibers terminating in the upper medial labia majora. The genitofemoral nerve originating from L1–2 runs over the psoas muscle branching to supply the deeper labia majora, the dartos muscle, and the vestigial cremaster muscle. The sacral plexus (the posterior femoral cutaneous nerve) originates from posterior sacral S–2 and anterior S2–3, dividing into several rami called the *perineal branches*. They supply the medial labia majora.

The innervation of the clitoris is through the terminal branch of the pudendal nerve, originating from the sacral plexus and terminating in branches to the glans, corona, and prepuce. The pudendal nerve originates primarily from S2–3, with some from S1 (Krantz, 1982). The terminal nerve is the dorsal nerve of the clitoris (Krantz, 1958, 1982).

There are neuropeptide and neurotransmitter factors involved in the neurophysiology and neuropharmacology of the female external genitalia, but their specific roles in female excitement and arousal are poorly understood. Nerve fibers containing VIP, substance P, enkephalins, and somatostatin have been reported in the female mammalian urogenital tract by immunochemistry and immuno-histochemistry (Alm, Alumets, Hakanson, Owman, Sjoberg, Sundler, & Walles, 1980; Fahrenkrug, Palle, Jorgensen, & Ottsen, 1989; Goldstein, deTejada, Krane, Ottsen, Fahrenkrug, & Wagner, 1985; Larsson & Fahrenkrug, 1977; Meyerson, 1988; Ottsen, Sondergaard, & Fahrenkrug, 1983). VIP and substance P are found in relation to smooth muscle, blood vessels, and epithelial cells, whereas enkephalin is found in nerve endings in ganglia. Ottsen, Sondergaard, and Fahrenkrug (1983) studied these four substances *in vitro* and reported that substance P caused a dose-dependent smooth muscle contraction in uterine, cervical, and tubal specimens, which was blocked in a dose-dependent fashion by VIP, while somatostation, met-enkephalin, and leu-enkephalin had neither a stimulatory nor an inhibitory effect.

Female Genital Hemodynamics

Interestingly, the controversies regarding male erectile mechanisms also apply to the female, with similar confusions. The literature on the CCP of the vagina and clitoris is scanty. What there is agrees that "the structure is highly vascular, with blood spaces (lacunae), surrounded by solid walls (trabeculae)" (Danesino & Martella, 1976). Danesino and Martella (1976) reported on their examinations of the "erectile organs" in ten human subjects, ranging from a nine-month-old fetus to an adult of 84 years. Their study was published in 1955 in Italian in Archivo di Obstetricia e Ginecologia; the article is either confusing to begin with or has lost something in the translation. It describes the architecture of the erectile tissue at different ages and confidently defines lacunae, trabeculae, helicine arteries, feeding or nutrient arteries, and arteriovenous anastomoses. There is mention of some "invaginations," which are not blockage devices and disappear in adults, and subintimal longitudinal muscular structures that function as ball-valves and are important in the hemodynamics of both arteries and veins. There are also myoepithelial sponge cells that act to occlude vessels, as well as a proposed role for the tunica albuginea. Regardless of these specifics, the conclusion is that there is increased arterial flow, partially due to inhibition of arterial blockage mechanisms and decrease in venous outflow, which, in turn, is due in part to contraction of venous blockage mechanisms.

The erectile tissue, as noted above, includes the vulva, the vagina, the surrounding vasculature, and the clitoris. The labia minora have been observed by Masters and Johnson (1966) to increase in diameter by two to three times during sexual excitement. The clitoris undergoes a vasocongestive response that Masters and Johnson observed through the colposcope, including a microscopic tumescent component and a macroscopic clinically observable component. When the macroscopic reaction occurs, it ranges from barely observable to a twofold expansion of the glans. Kobelt (Lowry, 1978) gives the most convincing description of clitoral-bulbar erection. This description includes the glans, the pars intermedia, the bulbs of the vestibule, and the whole "sponge-like network of the vagina." Kobelt also speculates on how the perineal muscles aid in both erection and positioning of the glans. Sherfey (1972) has also speculated extensively on how these various structures function. However, only Masters and Johnson have reported extensive observations, and no one has made the appropriate measurements to evaluate any hypothesis. In fact, Wagner and Sjostrand (1988) are unaware of any physiologic or pharmacologic studies of clitoral tumescence. Masters and Johnson's observation of vaginal lubrication resulting from the vascular response was described as a "transudation-like" material (i.e., clear viscous fluid), as the result of marked dilatation of the venous plexi that encircle the entire vaginal barrel (Masters & Johnson, 1966). During the arousal process, the vagina increases up to 50% in length and diameter. Pelvic vasocongestion occurs as the physiological response that is the basis of female excitement, and any malfunction of that mechanism results in disorder or disease, as will be discussed under pathophysiology. Vaginal lubrication and vulvar-clitoral tumescence are the consequences of the vasocongestion, together with muscular tension underlying female sexual arousal in the external genitalia. The signs of extragenital arousal, such as changes in the breast and the skin flush that is similar to that of the male, are from the generalized response that accompanies both male and female sexual arousal and will therefore not be specifically covered in this chapter.

Summary

As noted at the beginning of the chapter, the female arousal disorder, FSAD, is based on a four-part description of the human sexual response cycle—appetitive, excitement, orgasm, and resolution—following Masters and Johnson (1966), as modified to include Kaplan's (1983) descriptions of the desire disorders. Thus, the excitement phase is accompanied by reflex vasodilation, swelling of the labia and circumvaginal tissues, heightened labial coloring, and increased lubrication or wetness. The lubrication is a transudate from the circumvaginal vasculature. Arteriorlar dilation is activated by spinal cord centers at two loci, S2–4 and T11–L2. Excitement can be enhanced or inhibited by supraspinal mechanisms.

As in discussing the male, I have not reviewed the female hormonal physiology—for reasons that are basically similar. However, the effects of estrogen on vaginal lubrication are important in the assessment and treatment of FSAD, and they will be discussed in the sections below.

One reason there is less literature about female sexual response is that much of the animal experimentation in the female relates to lordosis, and very little has been done to investigate vasocongestive or neuromuscular reflexes that may relate to FSAD. Lordosis is a fascinating rodent sexual behavior, but is not at all clear what, if anything, it has to do with human female sexual behavior. Therefore, I will not use any of those data in my attempt to describe human sexual behavior here.

PATHOPHYSIOLOGY

Male Erectile Disorder

Male erectile disorder (MED) (or *impotence,* as it is more commonly called in the literature) has many pathophysiological etiologies, some more common than others. Table 5.2 is an "A–Z" listing with some selected examples. The following section discusses some important or otherwise informative entries from that listing.

Organ System Failure

Diabetes mellitus (DM) is a common cause of MED (Ando, Rubens & Rottiers, 1985; El-Bayoumi, El-Sherbini, & Mostafa, 1984; Faerman, Glocer, Gox, Jadzinsky, & Rapaport, 1974; Forsberg, Hojerback, Olsson, & Rosen, 1989; Kaiser & Korenman, 1988; Kolodny, Kahn, Goldstein, & Barnett, 1974; Lin & Brad-

Table 5.2. Pathophysiological Etiologies of Male Erectile Disorder

Aging	Anatomic defects of penis, chordee, Peyronie's disease
Congenital	Absent phallus, diphallus, hypospadius, spina bifida, Kleinfelter's syndrome, testicular agenisis
Drug abuse	Alcohol, opiates, barbiturates, cocaine, marijuana
Endocrinologic	Acromegaly, Addison's disease, adrenal neoplasias, chromophobe, adenomas, hypogonadism (primary and secondary) infantism, myxedema (hypothyroid), hyperthyroidism, hypogonadal androgen deficiency, testicular disease, pituitary insufficiency, hyperprolactinemia
Infection	Prostatitis, penile skin infection
Neurogenic	Multiple sclerosis, amyotrophic lateral sclerosis, peripheral neuropathies, general paresis, tabes dorsalis, temporal lobe lesion, pernicious anemia, nutritional deficiencies, spinal cord injury or disease, Parkinson's disease, brain tumor, lumbar disc disease
Organ system failure	Cardiac, respiratory, diabetes mellitus, hypertension, cardiovascular disease, angina, arteriosclerosis, postmyocardial infarction, chronic renal failure, chronic lung disease, scleroderma
Pharmacologic	Phenothiazines, butyrophenoes, thiothixenes, antidepressants, antihypertensives, disulfiram, estrogens
Surgical complication	Lumbar sympathectomy, perineal prostatectomy, aortofemoral bypass, abdominoperineal resection
Toxicological	Lead and herbicides
Traumatic	Castration, pelvic fracture, penile trauma, ruptured intervertebral disc
Urological	Peyronie's disease, hydrocele, varicocele, phimosis, priapism, elephantiasis
Vasculogenic	Vascular disease of terminal aorta, iliac arteries

ley, 1985; Maatman, Montague, & Martin, 1987; Martin, 1981; Miccoli, Giampietro, Tognarelli, Rossi, Giovannitti, & Navalesi, 1987; Nofzinger & Schmidt, 1990; Renshaw, 1975; Rubin & Babbott, 1958; Zorgniotti, 1985). We can "go to school" regarding MED by understanding the various ways in which DM causes MED, including examples of "vasculogenic" and "neurogenic" pathophysiology. First, it is important to understand the magnitude of this problem. In diabetic men, impotence is more common than either retinopathy or nephropathy, and a 1980 estimate suggests that between 2 and 2.5 million American diabetic men suffer from sexual dysfunction (Goldstein, Siroky, & Krane, 1983). As has been described above, erection requires an intact, unimpeded, functioning arterial-venous network that performs in a fashion that is as yet to be fully understood—but basically the process can be summarized as an increased arterial inflow and some venous restriction. The vascular pathology that plays a major role in the pathogenesis of MED in DM is due to a convergence of factors that all contribute to a high impediment of blood flow in the arterial bed of the penis. It includes both small-vessel disease (Faerman, Glocer, Gox, Jadzinsky, & Rapaport, 1974) and large-vessel disease (May, DeWeese, & Rob, 1969; Michal, Kramar, & Pospichal, 1974). DM's known effects on neural mechanisms are clearly a source of the MED associated with this disease. Perineal electromyography (EMG) (Goldstein, Siroky, & Krane, 1983) demonstrated characteristics of peripheral denervation, including neuropathic potentials and a decreased interference pattern. Sacral latency (bulbocavernosus reflex latency) testing revealed abnormal values indicative of pudendal sensory diabetic neuropathy in 75% of the patients tested (Lin & Bradley, 1985; Vacek & Lachman, 1977). Postmortem analysis of CCP tissue shows nerve damage not seen in potent nondiabetic subjects (Faerman, Vilar, Rivarola, Rosner, Jadzinsky, Fox, Lloret, Bernstein-Hahn, & Saraceni, 1972). Cystometrography showed detrusor areflexia (i.e., no reflex bladder contractions) in 75% of impotent diabetic men tested (Ellenberg, 1971). No significant

hormonal differences have been found between impotent diabetic patients and potent nondiabetic controls in luteinizing hormone, follicle stimulating hormone, prolactin, testosterone, or estradiol (Faerman et al., 1972; Goldstein et al., 1983; Kolodny et al., 1974).

Scleroderma is a disease of the connective tissue manifested primarily by a thickening of the skin but also involving fibrotic changes in other organ systems. It has been demonstrated to have a pathological effect on the microangioarchitecture discussed above. A large number of male patients will develop an erectile disorder at some stage in the disease. Rossman and Zorgniotti (1989) reported three cases in which corpus cavernosum biopsies were obtained. The histologic review of these specimens showed extensive replacement of smooth muscle tissue by connective tissue and marked vascular fibrosis. Although all three had a penile brachial index (PBI) in the normal range, a unilateral selective arteriogram in one patient showed atresia of the internal pudendal artery and nonvisualization of the cavernous artery, and another patient showed diminished arterial inflow on measurement of penile blood pressure by Doppler ultrasound.

Chronic renal failure, both before and after hemodialysis, is associated with a high incidence of MED (De-Nour, 1978; Levy, 1973; Milne, Golden, & Fibus, 1977; Wagner & Green, 1981b). In uremia, serum testosterone is decreased; there is testicular atrophy with loss of Leydig cells, and luteinizing hormone is increased. Evidence of disturbances of the hypothalamo-pituitary-gonadal axis with elevated prolactin has also been reported. About 50% of uremic patients are impotent, and 38–80% of patients on dialysis have erectile difficulty. Renal transplant, if a second transplant is required, carries about a 65% incidence of MED (Goldstein, Siroky, & Krane, 1983; De-Nour, 1978; Levy, 1973; Milne, Golden, & Fibus, 1977; Wagner & Green, 1981). Interestingly, contrary to speculations that MED seen with heart transplantation patients is secondary to the immunosuppressive treatment required erectile dysfunction in renal transplant patients often disappears during immunosuppression (Wagner & Green, 1981).

Chronic lung disease also is related to MED. It is seen in chronic bronchitis, asthma, and emphysema, yet is believed not to relate to pulmonary pathophysiology but rather to interpersonal problems associated with these disorders (Wagner & Green, 1981b).

Other organ system failures involving MED include cancer (Bachers, 1985), radiation therapy (Goldstein et al., 1983), chronic liver disease (Howard & Rees, 1976), lupus (SLE) (Hierons, 1971), arthritis (Currey, 1970; Hamilton, Lodge, & Hawkins, 1974), and arteriosclerosis and other cardiac conditions (Wagner & Metz, 1981).

Vasculogenic

Although much of the modern treatment of impotence relates to the physiology of the erectile tissue discussed above, the specific pathophysiological changes involved are still not known. Sidi (Sidi et al., 1988) defines impotence as the inability to achieve or sustain intracavernous pressure of 90–100 mm of Hg, the pressure he says is needed to achieve and sustain sufficient penile rigidity to permit intromission. The vasculogenic pathophysiologic processes leading to impotence basically amount to a failure to fill or store vascular volume. Failure to fill the CCP with blood can be caused by any disease that restricts blood through the hypogastric-cavernous arterial tree (Michal, 1982; Virag, Bouilly, & Frydman, 1985). The major diseases in this category are small- or large-vessel atherosclerotic disease (Mackey, 1986), diabetes-associated small-vessel disease (Faerman et al., 1974; Zorgniotti, 1985), and pelvic trauma effecting the pudendal or common penile arteries. These conditions may cause a slower rate of increase in intracavernous pressure, prolonging the time to achieve adequate pressure. A slowly developing partial erection is characteristic of vasculogenic impotence. Failure to store results from conditions that interfere with the expansion of the sinusoidal spaces, resulting in a partial erection (which improves

with upright posture, because this position increases venous pressure). Diseases that lead to fibrosis, such as Peyronie's disease, or conditions that damage the endothelium, such as smoking, diabetes, hypertension, or hyperlipidemia, can interfere with the ability to store blood.

Obviously, from the success of agents that act on smooth muscles when injected intracavernously, much of the pathophysiology of "vasculogenic" impotence has to do with the microangioarchitecture elaborated above. The failure of some surgical approaches to treatment (discussed below) are due to the fact that the pathology is "distal" or intracavernosal, rather than associated with occlusion in the proximal vasculature.

Neurogenic

Under this heading I will be discussing what might be referred to as primary neurogenic etiologies, as opposed to secondary ones resulting from either a nonneurological disease (such as diabetes mellitus, discussed previously) or iatrogenic causes (such as neural injury during surgery).

MED may result from a spinal cord injury or disease (Cibeira, 1970; Chigier, 1977; Geiger, 1979; Griffith, Tomko, & Timms, 1973; Higgins, 1979; Jochheim & Wahle, 1970; Kennedy & Over, 1990; Larsen & Hejgaard, 1984; Taylor & Coolican, 1988; Tsuji, Nakajima, Morimoto, & Nounaka, 1961; Zeitlin, Cottrell, & Lloyd, 1957). The incidence and degree of erectile function is mostly dependent on the completeness and level of the spinal lesion. Patients with incomplete lesions or injuries to the upper part of the cord frequently have the capacity to have reflexogenic erections, triggered by stimuli intentionally or accidently applied to a number of sites, including the abdomen, perineum, thighs, or directly to the genitalia. These erections are of varying hardness and duration. Lesions below T12 usually are associated with only CCP, with those above that level involving both CCP and CSP. The higher the lesion, the greater the chance of reflex erection (Talbot, 1955; Torrens,

1983; Tsuji et al., 1961). About 25–30% of patients with a lesion to the lower spinal cord, including the conus and cauda equina, are still able to have what have been referred to as psychogenic erections (Bors & Comarr, 1960). Any condition affecting the cord may result in MED. Transverse myelitis and anterior spinal artery thrombosis have a profound effect, while subacute combined degeneration has not been found to result in MED. Other processes reported to induce MED include tabes dorsalis, syringomyelia, myelodysplasia, spinal abscess, and arachnoiditis (Torrens, 1983).

Another common cause of MED is multiple sclerosis (MS). In spite of the widespread demyelination that may occur with MS, the cord is the most common site responsible for MED in these patients. MED is the presenting symptom in 3% of MS patients, becomes more common in later stages of the disease, and is positively related to bowel and bladder symptoms. This suggests that the pathology is an anterior spinal cord disturbance. The speculation is that descending reticulospinal fibers are interrupted by plaques prior to their termination in the lateral or intermediolateral cord (Vas, 1969).

Peripheral neuropathy as a cause for MED is usually among the sequelae of problems covered elsewhere in this section: diabetes mellitus or surgical injuries. Lumbar disk prolapse has been associated with impotence, presumably by compromising the peripheral nerve (Torrens, 1983).

Temporal lobe epilepsy (TLE) has been frequently associated with MED (Blumer & Walker, 1967; Ellison, 1982; Shukla, Srivastava, & Katiyar, 1979; Taylor, 1971). The MED that occurs between seizure episodes is consistent with or related to the global hyposexuality seen with this disorder. The TLE may be from a number of etiologies, including trauma, tumor, or even calcification (Hierons, 1971). Although there have been associations made between generalized epilepsy and MED (Jensen, Jensen, Sorensen, Bjerre, Rizzi, Sorensen, Klysner, Brinch, Jespersen, & Nielsen, 1990; Saunders & Rawson, 1970; Toone, Edeh, Nanjee, & Wheeler, 1989) recent attempts have failed to show a connection when a control group was selected with patients of similar severity of illness, types of treatment, and psychosocial status (Jensen et al., 1990).

Aging

The most frequent cause of MED in elderly men is comorbid disease or the sequelae of treatment of such disease. In a recent study (Mulligan & Katz, 1989) of 121 male veterans, with a mean age of 68, presenting with "geriatric erectile failure," the conclusion was that 87% had a "discernable organic cause," primarily of neurovascular origin. In this study, using nocturnal penile tumescence (NPT) methodology, 66% had no nocturnal erections, and no patient broke all three bands on snap-guage testing for rigidity. By using a combination of history, physical exam, and a variety of diagnostic procedure, the authors concluded that 21.1% of these geriatric erectile failures were of vascular etiology, 27.6% of neuropathic etiology, and 30.3% "multifactorial." General medical history and physical examination revealed a high prevalence of vascular or neurologic disease (Mulligan & Katz, 1989).

Aging brings on changes in the sexual response cycle, presumably based solely on the normal aging process. These changes include an increased length of time to achieve an erection, a longer plateau phase, more rapid detumescence, and a longer refractory period (Masters & Johnson, 1966). There is also a small progressive decrease in the number and duration of NPT episodes with aging (Karacan & Howell, 1988). These factors suggest that there is some organic basis for altered sexual performance with age and that it is not entirely due to social, psychological, or health-related variables.

Kempczinski (1979), on the basis of a number of variables of blood flow (PSP, PSBG, PBI, penile waveform analysis, and postreactive hyperemia) concluded that age exerted an inevitable deleterious influence on penile blood flow, suggesting an age-related atherosclerotic narrowing of the pelvic vasculature, which, in advanced cases, may cause impotence. With age, first the CSP and later the CCP undergo fibro-elastosis of the trabeculae followed by progressive sclerosis of the small arteries and veins, which may be related to the increased incidence of MED in aging men.

Pharmacologic

Under this category it is important to look at illicit drugs as well as prescription medications. Drugs of abuse include a variety of compounds used in an addictive or "recreational" fashion, and these agents are a major cause of MED. They include alcohol, marijuana, stimulants, sedatives, and narcotics.

Acute alcohol intoxication impairs erectile ability because of its sedating effects and its vasodilatory properties. Chronic alcohol abuse affects erectile abilities through its damaging effects on central neural structures, peripheral nerves, and endocrine balance. Chronic alcoholism can affect potency directly by decreasing testosterone and suppressing gonadotropins and indirectly by cirrhotic-induced hormonal changes. The reported incidence of MED in heroin addicts ranges from 28% to 43%; in methadone maintenance patients, 40–50% (Segraves, Madsen, Carter, Davis, 1985).

Prescription medications are a major source of iatrogenic impotence. Antihypertensives and cardiovascular drugs may interfere with the neurovascular response to stimulation by their effect on autonomic innervation, including that involving the intracorporeal sinusoids, or they may decrease blood pressure in diseased cavernous arteries. Antihypertensives are especially troublesome with regard to MED. Some examples (and the approximate percentage of cases affected) include methyldopa (25%), reserpine (3–33%), guanethidine (24%), clonidine (4–41%), propanolol (13%) (Segraves et al., 1985). Psychiatric drugs, including antidepressants, antipsychotics, and anxiolytics, may decrease libido and/or antagonize neurotransmitters, possibly by anticholinergic effects. Examples include mellaril, trazadone, imipramine, and protriptyline.

In this section I have limited both the number of specific examples and the relevant references. In recent years there have been numerous reviews on the subject of drugs and sexual dysfunction, but a particularly valuable source is the chapter of Segraves et al., (1985) that specifically reviews MED, citing 335 references. Table 5.3 is modified from that chapter and gives a more expanded list of examples.

Surgical Complications

A major source of iatrogenic impotence is as an adverse byproduct of surgical procedures. Although there is an apparently high incidence of psychogenic impotence in these patients, there is clearly a chance of compromising innervation and/or vascular hemodynamics, especially in pelvic-perineal surgical procedures. A partial listing, as well as suggested mechanisms, can be seen in Table 5.4. Some specific examples, as well as supporting references, are prostatectomy (Bergman, Nilsson, & Petersen, 1979; Catalona & Bigg, 1990; Finkle & Taylor, 1981; Hansen, Ertekin, Larsson, & Pedersen, 1989; Hauri, Knonagel, & Konstantinidis, 1989; Pontes, Huben, & Wolf, 1985; Stief, Bohren, Gall, Scherb, & Altwein, 1988; Surya, Provet, Dalbagni, Johanson, & Brown, 1988; Walsh & Mostwin, 1984), cystectomy (Bergman, Nilsson, & Petersen, 1979; Walsh & Mostwin, 1984), proctectomy (Corman, Veidenheimer, & Coller, 1978), abdominoperineal resection (Bernstein & Bernstein, 1966; Bernstein & Long, 1959; Stahlgren & Ferguson, 1958), rectal excision (Bernstein & Bernstein, 1966; Goligher, 1951), rectosigmoid surgery (Hellstrom, 1988), and aortoiliac reconstruction (Goldstein et al., 1983; Hallbook & Holmquist, 1970; May, DeWeese, & Rob, 1969; Sabri & Cotton, 1971).

Bilateral lesion of the ansa lenticularis extending into the hypothalamus, thalamus, and perifornical region (for relief of hyperkinetic behavior) has been reported to produce erectile failure (deGroat & Steers, 1988; Meyers, 1963). Neurosurgical procedures dealing with cervical spondylosis, cervical or lumbar disk degeneration, or tumors have been associated with MED (Goldstein et al., 1983), and in those cases in-

Table 5.3. Sexual Side Effects of Drugs

DRUG	DOSE (MG/DAY)	ERECTILE FAILURE*
HYPOTENSIVE AGENTS		
Hydrochlorothiazide	100	9%
Chlorthalidone	100	+
Bendrofluazide	10	36%
Spironolactone	50–400	4–30%
Alpha-methyldopa	500–4000	20%
Reserpine	0.5–1	46%
Guanethidine	33–95	24%
Clonidine	0.5–1.8	4–41%
Propranolol	320	13.8
Oxprenolol	160	0
Atenolol	50–100	+
Pindolol	30	+
Hydralazine	50–100	+
Phenoxybenzamine	30–50	0
Guanoxan	30–31	20–35%
Guanoclor	?	15%
Bethanidine	31–52	20–67%
Debrisoquine	40	0
Prazosin	3–20	+
Indoramin	60	0
PSYCHIATRIC DRUGS		
Thioridazine	30–2400	44%
Chlorpromazine	400–100	0
Chlorprothixine	300	0
Mesoridazine	60	0
Fluphenazine	25/2 weeks	+
Thiothixine	20	+
Perphenazine		0
Trifluoperazine		0
Butaperazine		0
Butyrophenones		0
Phenelzine	60–75	+
Pargyline	50	0
Mebanazine	20	0
Iproniazid	50–100	0
Isocarboxazid	20–40	0
Imipramine	75–150	+
Chlomipramine	50–300	+
Amoxapine	75–150	?
Amitriptyline	75–150	
Protriptyline	20	+
Desmethylimipramine	150–225	+
Lithium	0.5–0.9meg/liter	+
Clorazepate	15 mg	0
Diazepam	15 mg	0
Chlordiazepoxide	30 mg	?

*O, No reported effect; +, reported effect.
Modified from Segraves, Madsen, Carter, & Davis, 1985 (Tables 1 and 2).

volving the sacral cord sacral latency, testing revealed abnormality (Siroky, Sax, & Krane, 1979). Sacral rhizotomy, which involves complete bilateral section of the anterior and posterior roots of S2–4, results in a high incidence of MED (Goldstein et al., 1983).

Endocrinologic Factors

"The incidence of hormonal dysfunction as a cause of impotence remains controversial" (Baskin, 1989, p. 446). Baskin reported on the endocrinologic evaluation of 600 patients with impotence. Subjects were screened for previously diagnosed endocrine disorders, drug abuse history, and diabetes. In this sample, more than 30% had a hormonal abnormality: primary testicular failure (14%), hypothalamic-pituitary dysfunction (13%), hypothyroidism (6%), and hyperprolactinemia (3%). Primary testicular failure was diagnosed in patients with

Table 5.4. Nonpharmacologic Iatrogenic Impotence

MECHANISM	AFTER THERAPY OR TREATMENT
Arterial vascular	
Large vessel	Aortoiliac reconstruction
	Renal transplantation
	Pelvic surgery
	Uncontrolled pelvic hemorrhage treatment
Small vessel	Pelvic radiation therapy
Venous vascular	Priapism treatment
Neurologic	
Central	Bilateral ansotomy
Supprasacral or sacral	Lumbar laminectomy
Peripheral	
Infrasacral	Sacral rhizotomy
	Abdominoperineal resection
Autonomic	Radical cystectomy
	Radical prostatectomy
Somatic	Pudendal neurectomy
Endocrinologic	
Hypergonadotropic Hypogonadism	Bilateral orchiectomy
Hypogonadotropic Hypogonadism	Pituitary resection
	Hemodialysis
Mechanical	Partial penectomy
	Hypospadias repair
Psychologic	Transurethal resection of the prostate

Adapted from Goldstein, Siroky, & Krane, 1983, Table 11-1.

a low or low-normal serum testosterone with increased gonadotropins. Patients with low testosterone and no rise in gonadotropins were diagnosed with hypothalamic-pituitary dysfunction. Patients were diagnosed as hypothyroid who had an elevated TSH, with or without low thyroxine. In this group of occult hypothyroidism, impotence was the earliest symptom of the endocrine disorder. Although the patients with hyperprolactinemia showed no other symptoms, patients with more than 20ng/ml of PRL were found to have pituitary microadenomas. In this group of patients presenting with impotence, 5% (30 of 600) had more than one abnormality.

Although a number of studies have documented a decline in mean serum testosterone with age, not all elderly men show such a decline. Chronic illness, medications, obesity, alcohol intake, and environmental stress all affect plasma testosterone, complicating studies of the elderly. Although there may be a modest rise in serum PRL levels with age, it is not sufficient to produce a hypogonadal state and thus unlikely to cause impotence in the elderly (Harman & Nankin, 1985).

Urologic

Priapism is a persistent erection of the penis that lasts longer than 4–6 hours. It can be caused by thromboembolic, neurogenic, and pharmacological factors, and it may lead to MED (Lue & McAninch, 1988). Priapism may induce cavernous fibrosis and thereby mechanical impotence, and it is sometimes necessary to use infusion cavernography to differentiate abnormal venous drainage from such a fibrotic mechanical etiology. The surgical correction of priapism, which involves creating an anastomosis between the saphenous vein and the CCP, or creating a surgical window between the CCP and the CSP, or coring the septum between the glans and CCP, may impair venous outflow and lead to MED (Goldstein et al., 1983).

Other potential urologic disorders associated with MED include fracture of the penis (Perr, 1977; Tiong, Taylor, England, & Hirsch, 1988),

rupture of the CCP (Joos, Kunit, & Frick, 1985), varicocele (Comhaire & Vermeulen, 1975; Pryor & Howards, 1988), vanishing penis syndrome (Badejo, 1989), and Peyronie's disease (O'Donnell, Leach, & Raz, 1983; Pryor, 1988; Willscher, 1983).

Female Sexual Arousal Disorder

The pathophysiology of female sexual arousal disorder (FSAD) involves any interference with the mechanisms that produce the lubrication-swelling response in the female. Similar to the male, this would involve basically any neurogenic, vasculogenic, or hormonal problem that would interfere with the underlying mechanisms facilitating the lubrication-swelling response. As with the male, the autonomic nervous system, especially the parasympathetic division, must not be compromised. However, the vasocongestive phase of the female sexual response cycle has been said to more resistant to illness and drugs (Kolodny, 1971). It has been suggested that the anatomic structures involved are simpler and that a complex hemodynamic high-pressure system in the genitals is not essential (Kaplan, 1974). According to Kaplan, although female excitation is also ultimately under control of the cortex, this disorder is less common in females; if a woman develops a sexual dysfunction, she is much more likely to lose interest in sex or have orgasm difficulties (Kaplan, 1983).

Aging and Cycling (Endocrinologic)

As with men, female sexual activity decreases with age, declining to its lowest by the early 70s (Gupta, 1990). The lack of availability of male partners is a major problem for elderly women (of course, this is a psychosocial issue, not a pathophysiological one). Again, comorbid disease and treatment of such disease are major problems for women as well as men.

The excitement stage of the EPOR model, like the vasocongestive processes in the male, is affected by the normal aging process. The appearance of vaginal lubrication slows from 10–15 seconds to up to 5 minutes or more in postmenopausal women. The capacity of the vaginal barrel to lengthen and increase in transcervical diameter decreases and is delayed (Gupta, 1990). There is decreased incidence of skin flush, decrease in muscle tension, distention of the urinary meatus, lack of increase in breast size with stimulation, delay in reaction time of the clitoris, slowing or absence of Bartholin gland secretion, and decreased congestion in the outer third of the vagina (Masters & Johnson, 1966; Wagner & Levin, 1978).

In order for the vasocongestion and lubrication response to occur, the vagina must be supplied with adequate levels of estrogen. Therefore, the factors of age and menstrual cycle are interwoven with hormone balance and endocrinological functioning, all of which must be operating together for a normal response

When estrogen is deficient, there is atrophy of the vaginal endothelium, which transmits the transudate, and the underlying vasculature. The most common cause of estrogen deficiency is menopause, whether it occurs as a part of normal aging or by surgical oophorectomy. The postmenopausal ovary and adrenal gland may not produce sufficient estrogen to support the lubrication response. Vaginal blood flow in menopausal women has been reported to decrease with age (Tsai, Semmens, Semmens, Lam, & Lee, 1987), as studied by the use of a warmed thermistor (Wagner & Levin, 1978), and to increase with estrogen replacement therapy (Semmens & Wagner, 1982). Sarrel (1990) has used Doppler techniques to study vulvar blood flow, reporting a 50% increase with estradiol treatment.

Investigators (Levin & Wagner, 1978, 1980; Semmens & Semmens, 1984; Wagner & Levin, 1978) have written frequently and at times passionately about the importance of addressing the problems of aging and female sexual function, including FSAD, noting that the neurovascular changes of aging can affect lubrication and lead to vaginal dryness. They have noted that, anatomically, the menopausal female's vaginal tissues are thinner and the vaginal barrel is shortened. Coitus despite vaginal dryness can result in urethritis, hemorrhagic cystitis, submucosal

hemorrhage, laceration, and excoriation of the vaginal wall. Vaginal circulation, the quantity of secretions, the vaginal pH, and the electropotential of the cells to the transudate fluids and electrolytes are all adversely affected by menopause and can be reversed by estrogen replacement. However, Semmens and Semmens (1984) have reported that it may take 18–24 months for cellular function to return to normal with hormonal replacement treatment in menopausal women.

Organ System Failure

As with MED, the underlying hemodynamics in the female excitement response are vulnerable to the vasculogenic, neurogenic, and hormonal effects that occur as a sequela of diabetes mellitus. In fact, as is the case with males, autopsy evidence in diabetic females shows evidence of clitoral nerve degeneration, blood vessel damage, and hyperargentophilia of neural fibers in the clitoris (Prathar, 1988). The neuropathy of the sensory nerves can clearly lead to problems in achieving sexual excitement. There have been reports about sexual dysfunction in diabetic females (Jensen, 1981; Kolodny, 1971), but only Tyrer, Steel, Ewing, Bancroft, Warner and Clarke (1983) looked specifically at symptoms relating to FSAD. An unexplained finding showed that in questions relating specifically to sexual arousal and vaginal lubrication, the diabetic women showed a significantly different distribution for vaginal lubrication, with more in the worst and the best categories. The assessment of diabetic neuropathy based on cardiovascular reflex testing did not show a clear association with FSAD-related symptoms.

Looking specifically at DSM-III diagnoses, Andersen et al. found a statistically significant increase in inhibited sexual excitement in 41 women newly diagnosed with gynecologic cancer (Andersen, Lachenbruch, Andersen, & de Prosse, 1986). Assessment of sexual response cycle disruption indicated a specific problem in the sexual excitement phase in these patients.

Two other medical disorders that may diminish female excitement are chronic liver disease and chronic renal disease. Chronic liver disease can lead to insufficient conjugation of estrogen. Chronic renal disease with concomitant uremic neuropathy can affect the pelvic autonomic system, interfering with arousal through diminished lubrication and vasocongestion.

Neurogenic

Any disease process that interferes with the nerves mediating the vasocongestive reflexes can cause FSAD. Such processes include multiple sclerosis, alcoholic neuropathy, tabes dorsalis, amyotrophic lateral sclerosis, syringomyelia, myelitis, severe malnutrition, vitamin deficiencies, primary autonomic degeneration, and traumatic paraplegia (Kaplan, 1983). In multiple sclerosis (Lundberg, 1978), sexual difficulties may be the first manifestation of the disease. Patches of demyelinization in the spinal cord interfere with genital reflexes and result in diminished lubrication and/or absent clitoral sensitivity. Alcoholic neuropathy can cause similar problems (Kaufman, 1983). Head trauma, cerebrovascular accidents, or brain tumors can cause direct injury to cerebral centers, or (in the specific case of pituitary tumors) also increase prolactin levels (Kaufman, 1983).

FSAD, like MED, may result from spinal cord injury or disease. In spinal cord injuries, FSAD has not been well studied (Willmuth, 1987). Self-report information from small samples of women suggest that most, but not all, continue to lubricate. Bregman (1975) reported that 27 of 31 women continued to lubricate during their sexual activity. Lubrication may still occur, with its psychogenic or reflexogenic components, at all levels with incomplete cord lesions. When the injury is between T10–T12, neither reflex nor psychogenic lubrication occurs. If the lesion is below T12 and the sympathetic innervation is intact, psychogenic lubrication is possible. In high complete lesions (T9 or above) only reflex lubrication can be elicited. Reflex congestion of the genitals from, for instance, washing the genitals, occurs in female paraplegics with injuries above T10. The sensations felt by female paraplegics with complete lesions above T10 are not the same as before the injury; they are described as either a sensation of having a full bladder or a burning feeling in the urethra. There are no sensations during excitation with lesions from T10–12, but much attenuated ones for injuries below T12. Of the two women in Fitzpatrick's (1974) study, one reported "sensation of clitoral tumescence," while the other woman reported no awareness of genital arousal. The clitoral retraction of the plateau phase has been elicited by masturbation in complete lesions above T10, indicating that that particular phenomenon involves sacral parasympathetic innervation. Lesions above T6 cause autonomic hyperreflexia, headaches, and bradycardia during plateau stimulation (Berard, 1989). The only case of a spinal cord injury, male or female, where the complete sexual response cycle was observed (using the methods outlined in HSR; Masters & Johnson, 1966) was in a woman. Postinjury breast stimulation produced arousal and orgasm without significant vaginal lubrication or pelvic vasocongestion (Willmuth, 1987).

Pharmacologic

Antihistamines, anticholinergics, antihypertensives, and psychotropic drugs all can cause vaginal dryness (Kaufman, 1983). To the degree that the neurophysiology is comparable to MED, the extensive literature mentioned above would suggest that these drugs could also result in FSAD. However, to the best of my knowledge, there is no literature to support this thesis.

Surgical Complication

FSAD has been reported following vaginal hysterectomy (Crain & Jackson, 1975). Looking specifically at DSM-III diagnoses, Anderson reported that follow-up analyses showed a significant increase in inhibited sexual excitement in women treated for *in situ* vulvar cancer (Andersen, Turnquist, LaPolla, & Turner, 1988). The statement above in regard to the pharmacologic pathophysiology of FSAD in relation to MED applies here as well.

ASSESSMENT AND DIAGNOSIS OF SEXUAL AROUSAL DISORDERS

Male Erectile Disorder

Sexual History

Erectile failure is often confused with ejaculatory dysfunction, infertility, or decreased libido. It is important to establish the onset—whether it was abrupt or gradual, situational (e.g., different partners, masturbation, morning erections), persistent, or intermittent. The quality of the erections must also be determined. History should include risk factors for diseases such as peripheral vascular disease, atherosclerotic heart disease, or CVA which can be associated with vasculogenic impotence. Risk factors include obesity, lack of physical exercise, diabetes, hypertension, hyperlipidemia, cigarette smoking, drugs, and trauma. Men with hormonal abnormalities usually report decreased libido. Testosterone deficiency and hyperprolactinemia are the most common disorders. Hyperprolactinemia associated with pituitary tumor may cause vision changes, headaches, and/or gynecomastia, with or without galactorrhea.

Physical Examination

Physical examination for vascular impotence includes skin changes in the lower limbs, palpation of peripheral pulses, auscultation for bruits over arterial vessels, and palpation for fibrosis. The examination of peripheral pulses is part of a routine physical examination. Canning, Bowers, Lloyd, and Cottrell (1963) reported results from palpation of the penile pulse in 451 patients. All 31 patients without a palpable pulse were "totally impotent or had had a decrease in potency." The physical examination for neurogenic impotence includes testing for the function of the sacral cord and its peripheral nerves by assessing genital and perineal sensations, tone, and reflexes (voluntary anal sphincter contraction, anal wink reflex). The physical examination for endocrinopathies includes observing for female body habitus, abnormalities in secondary sex characteristics, and absence of or atrophy of soft testicles.

Nocturnal Penile Tumescence

Nocturnal penile tumescence (NPT) is the godfather of assessment devices for MED and is therefore the focus of much attention (Allen & Brendler, 1988; Bohlen, 1981; Campbell, Reynolds, Jennings, Thase, Frank, Howell, & Kupfer, 1987; Casey, 1979a, 1980; Dhabuwala, Ghayad, Smith, & Pierce, 1983; Fisher, Schiavi, Edwards, David, Reitman, & Fine, 1979; Hursch, Karacan, & Williams, 1972; Karacan, Williams, Guerrero, Salis, Thornby, & Hursch, 1974; Lamid, 1985; Lavoisier, Proulx, Courtois, DeCaruffel, & Durand, 1988; Marshall, Morales, & Surridge, 1982; Morales, Condra, & Reid, 1990; Procci & Martin, 1984; Rosen, Goldstein, Scoles, & Lazarus, 1986; Schiavi 1986, 1988; Thase, Reynolds, Jennings, Berman, Houck, Howell, Frank, & Kupfer, 1988; Thase, Reynolds, Jennings, Frank, Howell, Houck, & Kupfer, 1987; Wasserman, Pollak, Spielman, & Weitzman, 1980; Wincze, Bansal, Malhotra, Balko, Susset, & Malamud, 1988; Zuckerman & Neeb, 1981). From the outset, there have been two centers, one led by Fisher (Fisher, Schiavi, Lear, Edwards, Davis, & Witkin, 1975) and the other by Karacan (Karacan & Howell, 1988), although it is Karacan who is credited with suggesting its use in the assessment of MED (Karacan, 1970; Schiavi, 1988). The problem with such a popular device is its potential for misuse. In some instances, undue emphasis has been placed on NPT for distinguishing between psychogenic and organic etiology. As will be discussed below, since there are both false positives and false negatives, NPT should be used in conjunction with other tests in the comprehensive assessment of MED.

NPT is the monitoring of erections occurring

in close temporal relationship to the rapid eye movement phase of sleep (REM). During REM, 3–5 erections occur, lasting 20 minutes to 1 hour 30 minutes. NPT decreases with age, from 6 episodes in adolescence to 3 episodes in men above 70 years of age (Fisher et al., 1975; Hursch et al., 1972). According to Schiavi (1988), in spite of the extensive literature noted above, only two studies had been done to assess the diagnostic validity of the test itself. Marshall, Surridge, and Delva (1981) found increased accuracy if maximum frequency of nocturnal erection (95%) formed the basis of a decision rule rather than maximum increase in circumference (80%). Schiavi, Fisher, Quadland, and Glover (1985) assessed the sensitivity (false negatives), specificity (false positives), and efficiency of NPT decision rules for discriminating organic from psychogenic impotence. A number of studies have found abnormal NPT in the apparent absence of medical illness, and Schiavi and Fisher (Schiavi, Fisher, White, Beers, & Szechter, 1984) believe that at least some of these NPT abnormalities have a psychological etiology. Goldstein has reported on patients with vascular impotence who have abnormal NPT protocols (Goldstein, Siroky, Nath, McMillian, Menzoian, & Krane, 1982). The fundamental problem is that there is a paucity of evidence linking the physiology of NPT to erotically induced erections. A major source of error is due to the fact that sleep apnea, leg movements, or other sleep related disturbances can result in NPT abnormalities that are not diagnostic of MED (Pressman, DiPhillipo, Kendrick, Conroy, & Fry, 1986). Polysomnographic information is essential to a thorough analysis of NPT data. NPT evaluations that do not also measure rigidity (Bradley, Timm, Gallagher, & Johnson, 1985) are also incomplete. After a thorough review, Schiavi (1988) is unwilling to formulate specific NPT cutoffs, emphasizing the importance of clinical experience in interpreting these data. Inexpensive alternatives for measuring NPT include postage stamps and a snap-guage (Allen, Ellis, Carroll, Baltish, & Bagley, 1989; Anders, Bradley, & Krane, 1983).

Penile-Brachial Index (PBI)

In normal male subjects, the penile systolic pressure always exceeds the brachial systolic pressure (Abelson, 1975; Britt, Kemmerer, & Robison, 1971; Gaskell, 1971). Penile and digital pulse contours are "remarkably similar" (Kempczinski, 1979). These findings form the basis for the penile-brachial index (PBI) (Engle, Burnham, & Carter, 1978; Kempczinski, 1979). After locating the penile arterial pulsations on the lateral surfaces of the CCP with a Doppler ultrasound probe, a pneumatic cuff is applied at the base of the penis, and penile systolic pressure (PSP) is measured. The PSP divided by the brachial systolic pressure is reported as the PBI. Engle, Burnham, and Carter (1978) first reported that patients with normal potency had a PBI ≥ 0.833. Based on results from 106 patients, Kempczinski (1979) determined that a normal PBI was > 0.75 and an abnormal PBI < 0.60. Sidi, Koleilat, and Fraley (1988) reported that a PBI < 0.6 indicates vasculogenic impotence, a PBI > 0.85 is normal, and a PBI between 0.6 and 0.85 is inconclusive. One of the criticisms of penile blood pressure testing is that a nonspecific Doppler signal can originate from arteries other than the one intended. Moreover, because these measurements are on a flaccid penis, they do not reflect the hemodynamics of erection. The latter criticism is the rationale for combining this test with other procedures that involve erection (Abber, Lue, McClure, & Williams, 1985; Lakin & Montague, 1989).

Penile Pneumoplethysmography

Penile pneumoplethysmography is performed by inflating a pneumatic cuff containing a transducer around the base of the penis and measuring waveforms generated by arterial pulsation. Amplitudes and shapes of the waveforms are measured. Kempczinski (1979) also reported on penile volume waveforms recorded on a "pulse volume recorder" and graded as good, fair, and poor in comparison to the digital waveform, both in relation to contour and amplitude. A good waveform shows a brisk upstroke, a sharp systolic peak, a slower downstroke, and occasionally a dicrotic notch. A poor waveform shows both a marked decrease in amplitude and an extreme flattening of the contours. Poor waveforms were seen only in patients more than 40 years old, with a trend toward more abnormal waveforms in older impotent patients. Criticisms of this test are that is measures arterial flow in the entire penis and is not specific for a particular artery.

Papaverine Test (PT)

Intracavernous injection of papaverine has been used as a diagnostic test for vasculogenic impotence (Abber et al., 1985). A papaverine test (PT) is performed by injecting 60 mg of papaverine in 20ml of saline into the dorsolateral CCP with the patient supine and a rubber band constricting the base of the penis for two minutes postinjection. The test was considered abnormal if the onset of full erection took more than 10 minutes and if the duration of erection was less than one hour. Erection cavernography performed in 15-PT abnormal patients confirmed a diagnosis of penile venous insufficiency in 80% of the cases (Lin, Liu, Yu, Chang, Yeh, & Kuo, 1989). This test by itself is not conclusive. The response may vary according to dose, test conditions, testing environment, and degree of anxiety. Men with minor vascular abnormalities may respond with a normal erection (Buvat, Buvat-Herbaut, Dehaene, & Lemaire, 1986). The addition of measuring the angle between the penis and vertical axis of the standing patient to PT adds additional diagnostic value to the test (Wespes, Delcour, Rondeux, Struyven, & Schulman, 1987). Pharmacocavernometry (Bennett & Garofalo, 1989; Desai & Gingell, 1988; Dickinson & Pryor, 1989; Stief, Diederichs, Benard, Bosch, Lue, & Tanagho, 1988) is a modification of the PT that involves combining it with the artificial perfusion erection procedure used to study penile hemodynamics (Newman, Northup, & Devlin, 1964). It is the basis for dynamic infusion cavernography (described below).

Duplex Ultrasound/Doppler Scanning

A 10 MHz high-resolution ultrasound probe is used to image the corpora (CCP, CSP), tunica albuginea, dorsal penile artery, and cavernous arteries. A pulsed Doppler is used to measure arterial blood flow. The measurements include changes in the luminal diameter of the vessels and the peak flow velocity. A normal arterial response to the injection of 30–60 mg of papaverine is a concentric pulsation of a thin-walled artery, a 75% increase in luminal diameter, and a peak flow velocity of >30 cm/second (1.0 kHz) with a rigid erection of more than 90 degrees lasting more than 30 minutes (Benson & Vickers, 1989; du Plessis, Bornman, Koch, & Van Der Merwe, 1987; Gall, Bahren, Stief, Scherb, & Sparwasser, 1988; Lin, Hsu, Chen, Wang, & Tsai, 1988; Lue, Hricak, Marich, & Tanagho, 1985; Shabsigh, Fishman, Quesada, Seale-Hawkins, & Dunn, 1989; Velcek, Sniderman, Vaughan, & Sos, 1980; Vyas, Pierce, & Dhabuwala, 1985). Sidi, Koleilat, and Fraley (1988) used this test in more than 100 patients and observed that there were false negatives in anxious patients, probably due to vasoconstriction from adrenergic discharge. A normal increase in arterial diameter without an increase in peak flow velocity may mean obstruction in a large proximal vessel. Significant diastolic anterograde flow in the cavernous arteries after papaverine injection may be associated with venous incompetence.

Selected Arteriography

Selected internal pudendal angiography is an invasive test performed on candidates for percutaneous transluminal angioplasty or arterial reconstructive procedures. A femoral arterial puncture is performed (on an outpatient basis) under local anaesthesia, including the optional use of intravenous sedation. These procedures have been markedly improved by the introduction of pharmacoarteriography (Bahren, Gall, Scherb, Stief, & Thon, 1988; Delcour, Vandenbosch, Wespes, Delatte, & Struyven, 1988; Forsberg, Ekelund, Hederstrom, & Olsson, 1988;

Gall, Bahren, Scherb, Stief, & Thon, 1988). A nonionic (to minimize pain) contrast solution is injected after intracavernous papaverine and phentolamine have been injected, to maximize arterial dilation and flow. Pathology can be observed from the aorta to the cavernous arteries. Pathological findings include direct signs, such as actual absence of an artery, arterial amputation, arterial stenosis, and arterial hypotrophy, as well as indirect signs such as compensatory injection of opposite-side deep artery, cavernogram truncated at level of amputation of deep artery, and contralateral compensatory hypertrophy (Ginestie, 1980). A recent study (Rosen, Greenfield, Walker, Grant, Guben, Dubrow, Bettman, & Goldstein, 1990) found that in 195 patients suspected of arteriogenic impotence, disease was mostly localized to the cavernous arteries, as opposed to earlier findings of pathology in the inflow and proximal arteries (including the hypogastric and internal pudendal). Marked variation in the origin of the internal pudendal artery was also mentioned.

Bilateral hypogastric arteriography (Lin et al., 1989) is performed using heavy sedation and local anaesthesia. The arterial catheter is introduced through the femoral artery, with the tip placed in the anterior trunk of the hypogastic artery. After an erection is obtained using the PT procedure, contrast medium is injected at 2ml/sec and films taken every two seconds for 30 seconds.

Cavernography

Corpus cavernography has been used to evaluate structural abnormalities leading to MED. Cavernometry involves saline perfusion with manometric monitoring of blood flow and observation of tumescence/erection. Cavernography-cavernometry involves perfusion of the CCP with simultaneous recording of the intracavernous pressure and visualization of penile vascular anatomy. A needle is inserted in each CCP, and intracavernous pressure is recorded through one needle while a contrast medium is infused through the other needle in increments, until a full rigid erection is obtained. Measure-

ments include the flow rate required to reach and maintain erection and intracavernous pressure. Maintenance flow rate is the most significant criterion in determining the presence of abnormal venous leakage. During the procedure, radiographs show the CCP and the penile venous network. Prior to full rigidity, the circumflex system, emissary veins, dorsal veins, and vesicoprostatic plexus opacity can be distinguished. With full rigidity, the prostatic plexus is not easily seen, and the penile veins are obscured by the filled CCP, CSP, and glans. As the penis is filling during cavernography-cavernometry, intracavernous pressure remains low, while penile diameter initially increases. Penile diameter reaches a maximum before full rigidity occurs. In young healthy volunteers, the rate of flow for induction of erection (FIE) ranges from 80 to 140 ml/min, the flow required to maintain erection (FME) ranges from 15 to 50 ml/min, the maintenance index (FME/FIE) is 0.32, mean control intracavernous pressure is 14mm Hg, and during erection the mean intracavernous pressure is 140mm Hg. A maintenance index of greater than 0.4–0.5 is considered a sign of abnormal venous leakage (Delcour & Struyven, 1988; Delcour, Wespes, Schulman, & Struyven, 1988; Fetter, Yunen, & Dodd, 1963; Fitzpatrick, 1980; Gray, Grosman, St. Louis, & Leekam, 1984; Netto Junior, Reinato, Cara, & Claro, 1990; Reiss, 1988; Stief & Wellerauer, 1989; Stief, Wetterauer, & Sommerkamp, 1989; Velcek & Evans, 1982; Wespes, Delcour, Struyven, & Schulman, 1984).

A modification of cavernography involves the injection of papaverine. Following the routine cavernography procedure, 60mg of papaverine is injected through one of the indwelling needles after a tourniquet has been placed at the base of the penis. The corpus injected is squeezed to distribute the drug to both corpora. After 5 minutes the tourniquet is released, and at 10 minutes postinjection the standard perfusion procedure is performed. Risk of priapism is reduced by using moderate doses of papaverine and clearance of the corpora following the procedure. If erection persists for longer than two hours, a clearance puncture of the cavernous bodies can be performed, together with intra-cavernous injection of noradrenaline (0.025mg) (Bookstein, Fellmeth, Moreland, & Lurie, 1988; Bookstein, Valji, Parsons, & Kessler, 1987; Buvat, Lemaire, Dehaene, Buvat-Herbaut, & Guieu, 1986; Fuchs, Mehringer, & Rajfer, 1989; Lue, Hricak, Schmidt, & Tanagho, 1986; Malhotra, Balko, Wincze, Bansal, & Susset, 1986; Puyau, Lewis, Balkin, Kaack, & Hirsch, 1987; Reiss, 1989a; Stief, Wetterauer, & Sommerkamp, 1989).

Bulbocavernosus Reflex (BCR)

Evoked bulbocavernosus reflex latency measurement provides information regarding the integrity of the somatic sacral reflex (Blaivas, O'Donnell, Gottlieb, & Labib, 1980; Devathasan, Cheah, & Puvanendran, 1984; Ertekin & Reel, 1976; Gallai & Mazzotta, 1986; Mehta, Viosca, Korenman, & Davis, 1986; Sarica & Karacan, 1987; Wabrek, 1985). This test has evolved from physical to electrical stimulation techniques, but basically it involves the delivery of a stimulus to the glans or shaft of the penis and recording the motor response with an electromyographic needle electrode placed in the bulbocavernosus muscle. The normal response is bilateral, because the BCR is similar to the crossed polysynaptic specialized reflex pathway seen in the blink reflex (Goldstein, 1988). An abnormal study is a latency of more than 42/msec (Krane & Siroky, 1980; Siroky, Sax, & Krane, 1979).

Dorsal Penile Nerve (DPN) Conduction Velocity

DPN conduction velocity measurements provide information on somatic sensory penile innervation (Gerstenberg & Bradley, 1983; Lin & Bradley, 1985). This test is performed by either directly stimulating the DPN at the glans and recording at the base of the penis (Lin & Bradley, 1985) or by stimulating at those two sites, recording the BCR latency, finding the difference between the two, and dividing by the difference in distance between stimulating electrodes. In the latter case, the normal conduction velocity is reported as between 21.4–29.1 m/sec (Kaneko & Bradley, 1987). The direct recording produces a mean compound action potential of 12 microvolts and a conduction velocity of 33 m/sec (Bradley, Lin, & Johnson, 1984).

Pudendal Evoked Potential

Pudendal somatosensory evoked potential testing (Fitzpatrick, Graber, Hendricks, Balogh, & Wetzel, 1986; Fitzpatrick, Hendricks, Graber, Balogh, & Wetzel, 1989; Ertekin, Akyurekli, Gurses, & Turgut, 1985; Goldstein, 1988; Haldeman, Bradley, & Bhatia, 1982; Haldeman, Bradley, Bhatia, & Johnson, 1982, 1983; Kaplan, 1981; Pinto & Sister, 1989; Tackman, Porst, & vanAhlen, 1988) provides information on peripheral, sacral, and suprasacral sensory somatic penile innervation. This test involves adapting standard evoked potential techniques to this specialized indication. The pathway studied is dependent on the site of stimulation. A better generic term for this area of assessment might be *genital evoked potentials*. Using a catheter, the evoked potential can be measured from intraurethral sites; it is different from that recorded from stimulation of the penile shaft (Ponchietti, Tosto, Boncinelli, & Raugei, 1985; Sarica & Karacan, 1986a; Sarica, Karacan, Thornby, & Hirshkowitz, 1986). These intraurethral studies may be measuring more of the pathway from the cavernous nerves or plexus and/or pelvic plexus. These studies provide objective neurophysiologic information about the genital afferent nerve pathway, both peripheral and central, and thus add much to the evaluation of neurogenic impotence.

Penile Biothesiometry

Sensory integrity of the DPN is evaluated either crudely (with a tuning fork) or with a biothesiometer, which measures vibratory proprioception. Goldstein has used this test in impotent patients and reports that a large number of them reveal vibratory impairment (Goldstein, 1988).

Autonomic Nerve Function Tests

Autonomic innervation of the penis can be assessed indirectly by bladder testing, due to shared pathways. Bethanechol chloride denervation tests showing a hypotonic or areflexic bladder may indirectly signal injury to penile parasympathetic innervation. Kempczinski (1979) suggests that cystometry, especially in diabetes mellitus (Ellenberg, 1971), can distinguish between vasculogenic and neurogenic etiologies. It is important to note that objective measurement via cystometrography and bethanecol testing detects only parasympathetic injuries involving their sacral roots, the parapelvic-pararectal plexus and paravesical plexus, and does not detect distal lesions involving the prostatic or corporal plexuses (Goldstein, Siroky, & Krane, 1983). Detrusor areflexia and positive bethanecol supersensitivity strongly suggest parasympathetic denervation as a part of the pathophysiology.

Xenon (133Xe) Washout

The disappearance of the inert gas xenon-133 from an injected organ, referred to as *washout,* relies directly and solely on the blood flow to and from that site. Penile xenon-133 washout test (XWT) (Haden, Katz, Mulligan, & Zasler, 1989; Lin, et al., 1989; Nseyo, Wilbur, Kang, Flesh, & Bennett, 1984) involves subcutaneous injection of 0.1 ml (1–2mCi) of xenon-133 dissolved in saline at the level of the coronal sulcus, and then monitoring for 20 minutes with gamma camera. $T^{1/2}$ is the half-time for 50% of the radioactivity to disappear, and the flow rate (Q) is then calculated. This procedure works well because xenon-133 is a highly diffusible tracer that binds loosely to hemoglobin, with 95% being expired in one circulation through the alveoli of the lungs. Based on this preliminary study with a control group of three healthy males, Nseyo et al. (1984) suggested that the normal range for

penile blood flow (Q) values is 6–15cc/100g tissue/minute and $T^{1/2}$ normal range is 3–8 minutes. Lin et al. (1989), reporting on 10 young (24±4.9 years) and 11 older (58±7.3 years) subjects undergoing XWT by the technique and calculations suggested by Nseyo et al. (1984), arrived at a cutoff clearance time ($T^{1/2}$) of >7.5 minutes and Q <6 ml/100g tissue/minute. Bilateral hypogastric arteriography in 10 XWT abnormal impotent patients, and surgical correction of abnormal curvature on another 5 XWT abnormal patients, confirmed penile arterial insufficiency (PAI) in 100% of the cases. Lin points out the important fact that since the xenon-133 is injected in the penile subcutaneous tissue, and it is only in this tissue that clearance is measured, XWT will not demonstrate insufficiency or occlusion in the deep penile artery.

Isotope Phallography

This technique involves injecting Technetium 99m-labeled serum albumin in an antecubital vein and using a gamma camera to measure the activity over the aorto-iliac region, the internal iliac arteries, and the penis. A delay time for transit of the isotope from the aorto-iliac region to the penis is calculated. A transit time greater than 2.5s is abnormal. In patients in whom dynamic cavernography had failed to detect venous leakage and who had a poor clinical response to papaverine, phallography was able to identify arterial insufficiency (Eardley, Vale, Holmes, Patel, Kirby, & Lumley, 1990).

Nuclear Penogram

Diagnostic technology in the rapidly expanding field of treating impotence must at times become inventive in the creation of new procedures. Since pharmacological treatment of impotence by the injection of intracavernosal agents is now fairly common, it would be useful to be able to obtain an image of the response to these treatment modalities. The nuclear penogram (NP) (Chaudhuri, Fink, Burger, Netto, & Palmer, 1990; Fanous, Jevtich, Chen, & Edson, 1982) is a new technique in which 5–10 mCi of Tc-99m-labeled autologous red blood cells is injected intravenously to obtain an image and quantitative measure of penile blood volume changes that occur with a pharmacologically induced penile erection.

Hormonal Blood Levels

Baskin (1989) writes about the importance of doing a thorough endocrinologic evaluation of MED. This is contrary to what he feels is the current opinion: that it is unimportant to measure serum hormones in evaluating impotence. In a study of 600 patients presenting with impotence, he drew fasting AM blood samples for follicle-stimulating hormone (FSH), luteinizing hormone (LH), testosterone, prolactin (PRL), thyroxine (T4), and thyroid-stimulating hormone (TSH). Serum samples were drawn 30 minutes apart and pooled in order to dampen the effect of LH and testosterone spikes due to their pattern of episodic release. An androgen quotient (AQ) was calculated by multiplying LH by FSH and dividing by testosterone. Subjects were screened for previously diagnosed endocrine disorder, drug abuse history, or diabetes. In this sample, 32% had a hormonal abnormality. Primary testicular failure was diagnosed in patients with a low or low-normal serum testosterone with increased gonadotropins (an AQ>.19). Hypothalamic-pituitary dysfunction was diagnosed when serum testosterone was low and serum gonadotropins where low or normal (AQ<0.19) Baskin (1989) explained the use of his AQ with a discussion of the feedback relationship between the testosterone and gonadotropins. Patients with a high AQ more often than not did not have low testosterone. Their relative increase in gonadotropins, Baskin believes, justifies labeling them as suffering from primary testicular deficiency, and this group did in fact benefit most from testosterone replacement. A normal AQ in patients with low testosterone reflects a lack of rise in gonadotropins. Therefore, the problem is labeled *hypothalamic-pituitary dysfunction* and does

not respond to testosterone replacement. Thus, a high AQ was more predictive of response to testosterone than serum testosterone levels themselves.

There was a 6% incidence in this group of occult hypothyroidism, where impotence was the earliest symptom. Although patients with hyperprolactinemia showed no other symptoms, seven patients with more than 20 ng/ml of PRL were found to have pituitary microadenomas.

Other studies assessing hormones in MED include testosterone (Legros, Franchimont, Palem-Vliers, & Servais, 1973; Raboch, Mellan, & Starka, 1975; Wayrence & Swyer, 1974), LH, FSH, (Legros et al., 1973), and PRL (Modebe, 1989; Rao, Rao, Gupta, Sialy, & Vaidyanathan, 1981).

Apomorphine Injection

Lal, Laryea, Thavundayil, Vasavan Nair, Negrette, Ackman, Blundell, and Gardiner (1987) have described the use of apomorphine as a diagnostic test in the treatment of impotence. Eight patients presenting with impotence were screened for psychological or vascular etiologies. Apomorphine induced a full erection in four of the eight subjects, with tumescence measured by mercury strain gauge. Both responders and failures developed side effects, including nausea and sweating. Lal concluded that apomorphine may provide a diagnostic and predictive test to identify a subgroup of impotent patients with impaired central dopamine function.

Female Sexual Arousal Disorder

The amount of data on FSAD assessment (compared to MED assessment) is small. Perhaps the most succinct statement on this area is in the title of a paper by Hoon (1984): "Physiologic Assessment of Sexual Response in Women: The Unfulfilled Promise." Although there has been much effort and some pioneering work, including that of one of the editors of this book (Sintchak & Geer, 1975), there have not yet emerged any established physiological assessment techniques in the diagnosis and evaluation of FSAD.

Sexual History

This is the single most frequently used "measurement" device for FSAD. Questionnaires and scales of variable reliability are employed. Dennerstein and Burrows (1982), testing the efficacy of hormone replacement in women undergoing surgically related menopause, used an ordinal scale from an interview that sought details of female sexual excitement, including spontaneous vaginal lubrication during coitus. Andersen, Turnquist, LaPolla, and Turner (1988) assessed the sexual response cycle by phase. The excitement phase was measured by a five-point scale rating the frequency of current difficulties and, secondly, the Sexual Arousability Index (SAI). The latter instrument (Hoon, Hoon, & Wincze, 1976), is probably the most widely used assessment scale. It includes 28 sexual/erotic experiences that subjects rate on a seven-point scale, ranging from −1 (to indicate an adverse affect on sexual arousal) to +5 (when an activity always results in sexual arousal) in terms of concurrent activity. In an earlier study of newly diagnosed gynecologic cancer patients (Andersen, Lachenbruch, Andersen, & de Prosse, 1986), the investigators specifically identified the female excitement phase as disrupted using several methods, but the SAI was identified as the relevant measure by follow-up univariate analyses. FSAD has not been specifically studied in spinal cord-injured women, but some related questions have been asked, again by interview technique (Willmuth, 1987).

Physical Exam

On pelvic examination, a dry pale vaginal mucosa is indicative of estrogen deficiency. A microscopic examination for cytology of the vaginal smear, sometimes referred to as the *maturation index* (Semmens & Semmens, 1984),

can provide an estimate of adequate estrogen levels.

Vaginal/Labial Tumescence Measurement

Geer has been a pioneer in this area and continues to contribute to its development (Geer, 1975, 1976, 1980, 1983; Geer & Fuhr, 1976; Geer & Quartararo, 1976b; Korff & Geer, 1983; Messe & Geer, 1985; O'Donohue & Geer, 1985; Sintchak & Geer, 1975; Stock & Geer, 1982). The vaginal photometer is the instrument most commonly referred to (Hatch, 1981; Henson, Rubin, & Henson, 1979a; Rosen & Beck, 1988). The basic principle of vaginal photometry is the use of a probe with a light source and a photocell to reflect changes in the amount of light backscattered to the photocell, as an indirect measure of vasoengorgement (due to differences in the transparency of engorged and nonengorged vaginal tissues). Vaginal pulse amplitude (VPA) and vaginal pulse volume (VBV) are the two basic measurements. The VPA reflects the arrival of the pulse wave in the cardiac cycle and assesses more short-term changes in vasocongestion, whereas VPV reflects the slow changes in the pooling of blood in the vaginal tissues. Arguments have been made concerning which is the better measure (Heiman, 1977; Henson, Rubin, & Henson, 1979b), but according to Rosen and Beck (1988), the VPA is most used in practice. Other measures include vaginal (Fugl-Meyer, Sjogren, & Johansson, 1984) and labial temperature devices (Henson & Rubin, 1978; Henson, Rubin, & Henson, 1979a; Henson, Rubin, Henson, & Williams, 1977; Jovanovic, 1971; Wincze, Hoon, & Hoon, 1977), and thermography (Abramson, Perry, Seeley, Seeley, & Rothblatt, 1981). These instruments continue to be used to study the physiology of female sexual response; as more is learned, they may play a greater role in the diagnosis and evaluation of FSAD.

The xenon washout technique described above for MED assessment has been used in females (Wagner & Ottesen, 1980), but not to study patients with FSAD.

Autonomic Nerve Function Tests

Cardiovascular autonomic nerve function tests have been used to evaluate FSAD. The tests used were noting heart rate responses to the Valsalva maneuver, deep breathing, and standing up; and blood pressure responses to sustained hand grip and posture. A study of these tests in 80 diabetic females (Tyrer et al., 1983) did not reveal a clear association between diabetic neuropathy and the symptoms of FSAD.

Oxygen Electrode

This technique for assessing female arousal was developed by Levin and Wagner (1978, 1980). In this procedure, a heated oxygen electrode for measuring P_{O_2} is placed on the vaginal wall, and the power needed required to maintain the heat setting at 43° C is used as an index of qualitative changes in local blood flow and content, since both affect heat loss from the electrode. The energy required to maintain a constant heat setting is related to the thermal conductivity of the underlying tissues and is measured in milliwatts. Semmens and Semmens (1984) used this technique to assess estrogen replacement therapy in menopausal women, reporting decreased heat requirements in postmenopausual women and significant rises in heat requirements with treatment.

Vaginal Secretions and Cytology

The transudate produced by the vasocongestive response involved in female excitement and arousal can be studied for its quantity, electrolyte content, and pH. The levels of sodium, potassium, and chloride ions in vaginal secretions have been shown to approach plasma levels with the increased transudation involved in sexual arousal and orgasm. Vaginal pH is measured at multiple sites in the vagina, including the right and left fornices as well as sites anterior, posterior, and midvagina. A glass electrode containing a reference electrode connected to a standard pH meter is utilized in this assessment technique. The normal pH of vaginal secretions is acidic in the range of 3.5–4.0. These levels have been found to be elevated in menopausal women and to respond to hormonal replacement therapy. In addition, the amount of vaginal secretion can be measured. Using preweighed, commercially available tampons, Semmens and Semmens (1984) found an increase of 2.5 g within three months of initiating hormone replacement treatment in menopausal women. This increase in quantity of secretions was paralleled by an increase in potassium ions, which is interpreted to mean an increase in transudation through the walls of the vagina.

Transvaginal Electropotential Difference Measurement

Semmens and Semmens (1984) reported on the use of transvaginal electropotential difference measurement in menopausal females. This test demonstrates the capacity of the vaginal epithelial cells to transudate fluid and electrolytes. In normal menstruating women, the values are 34.0–36.0 mv. In menopausal females in the estrogen-deprived state, the average value was approximately half the normal, or 19.4 mv. A significant continuous rise in transvaginal electropotential difference is seen with estrogen replacement treatment, reaching 33.8 mv in 18 months.

Hormone Blood Levels

FSAD may be diagnosed by changes in serum estrogen levels, including 17 Beta estradiol and estrone, and/or serum gonadotropins, including FSH and LH. Semmens and Semmens (1984) have reported decreased serum estrogen levels and elevated serum gonadotropin levels in menopausal patients, returning to normal levels with replacement therapy.

THERAPY FOR SEXUAL AROUSAL DISORDERS

Male Erectile Disorder

Arterial Reconstruction

Aortoiliac occlusive disease has been recognized as a cause of MED since 1923 (Forsberg, Olsson, & Neglen, 1982; Iwai, Sato, Muraoka, Sakurazawa, Kinoshita, Inoue, Endo, & Yoshida, 1989; Nagler & Blaivas, 1987). The proximal arterial pathology is located in either the distal aorta, the common iliac, or the proximal internal iliac arteries. The basic intent is to improve blood flow to the internal pudendal and penile arteries. Methods include internal iliac endarterectomy, transluminal balloon angioplasty (Valji & Bookstein, 1988), aortobifemoral graft anastomoses, and iliacohypogastric anastomoses (Padma-Nathan & Goldstein, 1988).

When vascular insufficiency is due to lesions in the internal pudendal artery or its branches, revascularization directly to the CCP is attempted (Casey, 1979b; Kedia, 1981; Michal, Kramar, & Pospichal, 1974). Early attempts included directly anastomosizing the inferior epigastric artery to the tunica albuginea of the CCP (Michal, Pospical & Blazkova, 1980; Padma-Nathan & Goldstein, 1988), as well as using the saphenous vein interposed between the inferior epigastric or femoral arteries and the corporal bodies (Hawatmeh, Houttuin, Gregory, & Purcell, 1983; Zorgniotti, Rossi, Padula, & Makovsky, 1980). The results of these earlier techniques were poor (Nagler & Blaivas, 1987; Wagner, 1981). Distal penile revascularization procedures involve anastomosing the inferior epigastric artery to the deep dorsal artery (Michal, Kramar, Hejhal, & Firt, 1980) or the cavernous artery (Padma-Nathan & Goldstein, 1988). The latter has a much better success rate, approaching 80% in selected cases (Padma-Nathan & Goldstein, 1988). This approach requires microsurgical techniques (Valji & Bookstein, 1988).

Venous Surgical Approaches

Venous surgery to improve erection by decreasing venous outflow has been tried (Lue, 1988). Approaches include ligating the deep dorsal vein or closure of fistula, if found (Wagner, 1981). A more recent approach involves detachable balloons and coils (Courtheoux, Maiza, Henriet, Vaislic, Evrard, & Theron, 1986). Of the 12 patients followed for up to two years, 11 returned to a "normal sexual life," and posttreatment cavernosograms and plethymograms showed specific improvement.

Intracavernous Injection Therapy

Intracavernous pharmacotherapy has revolutionized the treatment of MED. Since Brindley's dramatic demonstration at the 1983 meeting of the American Urologic Association, this procedure has undergone explosive growth (Castillo, Rodriguez, Gutierrez, & Cartagena, 1985; Duffy, Sidi, & Lange, 1987; Kabalin & Kessler, 1989b; Kiely, Ignotus, & Williams, 1987; Siraj & Akhtar, 1989; Szasz, Stevenson, Lee, & Sanders, 1987; Virag, 1985; Watters, Keogh, Earle, Carati, Wisniewski, Tulloch, & Lord, 1988; Zenico, Zoli, & Maltoni, 1989; Zorgniotti, 1986). The most common regimen involves either papaverine alone (usually 30 mg/ml) (al-Juburi & O'Donnell, 1990b; Dhabuwala, Kerkar, Bhutwala, Kumar, & Pierce, 1990; Gilbert, Gillatt, Desai, & Gingell, 1990; Goldstein, Payton, & Padma-Nathan, 1988; Mooradian, Morley, Kaiser, Davis, Viosca, & Korenman, 1989) or a mixture of papaverine and phentolamine (usually 25 mg/ml of papaverine with 0.83 mg/ml of phentolamine) (Gasser, Roach, Larsen, Madsen, & Bruskewitz, 1987; Robinette & Moffat, 1986; Stief & Wetterauer, 1988; Turner, Althof, Levine, Risen, Bodner, Kursh, & Resnick, 1989; Zentgraf, Baccouche, & Junemann, 1988). The alpha-adrenergic blocking agent phenoxybenzamine has also been used, sometimes in combination with other agents. However, because of a possible carcinogenic side effect, it is not available in the United States (Zorgniotti & Lue, 1988). More recently, prostaglandin E1 has been introduced (Porst, vanAhlen, Block, Halbig, Hautmann, Lochner-Ernst, Rudnick, Staehler, Weber, Weidner, et al., 1989; Reiss, 1989a; Roy & Ratnam, 1990; Sarosdy, Hudnall, Erickson, Hardin, & Novicki, 1989; Schramek, Dorninger, Waldhauser, Konecny, & Porpaczy, 1990; Schramek & Waldhauser, 1989; Stackl, Hasun, & Marberger, 1988). The most rapidly spreading technique is the pharmacoinjection program (PIP), in which the patient is instructed in the use of the ultrafine 30 gauge needle injection in the lateral aspect of the CCP so that he can perform the procedure at home. Another intracavernous procedure is office treatment with papaverine injections every two to three weeks, for at least three injections. These programs have experienced rapid proliferation. Of course, there are complications, including iatrogenic priapism, and there are many failures for a variety of reasons (Fuchs & Brawer, 1989; Levine, Althof, Turner, Risen, Bodner, Kursh, & Resnick, 1989; Virag, 1985). Nonetheless, this technique appears to be becoming a routine urological practice. The outcome of 62 patients who were followed for 3 to 21 months, as well as the expressed difficulties with the therapy, are illustrated in Figure 5.9.

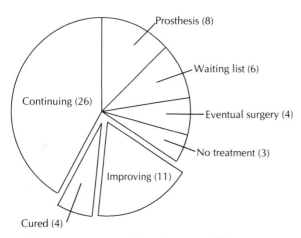

Figure 5.9. Outcome and complications of PIP programs (modified from Watters, Keogh, Earle, Carati, Wisniewski, Tulloch, & Lord, 1988, Figures 1 and 3).

Implants and Prostheses

Surgical implantation of prostheses has been attempted for 50 years, but early attempts with bone and cartilage were largely unsuccessful. There is now a wide variety of synthetic devices available (Bias, Leverett, Parry, & Halverstadt, 1975; Furlow, 1979; Finney, 1983; Gee, McRoberts, Raney, & Ansell, 1974; Hrebinko, Bahnson, Schwentker, & O'Donnell, 1990; Jonas, 1983; Kabalin & Kessler, 1989a, 1989b; Kirschenbaum & Mitty, 1988; Lash, 1968; Loefler & Iverson, 1976; Merrill, 1988; Montague, 1979; Mulcahy, 1988; Pearman, 1967; Small, 1983; Timm, Frohrib, & Bradley, 1976). The semirigid prosthesis consists of a pair of silicone rods that are intended to occupy the entire length of the CCP. They are supplied in two diameters and a variety of lengths. They have a low incidence of failure but do not detumesce, making them somewhat of a problem in terms of concealment (Sidi, Koleilat, & Fraley, 1988). The inflatable prosthesis first tried by Scott, Byrd, Karacan, Olsson, Beutler, and Attia (1979) in 1973 is now made of either silicone or polyurethane. Many improvements have been attempted to overcome mechanical problems. The newer implants consist of three components: inflatable cylinders, an indwelling reservoir placed near the bladder, and a pump placed in the scrotum. Although these devices have had numerous surgical and device-related problems, they do increase in girth during erection and have a more natural appearance in the flaccid state (Sidi, Koleilat, & Fraley, 1988). The surgical procedure involves exposing the CCP, incising the tunica albuginea, using metal dilators to create a tunnel, and placing the implant (Figure 5.10). Complications include infection, extrusion of the implant, and mechanical failure. Although there are no ideal prostheses, Sidi, Koleilat and Fraley (1988) state that a "high percentage" of patients and their partners are satisfied with the devices, and these investigators feel that prostheses will remain one of the primary surgical options for the treatment of impotence.

The newest type of prostheses are suction

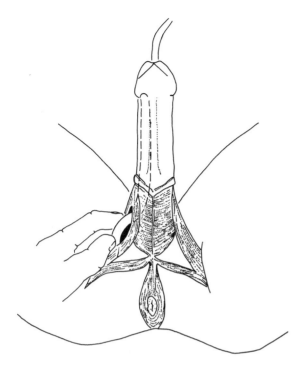

Figure 5.10. Penile implantation (modified from Nagler & Blaivas, 1987, Figure 9.8).

devices. By applying negative pressure to the penile shaft, an erection can be induced by the blood that fills the CCP, which can then be maintained with sufficient rigidity for coitus by use of a tourniquet at the base of the penis (Figure 5.11). Short-term complications reported thus far include signs of some trauma such as ecchymoses, skin petechiae, and swelling (Sidi, Koleilat, & Fraley, 1988). The Synergist Erection System (SES) (al-Juburi & O'Donnell, 1990a) was reported to be successful in a six-month clinical trial in 73% of the 44 men trying it. They were able to maintain an erection for an average of 30 minutes, with 88% reporting either very good or satisfactory quality of the erection. Two female partners reported traumatization of the vagina, and the major male complaint was poor penile sensitivity. Despite these drawbacks and technical complaints such as difficulty in sizing, it is noteworthy that 13 of the 44 patients in the trial had previously tried a pharmacological injection program, and only two of

these patients did not prefer the SES over that form of treatment.

Endocrine Therapy

Hormonal treatment of MED was at one time the most common and successful treatment (Nagler & Blaivas, 1987). Specific hypogonadal states (whether due to gonadal, pituitary, or hypothalamic causes) can be readily diagnosed by laboratory tests and treated with appropriate replacement therapy (Davidson, Camargo, & Smith, 1979; Green, 1981; Pogach & Vaitukaitis, 1983). The early enthusiasm for treatment of MED with testosterone, sometimes with little or no true work-up, has been tempered by the poor result of outcome studies (Green, 1981). Luteinizing hormone releasing hormone (LHRH) (Benkert, Hordan, Dahlen, Schneider & Gammel, 1975; Davies, Mountjoy, Gomez-Pan, Watson, Hanker, Besser, & Hall, 1976; Ehrensing, Kastin, & Schally, 1981; Green, 1981) and oxytocin (Green, 1981; Morales, Condra, Owen, Fenemore, & Surridge, 1988) have been tried but have not yet been used widely.

Baskin (1989) has recently described a more sophisticated and careful treatment of a number

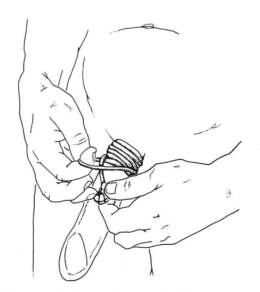

Figure 5.11. Suction prosthesis (modified from al-Juburi & O'Donnell, 1990a, Figure 2).

of MED patients diagnosed with a hormonal abnormality. Primary testicular failure diagnosed in patients with low or low-normal serum testosterone with increased gonadotropins was treated with testosterone enathanoate 200 mg q two weeks, and 55% were reported to have "had a correction of their impotence." Hypothalamic-pituitary dysfunction was diagnosed when serum testosterone was low and serum gonadotropins were low or normal. In these patients, the response rate (17%) to testosterone replacement was not better than that seen in patients with all-normal laboratory values (13%), which was considered to be a placebo response. Patients were diagnosed as hypothyroid who had an elevated TSH with or without low T4. Treatment with levothyroxine sodium, sufficient to lower TSH to normal, corrected impotence in the "majority" of these patients. Patients with hyperprolactinemia showed no other symptoms and were treated successfully with bromocriptine mesylate. Patients with > 20ng/ml of PRL were found to have pituitary microadenomas, but only two required surgical removal by transphenoidal hypophysectomy. In the 5% of the patients (30 of 600) who had more than one abnormality, patients with either hypothyroid disease or hyperprolactimeia did not respond to testosterone replacement until their other hormonal abnormality had been corrected.

Yohimbine

Yohimbine is an indole alkaloid that is a presynaptic alpha-2 receptor blocker. It has long been discussed as an aphrodisiac and 20 years ago was used in combination with testosterone, with mixed results (Green, 1981). Recent animal investigations (Chambers & Phoenix, 1989; Clark, Smith, & Davidson, 1984, 1985a, 1985b; Danjou, Alexandre, Warot, Lacomblez, & Puech, 1988; Peters, Koch, & Blythe, 1988; Sala, Braida, Leone, Calcaterra, Monti, & Gori, 1990) have renewed interest in its possible role in the treatment of MED (Danjou et al., 1988; Morales, Surridge, & Marshall, 1981; Nakatsu, Condra, Fenemore, Surridge, & Morales, 1985;

Morales, Condra, Owen, Surridge, Fenemore, & Harris, 1987; Quadraccia, Salvini, Corani, & Pizzi, 1988; Reid, Morales, Harros, Surridge, Condra, Owen, & Fenemore, 1987; Robinson, (1987); Susset, Tessier, Wincze, Bansal, Malhotra, & Schwacha, 1989).

Bromocriptine

Although, in general, bromocriptine has not proven to be successful in the treatment of MED (Ambrosi, Bara, Travaglini, Weber, Peccoz, Rondena, Elli, & Faglia, 1977; Benkert, 1980; Cooper, 1977), Lal et al. (1987) reported that by using apomorphine as a diagnostic screen as described above, three patients were placed on low-dose bromocriptine (max 2.5–3.75 mg/day), showed full erectile capability, and resumed intercourse within two weeks. Lal suggests that previous failures may have been related to dosage and/or patient selection; he feels that there is probably a subgroup of impotent patients with impaired central dopamine function who may respond to low doses of bromocriptine or other dopamine receptor agonists.

Nitroglycerine Paste

Nitroglycerine paste allows the use of a powerful smooth-muscle relaxant without the disadvantage of invasive administration. Initial tests have been encouraging, but it appears unlikely that this agent will mount a serious challenge to the popular PIP programs (Claes & Baert, 1989; Heaton, Morales, Owen, Saunders, & Fenemore, 1990; Morales, Condra, Owen, Fenemore, & Surridge, 1988; Negelev, 1990; Owen, Saunders, Harris, Fenemore, Reid, Surridge, Condra, & Morales, 1989).

Female Sexual Arousal Disorder

Hormone Replacement

The damaging effects of estrogen deficiency on the vagina can be reversed by topical vaginal cream or oral administration of premarin. The risk/benefit ratio involves the possible increased incidence of endometrial cancer, although the risk can be minimized with cyclic progesterone supplementation and frequent examinations. Sarrel (1990) reported that the use of a 0.1 mg transdermal estrogen patch was useful in treating problems with vaginal dryness. Dennerstein and Burrows (1982) found that within two months, ethinyl estradiol hormone replacement treatment in menopausal women (65-year-old women, postoophorectomy) experienced significantly increased sexual excitement, including spontaneous vaginal lubrication during coitus, as measured by subjective report. Semmens and Semmens (1984) have reported the use of hormone replacement to improve sexual function in menopausal women, including vaginal circulation, quantity of secretions, pH, and the electropotential of the cells to transudate fluids and electrolytes—all of which improved significantly or returned to premenopausal levels during the 24-month course of treatment.

Treatment studies using androgens are complicated by poor distinctions between low sexual desire and FSAD. In general, however, these treatments do not look promising (Carney, Bancroft, & Mathews, 1978; Dow & Gallagher, 1989).

Other Medications

Naloxone has been tried in an attempt to raise female arousal, without success (Brady & Bianco, 1980).

Pubococcygeal (PC) Muscle Exercises

Kegel (1984a) described his now well-known pubococcygeus exercises for the nonsurgical treatment of stress incontinence. However, several patients reported that they had increased awareness of their genital sensations, and some even reported an increase in their ability to attain orgasm (Kegel, 1952b). Kegel (Kegel, 1948a, 1948b, 1952a, 1952b) documented specifically that in patients using his Perineometer, voluntary vaginal contractions showed increased intravaginal pressure and that an exercise program could improve that effect. Kegel (1952a) and others (Graber & Kline-Graber, 1978, 1980; Graber, Kline-Graber, & Golden, 1981) have reported that an exercise program using the Perineometer and designed to improve PC condition resulted in an improvement in women with primary coital anorgasmia. Messe and Geer (1985), however, question whether that specific dependent variable (intravaginal pressure change) is relevant to sex therapy treatment outcome. They acknowledge that Kegel's exercises have been demonstrated to increase intravaginal pressure with consistent practice (Graber, Kline-Graber, & Golden, 1981; Kegel, 1952a; Levitt, Konovsky, Freese, & Thompson, 1979), but felt that vaginal pulse amplitude (VPA), a widely used measure of genital arousal in women (Geer, 1976; Hoon, Hoon, & Wincze, 1976), was a more clinically relevant measure of the arousal-enhancing effects of Kegel's exercises. Therefore, they designed a study to test the effect of brief vaginal exercise on VPA. Vaginal contractions did increase in both VPA and subjective arousal measures over nontensing control conditions. This finding supports the suggestion that tensing the circumvaginal musculature enhances sexual arousal. Baseline conditions were less arousing than tensing, which was less arousing than just fantasy. However, tensing and fantasy together produced the most arousal. The study quite correctly states that it is the first experimental support for the hypothesis that Kegel exercises can enhance sexual arousal and "suggests that the prescription of Kegel's exercises to sexually dysfunctional women is also likely to be appropriate" (Messe & Geer, 1985, p. 26).

CONCLUSIONS

The diagnosis and treatment of sexual arousal disorders has come a long way in a short time. It currently seems that, at times, the therapeutic tail is wagging the scientific body of knowledge. In the studies reported here, there are often wide variances in outcome criteria. Also, serious methodological criticisms of the studies can often be raised, including absence of a placebo control, small sample size, and inadequate measures of successful treatment. However, the enthusiasm for these new treatment techniques is advancing our scientific understanding of sexual behavior (albeit predominately that of the male). In this area, as in most others, the diagnosis and treatment of female excitement disorders unfortunately lags far behind, and there is little evidence of a change in this situation.

Given the range of pathophysiology in the sexual arousal disorders, it is recommended that as part of the initial assessment, the person seeking treatment for MED be referred to an urologist (or a gynecologist in the case of FSAD) for any assessment and/or treatment discussed in this chapter.

REFERENCES

Abber, J. C., Lue, T. F., McClure, R. D., & Williams, D. (1985). Diagnostic tests for impotence: A comparison of papaverine injections with the penile brachial pressure index and nocturnal penile tumescence. Part 2. *Journal of Urology, 133*(4), 188A.

Abelson, D. (1975). Diagnostic value of the penile pulse and blood pressure: A doppler study of impotence in diabetics. *Journal of Urology, 113,* 636–639.

Abramson, P. R., Perry, L. B., Seeley, T. T., Seeley, D. M., & Rothblatt, A. B. (1981). Thermographic measurement of sexual arousal: A discriminant validity analysis. *Archives of Sexual Behavior, 10*(2), 171–176.

al-Juburi, A. Z., & O'Donnell, P. D. (1990a). Synergist erection system: Clinical experience. *Urology, 35*(4), 304–306.

al-Juburi, A. Z., & O'Donnell, P. D. (1990b). Follow-up outcome of intracavernous papaverine. *Journal of the Arkansas Medical Society, 86*(10), 383–385.

Allen, J., Ellis, D. J., Carroll, J. L., Baltish, M. R., & Bagley, D. H. (1989). Snap-gauge band vs. multidisciplinary evaluation in impotence assessment. *Urology, 34*(4), 197–199.

Allen, R. P., & Brendler, C. B. (1988). Nocturnal penile tumescence predicting response to intracorporeal pharmacological erection testing. *Journal of Urology, 140*(3), 518–522.

Alm, P., Alumets, J., Hakanson, R., Owman, Ch., Sjoberg, N. O., Sundler, F., & Walles, B. (1980). Origin and distribution of VIP (Vasoactive Intestinal Polypeptide) nerves in the genito-urinary tract. *Cell and Tissue Research, 205,* 337–347.

Ambrosi, B., Bara, R., Travaglini, P., Weber, G., Peccoz, P. B., Rondena, M., Elli, R., & Faglia, G. (1977). Study of the effects of bromocriptine on sexual impotence. *Clinical Endocrinology, 7,* 417–421.

Anders, E. K., Bradley, W. E., & Krane, R. J. (1983). Nocturnal penile rigidity measured by the snap-gauge band. *Journal of Urology, 129,* 964–966.

Andersen, B. L., Lachenbruch, P. A., Andersen, B., & de Prosse, C. (1986). Sexual dysfunction and signs of gynecologic cancer. *Cancer, 57,* 1880–1886.

Andersen, B. L., Turnquist, D., LaPolla, J., & Turner, D. (1988). Sexual functioning after treatment of in situ vulvar cancer: Preliminary report. *Obstetrics and Gynecology, 71*(1), 15–19.

Ando, S., Rubens, R., & Rottiers, R. (1985). Endocrine testicular function in male diabetics. *Journal of Endocrinological Investigation, 8*(suppl 2), 103–109.

APA. (1987). *Diagnostic and statistical manual of mental disorders* (3rd ed., rev.). Washington, DC: Author.

Aronson, L. R., & Cooper, M. L. (1967). Penile spines of the domestic cat: Their endocrine-behavior relations. *Anatomical Record, 157,* 71–78.

Aronson, L. R., & Cooper, M. L. (1968). Desensitization of the glans penis and sexual behavior in cats. In M. Diamond (Ed.), *Perspectives in reproduction and sexual behavior* (pp. 51–82). Bloomington, IN: Indiana University Press.

Bachers, E. S. (1985). Sexual dysfunction after treatment for genitourinary cancers. *Seminars in Oncology Nursing, 1*(1), 18–24.

Badejo, O. A. (1989). Vanishing penis syndrome: The life experience. *Panminerva Med, 31*(4), 198–201.

Bahren, W., Gall, H., Scherb, W., Stief, C., & Thon, W. (1988). Arterial anatomy and arteriographic diagnosis of arteriogenic impotence. *Cardiovascular and Interventional Radiology, 11*(4), 195–210.

Baskin, H. J. (1989). Endocrinologic evaluation of impotence. *Southern Medical Journal, 82*(4), 446–449.

Benkert, O. (1980). Pharmacotherapy of sexual impotence in the male. *Modern Problems in Pharmacopsychiatry, 15,* 158–173.

Benkert, O., Hordan, R., Dahlen, H. G., Schneider, H. P. G., & Gammel, G. (1975). Sexual impotence: A double-blind study of LHRH nasal spray versus placebo. *Neuropsychobiology, 1,* 203–210.

Bennett, A. H., & Garofalo, F. A. (1989). Enhanced cavernometry: Procedure for the diagnosis of venogenic impotence. *British Journal of Urology, 64*(4), 420–422.

Benson, C. B., & Vickers, M. A. (1989). Sexual impotence caused by vascular disease: Diagnosis with duplex sonography. *American Journal of Roentgenology, 153*(6), 1149–1153.

Benson, G. S. (1988). Male sexual function: Erection, emission, and ejaculation. In E. Knobil & J. Neill (Eds.), *The physiology of reproduction* (pp. 1121–1136). New York: Raven Press.

Berard, E. J. J. (1989). The sexuality of spinal cord injured women: Physiology and pathophysiology. A review. *Paraplegia, 27,* 99–112.

Bergman, B., Nilsson, S., & Petersen, I. (1979). The effect on erection and orgasm of cystectomy, prostatectomy and vesiculectomy for cancer of the bladder: A clinical and electromyographic study. *British Journal of Urology, 51,* 114–120.

Bernstein, W. C., & Bernstein, E. F. (1966). Sexual dysfunction following radical surgery for cancer of the rectum. *Diseases of the Colon & Rectum, 9,* 328–332.

Bernstein, W. C. & Long, D. M., Jr. (1959). Is sexual dysfunction following radical surgery for cancer of the rectum and signoid colon a justifiable complication? *Proceedings of the Royal Society of Medicine, 52,* 77–81.

Bertolini, A., Gessa, G. L., Vergoni, W., & Ferrari, W. (1968). Induction of sexual excitement with intraventricular ACTH: Permissive role of testosterone in the male rabbit (Part II). *Life Sciences,* 1203–1206.

Bias, H. I., Leverett, C. L., Parry, W. L., & Halverstadt, D. B. (1975). Implantable penile prostheses in impotent males. *Urology, 5*(2), 224–226.

Blaivas, J. G., O'Donnell, T. F., Jr., Gottlieb, P., & Labib, K. B. (1980). Measurement of bulbocavernosus reflex latency time as part of a comprehensive evaluation of impotence. In A. W. Zorgniotti (Ed.), *Vasculogenic impotence* (pp. 49–65). Springfield, IL: Charles C. Thomas.

Blumer, D. (1970). Hypersexual episodes in temporal lobe epilepsy. *American Journal of Psychiatry, 126,* 1099–1106.

Blumer, D., & Walker, A. E. (1967). Sexual behavior in temporal lobe epilepsy. *Archives of Neurology, 16,* 37–43.

Bohlen, J. G. (1981). Sleep erection monitoring in the evaluation of male erectile failure. *Urologic Clinics of North America, 8*(1), 119–133.

Bookstein, J. J., Fellmeth, B., Moreland, S., & Lurie, A. L. (1988). Pharmacoangiographic assessment of the corpora cavernosa. *Cardiovascular and Interventional Radiology, 11*(4), 218–224.

Bookstein, J. J., Valji, K., Parsons, L., & Kessler, W. (1987). Penile pharmacocavernosography and cavernosometry in the evaluation of impotence. *Journal of Urology, 137*(4), 772–776.

Booth, A. M., Roppolo, J. R., & deGroat, W. C. (1986). Distribution of cells and fibers projecting to the penis of the cat. *Society of Neurology Abstracts, 12,* 1056–1056.

Bors, E., & Comarr, A. E. (1960). Neurological disturbances of sexual function with special reference to 529 patients with spinal cord lesions. *Urological Survey, 10,* 191–222.

Bradley, W. E., Timm, G. W., Gallagher, J. M., & Johnson, B. K. (1985). New method for continuous measurement of nocturnal penile tumescence and rigidity. *Urology, 26*(1), 4–9.

Bradley, W. F., Lin, J. T. Y., & Johnson, B. (1984). Measurement of the conduction velocity of the dorsal nerve of the penis. *Journal of Urology, 131,* 1127–1129.

Brady, J. P., & Bianco, F. C. (1980). Endorphins: Naloxone failure to increase sexual arousal in sexually unresponsive women: A preliminary report. *Biological Psychiatry, 15*(4), 627–631.

Bregman, S. (1975). *Sexuality and the spinal cord injured woman* (pp. 1–24). Minneapolis: University of Minnesota Medical School and Sister Kenny Institute.

Brindley, G. S. (1988). The Ferrier lecture, 1986. The actions of parasympathetic and sympathetic nerves in human micturition, erection and seminal emission, and their restoration in paraplegic patients by implanted electrical stimulators. *Proceedings of the Royal Society of London, Series B, 235*(1279), 111–120.

Britt, D. B., Kemmerer, W. T., & Robison, J. R. (1971). Penile blood flow determination by mercury strain gauge plethysmography. *Investigative Urology, 8*(6), 673–678.

Buvat, J., Buvat-Herbaut, M., Dehaene, J. L., & Lemaire, A. (1986). Is intracavernous injection of papaverine a reliable screening test for vascular impotence? *Journal of Urology, 135*(3), 476–478.

Buvat, J., Lemaire, A., Dehaene, J. L., Buvat-Herbaut, M., & Guieu, J. D. (1986). Venous incompetence: Critical study of the organic basis of high maintenance flow rates during artificial erection test. *Journal of Urology, 135*(5), 926–928.

Caggiula, A. R., Antelman, S. M., & Zigmond, M. J. (1973). Disruption of copulation in male rats after hypothalamic lesions: A behavioral, anatomical and neurochemical analysis. *Brain Research, 59,* 273–287.

Calaresu, F. R., & Mitchell, R. (1969). Short communications. Cutaneous mechanoreceptors in the glans penis of the rat. *Brain Research, 15,* 295–297.

Campbell, B., Good, C. A., & Kitchell, R. L. (1954). Neural mechanisms in sexual behavior. I. Reflexology of sacral segments. *Proceedings of the Society for Experimental Biology and Medicine, 86,* 423–426.

Campbell, P. I., Reynolds, C. F., III, Jennings, J. R., Thase, M., Frank, E., Howell, J., & Kupfer, D. J. (1987). Reliability of NPT scoring and visual estimates of erectile fullness. *Sleep, 10*(5), 480–485.

Canning, J. R., Bowers, L. M., Lloyd, F. A., & Cottrell, T. L. C. (1963). Genital vascular insufficiency and impotence. *Surgical Forum, 14,* 298–299.

Carney, A., Bancroft, J., & Mathews, A. (1978). Combination of hormonal and psychological treatment for female sexual unresponsiveness: A comparative study. *British Journal of Psychiatry, 132,* 339–346.

Carvalho, T. L. L., Hodson, N. P., Blank, M. A., Watson, P. F., Mulderry, P. K., Bishop, A. E., Gu, J., Bloom, S. R., & Polak, J. M. (1986). Occurrence, distribution and origin of peptide-containing nerves of guinea-pig and rat male genitalia and the effects of denervation on sperm characteristics. *Journal of Anatomy, 149,* 121–141.

Casey, W. C. (1979a). Phallography: Technique and results of nocturnal tumescence monitoring. *Journal of Urology, 122,* 752–753.

Casey, W. C. (1979b). Revascularization of corpus cavernosum for erectile failure. *Urology, 14*(2), 135–139.

Casey, W. C. (1980). Phallography: Technique pitfalls and interpretation. In A. W. Zorgniotti & G. Rossi (Eds.), *Vasculogenic impotence* (pp. 83–93). Springfield, IL: Charles C. Thomas.

Castillo, J., Rodriguez, H. Y., Gutierrez, I. Z., & Cartagena, R. (1985). Intracavernous injection of two vasoactive drugs for impotence: The buffalo experience (Part 2 abstract). *Journal of Urology, 133*(4), 190A.

Catalona, W. J., & Bigg, S. W. (1990). Nerve-sparing radical prostatectomy: Evaluation of results after 250 patients. *Journal of Urology, 143*(3), 538–543.

Chambers, K. C., & Phoenix, C. H. (1989). Apomorphine, deprenyl, and yohimbine fail to increase sexual behavior in rhesus males. *Behavioral Neuroscience, 103*(4), 816–823.

Chaudhuri, T. K., Fink, S., Burger, R. H., Netto, I. C., & Palmer, J. D. (1990). Nuclear penogram: Noninvasive technique to monitor and record effect of pharmacologically-induced penile erection in impotence therapy [letter]. *Urology, 35*(1), 98–98.

Chigier, E. (1977). Sexual rehabilitation of the young paraplegic. *Israel Rehabilitation Annual, 55,* 60.

Chung, S. K., McVary, K. T., & McKenna, K. E. (1988). Sexual reflexes in male and female rats. *Neuroscience Letters, 94*(3), 343–348.

Cibeira, J. B. (1970). Some conclusions on a study of 365 patients with spinal cord lesions. *Paraplegia, 7,* 249–254.

Claes, H., & Baert, L. (1989). Transcutaneous nitroglycerin therapy in the treatment of impotence. *Urologia Internationalis, 44*(5), 309–312.

Clark, J. T., Smith, E. R., & Davidson, J. M. (1984). Enhancement of sexual motivation in male rats by yohimbine. *Science, 225,* 847–849.

Clark, J. T., Smith, E. R., & Davidson, J. M. (1985a). Evidence for the modulation of sexual behavior by a-adrenoceptors in male rats. *Neuroendocrinology, 41,* 36–43.

Clark, J. T., Smith, E. R., & Davidson, J. M. (1985b). Testosterone is not required for the enhancement of sexual motivation by yohimbine. *Physiology and Behavior.*

Clark, T. K. (1975). Sexual inhibition is reduced by rostral midbrain lesions in the male rat. *Science, 190,* 169–171.

Comhaire, F., & Vermeulen, A. (1975). Plasma testosterone in patients with varicocele and sexual inadequacy. *Journal of Clinical Endocrinology and Metabolism, 40,* 824–829.

Conti, G. (1952). The erection of the human penis and its morphologico-vascular bases. *Acta Anatomica, 14,* 217–262.

Conti, G., & Virag, R. (1989). Human penile erection and organic impotence: Normal histology and histopathology. *Urologia Internationalis, 44*(5), 303–308.

Cooper, A. J. (1977). Bromocriptine in impotence. *Lancet,* 567–567.

Corman, M. L., Veidenheimer, M. C., & Coller, J. A. (1978). Impotence after protectomy for inflammatory disease of the bowel. *The American Society of Colon Rectal Surgeons, 21*(6), 418–419.

Cottrell, D. F., Iggo, A., & Kitchell, R. L. (1978). Electrophysiology of the afferent innervation of the penis of the domestic ram. *Journal of Physiology, 283,* 347–367.

Courtheoux, P., Maiza, D., Henriet, J-P., Vaislic, C. D., Evrard, C., & Theron, J. (1986). Erectile dysfunction caused by venous leakage: Treatment with detachable balloons and coils. *Radiology, 161*(3), 807–809.

Crain, G. A., & Jackson, P. (1975). Sexual life after vaginal hysterectomy. *British Medical Journal,* 97–97.

Currey, H. L. F. (1970). Osteoarthritis of the hip joint and sexual activity. *Annals of the Rheumatic Diseases, 29,* 488–493.

Dail, W. G., Hamill, R. W., & Minorsky, N. (1986). Further evidence of a cholinergic mechanism in the function of the corpora cavernosa penis (Abstract). *Society of Neuroscience Abstracts, 12,* 900.

Dail, W. G., Jr., & Evan, A. P., Jr. (1974). Experimental evidence indicating that the penis of the rat is innervated by short adrenergic neurons. *American Journal of Anatomy, 141,* 203–218.

Danesino, V., & Martella, E. (1976). Modern conceptions of corpora cavernosa function in the vagina and clitoris. In T. P. Lowry & T. S. Lowry (Eds.), *The clitoris* (pp. 75–86). St. Louis: Green.

Danjou, P., Alexandre, L., Warot, D., Lacomblez, L., & Puech, A. J. (1988). Assessment of erectogenic properties of apomorphine and yohimbine in man. *British Journal of Clinical Pharmacology, 26*(6), 733–739.

Davidson, J. M., Camargo, C. A., & Smith, E. R. (1979). Effects of androgen on sexual behavior in hypogonadal men. *Journal of Clinical Endocrinology and Metabolism, 48*(6), 955–958.

Davies, T. F., Mountjoy, C. Q., Gomez-Pan, A., Watson, M. J., Hanker, J. P., Besser, G. M., & Hall, R. (1976). A double blind cross over trial of gonadotrophin releasing hormone (LHRH) in sexually impotent men. *Clinical Endocrinology, 5,* 601–607.

deGroat, W. C., & Booth, A. M. (1980). Physiology of male sexual function (Part 2). *Annals of Internal Medicine, 92,* 329–331.

deGroat, W. C., & Steers, W. D. (1988). Neuroanatomy and neurophysiology of penile erection. In E. A. Tanagho, T. F. Lue, & R. D. McClure (Eds.), *Contemporary management of impotence and infertility* (pp. 3–27). Baltimore: Williams & Wilkins.

Delcour, C., & Struyven, J. (1988). Techniques for performing cavernosometry and cavernosography. *Cardiovascular and Interventional Radiology, 11*(4), 211–217.

Delcour, C., Vandenbosch, G., Wespes, E., Delatte, P., & Struyven, J. (1988). Pudendal arteriography. *Acta Urologica Belgica (Bruxelles), 56*(2), 308–314.

Delcour, C., Wespes, E., Schulman, C., & Struyven, J. (1988). Techniques for performing cavernosometry and cavernosography. *Acta Urologica Belgica (Bruxelles), 56*(2), 290–298.

Dennerstein, L., & Burrows, G. D. (1982). Hormone replacement therapy and sexuality in women. *Clinics in Endocrinology and Metabolism, II*(3), 661–679.

De-Nour, A. K. (1978). Hemodialysis: Sexual functioning. *Psychosomatics, 19*(4), 229–235.

Desai, K. M., & Gingell, J. C. (1988). Saline-induced artificial erection without papaverine: A potential source of error in diagnosing cavernosal venous leakage. *British Journal of Urology, 62*(2), 176–178.

Devathasan, G., Cheah, J. S., & Puvanendran, K. (1984). The bulbocavernosus reflex in diabetic impotence. *Singapore Medical Journal, 25*(3), 181–183.

Dhabuwala, C. B., Ghayad, P., Smith, J. B., Jr., & Pierce, J. M. (1983). Penile calibration for nocturnal penile tumescence studies. *Urology, 22*(6), 614–616.

Dhabuwala, C. B., Kerkar, P., Bhutwala, A., Kumar, A., & Pierce, J. M. (1990). Intracavernous papaverine in the management of psychogenic impotence. *Archives of Andrology, 24*(2), 185–191.

Dickinson, I. K., & Pryor, J. P. (1989). Pharmacocavernometry: A modified papaverine test. *British Journal of Urology, 63*(5), 539–545.

Dickinson, R. L. (1949). *Human sex anatomy* (2nd ed.). Baltimore: Williams & Wilkins.

Dorr, L. D., & Brody, M. J. (1967). Hemodynamic mechanisms of erection in the canine penis. *American Journal of Physiology, 213*(6), 1526–1531.

Dow, M. G., & Gallagher, J. (1989). A controlled study of combined hormonal and psychological treatment for sexual unresponsiveness in women (Part 3). *British Journal of Clinical Psychology, 28*, 201–212.

Dua, S., & Maclean, P. D. (1964). Localization for penile erection in medial frontal lobe. *American Journal of Physiology, 207*, 1425–1434.

Duffy, L. M., Sidi, A. A., & Lange, P. H. (1987). Vasoactive intracavernous pharmacotherapy— the nursing role in teaching self-injection therapy. *Journal of Urology, 138*, 1198–1200.

du Plessis, D. J., Bornman, M. S., Koch, Z., & Van Der Merwe, C. A. (1987). Penile ultrasonography in impotence. *South African Journal of Surgery, 25*, 69–71.

Eardley, I., Vale, J., Holmes, S., Patel, A., Kirby, R. S., & Lumley, J. S. P. (1990). Pharmacocavernometry in the assessment of erectile impotence. *Journal of the Royal Society of Medicine, 83*(1), 22–24.

Ehrensing, R. H., Kastin, A. J., & Schally, A. V. (1981). Behavioral and hormonal effects of prolonged high doses of LHRH in male impotence. *Peptides, 2*(1), 115–121.

Eibergen, R. D., & Caggiula, A. R. (1973). Ventral midbrain involvement in copulatory behavior of the male rat. *Physiology and Behavior, 10*, 435–441.

El-Bayoumi, M., El-Sherbini, O., & Mostafa, M. (1984). Impotence in diabetics: Organic versus psychogenic factors. *Urology, XXIV*(5), 459–463.

Ellenberg, M. (1971). Impotence in diabetes: The neurologic factor. *Annals of Internal Medicine, 75*, 213–219.

Ellison, J. M. (1982). Alterations of sexual behavior in temporal lobe epilepsy. *Psychosomatics, 23*(5), 499–509.

Engle, G., Burnham, S. J., & Carter, M. F. (1978). Penile blood pressure in the evaluation of erectile impotence. *Fertility and Sterility, 30*(6), 685–690.

Ertekin, C., Akyurekli, O., Gurses, A. N., & Turgut, H. (1985). The value of somatosensory-evoked potentials and bulbocavernosus reflex in patients with impotence. *Acta Neurologica Scandinavica, 71*(1), 48–53.

Ertekin, C., & Reel, F. (1976). Bulbocavernosus reflex in normal men and in patients with neurogenic bladder and/or impotence. *Journal of the Neurological Sciences, 28*, 1–15.

Faerman, D. I., Glocer, L., Gox, D., Jadzinsky, M. N., & Rapaport, M. (1974). Impotence and diabetes—histological studies of the autonomic nervous fibers of the corpora cavernosa in impotent diabetic males. *Diabetes, 23*, 971–976.

Faerman, I., Vilar, O., Rivarola, M. A., Rosner, J. M., Jadzinsky, M. N., Fox, D., Lloret, A. P., Bernstein-Hahn, L., & Saraceni, D. (1972). Impotence and diabetes—studies of androgenic function in diabetic impotent males. *Journal of Diabetes, 21*(1), 23–30.

Fahrenkrug, J., Palle, C., Jorgensen, J., & Ottesen, B. (1989). Regulatory peptides in mammalian urogenital system. *Experientia Supplement, 56*, 362–381.

Fanous, H. N., Jevtich, M. J., Chen, D. C. P., & Edson, M. (1982). Radioisotope penogram in diagnosis of vasculogenic impotence. *Urology, 20*, 499–502.

Fetter, T. R., Yunen, J. R., & Dodd, G. (1963). Application of cavernosography in the diagnosis of lesions of the penis. *American Journal of Roentgenology, 90*(1), 169–175.

Finkle, A. L., & Taylor, S. P. (1981). Sexual potency after radical prostatectomy. *Journal of Urology, 125*, 350–352.

Finney, R. P. (1983). Finney flexirod penile prosthesis. In R. J. Krane, M. B. Siroky, & I. Goldstein (Eds.), *Male sexual dysfunction* (pp. 243–252). Boston: Little, Brown.

Fisher, C., Schiavi, R., Edwards, A., Davis, D. M., Reitman, M., & Fine, J. (1979). Evaluation of nocturnal penile tumescence in the differential diagnosis of sexual impotence. *Archives of General Psychiatry, 36*, 431–437.

Fisher, C., Schiavi, R., Lear, H., Edwards, A., Davis, D. M., & Witkin, A. P. (1975). The assessment of nocturnal r.e.m. erection in the differential diagnosis of sexual impotence. *Journal of Sex & Marital Therapy, 1*(4), 277–289.

Fitzpatrick, D., Graber, B., Hendricks, S. E., Balogh, S., & Wetzel, M. W. (1986). Habituation of cortical evoked potentials produced by tibial or dorsal penile nerve stimulation. *Society of Neuroscience Abstracts, 12*, 336–336.

Fitzpatrick, D., Hendricks, S. E., Graber, B.,

Balogh, S. E., & Wetzel, M. (1989). Somatosensory evoked potentials elicited by dorsal penile and posterior tibial nerve stimulation. *Electroencephalography and Clinical Neurophysiology, 74,* 95–104.

Fitzpatrick, T. (1980). The venous drainage of the corpus cavernosum and spongiosum. In A. W. Zorgniotti & G. Rossi (Eds.), *Vasculogenic impotence* (pp. 181–184). Springfield, IL: Charles C. Thomas.

Fitzpatrick, W. F. (1974). Sexual function in the paraplegic patient. *Archives of Physical Medicine and Rehabilitation, 55,* 221–227.

Forleo, R., & Pasini, W. (1980). *Medical sexology— the Third International Congress.* Littleton, MA: PSG Publishing Co.

Forsberg, L., Ekelund, L., Hederstrom, E., & Olsson, A. M. (1988). Pharmacoangiography of the penile arteries. *Urologic Radiology, 10*(3), 132–135.

Forsberg, L., Hojerback, T., Olsson, A. M., & Rosen, I. (1989). Etiologic aspects of impotence in diabetes. *Scandinavian Journal of Urology and Nephrology, 23*(3), 173–175.

Forsberg, L., Olsson, A. M., & Neglen, P. (1982). Erectile function before and after aorto-iliac reconstruction: A comparison between measurements of Doppler acceleration ratio, blood pressure and angiography. *Journal of Urology, 27,* 379–382.

Fuchs, A. M., Mehringer, C. M., & Rajfer, J. (1989). Anatomy of penile venous drainage in potent and impotent men during cavernosography. *Journal of Urology, 141*(6), 1353–1356.

Fuchs, M. E., & Brawer, M. K. (1989). Papaverine-induced fibrosis of the corpus cavernosum. *Journal of Urology, 141*(1), 125–125.

Fugl-Meyer, A. R., Sjogren, K., & Johansson, K. (1984). A vaginal temperature regulation system. *Archives of Sexual Behavior, 13*(3), 247–260.

Furlow, W. L. (1979). Inflatable penile prosthesis: Mayo Clinic experience with 175 patients. *Urology, 13*(2), 166–171.

Gall, H., Bahren, W., Scherb, W., Stief, C., & Thon, W. (1988). Diagnostic accuracy of Doppler ultrasound technique of the penile arteries in correlation to selective arteriography. *Cardiovascular and Interventional Radiology, 11*(4), 225–231.

Gall, H., Bahren, W., Stief, C. G., Scherb, W., & Sparwasser, C. (1988). Diagnosis of vasculogenic impotence. Comparing investigations by Doppler sonography and angiography. *Acta Urologica Belgica (Bruxelles), 56*(2), 246–251.

Gallai, V., & Mazzotta, G. (1986). Electromyographical studies of the bulbo-cavernosus reflex in diabetic men with sexual dysfunction. *Electromyography & Clinical Neurophysiology, 26,* 521–527.

Gaskell, P. (1971). The importance of penile blood pressure in cases of impotence. *Canadian Medical Association Journal, 105,* 1047–1051.

Gasser, T. C., Roach, R. M., Larsen, E. H., Madsen, P. O., & Bruskewitz, R. C. (1987). Intracavernous self-injection with phentolamine and papaverine for the treatment of impotence. *Journal of Urology, 137*(4), 678–680.

Gee, W. F., McRoberts, W., Raney, J. O., & Ansell, J. S. (1974). The impotent patient: Surgical treatment with penile prosthesis and psychiatric evaluation. *Journal of Urology, 111,* 41–43.

Geer, J. H. (1975). Direct measurement of genital responding. *American Psychologist, 40,* 415–418.

Geer, J. H. (1976). Genital measures: Comments on their role in understanding human sexuality. *Journal of Sex & Marital Therapy, 2*(3), 165–172.

Geer, J. H. (1980). Measurement of genital arousal in human males and females. In I. Martin & P. H. Venables (Eds.), *Techniques in psychophysiology* (pp. 431–458). New York: Wiley.

Geer, J. H. (1983). Measurement and methodological considerations in vaginal photometry (Abstract). *International Academy of Sex Research, 21.*

Geer, J. H., & Fuhr, R. (1976). Cognitive factors in sexual arousal: The role of distraction. *Journal of Consulting & Clinical Psychology, 44*(2), 238–243.

Geiger, R. C. (1979). Neurophysiology of sexual response in spinal cord injury. *Sexuality and Disability, 2*(4), 257–266.

Gerstenberg, T. C., & Bradley, W. E. (1983). Nerve conduction velocity measurement of dorsal nerve of penis in normal and impotent males. *Urology, 21*(1), 90–92.

Gilbert, H. W., Gillatt, D. A., Desai, K. M., & Gingell, J. C. (1990). Intracorporeal papaverine injection in androgen deprived men. *Journal of the Royal Society of Medicine, 83*(3), 161–161.

Ginestie, J. F. (1980). Pudendal angiography. In A. W. Zorgniotti & G. Rossi (Eds.), *Vasculogenic impotence* (pp. 125–142). Springfield, IL: Charles C. Thomas.

Goldstein, I. (1983). Neurologic impotence. In R. J. Krane, M. B. Siroky, & I. Goldstein (Eds.), *Male sexual dysfunction* (pp. 193–201). Boston: Little, Brown.

Goldstein, I. (1988). Evaluation of penile nerves. In E. A. Tanagho, T. F. Lue, & R. D. McClure (Eds.), *Contemporary management of impotence and infertility* (pp. 70–83). Baltimore: Williams & Wilkins.

Goldstein, I., deTejada, I. S., Krane, R. J., Ottesen, B., Fahrenkrug, J., & Wagner, G. (1985). Changes in corporal vasoactive intestinal polypeptide (VIP) concentration following pelvic nerve stimulation (Abstract). *Journal of Urology, 133*(4), 218A.

Goldstein, I., Payton, T., & Padma-Nathan, H. (1988). Therapeutic roles of intracavernosal papaverine. *Cardiovascular and Interventional Radiology, 11*(4), 237–239.

Goldstein, I., Siroky, M. B., & Krane, R. J. (1983). Impotence in diabetes mellitus. In R. J. Krane, M. B. Siroky, & I. Goldstein (Eds.), *Male sexual dysfunction* (pp. 77–86). Boston: Little, Brown.

Goldstein, I., Siroky, M. B., Nath, R. L., McMillian, T. N., Menzoian, J. O., & Krane, R. J. (1982). Vasculogenic impotence: Role of the pelvic steal test. *Journal of Urology, 128*, 300–306.

Goligher, J. C. (1951). Sexual function after excision of the rectum. *Proceedings of the Royal Society of Medicine, 44*, 824–828.

Graber, B., & Kline-Graber, G. (1979). Female orgasm: Role of pubococcygeus muscle. *Journal of Clinical Psychiatry, 40*(8), 348–351.

Graber, B. and Kline-Graber, G. (1980). Pathophysiology of pubococcygeus muscle. In R. Forleo & W. Pasini (Eds.), *Medical sexology* (pp. 267–272). Littleton, MA: PSG Publishing Co.

Graber, B., & Kline-Graber, G. (1981). Research criteria for male erectile failure. *Journal of Sex & Marital Therapy, 7*(1), 37–48.

Graber, B., Kline-Graber, G., & Golden, C. J. (1981). A circumvaginal muscle nomogram: A new diagnostic tool for evaluation of female sexual dysfunction. *Journal of Clinical Psychiatry, 42*, 157–161.

Gray, H. (1985). *Anatomy of the human body* (30th ed.). Philadelphia: Lea & Febiger.

Gray, R., Grosman, H., St. Louis, E. L., & Leekam, R. (1984). The uses of corpus cavernosography. A review. *Journal of the Canadian Association of Radiologists, 35*(4), 338–342.

Green, R. (1981). Endocrine therapy of erectile fail-

ure. In G. Wagner & R. Green (Eds.), *Impotence* (pp. 143–148). New York: Plenum.

Griffith, E. R., Tomko, M. A., & Timms, R. J. (1973). Sexual function in spinal cord-injured patients: A review. *Archives of Physical Medicine and Rehabilitation, 54*, 539–542.

Griffith, E. R., Trieschmann, R. B., Hohmann, G. W., Cole, T. M., Tobis, J. S., & Cummings, V. (1975). Sexual dysfunctions associated with physical disabilities. *Archives of Physical Medicine and Rehabilitation, 56*, 8–13.

Gu, J., Lazardes, M., Pryor, J. P., Blank, M. A., Polak, J. M., Morgan, R., Marangos, P. J., & Bloom, S. R. (1984). Decrease of vasoactive intestinal polypeptide (VIP) in the penises of impotent men. *Lancet, 2*(8398), 315–318.

Gupta, K. (1990). Sexual dysfunction in elderly women. *Clinics in Geriatric Medicine, 6*(1), 197–203.

Haden, H. T., Katz, P. G., Mulligan, T., & Zasler, N. D. (1989). Penile blood flow by xenon-133 washout. *Journal of Nuclear Medicine, 30*(6), 1032–1035.

Haldeman, S., Bradley, W. E., & Bhatia, N. (1982). Evoked responses from the pudendal nerve. *Journal of Urology, 128*(5), 974–980.

Haldeman, S., Bradley, W. E., Bhatia, N. N., & Johnson, B. K. (1982). Pudendal evoked responses. *Archives of Neurology, 39*, 280–283.

Haldeman, S., Bradley, W. E., Bhatia, N. N., & Johnson, B. K. (1983). Cortical evoked potentials on stimulation of pudendal nerve in women. *Urology, 21*(6), 590–593.

Hallbook, T., & Holmquist, B. (1970). Sexual disturbances following dissection of the aorta and the common iliac arteries. *Journal of Cardiovascular Surgery, 4*, 255–260.

Hamilton, A., Lodge, M. M., & Hawkins, C. (1974). Sex and arthritis. *Reports on Rheumatic Diseases, 53*.

Hansen, M. V., Ertekin, C., Larsson, L. E., & Pedersen, K. (1989). A neurophysiological study of patients undergoing radical prostatectomy. *Scandinavian Journal of Urology and Nephrology, 23*(4), 267–273.

Harman, S. M. and Nankin, H. R. (1985). Alterations in reproductive and sexual function: Male. In R. Andres, E. L. Bierman, & W. R. Hazzard (Eds.), *Principles of geriatric medicine* (pp. 337–353). New York: McGraw-Hill.

Hart, B. L., & Haugen, C. M. (1968). Activation of sexual reflexes in male rats by spinal implantation of testosterone. *Physiology and Behavior, 3,* 735–738.

Hatch, J. P. (1981). Psychophysiological aspects of sexual dysfunction. *Archives of Sexual Behavior, 10*(1), 49–64.

Hauri, D., Knonagel, H., & Konstantinidis, K. (1989). Radical prostatectomy in cases of prostatic carcinoma: The problem concerning erectile impotence. *Urologia Internationalis, 44*(5), 272–278.

Hawatmeh, I. S., Houttuin, E., Gregory, J. G. and Purcell, M. H. (1983). Vascular surgery for the treatment of the impotent male. In R. J. Krane, M. B. Siroky, & I. Goldstein (Eds.), *Male sexual dysfunction* (pp. 291–300). Boston: Little, Brown.

Heath, R. G. (1954). Definition of the septal region. In *Studies in schizophrenia* (pp. 1–5). Cambridge, MA: Harvard University Press.

Heath, R. G., John, S. B., & Fontana, C. J. (1968). The pleasure response: Studies by stereotaxic technics in patients. In N. Kune & E. Laska (Eds.), *Computers and electronic devices in psychiatry* (pp. 178–189). New York: Wiley Interscience.

Heath, R. G., & Mickle, W. A. (1960). Evaluation of seven years' experience with depth electrode studies in human patients. In E. R. Ramey & D. S. O'Doherty (Eds.), *Electrical studies on the unanesthetized brain* (pp. 214–247). New York: Paul B. Hoeber.

Heaton, J. P., Morales, A., Owen, J., Saunders, F. W., & Fenemore, J. (1990). Topical glyceryltrinitrate causes measurable penile arterial dilation in impotent men. *Journal of Urology, 143*(4), 729–731.

Hedlund, H., & Andersson, K-E. (1985). Peptide effects on isolated human penile smooth muscle (Part 2, abstract). *Journal of Urology, 133*(4), 262A.

Heiman, J. R. (1977). A psychophysiological exploration of sexual arousal patterns in females and males. *Psychophysiology, 14*(3), 266–274.

Hellstrom, P. (1988). Urinary and sexual dysfunction after rectosigmoid surgery. *Annales Chirurgiae et Gynaecologiae, 77*(2), 51–56.

Henderson, V. E., & Roepke, M. H. (1933). On the mechanism of erection. *American Journal of Physiology, 106*, 441–448.

Henson, D. E., & Rubin, H. B. (1978). A comparison of two objective measures of sexual arousal of women (Abstract). *Behaviour Research and Therapy, 16*, 143–151.

Henson, C., Rubin, H. B., & Henson, D. E. (1979a). Women's sexual arousal concurrently assessed by three genital measures. *Archives of Sexual Behavior, 8*(6), 459–469.

Henson, D. E., Rubin, H. B., & Henson, C. (1979b). Analysis of the consistency of objective measures of sexual arousal in women. *Journal of Applied Behavioral Analysis, 12*, 701–711.

Henson, D. E., Rubin, H. B., Henson, C., & Williams, J. R. (1977). Temperature change of the labia minora as an objective measure of female eroticism. *Journal of Behavioral Therapy & Experimental Psychiatry, 8*, 401–410.

Herbert, J. (1973). The role of the dorsal nerves of the penis in the sexual behaviour of the male rhesus monkey. *Physiology & Behavior, 10*, 293–300.

Hierons, R. (1971). Impotence in temporal lobe lesions. *Journal of Neuro-Visceral Relations, Supplement 10*, 477–481.

Higgins, G. E., Jr. (1979). Sexual response in spinal cord injured adults: A review of the literature. *Archives of Sexual Behavior, 8*(2), 173–196.

Hoon, P. W. (1984). Physiologic assessment of sexual response in women: The unfulfilled promise. *Clinical Obstetrics and Gynecology, 27*(3), 767–780.

Hoon, E. F., Hoon, P. W., & Wincze, J. P. (1976). An inventory for the measurement of female sexual arousability: The SAI. *Archives of Sexual Behavior, 5*(4), 291–300.

Howard, D. J., & Rees, J. R. (1976). Long-term perhexiline maleate and liver function. *British Medical Journal, 1*, 123–133.

Hrebinko, R., Bahnson, R. R., Schwentker, F. N., & O'Donnell, W. F. (1990). Early experiences with the DuraPhase penile prosthesis. *Journal of Urology, 143*(1), 60–61.

Hulsebosch, C. E., & Coggeshall, R. E. (1982). An analysis of the axon populations in the nerves to the pelvic viscera in the rat. *Journal of Comparative Neurology, 211*(1), 1–10.

Hursch, C. J., Karacan, I., & Williams, R. L. (1972). Some characteristics of nocturnal penile tumescence in early middle-aged males. *Comprehensive Psychiatry, 13*(6), 539–548.

Iwai, T., Sato, S., Muraoka, Y., Sakurazawa, K., Kinoshita, H., Inoue, Y., Endo, M., & Yoshida, T. (1989). The assessment of pelvic circulation after internal iliac arterial reconstruction: A retrospective study of the treatment for vasculogenic impotence and hip claudication. *Japanese Journal of Surgery, 19*(5), 549–555.

Jamison, P. L., & Gebhard, P. H. (1988). Penis size increase between flaccid and erect states: An analysis of the Kinsey data. *Journal of Sex Research, 24,* 177–183.

Jensen, P., Jensen, S. B., Sorensen, P. S., Bjerre, B. D., Rizzi, D. A., Sorensen, A. S., Klysner, R., Brinch, K., Jespersen, B., & Nielsen, H. (1990). Sexual dysfunction in male and female patients with epilepsy: A study of 86 outpatients (Abstract). *Archives of Sexual Behavior, 19*(1), 1.

Jensen, S. B. (1981). Diabetic sexual dysfunction: A comparative study of 160 insulin treated diabetic men and women and an age-matched control group. *Archives of Sexual Behavior, 10*(6), 493–504.

Jevitch, M. J., Khawand, N. Y., & Vidic, B. (1990). Clinical significance of ultrastructural findings in the corpora cavernosa of normal and impotent men. *Journal of Urology, 143*(2), 289–293.

Jochheim, K.-A., & Wahle, H. (1970). A study on sexual function in 56 male patients with complete irreversible lesions of the spinal cord and cauda equina. *Paraplegia, 8,* 166–170.

Johnson, R. D., Kitchell, R. L., & Gilanpour, H. (1986). Rapidly and slowly adapting mechanoreceptors in the glans penis of the cat. *Physiology & Behavior, 37*(1), 69–78.

Johnston, P., & Davidson, J. M. (1972). Intracerebral androgens and sexual behavior in the male rat. *Hormones & Behavior, 3,* 345–357.

Jonas, U. (1983). Silicone-silver penile prosthesis. In R. J. Krane, M. B. Siroky, & I. Goldstein (Eds.), *Male sexual dysfunction* (pp. 267–274). Boston: Little, Brown.

Joos, H., Kunit, G., & Frick, J. (1985). Traumatic rupture of corpus cavernosum. *Urologia Internationalis, 40*(3), 128–131.

Jovanovic, U. J. (1971). The recording of physiological evidence of genital arousal in human males and females. *Archives of Sexual Behavior, 1*(4), 309–320.

Juenemann, K-P., Lue, T. F., Luo, J-A., Jadallah, S. A., Nunes, L. L., & Tanagho, E. A. (1987). The role of vasoactive intestinal polypeptide as a neurotransmitter in canine penile erection: A combined *in vivo* and immunohistochemical study. *Journal of Urology, 138*(4), 871–877.

Kabalin, J. N., & Kessler, R. (1989a). Penile prosthesis surgery: Review of ten-year experience and examination of reoperations. *Urology, 33*(1), 17–19.

Kabalin, J. N., & Kessler, R. (1989b). Experience with the Hydroflex penile prosthesis. *Journal of Urology, 141*(1), 58–59.

Kaiser, F. E., & Korenman, S. C. (1988). Impotence in diabetic men. *American Journal of Medicine, 85*(5A), 147–152.

Kaneko, S., & Bradley, W. E. (1987). Penile electrodiagnosis: Penile peripheral innervation. *Urology, 30*(3), 210–212.

Kaplan, H. S. (1974). The classification of the female sexual dysfunctions. *Journal of Sex & Marital Therapy, 1*(2), 124–138.

Kaplan, H. S. (1983). The comprehensive evaluation of the psychosexual disorders II. The psychosexual dysfunctions 2. Excitement phase disorders: Impotence and impaired female excitement. In H. S. Kaplan (Ed.), *The evaluation of sexual disorders: Psychological and medical aspects* (pp. 224–239). New York: Brunner/Mazel.

Kaplan, P. E. (1981). A somatosensory evoked response obtained after stimulation of the contralateral pudendal nerve. *Electromyography and Clinical Neurophysiology, 21*(6), 585–587.

Karacan, I. (1970). Clinical value of nocturnal erection in the prognosis and diagnosis of impotence. *Medical Aspects of Human Sexuality, 4,* 27.

Karacan, I., & Howell, J. W. (1988). Use of nocturnal penile tumescence in diagnosis of male erectile dysfunction. In E. A. Tanagho, T. F. Lue, & R. D. McClure (Eds.), *Contemporary management of impotence and infertility* (pp. 95–103). Baltimore: Williams & Wilkins.

Karacan, I., Williams, R. L., Guerrero, M. W., Salis, P. J., Thornby, J. I., & Hursch, C. J. (1974). Nocturnal penile tumescence and sleep of convicted rapists and other prisoners. *Archives of Sexual Behavior, 3*(1), 19–26.

Kaufman, S. A. (1983). The gynecologic evaluation of female excitement disorders. In H. S. Kaplan (Ed.), *The evaluation of sexual disorders* (pp. 122–127). New York: Brunner/Mazel.

Kedia, K. R. (1981). Vascular disorders and male erectile dysfunction—current status in diagnosis and management by revascularization of the corpora cavernosa. *Urologic Clinics of North America, 8*(1), 153–168.

Kegel, A. H. (1948a). The nonsurgical treatment of genital relaxation—use of the perineometer as an aid in restoring anatomic and functional structure. *Annals of Western Medicine & Surgery, 2,* 213–216.

Kegel, A. H. (1948b). Progressive resistance exercise in the functional restoration of the perineal muscles. *American Journal of Obstetrics & Gynecology, 56*(2), 238–248.

Kegel, A. H. (1952a). Stress incontinence and genital relaxation: A nonsurgical method of increasing the tone of sphincters and their supporting structures. *Ciba Clinical Symposia, 4*(2), 35–49.

Kegel, A. H. (1952b). Sexual functions of the pubococcygeus muscle. *Western Journal of Surgery, Obstetrics and Gynecology* (October), 521–524.

Kempczinski, R. F. (1979). Role of the vascular diagnostic laboratory in the evaluation of male impotence. *American Journal of Surgery, 138,* 278–282.

Kennedy, S., & Over, R. (1990). Psychophysiological assessment of male sexual arousal following spinal cord injury. *Archives of Sexual Behavior, 19*(1), 15–27.

Kiely, E. A., Ignotus, P., & Williams, G. (1987). Penile function following intercavernosal injection of vasoactive agents or saline. *British Journal of Urology, 59,* 473–476.

Kirschenbaum, A., & Mitty, H. A. (1988). Penile prosthesis. *Urologic Radiology, 10*(3), 160–165.

Kling, A. (1972). Effects of amygdalectomy on social-affective behavior in non-human primates. In B. E. Eleftheriou (Ed.), *Advances in behavioral biology* (Vol. 2, pp. 511–536). New York: Plenum.

Kluver, H. (1958). "The temporal lobe syndrome" Produced by bilateral ablations. In G. E. W. Woltensholme & M. E. O'Connor (Eds.), *Neurological basis of behavior* (pp. 175–182). Boston: Little, Brown.

Kluver, H., & Bucy, P. C. (1939). Preliminary analysis of functions of the temporal lobes in monkeys. *Archives of Neurology and Psychiatry, 42,* 979–1000.

Kolodny, R. C. (1971). Sexual dysfunction in diabetic females. *Diabetes, 20*(8), 557–559.

Kolodny, R. C., Kahn, C. B., Goldstein, H. H., & Barnett, D. M. (1974). Sexual dysfunction in diabetic men. *Diabetes, 23*(4), 306–309.

Korff, J., & Geer, J. H. (1983). The relationship between sexual arousal experience and genital response. *Psychophysiology, 20*(3), 121–127.

Krane, R. J., & Siroky, M. B. (1980). Studies on sacral-evoked potentials. *Journal of Urology, 124,* 872–876.

Krantz, K. E. (1958). Innervation of the human vulva and vagina. *Obstetrics and Gynecology, 12*(4), 382–396.

Krantz, K. E. (1959). The gross and microscopic anatomy of the human vagina. *Annals of the New York Academy of Sciences, 83*(2), 89–104.

Krantz, K. E. (1982). Anatomy of the female reproductive system. *Obstetrics & gynecologic diagnosis & treatment* (Chapter 2—pp. 14–57).

Kuo, D. C., Hisamitsu, T., & deGroat, W. C. (1984). A sympathetic projection from sacral paravertebral ganglia to the pelvic nerve and to postganglionic nerves on the surface of the urinary bladder and large intestine of the cat. *Journal of Comparative Neurology, 226,* 76–86.

Lakin, M. M., & Montague, D. K. (1989). Intracavernous injections of papaverine and phentolamine: Correlation with penile brachial index. *Urology, 33*(5), 383–386.

Lal, S., Laryea, E., Thavundayil, J. X., Vasavan Nair, N. P., Negrette, J., Ackman, D., Blundell, P., & Gardiner, R. J. (1987). Apomorphine-induced penile tumescence in impotent patients—preliminary findings. *Progress of Neuro-Psychopharmacological and Biological Psychiatry, 11,* 235–242.

Lamid, S. (1985). Nocturnal penile tumescence studies in spinal cord injured males. *Paraplegia, 24*(1), 26–31.

Langley, J. N., & Anderson, H. K. (1895). The innervation of the pelvic and adjoining viscera. *Journal of Physiology, 19,* 71–84.

Langley, J. N., & Anderson, H. K. (1896). The innervation of the pelvic and adjoining viscera. *Journal of Physiology, 20,* 372–406.

Larsen, E., & Hejgaard, N. (1984). Sexual dysfunction after spinal cord or cauda equina lesions. *Paraplegia, 22,* 66–74.

Larsson, K., & Sodersten, P. (1973). Mating in male rats after section of the dorsal penile nerve. *Physiology & Behavior, 10,* 567–571.

Larsson, L.-I., & Fahrenkrug, J. (1977). Vasoactive intestinal polypeptide occurs in nerves of the female genitourinary tract. *Science, 197,* 1374–1375.

Lash, H. (1968). Silicone implant for impotence. *Journal of Urology, 100,* 709–710.

Lavoisier, P. (1982). Rehabilitation for the circumvaginal musculature. In B. Graber (Ed.), *Circumvaginal musculature and sexual function* (pp. 88–92). Basel New York: Karger.

Lavoisier, P., Proulx, J., Courtois, F., DeCaruffel, F., & Durand, L-G. (1988). Relationship between perineal muscle contractions, penile tumescence, and penile rigidity during nocturnal erections. *Journal of Urology, 139,* 176–179.

Learmonth, J. R. (1931). A contribution to the neurophysiology of the urinary bladder in man. *Brain, 54,* 147–176.

Legros, J. J., Franchimont, P., Palem-Vliers, M., & Servais, J. (1973). FSH, LH and testosterone blood level in patients with psychogenic impotence. *Endocrinologia Experimentalis, 7,* 59–64.

Levin, R. J. (1981). The female orgasm—a current appraisal. *Journal of Psychosomatic Research, 25*(2), 119–133.

Levin, R. J., & Wagner, G. (1978). Haemodynamic changes of the human vagina during sexual arousal assessed by a heated oxygen electrode. *Journal of Physiology, 275,* 23–24.

Levin, R. J., & Wagner, G. (1980). Sexual arousal in women—which haemodynamic measure gives the best assessment? *Journal of Physiology, 302,* 22–22.

Levine, S. B., Althof, S. E., Turner, L. A., Risen, C. B., Bodner, D. R., Kursh, E. D., & Resnick, M. I. (1989). Side effects of self-administration of intracavernous papaverine and phentolamine for the treatment of impotence. *Journal of Urology, 141*(1), 54–57.

Levitt, E. E., Konovsky, M., Freese, M. P., & Thompson, J. F. (1979). Intravaginal pressure assessed by the kegel perineometer. *Archives of Sexual Behavior, 8*(5), 425–429.

Levy, N. B. (1973). Sexual adjustment to maintenance hemodialysis and renal transplantation: National survey by questionnaire: Preliminary report. *Transactions of the American Society for Artificial Internal Organs, 19,* 138–143.

Lewis, R. W. (1988). This month in investigative urology: Venous impotence. *Journal of Urology, 140*(6), 1560–1570.

Lierse, W. (1982). Blood vessels and nerves of the human penis. *Urologia Internationalis, 37*(3), 145–151.

Lin, J. T., & Bradley, W. E. (1985). Penile neuropathy in insulin-dependent diabetes mellitus. *Journal of Urology, 133,* 207–212.

Lin, M. C., Hsu, G. L., Chen, S. C., Wang, C. L., & Tsai, T. C. (1988). Role of Doppler ultrasound in the evaluation of penile hemodynamics in male impotence. *Taiwan I Hsueh Hui Tsa Chih, 87*(10), 960–965.

Lin, S. N., Liu, R. S., Yu, P. C., Chang, L. S., Yeh, S. H., & Kuo, J. S. (1989). Diagnosis of vasculogenic impotence: Combination of penile xenon-133 washout and papaverine tests. *Urology, 34*(1), 28–32.

Lisk, R. D. (1967). Neural localization for androgen activation of copulatory behavior in the male rat. *Endocrinology, 80,* 754–761.

Loefler, R. A., & Iverson, R. E. (1976). Surgical treatment of impotence in the male—an 18-year experience with 250 penile implants. *Plastic & Reconstructive Surgery, 58*(3), 292–297.

Lowry, T. P. (1978). *The classic clitoris . . . Historic contributions to scientific sexuality.* Chicago: Nelson-Hall.

Lue, T. F. (1988). Treatment of venogenic impotence. In E. A. Tanagho, T. F. Lue, & R. D. McClure (Eds.), *Contemporary management of impotence and infertility* (pp. 175–177). Baltimore: Williams & Wilkins.

Lue, T. F., Hricak, H., Marich, K. W., & Tanagho, E. A. (1985). Vasculogenic impotence evaluated by high-resolution ultrasonography and pulsed Doppler spectrum analysis. *Radiology, 155,* 777–781.

Lue, T. F., & McAninch, J. W. (1988). Priapism. In E. A. Tanagho, T. F. Lue, & R. D. McClure (Eds.), *Contemporary management of impotence and infertility* (pp. 201–210). Baltimore: Williams & Wilkins.

Lue, T. F., Hricak, H., Schmidt, R. A., & Tanagho, E. A. (1986). Functional evaluation of penile veins by cavernosography in papaverine-induced erection. *Journal of Urology, 135*(3), 479–482.

Lue, T. F., & Tanagho, E. A. (1987). Physiology of erection and pharmacological management of impotence. *Journal of Urology, 137,* 829–836.

Lue, T. F., & Tanagho, E. A. (1988a). Functional anatomy and mechanism of penile erection. In E. A. Tanagho, T. F. Lue, & R. D. McClure (Eds.), *Contemporary management of impotence and infertility* (pp. 39–50). Baltimore: Williams & Wilkins.

Lue, T. F., & Tanagho, E. A. (1988b). Hemodynamics of erection. In E. A. Tanagho, T. F. Lue, & R. D. McClure (Eds.), *Contemporary management of impotence and infertility* (pp. 28–38). Baltimore: Williams & Wilkins.

Lundberg, P. O. (1978). Sexual dysfunction in women with multiple sclerosis. In R. Forleo & W. Pasini (Eds.), *Medical sexology* (pp. 426–429). Littleton, MA: PSG Publishing Co.

Maatman, T. J., Montague, D. K., & Martin, L. M. (1987). Erectile dysfunction in men with diabetes mellitus. *Urology, 29*(6), 589–592.

Mackey, F. G. (1986). Sexuality in coronary artery disease—A problem-oriented approach. *Sex in Coronary Artery Disease, 80*(1), 58–72.

Maclean, P. D. (1966). Studies on the cerebral representation of certain basic sexual functions. In R. A. Gorski & R. E. Whelan (Eds.), *Brain and behavior* (Vol. 3, pp. 35–79). Los Angeles: University of California Press.

Maclean, P. D. (1989). The hypothalamus and emotional behavior. In W. Haymaker, E. Anderson, & W. J. H. Nauta (Eds.), *The hypothalamus* (pp. 659–678). Springfield, IL: Charles C. Thomas.

Maclean, P. D., & Delgado, J. M. R. (1953). Electrical and chemical stimulation of frontotemporal portion of limbic system in the waking animal. *Electroencephalography & Clinical Neurophysiology, 5,* 91–100.

Maclean, P. D., Denniston, R. H., & Dua, S. (1963). Further studies on cerebral representation of penile erection: Caudal thalamus, midbrain, and pons. *Journal of Neurophysiology, 26,* 273–293.

Maclean, P. D., Denniston, R. H., Dua, S., & Ploog, D. W. (1962). Hippocampal changes with brain stimulation eliciting penile erection. In *Physiologie de l'hippocampe* (pp. 491–510). Paris: Centre National de la Recherche Scientifique.

Maclean, P. D., Dua, S., & Denniston, R. H. (1961). Dien-mesencephalic loci involved in penile erection and seminal discharge. *Federation Proceedings, 20,* 331c.

Maclean, P. D., & Ploog, D. W. (1962). Cerebral representation of penile erection. *Journal of Neurophysiology, 25,* 29–55.

Malhotra, C. M., Balko, A., Wincze, J. P., Bansal, S., & Susset, J. G. (1986). Cavernosography in conjunction with artificial erection for evaluation of venous leakage in impotent men. *Radiology, 161*(3), 799–802.

Marshall, P., Morales, A., & Surridge, D. (1982). Diagnostic significance of penile erections during sleep. *Urology, 20*(1), 1–6.

Marshall, P., Surridge, D., & Delva, N. (1981). The role of nocturnal penile tumescence in differentiating between organic and psychogenic impotence: The first stage of validation. *Archives of Sexual Behavior, 10*(1), 1–10.

Martin, L. M. (1981). Impotence in diabetes: An overview. *Psychosomatics, 22*(4), 318–328.

Masters, W. H., & Johnson, V. E. (1966). *Human sexual response.* Boston: Little, Brown.

May, A. G., DeWeese, J. A., & Rob, C. G. (1969). Changes in sexual function following operation on the abdominal aorta. *Surgery, 65*(1), 41–47.

McConnell, J., Benson, G. S., & Wood, J. (1979). Autonomic innervation of the mammalian penis: A histochemical and physiological study. *Journal of Neural Transmission, 45,* 227–238.

McKenna, K. E., & Nadelhaft, I. (1985). Pudendal nerve reflexes in the male and female rat. *Society of Neuroscience Abstracts, 11,* 701.

McKenna, K. E., & Nadelhaft, I. (1986). The organization of the pudendal nerve in the male and female rat. *Journal of Comparative Neurology, 248,* 532–549.

Mehta, A. J., Viosca, S. P., Korenman, S. G., & Davis, S. S. (1986). Peripheral nerve conduction studies and bulbocavernosus reflex in the investigation of impotence. *Archives of Physical Medicine and Rehabilitation, 67*(5), 332–335.

Meisel, R. L., Lumia, A. R., & Sachs, B. D. (1980). Effects of olfactory bulb removal and flank shock on copulation in male rats. *Physiology & Behavior, 25,* 383–387.

Merrill, D. C. (1988). Clinical experience with the Mentor inflatable penile prosthesis in 301 patients. *Journal of Urology, 140*(6), 1424–1427.

Messe, M. R., & Geer, J. H. (1985). Voluntary vaginal musculature contractions as an enhancer of sexual arousal. *Archives of Sexual Behavior, 14*(1), 13–28.

Meyers, R. (1963). Central neural counterparts of penile potency and libido in humans and subhuman mammals. *Cincinnati Journal of Medicine,* 281–291.

Meyerson, B. (1988). Neuropeptides and sexual function. In J. M. A. Sitsen (Ed.), *Handbook of sexology* (Vol. 6, pp. 44–65). New York: Elsevier.

Miccoli, R., Giampietro, O., Tognarelli, M., Rossi, B., Giovannitti, G., & Navalesi, R. (1987). Prevalence and type of sexual dysfunctions in diabetic males: A standardized clinical approach. *Journal of Medicine, 18*(5-6), 305–321.

Michal, V. (1982). Arterial disease as a cause of impotence. *Clinics in Endocrinology and Metabolism, 11*(3), 725–748.

Michal, V., Kramar, R., Hejhal, L., & Firt, P. (1980). Aortoiliac occlusive disease. In A. W. Zorgniotti & G. Rossi (Eds.), *Vasculogenic impotence. Proceedings of the First International Conference on Corpus Cavernosum Revascularization* (pp. 203–215). Springfield, IL: Charles C. Thomas.

Michal, V., Kramar, R., & Pospichal, J. (1974). Femoro-pudendal bypass, internal iliac thromboendarterectomy and direct arterial anastomosis to the cavernous body in the treatment of erectile impotence. *Bulletin de la Société Internationale de Chirurgie (Brussels), 33,* 343–350.

Michal, V., Pospichal, J., & Blazkova, J. (1980). Arteriography of the internal pudendal arteries and passive erection. In A. W. Zorgniotti & G. Rossi (Eds.), *Vasculogenic impotence. Proceedings of the First International Conference on Corpus Cavernosum Revascularization* (pp. 169–179). Springfield, IL: Charles C. Thomas.

Milne, J. F., Golden, J. S., & Fibus, L. (1977). Sexual dysfunction in renal failure: A survey of chronic hemodialysis patients. *Psychiatry in Medicine, 8,* 335–345.

Mitchell, G. A. G. (1953). The thoracic part of the sympathetic system. In G. A. G. Mitchell (Ed.), *Anatomy of the autonomic nervous system* (pp. 237–256). London: E. & S. Livingston.

Modebe, O. (1989). Serum prolactin concentration in impotent African males. *Andrologia, 21*(1), 42–47.

Montague, D. K. (1979). Which penile prosthesis? Study provides some guidelines. *Hospital Practice, 14*(7), 19–25.

Mooradian, A. D., Morley, J. E., Kaiser, F. E., Davis, S. S., Viosca, S. P., & Korenman, S. C. (1989). Biweekly intracavernous administration of papaverine for erectile dysfunction. *Western Journal of Medicine, 151*(5), 515–517.

Morales, A., Condra, M., Owen, J. A., Fenemore, J., & Surridge, D. H. (1988). Oral and trunscutaneous pharmacologic agents for the treatment of impotence. In E. A. Tanagho, T. F. Lue, & R. D. McClure (Eds.), *Contemporary management of impotence and infertility* (pp. 175–185). Baltimore: Williams & Wilkins.

Morales, A., Condra, M., Owen, J. A., Surridge, D. H., Fenemore, J., & Harris, C. (1987). Is yohimbine effective in the treatment of organic impotence? *Journal of Urology, 137,* 1168–1172.

Morales, A., Condra, M., & Reid, K. (1990). The role of nocturnal penile tumescence monitoring in the diagnosis of impotence: A review. *Journal of Urology, 143*(3), 441–446.

Morales, A., Surridge, D. H., & Marshall, P. G. (1981). Yohimbine for treatment of impotence in diabetes. *New England Journal of Medicine, 305*(20), 1221.

Mulcahy, J. J. (1988). The Hydroflex self-contained inflatable prosthesis: Experience with 100 patients. *Journal of Urology, 140*(6), 1422–1423.

Mulligan, T., & Katz, P. G. (1989). Why aged men become impotent. *Archives of Internal Medicine, 149*(6), 1365–1366.

Nagler, H. M., & Blaivas, J. G. (1987). Impotence: Treatment. In J. P. Pryor & L. I. Lipshultz (Eds.), *Andrology* (pp. 148–182). London: Butterworth's.

Nakatsu, S. L., Condra, M., Fenemore, J., Surridge, D. H., & Morales, A. (1985). The pharmacokinetics of yohimbine in man. *Journal of Urology, 133*(4), 262A.

Negelev, S. (1990). Re: Topical nitroglycerin: A potential treatment for impotence [letter]. *Journal of Urology, 143*(3), 586.

Netto Junior, N. R., Reinato, J. A., Cara, A., & Claro, J. F. (1990). Cavernosometry: Corroboratory method to surgical treatment of impotence due to venous leakage. *Urology, 35*(1), 35–37.

Newman, H. F. (1983). Physiology of erection: Anatomic considerations. in R. J. Krane, M. B. Siroky, & I. Goldstein (Eds.), *Male sexual dysfunction* (pp. 1–8). Boston: Little, Brown.

Newman, H. F., Northup, J. D., & Devlin, J. (1964). Mechanism of human penile erection. *Investigative Urology, 1,* 350–353.

Nofzinger, E. A., & Schmidt, H. S. (1990). An exploration of central dysregulation of erectile function as a contributing case of diabetic impotence. *Journal of Nervous & Mental Disease, 178*(2), 90–95.

Nseyo, U. O., Wilbur, H. J., Kang, S. A., Flesh, L., & Bennett, A. H. (1984). Penile xenon (133Xe) washout: A rapid method of screening for vasculogenic impotence. *Urology, (23)*(1), 31.

Nunez, R., Gross, G. H., & Sachs, B. D. (1986). Origin and central projections of rat dorsal penile nerve: Possible direct projection to autonomic and somatic neurons by primary afferents of nonmuscle origin. *Journal of Comparative Neurology, 247,* 417–429.

O'Donnell, P., Leach, G., & Raz, S. (1983). Surgical treatment of Peyronie's disease. In R. J. Krane, M. B. Siroky, & I. Goldstein (Eds.), *Male sexual dysfunction* (pp. 225–242). Boston: Little, Brown.

O'Donohue, W. T., & Geer, J. H. (1985). The habituation of sexual arousal. *Archives of Sexual Behavior, 14*(3), 233–246.

Ottsen, B., Sondergaard, F., & Fahrenkrug, J. (1983). Neuropeptides in the regulation of female genital smooth muscle contractility. *Acta Obstetricia Gynecologia Scandinavica, 62,* 591–592.

Owen, J. A., Saunders, F., Harris, C., Fenemore,

J., Reid, K., Surridge, D., Condra, M., & Morales, A. (1989). Topical nitroglycerin: A potential treatment for impotence. *Journal of Urology, 141*(3), 546–548.

Padma-Nathan, H., & Goldstein, I. (1988). Arteriogenic impotence: C. Arterial reconstruction. In E. A. Tanagho, T. F. Lue, & R. D. McClure (Eds.), *Contemporary management of impotence and infertility* (pp. 163–174). Baltimore: Williams & Wilkins.

Pearman, R. O. (1967). Treatment of organic impotence by implantation of a penile prosthesis. *Journal of Urology, 97,* 716–719.

Perr, I. N. (1977). Traumatic impotence and the law—organic and psychologic factors. *Legal Aspects of Medical Practice,* 21–35.

Peters, R. H., Koch, P. C., & Blythe, B. L. (1988). Differential effects of yohimbine and naloxone on copulatory behaviors of male rats. *Behavioral Neuroscience, 102*(4), 559–564.

Pinto, L. C., & Sister, M. P. (1989). Pudendal cortical responses to male sexual dysfunction. *Clinical Evoked Potentials, 7*(1), 17–25.

Platzer, W., et al. (1978). Functional anatomy of the human vagina. In E. S. E. Hafez & T. N. Evans (Eds.), *The human vagina* (pp. 51–53). Amsterdam, NY/London: North-Holland Publishing Co.

Platzer, W., Poisel, S., & Hafez, E. S. E. (1978). Functional anatomy of the human vagina. In E. S. E. Hafez & T. N. Evans (Eds.), *The human vagina* (pp. 39–54). Amsterdam, NY/London: North-Holland Publishing Co.

Pogach, L. M., & Vaitukaitis, J. L. (1983). Endocrine disorders associated with erectile dysfunction. In R. J. Krane, M. B. Siroky, & I. Goldstein (Eds.), *Male sexual dysfunction* (pp. 63–76). Boston: Little, Brown.

Ponchietti, R., Tosto, A., Boncinelli, L., & Raugei, A. (1985). Our experience with sacral evoked potentials in impotence. *Acta Europaea Fertilitatis, 16*(5), 365–366.

Pontes, J. E., Huben, R. P., & Wolf, R. M. (1985). Sexual function in patients undergoing radical prostatectomy (Part 2). *Journal of Urology, 133*(4), 241A.

Porst, H., vanAhlen, H., Block, T., Halbig, W., Hautmann, R., Lochner-Ernst, D., Rudnick, J., Staehler, G., Weber, H. M., Weidner, W., et al. (1989). Intracavernous self-injection of prostaglandin E1 in the therapy of erectile dysfunction. *Vasa Supplementum (Bern), 28,* 50–56.

Prathar, R. C. (1988). Sexual dysfunction in the diabetic female: A review. *Archives of Sexual Behavior, 17*(3), 277–284.

Pressman, M. R., DiPhillipo, M. A., Kendrick, J. I., Conroy, K., & Fry, J. M. (1986). Problems in the interpretation of nocturnal penile tumescence studies: Disruption of sleep by occult sleep disorders. *Journal of Urology, 136*(3), 595–598.

Procci, W. R., & Martin, D. J. (1984). Preliminary observations of the utility of portable NPT. *Archives of Sexual Behavior, 13*(6), 569–580.

Pryor, J. P. (1988). Peyronie's disease and impotence. *Acta Urology Belgium, 56*(2), 317–321.

Pryor, J. L., & Howards, S. S. (1988). Variocele. In E. A. Tanagho, T. F. Lue, & R. D. McClure (Eds.), *Contemporary management of impotence and infertility* (pp. 247–264). Baltimore: Williams & Wilkins.

Puyau, F. A., Lewis, R. W., Balkin, P., Kaack, M. B., & Hirsch, A. (1987). Dynamic corpus cavernosography: Effect of papaverine injection. *Radiology, 164,* 179–182.

Quadraccia, A., Salvini, A., Corani, C., & Pizzi, P. (1988). Yohimbine plus intracavernous vasodilators in mild vasculogenic impotence. *Acta Urology Belgium, 56*(2): 272–278.

Raboch, J., Mellan, J., & Starka, L. (1975). Plasma testosterone in male patients with sexual dysfunction. *Archives of Sexual Behavior, 4*(5), 541–545.

Rao, K., Rao, M. S., Gupta, A. N., Sialy, R., & Vaidyanathan, S. (1981). Serum prolactin levels in male patients with erectile dysfunction. *Indian Journal of Medical Research, 74,* 412–414.

Reid, K., Morales, A., Harros, C., Surridge, D. H., Condra, M., Owen, J., & Fenemore, J. (1987). Double-blind trial of yohimbine in treatment of psychogenic impotence. *Lancet, 22,* 421–423.

Reiss, H. (1988). Improved technique for recording cavernosometries. *Urology, 32*(2), 115–118.

Reiss, H. (1989a). Use of prostaglandin E1 for papaverine-failed erections. *Urology, 33*(1), 15–16.

Reiss, H. (1989b). Re: Penile pharmacocavernosography and cavernosometry in the evaluation of impotence. *Journal of Urology, 142*(3), 830–831.

Reiss, H. F., Newman, H. F., & Zorgniotte, A. (1982). Artificial erection by perfusion of penile arteries. *Urology, 20*(3), 284–288.

Renshaw, D. C. (1975). Impotence in diabetics. *Diseases of the Nervous System, 36*(7), 369–371.

Robinette, M. A., & Moffat, M. J. (1986). Intracorporal injection of papaverine and phentolamine in the management of impotence. *British Journal of Urology, 58*(6), 692.

Robinson, B. W., & Mishkin, M. (1966). Ejaculation evoked by stimulation of the preoptic area in monkey. *Physiology and Behavior, 1,* 269–272.

Robinson, M. L., (1987). Yohimbine and psychogenic impotence. *Lancet 7,* 1088.

Rosen, M. P., Greenfield, A. J., Walker, T. G., Grant, P., Guben, J. K., Dubrow, J., Bettman, M. A., & Goldstein, I. (1990). Arteriogenic impotence: Findings in 195 impotent men examined with selective internal pudendal angiography (Part 2). *Radiology, 174*(3), 1043–1048.

Rosen, R. C., & Beck, J. G. (1988). *Patterns of sexual arousal: Psychophysiological processes and clinical applications.* New York: Guilford.

Rosen, R. C., Goldstein, L., Scoles, V., III, & Lazarus, C. (1986). Psychophysiologic correlates of nocturnal penile tumescence in normal males. *Psychosomatic Medicine, 48*(6), 423–429.

Rossman, B., & Zorgniotti, A. W. (1989). Progressive systemic sclerosis (scleroderma) and impotence. *Urology, 33*(3), 189–192.

Roy, A. C., & Ratnam, S. S. (1990). Re: Effects of prostaglandin E1 on penile erection and erectile failure [letter]. *Journal of Urology, 143*(1), 136–136.

Rubin, A., & Babbott, D. (1958). Impotence and diabetes mellitus. *Journal of the American Medical Association,* 498–500.

Sabri, S., & Cotton, L. T. (1971). Sexual function following aortoilliac reconstruction. *The Lancet* (December 4), 1218–1219.

Sachs, B. D., & Meisel, R. L. (1988). The physiology of male sexual behavior. In E. Knobil & J. Neill (Eds.), *The physiology of reproduction* (pp. 1264–1465). New York: Raven Press.

Sala, M., Braida, D., Leone, M. P., Calcaterra, P., Monti, S., & Gori, E. (1990). Central effect of yohimbine on sexual behavior in the rat. *Physiology and Behavior, 47,* (1), 165–173.

Sar, M., & Stumpf, W. E. (1973). Autoradiographic localization of radioactivity in the rat brain after the injection of 1,2-³H-testosterone. *Endocrinology, 92,* 251–256.

Sarica, Y., & Karacan, I. (1986). Cerebral responses evoked by stimulation of the vesico-urethral junction in normal subjects. *Electroencephalography and Clinical Neurophysiology, 65*(6), 440–446.

Sarica, Y., & Karacan, I. (1987). Bulbocavernosus reflex to somatic and visceral nerve stimulation in normal subjects and in diabetics with erectile impotence. *Journal of Urology, 138,* 55–58.

Sarica, Y., Karacan, I., Thornby, J. L., & Hirshkowitz, M. (1986). Cerebral responses evoked by stimulation of vesico-urethral junction in man: Methodological evaluation of monopolar stimulation. *Electroencephalography and Clinical Neurophysiology, 65*(2), 130–135.

Sarosdy, M. F., Hudnall, C. H., Erickson, D. R., Hardin, T. C., & Novicki, D. E. (1989). A prospective double-blind trial of intracorporeal papaverine versus prostaglandin E1 in the treatment of impotence. *Journal of Urology, 141*(3), 551–553.

Sarrel, P. M. (1990). Sexuality and menopause. *Obstetrics and Gynecology, 75*(4, Supp.), 26S–35S.

Saunders, M., & Rawson, M. (1970). Sexuality in male epileptics. *Journal of the Neurological Sciences, 10,* 577–583.

Schiavi, R. C. (1986). The role of NPT: Somatic versus psychological (Abstract). *National Institute of Diseased Diabetic Kidneys,* 1–3.

Schiavi, R. C. (1988). Nocturnal penile tumescence in the evaluation of erectile disorders: A critical review. *Journal of Sex & Marital Therapy, 14*(2), 83–97.

Schiavi, R. C., Fisher, C., White, D., Beers, P., & Szechter, R. (1984). Pituitary-gonadal function during sleep in men with erectile impotence and normal controls. *Psychosomatic Medicine, 46*(3), 239–254.

Schiavi, R. C., Fisher, C., Quadland, M., & Glover, A. (1985). Nocturnal penile tumescent evaluation of erectile function in insulin-dependent diabetic men. *Diabetologia, 28*(2), 90–94.

Schiavi, R. C., & White, D. (1976). Androgens and male sexual function: A review of human studies. *Journal of Sex & Marital Therapy, 2*(3), 214–228.

Schramek, P., Dorninger, R., Waldhauser, M., Konecny, P., & Porpaczy, P. (1990). Prostaglandin E1 in erectile dysfunction. Efficiency and incidence of priapism. *British Journal of Urology, 65*(1), 68–71.

Schramek, P., & Waldhauser, M. (1989). Dose-dependent effect and side-effect of prostaglandin E1 in erectile dysfunction. *British Journal of Clinical Pharmacology, 28*(5), 567–571.

Schwartz, N. B., & Kling, A. (1961). Effects of amygdalectomy on sexual behavior and reproductive capacity in the male rat. *Federation Proceedings, 20,* 335–335.

Scott, F. B., Byrd, G. J., Karacan, I., Olsson, P., Beutler, L. E., & Attia, S. L. (1979). Erectile impotence treated with an implantable, inflatable prosthesis. *Journal of the American Medical Association, 241*(24), 2609–2638.

Segraves, R. T., Madsen, R., Carter, C. S., & Davis, J. M. (1985). Erectile dysfunction associated with phramacological agents. In R. T. Segraves & H. W. Schoenberg (Eds.), *Diagnosis and treatment of erectile disturbances* (pp. 23–63). New York: Plenum.

Sem-Jacobsen, C. W. (1968). *Depth-electrographic stimulation of the human brain and behavior from fourteen years of studies and treatment of Parkinson's disease and mental disorders with implanted electrodes.* Springfield, IL: Charles C. Thomas.

Semans, J. H., & Langworthy, O. R. (1938). Observations on the neurophysiology of sexual function in the male cat. *Journal of Urology, 40,* 836–846.

Semmens, J. P., & Semmens, E. C. (1984). Sexual function and the menopause. *Clinical Obstetrics and Gynecology, 27*(93), 717–723.

Semmens, J. P., & Wagner, G. (1982). Estrogen deprivation and vaginal function in postmenopausal women. *Journal of the American Medical Association, 248*(4), 445–448.

Shabsigh, R., Fishman, I. J., Quesada, E. T., Seale-Hawkins, C. K., & Dunn, J. K. (1989). Evaluation of vasculogenic erectile impotence using penile duplex ultrasonography. *Journal of Urology, 142*(6), 1469–1474.

Sherfey, M. J. (1972). *The nature and evolution of female sexuality.* New York: Random House.

Shukla, G. D., Srivastava, O. N., & Katiyar, B. C. (1979). Sexual disturbances in temporal lobe epilepsy: A controlled study. *British Journal of Psychiatry, 134,* 288–292.

Sidi, A. A., Koleilat, N., & Fraley, E. E. (1988). Evaluation and treatment of organic impotence. *Investigative Radiology, 23*(10), 778–789.

Sintchak, G., & Geer, J. H. (1975). A vaginal plethysmograph system. *Psychophysiology, 12*(1), 113–115.

Siraj, Q. H., & Akhtar, M. A. (1989). Intracavernosal injection of pharmacological agents in the diagnosis and treatment of impotence. *Journal of the Philippine Medical Association, 39*(7), 172–176.

Siroky, M. B., & Krane, R. J. (1983). Neurophysiology of erection. In R. J. Krane, M. B. Siroky, &

I. Goldstein (Eds.), *Male sexual dysfunction* (pp. 9–20). Boston: Little, Brown.

Siroky, M. B., Sax, D. S., & Krane, R. J. (1979). Sacral signal tracing: The electrophysiology of the bulbocavernosus reflex. *Journal of Urology, 122,* 661–664.

Sjostrand, N. O., & Klinge, E. (1979). Principal mechanisms controlling penile retraction and protrusion in rabbits. *Acta Physiologica Scandinavica, 106,* 199–214.

Slimp, J. C., Hart, B. L., & Goy, R. W. (1978). Heterosexual, autosexual and social behavior of adult male rhesus monkeys with medial preoptic-anterior hypothalamic lesions. *Brain Research, 142,* 105–122.

Small, M. P. (1983). The small-carrion penile implant. In R. J. Krane, M. B. Siroky, & I. Goldstein (Eds.), *Male sexual dysfunction* (pp. 253–266). Boston: Little, Brown.

Stackl, W., Hasun, R., & Marberger, M. (1988). Intracavernous injection of prostaglandin E1 in impotent men. *Journal of Urology, 140,* 66–68.

Stahlgren, L. H., & Ferguson, L. K. (1958). Influence on sexual function of abdominoperineal resection for ulcerative colitis. *New England Journal of Medicine, 259*(18), 873–875.

Stief, C. G., Bohren, W., Gall, G., Scherb, W., & Altwein, J. E. (1988). Multidisciplinary evaluation in erectile dysfunction after radical prostatectomy. *International Urology and Nephrology (Budapest), 20*(6), 617–621.

Stief, C. G., Diederichs, W., Benard, F., Bosch, R., Lue, T. F., & Tanagho, E. A. (1988). The diagnosis of venogenic impotence: Dynamic or pharmacologic cavernosometry? *Journal of Urology, 140*(6), 1561–1563.

Stief, C. G., & Wellerauer, O. (1989). Quantitative and qualitative analysis of dynamic cavernosographies in erectile dysfunction due to venous leakage. *Urology, 34*(5), 252–257.

Stief, C. G., & Wetterauer, U. (1988). Erectile responses to intracavernosus papaverine and phentolamine: Comparison of single and combined delivery. *Journal of Urology, 140*(6), 1415–1416.

Stief, C. G., Wetterauer, U., & Sommerkamp, H. (1989). Intra-individual comparative study of dynamic and pharmacocavernography. *British Journal of Urology, 64*(1), 93–97.

Stock, W. E., & Geer, J. H. (1982). A study of fantasy-based sexual arousal in women. *Archives of Sexual Behavior, 11*(1), 33–47.

Surya, B. V., Provet, J., Dalbagni, G., Johanson,

K. E., & Brown, J. (1988). Experience with potency preservation during radical prostatectomy. Significance of learning curve. *Urology, 32*(6), 498–501.

Susset, J. G., Tessier, C. D., Wincze, J. Bansal, S. Malhotra, C., Schwacha, M. G., (1989). Effect of yohimbine hydrochloride on erectile impotence: A double-blind study. *Journal of Urology, 141*(6), 1360–1363.

Szasz, G., Stevenson, R. W. D., Lee, L., & Sanders, H. D. (1987). Induction of penile erection by intracavernosal injection: A double-blind comparison of phenoxybenzamine versus papaverine-phentolamine versus saline. *Archives of Sexual Behavior, 16*(5), 371–378.

Tackman, W., Porst, H., & vanAhlen, H. (1988). Bulbocavernosus reflex latencies and somatosensory evoked potentials after pudendal nerve stimulation in the diagnosis of impotence. *Journal of Neurology, 235*, 219–225.

Talbot, H. S. (1955). The sexual function in paraplegia. *73*(1), 91–100.

Taylor, D. C. (1971). Appetitive inadequacy in the sex behaviour of temporal lobe epileptics. *Journal of Neuro-Visceral Relations* (Suppl. 10), 486–490.

Taylor, T. K., & Coolican, M. J. (1988). Injuries of the conus medullaris. *Paraplegia, 26*(6), 393–400.

Thase, M. E., Reynolds, C. F., III, Jennings, J. R., Berman, S. R., Houck, P. R., Howell, J. R., Frank, E., & Kupfer, D. J. (1988). Diagnostic performance of nocturnal penile tumescence studies in healthy, dysfunctional (impotent), and depressed men. *Psychiatry Research, 26*(1), 79–87.

Thase, M. E., Reynolds, C. F., III, Jennings, J. R., Frank, E., Howell, J., Houck, P. R., & Kupfer, D. J. (1987). Do nocturnal penile tumescence recordings alter electroencephalographic sleep? *Sleep, 10*(5), 486–490.

Timm, G. W., Frohrib, D. A., & Bradley, W. E. (1976). Genitourinary prosthetics of the present and future. *Mayo Clinic Proceedings, 51*, 346–350.

Tiong, J. T., Taylor, A., England, E., & Hirsch, R. (1988). Fracture of the penis—review with case report. *Australian and New Zealand Journal of Surgery, 58*(5), 428–431.

Toone, B. K., Edeh, J., Nanjee, M. N., & Wheeler, M. (1989). Hyposexuality and epilepsy: A community survey of hormonal and behavioural changes in male epileptics. *Psychological Medicine, 19*(4), 937–943.

Torrens, M. J. (1983). Neurologic and neurosurgical disorders associated with impotence. In R. J. Krane, M. B. Siroky, & I. Goldstein (Eds.), *Male sexual dysfunction* (pp. 55–62). Boston: Little, Brown.

Tsai, C. C., Semmens, J. P., Semmens, E. C., Lam, C. F., & Lee, F. S. (1987). Vaginal physiology in postmenopausal women: pH value, transvaginal electropotential difference, and estimated blood flow. *Southern Medical Journal, 80*(8), 987–990.

Tsuji, I., Nakajima, F., Morimoto, J., & Nounaka, Y. (1961). The sexual function in patients with spinal cord injury. *Urologia Internationalis, 126*, 270–280.

Turner, L. A., Althof, S. E., Levine, S. B., Risen, C. B., Bodner, D. R., Kursh, E. D., & Resnick, M. I. (1989). Self-injection of papaverine and phentolamine in the treatment of psychogenic impotence. *Journal of Sex & Marital Therapy, 15*(3), 163–176.

Tyrer, G., Steel, J. M., Ewing, D. J., Bancroft, J., Warner, P., & Clarke, B. F. (1983). Sexual responsiveness in diabetic women. *Diabetologia, 24*, 166–171.

Vacek, J., & Lachman, M. (1977). Bulbokavernozni reflex u diabetiku s poruchou erektivity. Klinicka a elektromyograficka studie. *Casopis Lekaru Ceskych (Praha), 116*(3), 1014–1017.

Valji, K., & Bookstein, J. J. (1988). Transluminal angioplasty in the treatment of arteriogenic impotence. *Cardiovascular and Interventional Radiology, 11*(4), 245–252.

Vas, C. J. (1969). Sexual impotence and some autonomic disturbances in men with multiple sclerosis. *Acta Neurologica Scandinavica, 45*, 166–182.

Velcek, D., & Evans, J. A. (1982). Cavernosography. *Radiology, 144*, 781–785.

Velcek, D., Sniderman, K. W., Vaughan, E. D., Jr., & Sos, T. A. (1980). Penile flow index utilizing a Doppler pulse wave analysis to identify penile vascular insufficiency. *Journal of Urology, 123*, 669–673.

Virag, R. (1984). Artificial erection in diagnosis and treatment of impotence. *Urology, 24*(2), 157–161.

Virag, R. (1985). About pharmacologically induced prolonged erection. *Lancet, 1*(8427), 519–520.

Virag, R., Bouilly, P., & Frydman, D. (1985). Is impotence an arterial disorder? A study of arterial risk factors in 440 impotent men. *Lancet, 1*(8422), 181–184.

Vyas, P. R., Pierce, J. M., Jr., & Dhabuwala, C. B.

(1985). Doppler evaluation of penile blood vessels in the impotent male. *Journal of Urology, 133*(4), 187–187.

Wabrek, A. J. (1985). Bulbocavernosus reflex testing in 100 consecutive cases of erectile dysfunction. *Urology, 25*(5), 495–498.

Wagner, G. (1981a). Erection: Anatomy. In G. Wagner & R. Green (Eds.), *Impotence* (pp. 7–24). New York: Plenum.

Wagner, G. (1981b). Surgical treatment of erectile failure. In G. Wagner & R. Green (Eds.), *Impotence* (pp. 155–166). New York: Plenum.

Wagner, G. (1985). Mechanism of erection physiology and pathophysiology. In P. Kothari (Ed.), *Proceedings of World Congress of Sexology, Nov 5–8, 1985, New Delhi* (pp. 39–42). Bombay, India: Indian Association of Sex Educators.

Wagner, G., & Green, R. (1981). General medical disorders and erectile failure. In G. Wagner & R. Green (Eds.), *Impotence* (pp. 37–50). New York: Plenum.

Wagner, G., & Levin, R. J. (1978). Vaginal fluid. In E. S. E. Hafez & T. N. Evans (Eds.), *The human vagina* (pp. 121–137). New York: Elsevier/North-Holland Biomedical Press.

Wagner, G., & Metz, P. (1981). Arteriosclerosis and erectile failure. In G. Wagner & R. Green (Eds.), *Impotence* (pp. 63–72). New York: Plenum.

Wagner, G., & Ottesen, B. (1980). Vaginal blood flow during sexual stimulation. *Obstetrics & Gynecology, 56*(5), 621–624.

Wagner, G., & Sjostrand, N. O. (1988). Autonomic pharmacology and sexual function. In J. M. A. Sitsen (Ed.), *Handbook of sexology (Vol. 6): The pharmacology and endocrinology of sexual function* (pp. 32–43). New York: Elsevier.

Walsh, P. C., & Mostwin, J. L. (1984). Radical prostatectomy and cystoprostatectomy with preservation of potency. Results using a new nerve sparing technique. *British Journal of Urology, 56*(6), 694–697.

Wasserman, M. D., Pollak, C. P., Spielman, A. J., & Weitzman, E. D. (1980). The differential diagnosis of impotence—the measurement of nocturnal penile tumescence. *Journal of the American Medical Association, 20*, 2038–2042.

Watters, G. R., Keogh, E. J., Earle, C. M., Carati, C. J., Wisniewski, Z. S., Tulloch, A. G., & Lord, D. J. (1988). Experience in the mangement of erectile dysfunction using the intracavernosal self-injection of vasoactive drugs. *Journal of Urology, 140*(6), 1417–1419.

Wayrence, D. M., & Swyer, G. I. M. (1974). Plasma testosterone and testosterone binding affinities in men with impotence, oligospermia, azoospermia, and hypogonadism. *British Medical Journal, 1*, 349–351.

Wespes, E., Delcour, C., Rondeux, C., Struyven, J., & Schulman, C. (1987). The erectile angle: Objective criterion to evaluate the papaverine test in impotence. *Journal of Urology, 138*, 1171–1173.

Wespes, E., Delcour, C., Struyven, J., & Schulman, C. C. (1984). Cavernometry-cavernography: Its role in organic impotence. *European Urology, 10*(4), 229–232.

Wespes, E., & Schulman, C. C. (1984). Parameters of erection. *British Journal of Urology, 56*(41), 416–417.

Williams, L. P., & Warwick, R. (1980). *Gray's anatomy* (36th ed.). Philadelphia: Saunders.

Willmuth, M. E. (1987). Sexuality after spinal cord injury: A critical review. *Clinical Psychology Review, 7*, 389–412.

Willscher, M. K. (1983). Peyronie's disease. In R. J. Krane, M. B. Siroky, & I. Goldstein (Eds.), *Male sexual dysfunction* (pp. 87–100). Boston: Little, Brown.

Wincze, J. P., Bansal, S., Malhotra, C., Balko, A., Susset, J. G., & Malamud, M. (1988). A comparison of nocturnal penile tumescence and penile response to erotic stimulation during waking states in comprehensively diagnosed groups of males experiencing erectile difficulties. *Archives of Sexual Behavior, 17*(4), 333–348.

Wincze, J. P., Hoon, P., & Hoon, E. F. (1977). Sexual arousal in women: A comparison of cognitive and physiological responses by continuous measurement. *Archives of Sexual Behavior, 6*(2), 121–133.

Woolsey, C. N., Marshall, W. H., & Bard, P. (1942). Representation of cutaneous tactile sensibility in the cerebral cortex of the monkey as indicated by evoked potentials. *Bulletin of the Johns Hopkins Hospital, 70*, 399–441.

Zeitlin, A. B., Cottrell, T. L., & Lloyd, F. A. (1957). Sexology of the paraplegic male. *Fertility and Sterility, 8*, 337–344.

Zenico, T., Zoli, M., & Maltoni, G. (1989). Chemical prosthesis. *Acta Urologica Belgica (Bruxelles), 57*(1), 223–226.

Zentgraf, M., Baccouche, M., & Junemann, K. P. (1988). Diagnosis and therapy of erectile dysfunction using papaverine and phentolamine. *Urologia Internationalis, 43*, 65–75.

Zorgniotti, A. W. (1985). Vascular impotence and

diabetes: An update. *Practical Diabetology, 4*(2), 1–20.

Zorgniotti, A. W. (1986). Pharmacologic injection therapy. *Seminars in Urology, 4*(4), 233–235.

Zorgniotti, A. W., & Lue, T. F. (1988). Arteriogenic impotence: Intracavernous injection of papaverine and phentolamine. In E. A. Tanagho, T. F. Lue, & R. D. McClure (Eds.), *Contemporary management of impotence and infertility* (pp. 160–161). Baltimore: Williams & Wilkins.

Zorgniotti, A. W., Rossi, G., Padula, G., & Makovsky, R. D. (1980). Diagnosis and therapy of vasculogenic impotence. *Journal of Urology, 123,* 674–677.

Zuckerman, M., & Neeb, M. (1981). Nocturnal penile tumescence in diabetic and non-diabetic sexual dysfunction. (Unpublished).

CHAPTER 6

FEMALE SEXUAL AROUSAL DISORDER

Patricia J. Morokoff, University of Rhode Island

Lack of sexual arousal in women is a prevalent problem. Nearly half of a community sample of women reported difficulty becoming aroused (Frank, Anderson, & Rubinstein, 1978). Yet in spite of this prevalence, clinicians often prefer to conceptualize women with sexual problems as experiencing inhibited orgasm rather than inhibited arousal. Therapy outcome studies rarely focus on treatment of inhibited arousal, and clinical assessment of sexual arousal in women tends to be incomplete. The fact that diagnostic and treatment practices devalue such a widespread problem is contradictory and confusing.

One purpose of this chapter is to affirm that sexual arousal disorder in women is important and to discuss why it has often been deemphasized. Perhaps most central to research and treatment issues is the definition of sexual arousal disorder which will be discussed first. As will be seen, sexual arousal in women has been acknowledged very slowly within the field of treatment of sexual dysfunctions—just as arousal has only recently been recognized as appropriate for

women to experience in our society. Data on the incidence and prevalence of arousal difficulties in women substantiate the importance of this problem; these data are discussed next.

The next section of this chapter explores the etiology of arousal disorder, focusing on psychobiological life stages, intrapersonal issues, interpersonal relationship factors, societal determinants of inhibited arousal, and the presence of sexual abuse. These aspects of women's lives are so important that sexuality cannot be discussed without examining them. Psychobiological life stages are important because they involve psychosocial, hormonal, and reproductive organ changes that may strongly affect sexuality. Such changes occur during the menstrual cycle, pregnancy, the postpartum period, breast feeding, and menopause and thereafter. Intrapersonal, interpersonal, and cultural contexts are also crucial to women's experience of sexual arousal. The experiences of early relationships shape women's capacity to form relationships as adults. The quality of these relationships, especially with respect to their mutuality and noncoerciveness, are central to adult experiences of sexual arousal. Cultural norms prescribe a sexual gatekeeping function for women and equate sexual arousal with loss of control, lack of moral responsibility, and vulnerability. Childhood sexual abuse has clear-cut effects on sexuality; it is considered separately here because of its prevalence and importance. The convergence of these factors often leads sexual arousal to be experienced as an anxiety-provoking or dangerous experience for women, which may contribute to sexual arousal disorder.

In the next sections of this chapter, assessment and treatment of sexual arousal disorder are discussed. It is my purpose to present a conceptualization of sexual arousal in women that may form the basis for multimodal assessment strategies. If clinicians and researchers are to take sexual arousal disorder seriously, there must be reliable and valid ways to measure it. Finally, I discuss the available literature on the treatment of sexual arousal disorder in women and present some ideas on treatment. My conclusions focus on ways in which future research may facilitate the treatment of this disorder.

CHARACTERISTICS OF SEXUAL AROUSAL DISORDER

Definition

The most commonly used conceptualization of human sexual function divides sexuality into four phases: desire, arousal, orgasm, and resolution—as in the DSM-III-R (American Psychiatric Association, 1987). For the most part, sexual dysfunctions are associated with the desire, arousal, or orgasm phases.

Sexual arousal is defined both by a set of physiological responses and by a subjective psychological state. The physiological changes that occur during sexual arousal in women include genital tumescence, or vasocongestion of erectile tissue in the genitals; vaginal lubrica-

tion; and elevated heart rate, blood pressure, and respiration. These genital and autonomic nervous system changes have been carefully delineated by Masters and Johnson (1966). In addition to physiological arousal, a normal part of the arousal experience is a subjective awareness of sexual arousal. This awareness may include awareness of physical changes such as genital swelling and vaginal lubrication as well as a global sense of sexual pleasure and excitement.

Currently, the most commonly accepted definition of female sexual arousal disorder is that provided by the DSM-III-R. This definition reflects the dual nature of arousal, requiring that there be either (1) "persistent or recurrent partial or complete failure to attain or maintain the lubrication-swelling response of sexual excitement until completion of the sexual activity" or (2) "persistent or recurrent lack of a subjective sense of sexual excitement and pleasure in a female during sexual activity" (p. 294). Thus, a woman who does not experience either genital changes or subjectively perceived sensations of arousal, even if vaginal lubrication or other physical signs of arousal are present, may be considered to have a sexual arousal disorder. As a final criterion, occurrence of the dysfunction must not be exclusively during the course of another disorder, such as depression. Because arousal has a dual nature, there may be a discordance between the two components.

The definition of female arousal disorder proposed in the DSM-III-R is different from the one proposed in the DSM-III and also from previous conceptualizations, as will be discussed below. In fact, our understanding of what constitutes an arousal disorder in women has probably undergone more change than for any other sexual diagnosis. Most likely, this reflects society's ambivalence over the true nature of women's sexuality. It is thus appropriate to discuss how we have arrived at our current conceptualization.

Masters and Johnson (1970), in their important book on treatment of sexual dysfunctions, proposed no category of arousal deficiency for women. Women presenting for treatment were diagnosed with primary orgasmic dysfunction

(56%), situational orgasmic dysfunction (43%), or vaginismus (8%). It did not matter how aroused a woman would typically become: If she did not reach orgasm, she was diagnosed with an orgasmic disorder. As pointed out by Wakefield (1987), this diagnostic system produces an artificially high rate of women with an orgasmic disorder, since it includes women with both orgasm and arousal deficits. The diagnostic situation was virtually the opposite for men. Except for premature ejaculators, most men were diagnosed with an erectile dysfunction, in a category called *impotence* (or *erectile dysfunction*). These terms refer to an impairment in sexual arousal. Masters and Johnson also proposed a diagnosis of "ejaculatory incompetence," which refers to a condition in which a man does not reach orgasm/ejaculation during coitus despite having a full erection. Masters and Johnson describe this as a "relatively infrequent complication of male sexual function" (p. 359). If one looks at the set of men presenting with problems in either the arousal or the orgasm phase, 94% received some form of impotence diagnosis, and 6% were diagnosed with ejaculatory incompetence. This is in contrast to the 100% of women presenting with problems in either the arousal or the orgasm phase who were diagnosed with an orgasmic dysfunction—because no arousal dysfunction was conceptualized and therefore even considered.

The case has been made that these differences in diagnostic criteria are sex-biased (Wakefield, 1987). Wakefield identifies a logical bias, in that female orgasmic dysfunction is more broadly defined than male orgasmic dysfunction. This is because women are diagnosed based on orgasmic achievement, whereas men are diagnosed based on orgasmic ability. Thus, women who have never engaged in sexual activity could still be diagnosed with an orgasmic dysfunction because they have never reached orgasm. In contrast, men receive the diagnosis only if orgasm is not reached given an adequately stimulating situation. A clear conceptual distinction is made between male arousal and orgasm in Masters and Johnson's "impotence" and "ejaculatory incompetence" diagnoses. The definition of

ejaculatory incompetence specified that it was not appropriate to use unless the man had a firm erection during coitus. A second logical bias is that women who lack sexual arousal and orgasm are diagnosed with orgasmic dysfunction, whereas men who lack sexual arousal and orgasm are diagnosed with arousal dysfunction (impotence), as described above. For women, no matter what level of arousal was present in any sexual activity, if the end result was not orgasm, the problem was considered to be an orgasmic dysfunction. The result of the first bias is that women are more pathologized than men. The second bias also results in greater pathology for women, if one conceptualizes an orgasmic dysfunction as a more severe disorder than an arousal dysfunction.

Masters and Johnson's omission of an arousal-phase disorder for women may be based on a cultural view that makes it easier to conceptualize women as having orgasm problems and men as having predominantly arousal problems. It is instructive to consider why this might be so. Two explanations for this phenomenon may be proposed. One is that arousal is much easier to assess in men than women, so arousal deficits are easier to identify. Male arousal is easy to observe based on strength of erection. Female arousal cannot be easily observed. Although engorgement of the female genitals may be visually observable, one might have to know how a particular woman's genitals looked in an unaroused state to be sure of accuracy. The same measurement issue applies whether the assessor is the woman herself, her sexual partner, or a psychophysiological researcher. In addition, the relationship of genital tumescence to vaginal lubrication is not clear. Sometimes a woman might perceive herself to be ready for intercourse because she feels engorgement, but then find that she had very little vaginal lubrication. Orgasm, in contrast, is a more discernable event, at least for the woman herself. It may be in part for this reason that orgasm seemed to be a defining event for women's sexuality.

A second explanation for the diagnostic disparity between men and women rests on the fact that male impotence appears to be presented by

Masters and Johnson as a counterpart to female orgasmic dysfunction. I have argued (Morokoff, 1989) that there is an unstated cultural assumption that the woman who is capable of having intercourse is sexually aroused. Capacity for intercourse is clearly equivalent to sexual arousal in men (because an erection is necessary for penile penetration of the vagina). Applying the same reasoning to women leads one to believe that if a woman is engaging in intercourse, she is adequately aroused to potentially reach orgasm. Thus, if women who have intercourse do not reach orgasm, they must have an orgasmic dysfunction. Similar reasoning leads to the myth that a woman who truly doesn't want sex cannot be raped. Unfortunately, it is very much the case that sexual arousal is not necessary for intercourse to occur, and that many women may engage in intercourse to please their partners without being very aroused. The situation for men is different. Lack of erection results in a major sexual problem for a couple wishing to have intercourse, in that intercourse cannot occur. Lack of erection is clearly a separate problem from not ejaculating once intercourse is underway. For women, one cannot see a lack of arousal, and it has an indeterminate effect on whether intercourse occurs. From this perspective it might seem unclear that lack of arousal is a separate problem from lack of orgasm, suggesting that it does not need its own diagnostic category.

Despite differences between men and women in arousal's observability and its functional significance for intercourse, arousal in men and women is really very much the same. Both involve the same nervous system regulation, which differs for both from that required to trigger orgasm (Wagner & Green, 1981; Weiss, 1972). Both involve genital vasocongestion of erectile tissues. It is true that these tissues are configured differently and that lubrication differs between women and men, but otherwise the physiology is quite analogous. For both women and men, arousal most often precedes orgasm. It thus makes just as much sense to acknowledge an arousal phase (with its own disorder) for women as for men.

It is for these reasons that Kaplan (1974) introduced a category of general sexual dysfunction (*frigidity*). She described this disorder, which was distinguished from an orgasmic dysfunction, as involving little if any erotic pleasure from sexual stimulation and no sexual feelings. A woman with this disorder would not experience the physiological responses of sexual arousal. However, a problem with this diagnostic category was that it did not clearly distinguish arousal from desire-phase disorders.

These problems were corrected by the diagnosis proposed in the DSM-III (American Psychiatric Association, 1980) called *inhibited sexual excitement,* defined as follows:

> A. Recurrent and persistent inhibition of sexual excitement during sexual activity, manifested by: . . . In females, partial or complete failure to attain or maintain the lubrication-swelling response of sexual excitement until completion of the sexual act. B. A clinical judgment that the individual engages in sexual activity that is adequate in focus, intensity, and duration (p. 279).

This definition improves on Masters and Johnson's diagnostic system in two major ways. The first is that a distinction is made between an arousal disorder and an orgasmic disorder. Inhibited female orgasm is a separate category that may be diagnosed only when absence of orgasm follows a "normal sexual excitement phase during sexual activity that is judged by the clinician to be adequate in focus, intensity, and duration" (p. 279). The inhibited arousal categories are essentially equivalent for women and men, although they are written separately. The second important improvement is the requirement that there be the occurrence of sexual activity judged by the clinician to be adequate to produce arousal. It should be noted that the same criterion is also included in the inhibited orgasm category. As has been discussed, this is important because Masters and Johnson's orgasmic dysfunction diagnoses for women were based on whether a woman reached orgasm at all, not taking into account whether the opportunity had been adequate; these diagnostic categories were thus logically biased toward pathologizing women.

The DSM-III's arousal disorder diagnoses were still flawed, however, for both men and women, due to the fact that they focused exclusively on physiological response. Clinical and research evidence reveals that, especially in women, physiological response may not coincide with subjective experience (Morokoff, 1988a). It has been clinically observed that women may show signs of physiological arousal and yet be aware of no sensations of arousal at all (Morokoff, 1989). Under the DSM-III diagnostic criteria, such women would have been appropriately diagnosed with an orgasmic disorder, despite clear evidence that they had no sense of being sexually aroused at all. Research evidence points to a similar conclusion—that it is very possible for a woman to report no awareness of sexual arousal and yet show vaginal vasocongestive responses when measured psychophysiologically (Morokoff, 1988b).

Fortunately, this diagnostic problem has been corrected in DSM-III-R. The new diagnosis for female sexual arousal disorder retains the positive features of the category provided in DSM-III but adds that a disorder may be present if either physiological or subjective arousal is persistently lacking. Of course, the difficulties in adequately assessing subjective and physiological female sexual arousal remain. These will be addressed in the assessment section of this chapter.

Incidence and Prevalence

The difficulty in defining female arousal disorder has clear consequences for determining the incidence and prevalence of the disorder. A significant problem is that well-designed studies simply have not been conducted on the frequency with which women have difficulty becoming aroused. This is in part due to the fact that there was not a strong consensus that female arousal was important to measure—or, if important, measurable. For example, Kinsey, Pomeroy, Martin, and Gehbard (1953), in their landmark study of sexual behavior in the human female, did not attempt to assess arousal in women. Nowinski and LoPiccolo's (1979) General Information Form, designed to be an objective measure of sexual functioning, included specific questions on orgasm through masturbation, orgasm through caressing by mate, orgasm through intercourse, erectile problems before intercourse for men, and erectile problems during intercourse for men—but no questions on women's arousal were included. (It should be noted that items assessing frequency of arousal difficulties were added to this instrument after the 1979 report.)

For those who have attempted to measure arousal disorders, the same lack of consensus has led to great differences in the criteria used for assessing arousal disorders. This has contributed to widely varied estimates of the incidence of these disorders. In a community sample of "normal" women, 48% indicated "difficulty getting excited" (Frank, Anderson, & Rubinstein, 1978) on a self-report questionnaire. In the same study, 33% also indicated difficulty maintaining excitement. In another study, 7 out of 59 black women (12%) attending a gynecology clinic were diagnosed with an arousal-phase disorder (Levine & Yost, 1976). Semistructured interviews were conducted with the women by gynecologists. One of the seven women was diagnosed as having a primary excitement-phase disorder, and the other six were found not to have experienced sexual excitement for a period of time ranging from five months to four years. None of these women was currently experiencing orgasm. Interestingly, there were only three women (5%) diagnosed with an orgasmic disorder. The substantially lower rate than found by Frank et al. is probably attributable both to the fact that women were reporting on their sexual functioning face-to-face with a (probably white) gynecologist and to the fact that a diagnostic criterion was used, rather than a simple self-report of problems. It may be that the populations were not comparable in the studies by Frank et al. and Levine and Yost. Frank et al.'s population was a predominantly white, community sample, whereas Levine and Yost's sample consisted of black women attending a gynecology clinic. These differences, as well as quite different methods and criteria for determining arousal disorder, may explain the different results.

Among women presenting for sex therapy, 57% have been reported to experience sexual arousal disorders (Frank, Anderson, & Kupfer, 1976). Among female cancer patients referred for sexual evaluation, 11.4% were diagnosed by interview as having had an arousal-phase disorder (criteria for diagnosis unspecified), prior to their cancer diagnosis (Schover, Evans, & von Eschenbach, 1987). In this study, distinctions were drawn between lack of subjective arousal (3%), lack of physiological arousal (7%), and lack of both (1.4%). Following cancer diagnosis, these figures increased dramatically—to 36% with a physiological arousal disorder and 34% with both subjective and physiological disorders. On the other hand, Kaplan (1979) estimates from her clinical practice that female arousal disorder is relatively uncommon. She writes, "dysfunctions of the female excitement phase, i.e., the isolated inhibition of lubrication and swelling, is a relatively uncommon clinical syndrome, except as the result of such local physiologic factors as estrogen deficiency with senile vaginitis" (p. 19). It is probable that the discrepancies between these studies result from differential applications of diagnostic criteria. Some studies have employed classification categories that are too ambiguous to be helpful. For example, Bancroft and Coles (1976) recorded a category of "general unresponsiveness," applicable to 62% of women in their sample, which may include both arousal- and desire-phase difficulties.

Survivors of Sexual Abuse

The high reported rate of childhood sexual abuse makes it important to consider sexual dysfunctions among the group of women who have been so abused. In 1981, the National Incidence Study of the Department of Health and Human Services estimated a yearly rate of 0.7 cases of sexual abuse per 1,000 children. Retrospective studies among adults suggest much higher rates. A national survey reported by the Los Angeles Times in 1985 provided evidence that a quarter of all women have some sort of childhood sexual experience with an adult by age 18. This figure is consistent with Finkelhor's (1979b) research, which also indicated a one-in-four ratio for women who had suffered child sexual abuse. Among women who seek therapy services, the prevalence of an abuse history may be considerably higher. For example, Briere (1984) reported that 44% of women who received help in clinical settings had been sexually abused as children.

It might be expected that sexual arousal disorder and other sexual dysfunctions would be greater in women who have been sexually abused than women who have not. A number of studies have explored the prevalence of sexual problems in women with abuse histories. A review of 58 therapy cases in which the client had survived childhood sexual abuse were compared to a control sample of 100 therapy cases in which no abuse was reported (Meiselman, 1978). Among a subset of the survivor group who had been abused by their fathers, 87% had a current or previous sexual problem. Only 20% of the control group cases mentioned a sexual problem. A methodological problem with this study was that in the sexual abuse cases—but not the control cases—therapists were interviewed and allowed to seek more information from clients. To take this into account, the author also looked only at information presented at intake. The sexually abused women presented sexual problems at intake in 62% of cases, compared to 20% for the control women. In another study, 83 incest and rape victims were interviewed concerning sexual dysfunction (Becker, Skinner, Abel, & Treacy, 1982). At least one sexual problem was reported by 56% of the group. Of the dysfunctional incest survivors, 42% reported an arousal dysfunction. Arousal dysfunction was the second most reported problem, behind "fear of sex," which was reported by 75% of the dysfunctional women.

The most methodologically sound study conducted to date compared three groups of 30 women each: (1) a clinical group of women seeking therapy for problems associated with childhood molestation; (2) a nonclinical group consisting of women molested as children but who had never sought therapy and considered themselves to be well adjusted; and (3) a control group of women who had not been molested (Tsai, Feldman-Summers, & Edgar, 1979). Sexual responsiveness, the closest measure to sexual arousal, was significantly less for the clinical group than the nonclinical or control groups. A comparable result was found for frequency of orgasms. Results also indicated that the women in the clinical group had been molested for a longer period of time, that the frequency of abuse was higher, and that the abuse involved attempted intercourse more often than for women in the nonclinical group. The authors suggest that the differential abuse patterns may account for the differences between the clinical and nonclinical groups.

Jehu (1988) examined the types of sexual problems presented by sexually dysfunctional abuse survivors. A phobia or aversion to sex was presented by 59% of a sample of 51 women presenting with sexual dysfunctions at initial assessment. Impaired sexual arousal was presented by 49% of the women (a figure quite comparable to the 42% reported by Becker et al., 1982). Impaired orgasm was reported by 45%, dyspareunia by 27%, and vaginismus by 8%. Research with sexual abuse and assault survivors makes it clear that the prevalence of sexual arousal and other disorders, which is high in the general population, is especially high in this subgroup.

Conclusions

Clarification of the incidence of sexual dysfunctions in the population is important. To do it properly would require a large-scale study in which a random population sample is interviewed or administered a psychometrically valid questionnaire based on current diagnostic criteria. Clearly, the same classification system should be adopted across studies. As discussed by Spector and Carey (1990), models for such

epidemiologic research are available for other disorders. It is also important to determine accurately the proportion of women with an arousal-phase disorder among those who request sex therapy. The relative proportion of the various diagnoses may vary over time and need to reported regularly by those providing services. It would be helpful to report figures using previous diagnostic criteria as well as new ones, as these categories change. In addition, more information is needed on the frequency with which nondysfunctional women (e.g., women who do not meet the diagnostic criteria for an arousal-phase disorder) experience problems becoming aroused.

Subtypes of Sexual Arousal Disorder

Two important qualifiers of sexual arousal disorder are (1) whether the disorder is global or situational and (2) whether or not it is a lifelong problem (Schover, Friedman, Weiler, Heiman, & LoPiccolo, 1982). A global sexual arousal disorder would be one in which a woman is unable to experience physiological or subjective arousal in any situation. Thus, she would not be aroused during masturbation, with her husband, or with extramarital sexual partners. A situational arousal disorder is one in which arousal has been experienced in some situations and not others, such as when masturbating but not when having sex with a partner, or when having sex with one partner but not another. Lifelong disorder has also been referred to as *primary,* as contrasted with a *secondary* disorder (temporary). A lifelong or primary disorder is one that has always been present. Thus, a woman who had a lifelong, global sexual arousal disorder would never have experienced arousal under any circumstances in her life.

ETIOLOGY OF SEXUAL AROUSAL DISORDER

There are many possible causes of sexual arousal dysfunction, and these may be conceptualized on numerous levels. Etiological issues will be discussed first from the perspective of life stages. Various life stages that women experience have specific and significant effects on sexual arousal potential. This is due both to physiological changes that occur during these psychobiological stages and to life stresses and developmental demands that accompany them. It is difficult to discuss arousal difficulties without knowledge of whether a woman is pregnant, breast feeding, or postmenopausal. It is most desirable to be able to separate hormonal or other physiological effects from psychological predictors of sexual arousal, although our state of knowledge does not always permit this degree of specificity. The second causal perspective examined is the intrapersonal, based on childhood and adolescent development as well as adult personality characteristics. Third, one may conceptualize interpersonal causes that include both relationship factors and a partner's ability to provide adequate stimulation. Next, societal causes will be examined, focusing primarily on a feminist theoretical analysis. Finally, I will address effects of childhood sexual abuse.

Effects of Psychobiological Life Stages on Sexual Arousal

Menstrual Cycle Effects

Cyclic hormonal functioning occurs in women between the ages of 12 and 51, on average. This reproductive phase of life is thus a very important substratum to adult sexuality. The menstrual cycle presents a good starting point in examining effects of reproductive hormones, moods, symptoms, and life demands on sexual arousal. Estrogen levels vary markedly across the menstrual cycle. However, estrogen levels measured across the cycle have not been found to correlate with sexual arousal or any other measure of sexuality in women (Persky et al., 1978). In contrast, androgen levels have been found to be related to various measures of sexual response in women, including sexual arousal (Persky et al., 1982). These authors related measures of all three phases of the sexual response

cycle (desire, arousal, and orgasm) to testosterone and other androgen levels ascertained across the menstrual cycle. They found a significant relationship between testosterone level and sexual arousal as measured by sexual responsivity. It should be noted that the correlations in this study were based on the combined data of two groups of women: older, postmenopausal women and younger, premenopausal ones. Testosterone and other androgen levels vary across the menstrual cycle, with maximal levels around the time of ovulation (Lobotsky, Wyss, Segre, & Lloyd, 1964; Judd & Yen, 1973). Testosterone and androstenedione were found to increase 40% over the mean level at midcycle (Vermeulen & Verdonck, 1976).

Most studies of sexuality across the menstrual cycle have used sexual behavior as a dependent variable, but some have measured sexual arousal. A study of vaginal vasocongestion across menstrual cycle phases was conducted by Schreiner-Engel, Schiavi, Smith, & White (1981). Sexual arousal, measured by vaginal pulse amplitude in response to fantasy and an erotic audiotape, was significantly lower during the ovulation phase than the postmenstrual or premenstrual phases. No differences in subjective ratings of arousal were found across cycle phases. Similarly, Hoon, Bruce, and Kinchloe (1982), using three physiological measures of genital response, found no difference in sexual arousal across the menstrual cycle.

In another study, users and nonusers of birth control pills were evaluated for 11 weeks to test the hypothesis that there would be a decrease in sexual arousal during the luteal phase, as a result of progestogenic influences (Englander-Golden, Chang, Whitmore, & Dienstbier, 1980). Reverse cycle days may be calculated by counting backward from the first day of menstruation. This method of determining cycle phase is used because the length of the luteal phase of the cycle is thought to be less variable than the follicular phase. For nonusers of pills, peaks of arousal were identified on reverse cycle days 13, 2, and 1 and forward cycle day 4. These days correspond to pre- and postmenstrual peaks as well as midcycle peaks. The authors thus concluded that sexual arousal was lower in the luteal phase. All women were kept unaware of the fact that the study focused on menstrual cycle effects. To evaluate awareness, women were then asked retrospectively to rate their feelings during different phases of their last cycle. This methodology unfortunately confounds awareness of the study's purpose with retrospective versus prospective data collection. Retrospective (aware) reports showed a different pattern from prospective (unaware) ratings. Women remembered their highest sexual arousal during the luteal phase. Interestingly, women remembered their sexual arousal as higher than they had prospectively rated it.

The results of these studies are consistent with the conclusion that estrogen levels in premenopausal women do not determine capacity for sexual arousal. If this were the case, one would expect to observe the highest levels of sexual arousal at midcycle, when estrogen level is highest. Although Englander-Golden et al. (1980) did observe a midcycle peak in self-reported arousal, they also observed pre- and postmenstrual peaks in arousal. No other study has reported a midcycle peak in sexual arousal.

Although hormone levels may not directly predict sexual arousal levels, it is possible that mood and state of well-being, which appear to vary cyclically, may be related to some aspects of sexuality. Research has indicated that there is a midfollicular peak in feelings of well-being (Bancroft, 1984; Sanders, Warner, Backstrom & Bancroft, 1983; Gallant, Hamilton, Popiel, Morokoff, & Chakraborty, 1991). This appears to be related to increased sexual activity present at this cycle phase. Bancroft (1984, 1987) reports that about one-third of the variance in women's sexual feelings is attributable to variations in general well-being, based on findings that well-being is a strong predictor of a composite factor of sexuality (Bancroft, Sanders, Davidson, & Warner, 1983; Sanders et al., 1983). Similarly, a significant correlation was found between well-being (a factor that emerged from daily ratings of individual affective reactions) and sexual desire (Popeil, Alagna, & Morokoff, 1988). In the studies just cited, sexual arousal was not specifically mesured. An important issue is thus how sexual arousal relates to well-being. Sanders et al. (1983) measured "sexual interest," which reflected "interest in or desire for sexual expression or activity, i.e., 'sexual feelings' " (p. 491), as well as "sexual activity," which included frequencies of specific sexual behaviors. In Popeil et al.'s (1988) study, sexual desire and sexual behaviors were also rated on a daily basis by participants. Thus, the two studies to date that have examined sexuality and well-being have not looked at sexual arousal.

Other explanations have been advanced for the premenstrual peak in sexual arousal. One view is that as the luteal phase of the menstrual cycle progresses, there is an increase in pelvic congestion and edema. This baseline of elevated congestion results in greater spontaneous desire for sex, greater ease in becoming sexually aroused, and greater volume of vaginal lubrication (Sherfey, 1973). Sherfey has suggested that vaginal lubrication at this cycle phase has a different, more "slippery" consistency than at other cycle phases and is more copious. As will be discussed, the phenomenon of increased pelvic congestion may also facilitate sexual response during pregnancy. Another explanation for the premenstrual peak in sexual arousal is that testosterone levels, which are highest at midcycle, may have a delayed effect on sexual arousal potential. As pointed out by Bancroft (1984) testosterone replacement therapy for hypogonadal men takes one to two weeks to show signs of effects on sexuality. If this is the case for women also, these endogenous changes in testosterone level may not produce behavioral effects until late in the luteal phase. An explanation that is often offered for increased sexual behavior premenstrually is that women and their partners are preparing for abstinence during menstrual bleeding. While this argument adequately explains why women might choose to have sex premenstrually (if they know they will abstain during menstruation), it does not explain why they would be more aroused at this time.

The studies reported here represent a minority of those that have examined female sexuality across the menstrual cycle. This is because most researchers have not been interested in sexual arousal per se, perhaps due to measurement issues, and have focused primarily on sexual behavior. This represents a research flaw, because knowledge of sexual arousal helps us to interpret sexual behavior data. For example, if masturbation or intercourse frquency is low during a particular cycle phase, this may be explained by low reported levels of arousal during the same phase.

Pregnancy

One of the earliest studies of sexuality during pregnancy was conducted by Masters and Johnson (1966), who examined physiological response patterns of six study participants. Because pregnancy itself produces pelvic vasocongestion, the vasocongestive response of sexual arousal is altered. That is, when the genital organs are already vasocongested, sexual arousal may not produce as much of an increase as it would for a nonpregnant woman. Psychophysiological procedures for measurement of vasocongestion (see the section on assessment) have not been used during pregnancy, perhaps due to unknown effects on the fetus, so some information that would be helpful in understanding arousal during pregnancy is not available. However, Masters and Johnson were able to observe clear differences in genital changes during arousal between the pregnant and nonpregnant states. During the plateau phase of arousal, the orgasmic platform (vasocongestion in the outer third of the vagina) is so extensive that the "vaginal barrel appeared completely obtunded, with the lateral vaginal walls meeting in the midline in severe vasocongestive response to sexual tensions. The more advanced the state of pregnancy, the more severe the venous engorgement of the entire vaginal barrel, and the more advanced the secondary development of the orgasmic platform in response to sexual stimulation" (p. 148). Production of vaginal lubrication was found to increase by the end of the first trimester, continuing throughout the pregnancy. This response was reported by all the women and confirmed through objective measurement for four of the women. Problems with this research include that (1) the authors do not specify their methods and (2) data are reported for only a small sample, who may be unrepresentative.

Masters and Johnson also studied self-reports of changes in the sexuality of 111 women across their pregnancies. Unfortunately, measurement of arousal during pregnancy has suffered from the same problems just discussed in menstrual cycle phase research. Sexual arousal was not specifically assessed. Masters and Johnson assessed "level of eroticism" and "sexual performance," without defining these concepts. The general pattern was that nulliparous women (those who had not previously borne a child) in particular reported a reduced level of eroticism and sexual performance in the first trimester, followed by a marked increase in the second trimester (reportedly exceeding the prepregnant state), followed by a reduction in the third trimester. Parous women (those who had previously borne one or more children) did not tend to report as much decline in the first trimester, unless they had significant nausea and vomiting. It appears to be a very viable hypothesis that the decline in sexual feelings of the first trimester is correlated with reduced feelings of well-being or increased physical symptoms. Although this hypothesis needs to be rigorously assessed, it is anecdotally supported by women's reports of the reasons for their declining sexual feelings (Falicov, 1973). Frequently cited reasons included tiredness, heartburn, and nausea. In Falicov's study, a first-trimester decline in "eroticism" was reported, followed by relative improvement in the second trimester and some continued improvement in the early third trimester. However, other patterns of results have also been reported, typically showing significant reductions in enjoyment of sex (which may be conceptualized as arousal) during the third trimester. For example, Kenney (1973) reported little change in enjoyment during the first two trimesters, with reduced enjoyment for about half the sample in the third trimester. Kumar, Brandt, and Robson (1981) report that most participants showed some reduction in sexual enjoyment during pregnancy, which was most marked in the third trimester.

In summary, women's sexual enjoyment appears to decline during pregnancy, with some indication that this decline is partially reversed in the second trimester. The factors that most strongly account for this decline have not been determined. Research examining predictors of sexual arousal during pregnancy is clearly needed. Among the most important predictors would seem to be moods and physical symptoms. However, hormonal changes accompanying pregnancy, such as the extremely high levels of both estrogen and progesterone, may affect sexual desire and/or sexual arousal. Many women also have fears about the effects of sexual activity on the developing fetus; such fears could easily interfere with becoming aroused. For example, Falicov (1973) quotes one women in the first trimester: "I am not sexually fulfilled right now. I think my husband and I unconsciously are both concerned about harming the baby, even though we both know better. Not only do we make love less often now but also we spend less time at it." Another woman said, "I've been told that I should not fear harming the baby. However, this is fear that does exist and prevents me from enjoying sex. It seems like subconsciously I am holding back." If a woman spends less time with lovemaking or holds back during sex, thus preventing enjoyment, it seems likely that her experience of sexual arousal might be impaired. Finally, the high level of genital congestion and pressure caused by the developing fetus may produce a tonic level of stimulation, which in sexual situations will facilitate the potential for arousal, as discussed by Sherfey (1973). This phenomenon is similar to that discussed with respect to the luteal phase of the menstrual cycle. For example, the woman who experiences inhibited sexual desire may find herself more easily aroused during pregnancy because the tonic level of vasocongestion leads her to be in a more sexual mood more often.

Information on sexual arousal during pregnancy is incomplete. The specific effects on sexuality of pregnancy hormones; the physical changes of increased vasocongestion, edema, and pressure of the fetus; physical symptoms such as morning sickness; changes in body image; and hopes and fears concerning the baby's welfare and motherhood have not been adequately studied. This information is necessary to be able to counsel individual women and their partners concerning what to expect with respect to sexual functioning during pregnancy.

Postpartum and Breast Feeding

The period following childbirth combines a variety of factors, any or all of which may affect the arousal phase of sexual functioning. One factor is the hormonal environment. The period of time before normal cycling and menstrual bleeding returns is extremely variable among women. One of the major factors affecting the duration of this amenorrhoeic period is the duration of full-time breast feeding. When lactation is suppressed, ovulation may return as soon as 36 days postpartum (Perez, Vela, Masnick, & Potter, 1972). Ovarian cyclicity tends to continue to be suppressed as long as full-time breast feeding is continued, averaging over one year. Follicle stimulating hormone is suppressed and barely detectable during late pregnancy (Rolland, Lequin, Schellekens, & De Jong, 1975) but returns to normal cyclic levels within the first 30–100 days postpartum (Baird et al., 1979). Luteinizing hormone remains below the normal cyclic range for approximately the same time period and longer in lactating women (Baird et al., 1979). The prolactin response during pregnancy and the puerperium is well documented. Prolactin levels increase approximately 20-fold during pregnancy (Tyson, Hwang, Guyda, & Friesen, 1972). Following parturition and clearance of estrogens and other steroids from the placenta, prolactin levels drop dramatically, returning to levels only slightly higher than those of cycling, nonpregnant women (Noel, Suh, & Frantz, 1974). However, within ten minutes of the start of suckling, prolactin rises markedly. An 18-fold increase in plasma prolactin from before suckling to 10 minutes after has been observed, gradually diminishing to baseline levels over the following hours (Noel et al., 1974). During the period of full-time breast feeding, estrogen levels are below normal for a cycling, nonpregnant woman (Rolland et al., 1975).

The hormonal environment present following childbirth may be expected to have a negative impact on sexual functioning. Hyperprolactinemia has been associated with decreased sexual desire (Fava et al., 1983), less frequent self-initiated sexual activities, and less frequent orgasm than controls (Koppelman, Parry, Hamilton, & Alagna, 1985; Mastrogiacomo et al., 1984). The specific impact of elevated prolactin on sexual arousal in women has not been well studied, although taking bromocriptine (a prolactin antagonist produced significant improvement in one woman's sexual responsiveness (conceptualized as a measure of arousal) and vaginal lubrication, as reported by Weizman et al., 1983).

Estrogen deprivation experienced postpartum may also have a negative impact on some aspects of sexual arousal. It is clearly established that estrogen deprivation results in thinning of the vaginal mucosa and vaginal atrophy (Vasquez, Samaras, & Nezhat, 1982). Estrogen deprivation has also been shown to result in a decrease in vaginal pH and vaginal fluid, which can be reversed by exogenous estrogen administration (Semmens & Wagner, 1982). A significant relationship between vaginal lubrication during sexual arousal in the laboratory and estrogen (estradiol) concentration has been reported (Myers & Morokoff, 1986). It is unclear however, whether estrogen is directly related to the vasocongestive component of sexual arousal. Administration of estrogen produced improved ratings of sexual enjoyment in one study (Dennerstein, Burrows, Wood, & Hyman, 1980). However, Sherwin, Gelfand, and Brenner (1985) found that self-reported sexual arousal was no different in women receiving replacement estrogen than in controls, and less than in women receiving replacement testosterone. In psychophysiologically measured vaginal vasocongestion, no difference was found between postmenopausal (low-estrogen) women and premenopausal women (Myers & Morokoff, 1986). It is thus possible that estrogen

deprivation affects the vaginal lubrication component of sexual arousal but not the vasocongestive component.

Many nonhormonal factors may affect sexuality during the postpartum, including fatigue, stress associated with care of the newborn, stress associated with the transition to motherhood for first-time mothers or with caring for more than one child, episiotomy pain, amount of help with child care from the mother's partner, and conflicts between partners. A variety of predictors of postpartum loss of sexual enjoyment have been evaluated (Pertot, 1981). The most important factor was loss of sexual desire. Other factors included feeling less close to the partner since the birth, inability to discuss sexual problems, resuming sexual relations earlier than desired, feeling less attractive, lack of energy, and specific complaints about the partner. Pertot (1981) concludes that sexual enjoyment was more affected by relationship variables than was sexual desire—including specifically how much the husband helped with the baby, the manner in which the couple cope with disagreements, and whether the activities engaged in during sex are amenable to the woman. Again, it should be noted that sexual enjoyment is not necessarily synonymous with sexual arousal. Furthermore, while 28% of the sample reported a decrease in sexual enjoyment from before pregnancy to postpartum, an almost equally large group (21%) reported an increase in enjoyment. Pertot concludes that childbirth had more of a negative impact on sexual desire than on sexual enjoyment, and that for a couple who communicate well, cooperate in caring for the baby, and have appropriate sexual techniques, sexual enjoyment need not be impaired and may even be enhanced.

Menopause and Aging

Sexual arousal is affected by aging. As we look at the effects of aging, it becomes evident, however, that the arousal process is not one-dimensional; different aspects are affected differently. Physiological aspects of sexual arousal were compared in older and younger women by Masters and Johnson (1966). Clitoral tumescence did not differ between the two groups, but vasocongestion did. Older women had less labial vasocongestion, and vaginal vasocongestion developed more slowly than for younger women. The rate and amount of vaginal lubrication were also observed to diminish with age, although individual exceptions were noted. Despite these changes in rapidity of the sexual arousal response and extent of vasocongestion, the capacity for sexual arousal continues to be present in all age groups. Studies of sexual behavior also indicate that frequency of sexual intercourse declines in older women. Nevertheless, a significant number continue to be sexually active (Bretschneider & McCoy, 1988; Pfeiffer, Verwoerdt, & Davis, 1972; Pfeiffer, Verwoerdt, & Wang, 1968).

Menopause appears to have a negative effect on sexuality separate from aging (see Morokoff, 1988b, for a review of this literature). Several studies (Bottiglioni & DeAloysio, 1982; Cutler, Garcia, & McCoy, 1987; Hallstrom, 1977; McCoy & Davidson, 1985) have found that menopausal status is associated with decreased frequency of sexual activity, decreased desire, decreased frequency of orgasm, and decreased vaginal lubrication. The effects on the vasocongestive component of sexual arousal and global subjective perceptions of sexual arousal are not clear, however. Vaginal pulse amplitude (a measure of vasocongestion) in response to an erotic videotape was significantly lower for postmenopausal women than either younger or older premenopausal women (Morrell, Dixen, Carter, & Davidson, 1984). However, these results were not replicated by Myers and Morokoff (1986), who found no differences in vaginal vasocongestion between pre- and postmenopausal groups, as discussed previously. However, a difference in perceived sexual arousal was found, with hypoestrogenic women (postmenopausal women not taking replacement estrogens) reporting less sexual arousal than premenopausal women or postmenopausal women taking replacement estrogen. This result was primarily accounted for by reported lower perceived vaginal lubrication.

The postmenopausal hormone environment is a possible cause of changes in sexual response. Following menopause, estrogen levels (especially estradiol) are dramatically reduced. For women undergoing natural menopause, testosterone levels do not necessarily decline, although other androgens have been reported to decline (Judd, 1976). If a woman undergoes surgical menopause as a result of the removal of her ovaries (bilateral oophorectomy), a significant reduction in testosterone occurs, as the ovaries secrete testosterone even after natural menopause (Greenblatt, Oettinger, & Bohler, 1976). A double-blind hormone replacement study has indicated that among women who have had hysterectomy and bilateral oophorectomy, testosterone replacement produces significantly higher self-reported sexual arousal than placebo or estrogen administration (Sherwin, Gelfand, & Brenner, 1985). The superiority of testosterone to estrogen replacement has been further confirmed in a subsequent study (Sherwin & Gelfand, 1987). It is thus clear that testosterone is necessary for maintenance of normal levels of sexual arousal in women.

Intrapersonal Determinants of Sexual Arousal Disorder

Psychoanalytic Theory

Most psychological theories ascribe primary importance to childhood in determining major adult affective reactions such as sexuality and eroticism. Psychoanalytic theory has had the most to say about the development of gender and sexuality. This theory proposes that the basis for adult experiences of relationships (and specifically sexual relationships, including desire for a partner and capacity for sexual response) is the relationship with parents in the early years. Kaplan states:

> The apparent inability of some women to become aroused sexually, although they are adequately stimulated, is probably indicative of some underlying sexual conflict. When a woman is in conflict about sex, the arousal of erotic feelings also

evokes anxiety. Typically, she defends against such anxiety not only by avoiding the stimulation which will elicit her sexual response, but also by erecting defenses against the perception of her erotic feelings. She simply does not allow herself to feel sexually aroused (1974, p. 352).

Psychodynamic theory offers explanations for why this suppression of sexual feelings occurs.

The basis for adult sexuality is hypothesized to be the oedipal conflict. The traditional requirements for a girl's resolution of the oedipal complex are to repress her desire for her father, to identify with her mother, and to seek another male as her mate when she is an adult. However, girls do not resolve the oedipal conflict as quickly or with the same finality as boys. Chodorow (1978) presents an excellent discussion of the reasons for this difference. A boy's oedipal love for his mother is far more overwhelming and threatening than a girl's for her father, because for the boy it is an extension of his preoedipal relationship with his primary parent. The girl's preoedipal relationship with her father is much less intense than the boy's with his mother. Her oedipal love with her father is also not as exclusive and intense as the boy's with his mother, partly because it is not reciprocated as intensely by her father and partly because it is mitigated by her continued attachment to her mother. Because of this lack of intensity, it is not as threatening to her future attachments to men, and she is not as motivated to give up the attachment as radically. At the same time, her fear of retaliation from her mother is less intense, so once again she does not need to repress her oedipal love as much.

The consequence of a less completely resolved oedipal conflict is that girls retain very strong affective relations with their mothers and somewhat sexualized/idealized relations with their fathers. Furthermore, Chodorow asserts, a woman's relationship to men is likely to take its character from her relation to her mother as to her father. The girl's oedipal complex is thus characterized by continued preoedipal attachments, sexual oscillation in an oedipal triangle, lack of absolute change of love object, and lack of absolute oedipal resolution. Although most girls become heterosexual, most retain strong love relationships with women and have strong nonsexual emotional attachments. Furthermore, women do not repress affective needs as men do; they may be willing to accept limitations in their male partners in exchange for fulfillment of their need for caring and love—a need that is the legacy of unrepressed, intense mother/daughter relationship.

Women's desire to avoid rejection can lead to the suppression of aggressive feelings toward men, based in part on transfer of childhood feelings. This suppression of anger or hostility may be associated with diminished arousal: It is difficult to experience sexual arousal while warding off unconscious anger. Although research evidence is lacking, it is a viable hypothesis that the hostility inherent in sexual objectification and pornography may help to preserve the capacity for arousal in men who experience hostility toward women. For example, Stoller (1979) asserts that hostility generates and enhances sexual excitement. Later, Stoller wrote, "I find all pornography to be little perversions and probably all erotic daydreams as well" . . . (1985, p. 9). In the same chapter, Stoller asserts that the desire to humiliate is an essential theme in male-oriented erotica. Content analysis has supported the conclusion that coercion and sexual exploitation are prevalent themes in popular male-oriented erotica (Cowan, Lee, Levy, & Snyder, 1988).

Fear of her mother's jealous reactions may inhibit a woman's feelings of arousal. The child's success in winning her father (or, later, another man) may invoke feelings of guilt or fear over her mother's angry reactions. Such feelings may be compounded when women become more successful than their mothers. This is often the case today, in a time when gender roles have changed dramatically. Such changes often mean that a woman will have a career and family, whereas her mother had to sacrifice her own career in order to raise a family. Unconscious guilt over these career accomplishments may lead to sacrifices in other areas. Lerner (1988) has suggested, for example, that a woman may strike an unconscious bargain with herself, saying that it is okay for her to be successful at work as long as she experiences no sexual pleasure with her husband. A similar unconscious avoidance of sexual pleasure may take place when a girl perceives that her mother also avoids pleasure. Religious injunctions against sexuality may serve as the rationale for the message that sexual feelings are wrong, resulting in guilt.

Psychodynamic theory presents a wealth of potential hypotheses concerning adult sexuality. Among the main sources of empirical support for these theoretical predictions are case studies, such as those presented by Chasseguet-Smirgel (1970) and Lerner (1988), in which the therapist is able to provide evidence of the effects of unconscious wishes and desires. These theoretical predictions are difficult to test in nomothetic research, however, because of the need to assess material that is not conscious to the research participant. Although some researchers feel that this requirement makes the theory untestable, I prefer to view this as a challenge to the field of psychology. Researchers may accept the challenge of a careful operationalization of psychoanalytic constructs in order to link intrapsychic conflict and childhood experience to adult sexual functioning.

Research on Sex Guilt and Other Inhibitory Dispositions

Psychoanalytic theory predicts that violation of internal standards for sexual (or other) behavior will lead to guilt, which tends to inhibit sexual arousal. A questionnaire measure of sex guilt was developed by Mosher (1966). Extensive research has supported the construct validity of sex guilt and the validity of this measure (Mosher, 1979). Research on the relationship between sex guilt and subjective sexual arousal in women has produced mixed results, however. No significant relationship between sex guilt and sexual arousal in response to erotic films was reported by Mosher (1973). Similarly, no relationship was found between sex guilt and sexual arousal in response to erotic reading material

(Mosher & Greenberg, 1969). In other studies, however, a significant inverse relationship between sex guilt and sexual arousal has been found. For example, low-sex-guilt women reported more genital sensations after viewing films of masturbation than high-sex-guilt women, although rated sexual arousal did not differ (Mosher & Abramson, 1977). An inverse relationship between sexual arousal and sex guilt in women was also reported by Mosher and O'Grady (1975) and Mosher and White (1980).

One study has examined the relationship between physiologically measured sexual arousal and sex guilt (Morokoff, 1985). Women who were higher in sex guilt showed greater vaginal vasocongestion in response to an erotic videotape than women who were low in sex guilt. Preexposure to an erotic videotape also facilitated sexual arousal in response to a fantasy for high-sex-guilt women but not for low-sex-guilt women. In this study (interestingly), subjectively reported sexual arousal was inversely related to sex guilt.

A structural model of sexual arousal was tested by Green and Mosher (1985) who postulated that sex guilt and masturbation guilt would have both direct and indirect effects on subjective sexual arousal. They hypothesized that the personality dispositions of sex guilt and masturbation guilt, functioning as affective-cognitive structures, would inhibit sexual arousal directly. In addition, they hypothesized that sex guilt would inhibit the positive affects of excitement and joy and increase the negative affects of guilt, fear, and disgust. In turn, excitement and joy are hypothesized to amplify sexual arousal, while guilt, fear, and disgust are assumed to inhibit sexual arousal. This causal model was tested using structural modeling on 241 male and female undergraduates. Sexual arousal was elicited by four fantasy conditions. Results indicated that although the causal model fit the data extremely well, not all predictions from the model were supported. The model was best supported with respect to the predicted relationship between sex guilt and affective reactions to the fantasies, showing that higher sex guilt led to greater affective guilt, fear, and disgust—and less affective excitement and joy. The proposal that sex guilt would directly affect sexual arousal did not receive strong support, as a significant path between sex guilt and sexual arousal was found in only one of the four fantasy conditions. The proposal that sex guilt would indirectly influence sexual arousal through affect was also only partially supported. The proposal that positive affects amplify sexual arousal was supported, but not that negative affects inhibit sexual arousal. Thus, the only fully significant completed path from sex guilt to affect to sexual arousal involved the inhibitory effect of sex guilt on affective joy, which amplified sexual arousal. Effects of gender of participant on sex guilt were examined and found not to be significant. However, models were not tested separately for males and females.

The finding that negative affects do not inhibit sexual arousal is consistent with previously reported data indicating that women may be emotionally disturbed by erotic material, such as rape stimuli, and yet find it arousing (Schmidt, 1975). The relationship between joy and sexual arousal is of interest in light of the positive relationship between well-being and other aspects of sexuality. Although Green and Mosher's model focuses specifically on joy as the psychological affect of orgasm, it is possible that positive emotions (including constructs such as well-being) have a more general predisposing effect on women's potential to become aroused.

It seems that guilt or other inhibitory dispositions have complex effects on sexual arousal. I have hypothesized that sex guilt functions in a consistent manner with other inhibiting dispositions, such as those that (in combination with guilt) influence individuals to have fewer sexual experiences and report lower sexual "arousability." Inventory measures of sex guilt, sex experience, and sexual arousability all evidenced a similar pattern of relationship to sexual arousal, in which more inhibited women had greater vaginal vasocongestion in response to an erotic videotape than less inhibited women, but reported less subjective arousal (Morokoff, 1985). The processes by which guilt might have such direct effects, as well as indirect effects

through positive emotional states, need to be explored.

Research on Anxiety

Research has begun to suggest that under some conditions, anxiety may be facilitative of sexual arousal in women. Preexposure to an anxiety-evoking film before exposure to an erotic film produced greater arousal than preexposure to a relaxation-inducing film in sexually functional women (Hoon, Wincze, & Hoon, 1977). A recent study evaluated the effects of preexposure to an anxiety-evoking stimulus in sexually functional and dysfunctional women who were being treated for sexual problems (Palace & Gorzalka, 1990). None of the women were diagnosed with a sexual arousal disorder, although it was reported that low sexual arousal was a secondary complaint for four of the women. The results of the study indicated that for both the sexually functional and the dysfunctional group, preexposure to the anxiety stimulus resulted in greater vaginal blood volume increases than preexposure to a neutral travelogue. Both groups reported less subjective sexual arousal after anxiety preexposure than neutral preexposure. Similar results have also been reported in sexually functional men (Barlow, Sakheim, & Beck, 1983; Heiman & Rowland, 1983; Wolchik, Beggs, Wincze, Sakheim, Barlow, & Mavissakalian, 1980). Sexually dyfunctional men, on the other hand, have been shown to respond less after provocation of anxiety (Heiman & Rowland, 1983). Palace and Gorzalka (1990) hypothesize that sexual arousal experienced by women may consist of two components: a biological predisposition for physiological arousal and a conditioned cognitive expectancy for sexual arousal.

Other evidence does not support the facilitative effect of anxiety on sexual arousal. Beggs, Calhoun, and Wolchik (1987) reported that a sexual anxiety narrative did not result in as much sexual arousal as a sexual pleasure narrative. The methodology of this study differs from that of the Hoon et al. (1977) and the Palace and Gorzalka (1990) studies, in that an anxiety stimulus was not presented before a purely erotic stimulus, and in that the anxiety stimulus was individualized to each participant. Women were asked to provide reports of either a sexual anxiety experience or a pleasurable sexual experience or fantasy, which were then used verbatim as the stimuli. In the previous studies, the anxiety stimuli evoked fear of bodily harm. The sexual anxiety experiences described in Beggs et al.'s study included hurried timing (60%), negative affects such as anxiety, disgust, anger, and disappointment (95%), and lack of control over the situation (65%). This study confounds presence of these sexual anxieties with the strength of the erotic stimulus. The authors report that sexual arousal was described in 90% of the pleasurable stimuli and only 50% of the anxiety stimuli, while lack of sexual arousal was described in 30% of the anxiety stimuli and none of the pleasure stimuli. Such phenomena alone could account for less physiological sexual arousal. Nevertheless, it is plausible that different types of anxiety may have different effects. Anxiety associated with fear of bodily harm may be facilitative of sexual arousal, whereas anxiety associated with a poor sexual performance may be inhibiting of sexual arousal. Such a hypothesis is consistent with Mosher's (1980) involvement theory, to the extent that some types of anxiety may be consistent with sexual roles or scripts (especially if one assumes that sexual fantasies may include unconscious attempts to master childhood injuries), while other types of anxiety, such as that evoked by failure to perform, are not consistent with sexual scripts.

Interpersonal Determinants of Sexual Arousal Disorder

The most straightforward way in which relations with a partner impair a woman's sexual arousal are if the partner does not supply adequate sexual stimulation. A partner may be unwilling to spend time on building up sexual tension. This may involve beginning by caressing nongenital areas, then slowly moving to direct clitoral, vulval, and vaginal stimulation (manual or oral). Reasons why a male partner might avoid providing adequate stimulation may include lack of knowledge or experience with these activities, a definition of the masculine role that excludes giving a woman pleasure, feelings that the female genitals are dirty, or other conscious and unconscious reactions.

Apart from adequacy of stimulation, there are many interpersonal factors within a relationship that may make it difficult for a woman to become aroused. These are usually related to two factors: anger toward the partner and fear of rejection by the partner. Both anger and fear of rejection in women must be considered within the context of perceived dependency on the relationship. A woman's perception of her dependence on a relationship is produced both by her childhood and developmental experiences (already discussed) and the reality of women's status, which may make it difficult for her to support herself. The traditional sex role expectations for a woman include an attitude of submission toward her male partner. She is expected to be passive, both in major life decisions and in lovemaking. Dependency on the relationship leads women not only to experience guilt over unconscious anger (as previously discussed), but also to avoid expression of consciously experienced anger—and to resist engaging in activities that they fear will lead to rejection by the partner.

When a woman agrees to have sex even though she is angry with her partner, it is not surprising if she does not become aroused. Anger or unexpressed hostility may lead her to focus on negatives about her partner during lovemaking. This process may be very similar to that described by Kaplan (1979) in the etiology of inhibited sexual desire. Although the true source of resentment may remain unacknowledged, minor irritants or symbolic issues may become the focus of her attention as she attempts to become aroused. For example, she may remember household tasks that her husband has not yet done, or focus on some aspect of his appearance that is a turn-off. If major areas of conflict exist in the relationship, such as a career conflict or the decision whether to have another child, these may come to mind and interfere with lovemaking. Barlow has presented a model of sexual dysfunction that suggests that cognitive interference interacts with anxiety to produce inhibited excitement in men and women (Barlow, 1986). Most of the research on cognitive interference in sexual arousal has been done on men, but the theoretical analysis presented here is consistent with this model. Barlow (1986) emphasizes that the cognitive process in dysfunctional subjects "revolves largely around focusing on or attending to a task-irrelevant context" (p. 146).

Adherence to sex-role expectations may also make it difficult to become aroused. By society's norms, it is expected that the male will indicate when to have sex and will "be the aggressor" during sex. The woman's traditional role is to be receptive to his initiations, to participate in the sexual activities he wishes, and to stimulate him sexually. More recently, the media have produced a public awareness that women have sexual responses and can become aroused and reach orgasm, and these are now considered desirable by women and their partners. If women attempt to preserve their traditional role of being passive/receptive partners while at the same time trying to be sexually responsive themselves, sexual responsivity will often be impaired. The attempt to achieve these incompatible goals is, in my experience, a major problem in treatment of arousal disorders in women. The logic behind my view is that it is not possible simultaneously to respond primarily to a partner's needs and to respond oneself, because sexual arousal requires an intense self-directed focus, which is different from women's traditional other-focused role. It seems intuitively evident that one cannot focus all of one's attention on meeting someone else's sexual needs while becoming aroused. If a woman wishes always to be receptive when her partner initiates sex, she will be having sex a good portion of the time when she is not in the mood, is stressed, or otherwise would not have initiated it herself. Furthermore, resentment over being what one client described as "sperm receptacle" may easily carry over into other sexual

experiences that occur in what otherwise might have been a good time. The traditional female role promotes arousal disorders and other sexual disorders in women. It may be women's reluctance to express dissatisfaction with traditional role expectations for sexuality, and/or the fear of being rejected, that prevents women from realizing the incompatibility of demands to be both sexually responsive and a sexual caretaker.

The experience of physical or sexual abuse in the current relationship further amplifies the effects discussed above. If physical or emotional coercion is used to obtain sex, a woman is not a voluntary participant. Under such conditions she will employ whatever coping skills she may possess to endure the experience. The ability to focus on oneself, discussed in the preceding paragraph, presumes voluntary participation in the activity. If participation is anything less than completely voluntary, such integrated self-absorption, assumed by Mosher's involvement theory to be an essential aspect of sexual arousal (Mosher, 1980), is impossible.

Societal Determinants of Female Sexual Arousal Disorder

Traditional sex roles are reinforced by overtly expressed societal expectations and institutions. Feminist theory would suggest that socialization in this role has even more far-reaching consequences for sexual functioning in women than has been so far discussed. One consequence is that women are expected to internalize the ability to control sexuality. That is, women act as gatekeepers and control whether sexual activity will occur. This gatekeeping role may prevent unwanted sexual activity, but it makes full sexual expression difficult (Morokoff, 1990).

Being the gatekeeper suggests a willingness and an ability to turn off sexual feelings. This role is in contrast to expectations for men. Sex roles in our society allow full experience of sexual urges in men to be the norm. Men are believed to be unable to control their sexual urges—hence the need for external controls imposed by women. These norms are a part of the societal support for rape, because the woman who arouses a man without being prepared to "satisfy" him is held at least partially responsible for any subsequent sexual assault. Recently, a jury decided that a woman was not raped because her clothing was considered to be provocative. A man is not asked by society to restrain himself sexually if a woman has acted to arouse him (although he is generally expected to adhere to her limits), and he is believed to suffer unduly if he is aroused and not "allowed" to ejaculate. Women are considered able to turn themselves off sexually, are not believed to suffer any undue physical consequences, and furthermore are frequently required to turn off sexual activity in order to avoid extreme negative sanctions.

What are the specific consequences of the gatekeeper role for sexuality? This question can be addressed by considering how one can learn to turn oneself off sexually. An effective way is to remain turned off at all times. It is not uncommon that women, especially among the population requesting sex therapy, have never consciously experienced sexual arousal. Another method for maintaining the ability to turn oneself off sexually is to not let go fully during sexual activity. Not fully letting go involves the experience of partial arousal but the maintenance of a watchful eye on the proceedings and retention of a feeling of control over the sexual events occurring. This attitude is extremely functional for women, in that one can turn off sexual arousal very quickly if needed and one can track whether the experience is in one's larger self-interest—as it frequently is not, due to the risk of pregnancy or sexually transmitted diseases. This state of partial arousal, far from representing a dysfunction (as it is seen in diagnostic terms), may thus in actuality be quite functional. It is unlikely, however, that such conditions could permit a sufficient level of arousal for orgasm to occur. It should be clear that the cost of the gatekeeping role for sexual self-expression in women is extremely high.

Childhood Sexual Abuse

Childhood sexual abuse is prevalent, as previously discussed. Therefore, the effects of abuse may constitute a significant determinant of the high rates of sexual problems reported by women in our culture. Sexual activity between adult and child or older child and younger child always involves coercion, even when no threats are employed, because of age and status differences between the participants. The issue of why children cannot give informed consent to sex with adults has been addressed by Finkelhor (1979a). He points out that children lack information about sex and the social meaning of sexual relationships, that children are not experienced in judging the acceptability of a sexual partner, and that children do not know the course that sexual relationships are likely to take and how people will react to their involvement in a sexual relationship.

One of the messages transmitted to girls who are sexually abused by men is that men's sexual needs are more important than their own. Another message that may be transmitted is that it is necessary to have sex in order to survive, since the family's livelihood may rest on support from the offender. The basic sexual role that is learned is submission (Maltz & Holman, 1987). The way in which the effects of incest piggyback on the general effects of sexual socialization for girls is delineated by Maltz and Holman (1987). In addition to the teenage girls' normative feelings about sex—confusion, fear, guilt, isolation, and dependency—the incest victim often feels powerless because she has no control over sexuality. "Sex was learned as an act of physical submission. Because it was coercive, the sexual activity did not permit the victim to develop limit-setting and assertiveness skills. Abuse survivors often feel at a loss as to how to prevent sexual activity from occurring or how to interrupt it once it has begun" (pp. 51–52). Because women are expected to prevent unwanted sex (the gatekeeper role previously discussed), the additional burden of being unable to control sex means that incest survivors are likely to reexperience sexual exploitation. Hopelessness about sex is experienced, because survivors assume that sexual relating means being exploited, humiliated, and overwhelmed.

Survivors may assume that in order to get love, they must have sex (as in the early abuse experiences). This rigidly establishes sex as a chore that is a prerequisite for love. Sexual attention from another may represent being loved. It is thus a treatment goal that a survivor not feel she must engage in sex to secure her partner's love. For women who have a history of childhood sexual abuse, it may be impossible to engage in completely mutual and voluntary sex, because of the perceived need to comply with the demands of a partner.

Sexual arousal is often impaired in women who have been sexually abused, as was discussed in the section on the incidence and prevalence of sexual arousal disorder. As soon as a woman begins sexual activity, feelings of helplessness, anger, or guilt may surface. She may also experience flashbacks of the abuse, including sensations of pain and nausea, which interfere with sexual enjoyment and arousal. Because the survivor learned a sexual role within the context of submission and exploitation, she may be unable to focus on her own sexual needs and feelings. Thus, a woman's traditional role emphasizes focus on the partner's needs rather than her own, and self-focus is difficult even for women who have not been sexually abused. For the woman who has been sexually abused, sex was taught as a responsibility of the child to the more powerful other. Sex as a coerced duty to another is incompatible with a self-focus on pleasure.

Dissociation is a common defense used by children and adults who have been abused—"It is not really me, it is just my body that is having this experience" (Malinosky-Rummell & Hoier, 1991). Adult use of dissociation as a defense mechanism has been found to be significantly correlated with the presence of childhood stress. The highest level of adult dissociation was associated with victimization from both physical and psychological abuse during childhood (Sanders, McRoberts, & Tollefson,

1989). The most extreme form of dissociation, multiple personality disorder, has also been found to be strongly related to childhood sexual abuse. In a series of 100 MPD patients, 83% were found to have been sexually abused as children, and 75% had been physically abused (Putnam, Guroff, Silberman, Barban, & Post, 1986). If dissociation is triggered during sexual activity, ability to maintain arousal is clearly impaired. Someone who dissociates during sex may be able to react physiologically in response to ongoing sexual stimulation but will not feel sexually aroused in the dissociative state. This phenomenon again emphasizes the need to assess both subjective and physiological arousal.

Several common patterns of sexual expression have been identified in childhood abuse survivors. One is sexual promiscuity. Tsai et al. (1979) found that women in their clinical group had more numerous sexual partners than women in their nonclinical and control groups. Maltz and Holman (1987) suggest that survivors may learn that their sexual attention can give them power over men and so may try to demonstrate this power (either in the sense of having power over their own sexuality or in the sense of dominating another person) on their own. It has also been observed that survivors may withdraw from sex, perhaps in an effort to make up for sexual acts they felt were wrong, or (as described by Maltz and Holman) to buy their way back to heaven. Therapists in Meiselman's (1978) study reported that their clients tended to sexualize relationships and that the survivors had difficulty differentiating between sex and affection. Gordy (1983) has observed that survivors could either be sexual or affectionate with partners, but not both. She referred to this phenomenon as *splitting*. A related type of splitting is described by Jehu (1988), who reports that some survivors do not experience sexual difficulties in short-term sexual relationships but do in committed relationships. This may be because a committed relationship bears similarity to the early traumatic experience, and the demands of a partner in a committed relationship are more unavoidable than partner demands in a transient relationship. When such splitting occurs, sexual arousal with the committed partner (as well as sexual desire) may be inhibited.

Summary

In examining the causal factors for women's sexual arousal disorders discussed here, it is evident that physiological factors, the realistic demands of specific life stages, capacity for relationships based on childhood experience, relationships with partners, societal expectations, and the effects of sexual abuse all interrelate to impair a woman's full experience of sexual arousal. It is thus not surprising that so many women indicate difficulties in becoming aroused. It is important to acknowledge the normative component of sexual arousal difficulties so as not to pathologize this experience, while at the same time emphasizing that women do have the capacity for full sexual response and that limitations on sexual responsiveness do not need to be.

ASSESSMENT

Assessment of sexual arousal disorder in women has typically been deemphasized and incomplete. My objective here is to describe the assessment strategies currently available and to propose criteria for measurement of sexual arousal in women that would be appropriate for both clinical evaluation and research investigations. When assessing sexual arousal disorder, it is most important to keep in mind that sexual arousal is composed of both physical responses (vasocongestion and lubrication) and subjective responses, including a global sense of excitement and awareness of the physical changes. It is also crucial to keep in mind that arousal occurs in the context of feelings toward a specific partner.

Interview

In the clinical setting, assessment of sexual arousal disorder (and of all sexual dysfunctions) is most commonly accomplished through an interview. Where the goal is to treat this problem in a sex therapy format, it is imperative to involve the woman's partner, even in an initial evaluation. The advantage of interviewing both partners include (1) establishing the perspective that both partners are part of the problem and the solution, (2) having the opportunity to determine whether her partner corroborates the woman's report, (3) assessing the partner's sexual functioning, and (4) assessing relationship dynamics.

Presenting Complaint

First, it is important to gain a general knowledge of the nature of the presenting complaint. It is crucial to hear how the client herself describes the problem, as this will give clues for accurate diagnosis and for treatment. For example, if she describes vaginal dryness, even though she is otherwise stimulated, this presents a completely different picture from a woman who reports no genital sensations at all and a lack of awareness of the meaning of sexual arousal.

It is important to determine whether the problem has been lifelong or, if not lifelong, how long it has been present. For those women who experience a lack of all feelings of sexual arousal, sexual arousal disorder may well have been of lifelong duration. Other women will have experienced sexual arousal in the past but not at present, or currently in some situations but not in others. It is especially important to evaluate any biopsychological life-stage issues that were in play at the time lack of arousal began to be a problem. It is not uncommon to notice lack of arousal first during pregnancy or after the birth of a baby, during some phases of the menstrual cycle, or postmenopause. A question such as ''What was happening at the time the problem began?'' may reveal other important information, such as the death of a loved one, a divorce or other significant loss, marriage, or a career change. It is also relevant to assess why the client and her partner think this problem developed—again because their answers provide clues concerning treatment approaches.

Sexual Arousal

Interview assessment of a sexual arousal disorder must focus on three important aspects of sexual arousal: presence of vaginal vasocongestion, lubrication, and cognitive/emotional feelings of sexual arousal. Ideally, we would like to measure both the objective presence of lubrication and vasocongestion and the client's awareness of these. It is often not possible to make physiological measurements of arousal, but the interviewer may attempt to make this distinction by listening carefully to a woman's description of her physical response as well as to her partner.

1. Presence of genital vasocongestion. It is important to ask specific questions in order to assess whether genital changes are occurring. Oftentimes clients lack the specific knowledge to answer these questions fully, but their degree of awareness of genital changes can be informative. As discussed, the information gained in the interview will not evaluate genital vasocongestion itself, but only the client's awareness of this. The woman who is becoming aroused and is aware of that arousal should be able to describe some sensations of tumescence or swelling in the clitoral, labial, or vaginal areas. Her partner may be helpful in corroborating or providing additional information about his perception of this response.

2. Presence of vaginal lubrication. It is also important to ask specifically whether vaginal lubrication is adequate. When lubrication is inadequate, a woman may experience a feeling of vaginal dryness, irritation, or pain during attempted intercourse. When lubrication is not adequate, it may be difficult for her to sense vasocongestion, even when it is fully present, because of the feeling of dryness. Again, a partner may provide information concerning the amount of lubrication, from his perspective.

3. Presence of feelings of sexual arousal and excitement. It is important to assess whether the client experiences a feeling of sexual excite-

ment. Feeling sexually aroused may be heightened by an awareness of physical responses. Sexual arousal may be diminished if a lack of physical response is observed, as is the case for a man whose ardor is dampened when he observes his lack of an erection. In the same manner, a woman may check to see if she is lubricated, to validate her feelings of sexual arousal. However, feelings of arousal are important in and of themselves. They may be closely related to the experience of sexual fantasies during sex or feelings of love for the partner.

The General Sexual Relationship and Adequacy of Stimulation

It is always important to find out how often the couple typically has sex and what percentage of the time the problem occurs. It is a different picture if the couple has sex several times a week, with lack of arousal occuring half the time, than if the couple has sex every few months. Furthermore, it is very important to assess the adequacy of stimulation; if it has been inadequate, treatment will focus on helping the couple implement more effective stimulation techniques. Part of this assessment will involve questions about the length of foreplay and the type of foreplay activities in which the couple engages. A woman who does not wish to place demands on her partner may tolerate foreplay that is extremely limited and then blame herself for lack of arousal during intercourse. One of the best ways to elicit this type of information is to ask the couple to describe concretely a typical sexual experience. This description will also provide important information about emotional reactions the couple experience when they try to have sex.

It is also relevant to determine what type of contraception is used and whether the couple wishes to conceive. This is important because some contraceptives may be perceived to interfere with arousal, such as oral contraceptives or condoms. Additionally, conflicts over whether to attempt conception may inhibit sexual arousal for some women.

It should be emphasized that although this

discussion focuses specifically on the assessment of arousal and factors related to it, a sexual evaluation always requires assessment of all phases of the sexual response cycle—i.e., desire and orgasm as well as dyspareunia and sexual aversions or phobias (see other chapters in this volume for more information on assessment of these areas). In addition, assessment should be made of whether or not the woman's partner presents sexual symptoms.

Situational Arousal

It is relevant to determine the adequacy of the above components of sexual arousal in different situations. For example, a woman may report that she is able to become aroused with only certain types of stimulation. She may find manual stimulation arousing, but not intercourse; or she may find that she requires oral stimulation or breast stimulation in order to become aroused. It may also be the case that a woman can adequately arouse herself during masturbation but cannot become aroused by her partner's stimulation. It is thus important to assess the three components of arousal in each of these situations. When assessing arousal during masturbation, it is also important to find out how frequently she masturbates and how this has changed over time. Some clients are extremely reluctant to discuss masturbation, especially in front of the partner, and this may suggest areas of inhibition that are relevant for treatment. A comparable situation may exist if she has or has had other partners with whom she had no difficulty becoming aroused. The interpersonal and intrapersonal causes of arousal disorder previously discussed can provide important hypotheses to be tested when assessing the woman's psychosexual history and the quality of her present relationship.

Reliability and Validity of Interview Data

It is intuitively evident that self-reports of sexual behavior and sexual arousal may be biased. Women may be reluctant to tell an interviewer

that they are aroused by certain stimuli and thus underreport sexual arousal; conversely, they may be embarrassed to report that they are not aroused and so overreport their own arousal. If a woman is accompanying her symptomatic partner, she may wish to protect her privacy and therefore not disclose accurate information concerning her own sexual functioning. In addition, a woman may simply not remember how often she typically becomes aroused or to what intensity. Because interviews are necessarily retrospective, participants are often asked to indicate a typical or average response. This question may not evoke a typical but rather an outstanding example of response. That is, a woman may remember a salient instance that demonstrates why she feels there is a problem, such as a time in which she couldn't become aroused even after her partner provided lengthy stimulation, leading to an argument, but this instance may not necessarily be her average response. Personal salience may therefore be a significant determinant of what is remembered (Catania, Gibson, Chitwood, & Coates, 1990).

Partner corroboration serves as one potential validity check on the individual's self-report. Although the correlation between partners' reports of sexual activity has been studied (Clark & Wallin, 1964; Coates et al., 1988; Jacobson & Moore, 1981), the correlation between partners' reports of level of sexual arousal has not yet been investigated. Given the difficulty of accurately assessing sexual arousal level even for a woman herself, and the fact that the correlation between partners' reports of sexual activities tend to be low, it seems likely that partners' reports of arousal would be a weak validity check. It may nevertheless be of clinical interest to know that a partner perceives adequate vaginal lubrication when the woman herself feels no arousal.

Objective indices of sexual arousal might be expected to serve as a validity check on self-reports. As will be discussed, physiological measures of sexual arousal are available and have been studied in conjunction with subjective self-reports. A difficulty in conceptualizing physiological measures as a validity check on self-reports, however, is that both physiological measures and self-report measures of subjective experience are valid aspects of sexual response in their own right. For example, if a man says he feels 100% sexually aroused but can be demonstrated to have only a partial erection, we would not wish to say he is wrong and should not feel aroused. Similarly in women, if discrepancies between physiological measures and self-reports exist, the physiological measure is not necessarily the accurate one. An important use of physiological measures is in cases in which women report no arousal but physiologically demonstrate a sexual response. A woman may be very interested to learn of her potential for physical response.

Clinicians know that clients very often will not answer a question the same way when asked again. A woman may on one occasion say she has never become aroused when masturbating, but on another occasion describe an arousing experience she had as a teenager as a result of self-stimulation. Factors such as whether she is asked to disclose information when she is alone or when her partner is present may be important determinants of the reliability of her responses. The overall reliability of sexual arousal estimates has not been researched. It seems clear, however, that when a question evokes personal conflict, the reliability of the information given will suffer.

Psychophysiological Assessment of Sexual Arousal

Vaginal Vasocongestion

Various devices have been developed to measure vaginal vasocongestion, including the vaginal photoplethysmograph, labial thermistors, and vaginal thermistors. These instruments have been used primarily for research purposes rather than clinical assessment. Vaginal photoplethysmography is the most commonly used method for physiologically measuring the vasocongestive component of sexual arousal in women. The instrument is a tampon-shaped

hard plastic cylinder in which a light source and photoelectric transducer are embedded. The light source and photodetector are positioned in such a way that light cannot reach the photodetector when inserted in the vagina unless the light is back-scattered from the vaginal wall. It is inserted into the outer third of the vagina. The photoplethysmographic method had been successfully used to measure pulse and pooling of blood in other body areas (e.g., finger, forehead) before its adaptation to vaginal vasocongestion (Weinman, 1967). Changes in reflected or back-scattered light signal changes in the amount of blood in vaginal tissue, due to the differential optical properties of tissue engorged with blood (Semlow & Lubowsky, 1983). Two signals can be derived from the vaginal photoplethysmograph: vaginal pulse amplitude, which represents changes in the amount of blood entering tissues with each cardiac cycle, and vaginal blood volume, a measure of the pooling of blood in vaginal tissue (Geer, Morokoff, & Greenwood, 1974). Vaginal pulse amplitude is obtained by an AC-coupling of the photoplethysmograph and is derived by measuring the amplitude of the cardiac pulse wave. The frequency of this wave provides a measure of heart rate. DC-coupling of the photoplethysmograph permits evaluation of slower changes that are believed to represent pooling of blood (Rosen & Beck, 1988).

The first popularly used photoplethysmograph model included an incandescent light source and photocell (Sintchak & Geer, 1975). Several problems have emerged in the use of the photoplethysmograph. One issue is the instability of the photodetector and illuminating source; this problem was addressed by development of a photoplethysmograph employing an LED rather than incandescent light and phototransistors rather than a photocell (Hoon, Wincze, & Hoon, 1976). A second problem is that responses may not be reliable within or across recording sessions. This may in part be due to the inability to maintain a constant position of the probe within the vagina. Significant differences in amplitude of the pulse wave may be observed when the probe is rotated within the vagina. This undoubtedly results from differences in vascularization of the tissues being measured at each rotation. A third issue is movement artifact. Women must remain relatively still in order to avoid producing artifactual increases in the signal. Both the issues of reliability and movement artifact have been addressed by development of a probe that utilizes a fixed vaginal position and a circularly symmetrical light source (Armon, Weinman, & Weinstein, 1978). Completely circumferential backscattering was achieved by further modification of this design (Benoit, Borth, & Woolever, 1980). This probe has not been widely used in psychological research, probably because many psychological studies involve single recording sessions, so that the problem of repeatability is not salient.

A final problem, which can probably not be addressed as long as indirect measurement is employed, is the inability to calibrate vaginal vasocongestion. Although calibration of the light source may be made, pulse amplitude must be measured in voltage output or millimeters of pen deflection on polygraph paper rather than in absolute units. A similar problem exists in measuring penile vasocongestion, but the shape of the penis permits a meaningful measure of circumference or volume changes. No comparable measurement units are available for assessing female genital vasocongestion.

Despite measurement issues, the vaginal photoplethysmograph is the most accurate means currently available of measuring the vasocongestive component of sexual arousal in women (Rosen & Beck, 1988). It is also the most widely used psychophysiological measure of sexual arousal in women.

Other measures of genital vasocongestion that have been employed focus on measuring temperature changes. Thermistors mounted on a diaphragm (one kept at an elevated fixed temperature) have been used to determine changes in blood flow (Cohen & Shapiro, 1970). Thermistors have also been used to measure labial temperature change, an indication of increased labial vasocongestion (Henson, Rubin, Henson, & Williams, 1977; Henson, Rubin, & Henson, 1978). Clitoral temperature has been measured by thermistors (Javanovic, 1971), and thermography has been used to measure pelvic temperature—an indicator of pelvic vasocongestion (Abramson, Perry, Seeley, Seeley, & Rothblatt, 1981). Combinations of these measurement strategies have been used by some investigators, such as Gillan and Brindley (1979), who packaged two incandescent light sources, four photocells, and a heated thermistor in a vaginal probe.

Another strategy for measuring vaginal changes is the use of a heated electrode in conjunction with measurement of transcutaneous oxygen partial pressure (pO_2) (Levin & Wagner, 1977). A heated oxygen electrode kept at a set temperature is fitted into a suction holder, which attaches it to the vaginal wall. This allows measurement of temperature change as described above, as well as a measure of pO_2. Sexual stimulation has been shown to result in increased oxygenation of the vaginal tissue (Wagner & Levin, 1978).

Vaginal Lubrication

Measures of vaginal fluids lag behind measures of genital vasocongestion, despite the importance of this component of female sexual arousal. Research employing measures of vaginal lubrication are especially needed in assessing women at life stages in which estrogen depletion is expected. A device for measuring vaginal lubrication was developed by Shapiro, Cohen, DiBianco, & Rosen (1968), involving an electrode placed in a tampon saturated with hypotonic saline, with a reference electrode outside the vagina. A procedure for studying vaginal fluids was also developed by Semmens and Wagner (1982): Three pieces of washed, dried, and preweighed filter paper were placed in the middle third of the vagina to absorb vaginal secretions. These papers could then be removed, placed in special preweighed containers, and weighed to calculate the amount of fluid. Wagner and Levin (1977) describe a device in which filter papers are secured to a bar. Perhaps the simplest procedure is that described by Preti,

Huggins, and Silverberg (1979): tampons are weighed before and after vaginal containment. However, this measurement procedure cannot be used to assess continuous changes in lubrication level; it can only be used to measure the total amount of vaginal fluids during the period in which the tampon is inserted.

Reliability and Validity of Psychophysiological Measures of Sexual Arousal

Reliable measurement of vaginal responses in the sexually unaroused state is dependent on sampling the same vascular tissue bed each time measurements are made. For this reason, vaginal position is all-important when using a vaginal photoplethysmograph with a single fixed light source. Extremely different results may be obtained from one insertion to the next. This problem has been lessened by the development of probes utilizing a fixed vaginal position and a circular light source. The issue of reliability in the sexually aroused state is a complex one. One would not necessarily expect a woman to experience the same level of sexual arousal each time she observes the same erotic stimulus or imagines the same sexual fantasy. Thus, what is meant by *reliability* here is the reliability of the instrument in detecting whatever level of arousal is present. Since we have no independent means of determining what level of arousal is present, it is currently impossible to estimate this type of reliability.

Determination of the validity of physiologically measured arousal also presents complex issues. Several studies have employed multiple physiological measures of arousal, finding moderate consistency across measures. For example, Henson and Rubin (1978) recorded vaginal blood volume and labial temperature simultaneously. During erotic stimulation the intraindividual correlation coefficients between the two measures ranged between $r = .61$ and $r = .95$ for six out of eight participants. Vaginal pulse amplitude showed a similar relationship

with vaginal blood volume and labial temperature for most but not all participants (Henson, Rubin, & Henson, 1979).

Physiologically measured sexual arousal is often poorly correlated with self-reports of arousal. Comparing physiologically measured arousal and self-reports, Heiman (1980) reported correlation coefficients between $r = .40$ and $r = .44$. Similarly, Morokoff (1985) reported a correlation of $r = .42$ between these same measures taken while women watched either erotic or neutral videotapes. The wide range of responses elicited by watching either a neutral or an erotic videotape ensures that low correlations could not be attributed to a restricted response range. No significant correlation was found between the measures of arousal while women fantasized. A possible cause of low correlations is the fact that self-report measures are taken after the erotic stimulus is over, whereas physiological response is measured continuously during the erotic stimulus. To address this problem, Morokoff (1981) cued participants to use a lever to rate sexual arousal while viewing an erotic videotape. Combining those who watched an erotic videotape with those who watched a neutral tape during sexual arousal, correlation coefficients across participants ranged from $r = .56$ to $r = .72$. Wincze, Hoon, and Hoon (1977), using a continuous measure of subjective arousal, were unable to demonstrate a significant correlation between subjective and physiological measures. However, significant correlations for the two measures were found for five of the six participants in the study when correlations were calculated individually.

Lower-level correlations between physiological and self-report measures of sexual arousal may be interpreted in two ways. One is that these measures are not tapping the same underlying construct. Further research utilizing a multimethod assessment across arousing conditions is needed to establish discriminative or convergent validity for these constructs. Alternatively, it is possible that some women are not skilled in attending to physiological cues of arousal. For example, Korff and Geer (1983) reported that the correlation between subjective and physiological measures of sexual arousal is higher when women are given an instructional intervention to focus on bodily cues. For those who received these instructions, the average intraindividual correlation between subjective and genital indices of arousal was $r = .86$. For women in the control group receiving no instructions, the average intraindividual correlation was $r = .48$. It should be noted that although most correlation coefficients were statistically significant, especially in the instructional group, their magnitude may have been higher than in other studies because they were based on only 10 data points.

Heiman (1977) found a greater correlation between subjective and physiological arousal measures in men than in women. Study participants were cross-tabulated by categories of physiological arousal and by whether subjective arousal was reported. All men who showed high physiological arousal also reported feeling sexually aroused. However, only 58% of the women categorized as highly aroused by the physiological measure reported being aroused. Anatomical differences between men and women may make it easier for men to be aware of the kinesthetic sensations of sexual arousal. Furthermore, Morokoff (1985) found a significant difference in the correlation between subjective and physiological arousal during fantasy for sexually experienced and inexperienced undergraduate women. The more experienced women showed a stronger relationship between the two measures of arousal ($r = .48$) than the sexually inexperienced women ($r = -.13$). It should be noted that higher correlations for this group were not attributable to higher absolute levels of physiological arousal in the experienced group.

Clinical Uses of Psychophysiological Assessment

Psychophysiological measures of sexual arousal are rarely used in assessing women's sexual arousal. The paragraphs that follow discuss several areas in which psychophysiological assessment would add significantly to the diagnosis and treatment.

1. Documentation of women's sexual arousal in response to erotic stimuli or fantasy. This information is valuable in treating a woman who believes she cannot become aroused. The clinician is able to demonstrate physiological signs of arousal to her in spite of her subjective lack of arousal. This does not invalidate her subjective experience, but it gives her the important information that she is capable of physical response. This is especially useful if a woman believes there is something physically wrong preventing her from becoming aroused.

2. Determination of arousing fantasy themes. For women who are unable to fantasize, it may be helpful to use psychophysiological methods to help identify the fantasy themes that are the most arousing. For assessment purposes, the fantasy themes might be presented in written form first before asking a woman to imagine them herself. This procedure is similar to traditional biofeedback, except that here a cognitive rather than a physiological response is being shaped. This methodology is commonly used with men diagnosed with paraphilias, to help shape more normal fantasies. Such masturbatory reconditioning for women has been reported by Annon (1973), although without the use of physiological measures. The technique suggested here would enable women to discover what fantasies are most arousing.

Such a procedure was used in developing an inventory measure of fantasy themes, the Female Sexual Fantasy Questionnaire (FSFQ). Factor analysis ratings of fantasy themes produced five dimensions of sexual fantasy: genital, sensual, sexual power, sexual suffering, and forbidden sexual activity. Ratings of sexual arousal in response to these themes was significantly correlated with vaginal blood volume measured while women engaged in fantasy employing these themes (Meuwissen & Over, 1991).

3. Determination of amount of vaginal lubrication. Vaginal fluids can be measured in the resting state and following an effective arousing stimulus. Unfortunately, normative data on levels of vaginal fluids are not currently available. Normative information would be necessary in order to assess whether the client's level of lubrication is a significant contributor to a sexual arousal problem. As this information becomes available, measurement of lubrication will provide important diagnostic information. As has been discussed, vaginal dryness is often associated with periods of reduced estrogen levels, such as postpartum and postmenopause, when sexual problems are frequently reported.

4. Differential diagnosis of physiological versus psychogenic causes of an arousal dysfunction. Data to make such a differential diagnosis in women can be obtained through sleep studies in the same way it is routinely obtained by measures of nocturnal penile tumescence in men. It has been observed that women undergo phasic increases in vaginal pulse amplitude during REM sleep, comparable to penile changes during REM sleep (Abel, Murphy, Becker, & Bitar, 1979). Increased vaginal blood flow during REM periods has also been reported by Fischer et al. (1983). The existence of periods of vascular changes in the vagina and other genital areas (Karacan, Rosenbloom & Williams, 1970) suggest that this may be an appropriate methodology for assessing presence of vascular disorders (Rogers, Van de Castle, Evans, & Critelli, 1985). Physiologial causes of female sexual arousal disorders are not well understood. Lack of clarity in assessment of arousal may be standing in the way of better research in this area. Given the prevalence of arterial insufficiency in men with erectile problems (Jevtich, 1983), it is unlikely that physiological factors play no role in women's arousal difficulties. Further studies of this possibility must be undertaken, utilizing assessment of nocturnal vaginal tumescence.

Lack of understanding of physiological factors in sexual arousal disorder in women has also impaired understanding of the way in which physiological and psychological factors may interact. Even when physiological impairment is well documented, as in vascular problems secondary to diabetes in men, psychological factors such as stress may interact to determine whether erectile problems occur or not. Such interactions may be assumed to exist in women as well, although they have not been documented. Assessment of nocturnal vaginal tumescence in women with diseases that might affect vaginal vasocongestion would help to illuminate the interaction of physiological and psychological factors in the etiology of sexual arousal disorder in women.

Despite the important ways in which psychophysiological assessment contributes to our understanding of arousal disorders, it is still a limited tool. This is primarily because it is currently not possible to assess arousal during sexual activity with a partner. We are restricted to assessing arousal to sexual stimuli in a laboratory setting. The stimuli most commonly used to evoke sexual arousal are erotic videotapes, audiotapes, or slides. Although such stimuli are satisfactory for many research questions, they do not help to address changes in sexual arousal experienced during sex with a partner. Most clients, regardless of diagnosis, have the capability for arousal to erotic stimuli when they begin treatment (Morokoff & Heiman, 1980). Thus, pre-post evaluation of such stimuli does not provide information about treatment outcome unless arousal in response to erotic stimuli is a treatment goal. In order to demonstrate clinically relevant changes, it would be necessary to monitor arousal during actual lovemaking at home. If this could be done unobtrusively, it would be a marvelous addition to our current diagnostic capabilities. One clinically relevant aspect of sexuality that can be used in the laboratory to evoke sexual arousal is sexual fantasy. The drawback people often have difficulty relaxing enough to imagine a fantasy as they might at home during sex. Nevertheless, as discussed above, assessment of arousal during fantasy may provide important clinical information. Finally, assessment during sleep does not suffer from the above limitations; it should be undertaken more often.

Self-Report Instruments for Assessing Sexual Arousal

A comprehensive questionnaire measure should focus on both subjective awareness of sexual arousal and subjective awareness of physiological signs of arousal, such as genital sensations and vaginal lubrication.

State Measures of Subjective Sexual Arousal

Single-item ratings of sexual arousal have been employed in psychological research. A question such as "How sexually aroused do you feel now?" is rated on a seven-point Likert scale, from 1 (no sexual arousal at all) to 7 (very strong sexual arousal) (Morokoff, 1985; Mosher, 1973; Mosher & Abramson, 1977). Such questions are typically asked following a sexually arousing stimulus such as an erotic videotape or sexual fantasy. A variant is to ask the woman to rate the maximum arousal she experienced during this stimulus (Morokoff, 1985). Similarly, women have been asked to rate perceptions of genital sensations, breast sensations, and vaginal lubrication (Morokoff, 1985; Mosher, 1973; Mosher & Abramson, 1977; Myers & Morokoff, 1986). As pointed out by Mosher, Barton-Henry, and Green (1988), such single-item measures tend to be inadequate from a psychometric standpoint and may fail to sample the relevant domain of the construct.

Affective sexual arousal is based on a theoretical conceptualization of subjective sexual arousal as "an affect-cognition blend in consciousness of awareness of physiological sexual arousal and sexual affects or affect-cognition blends" (Mosher et al., 1988, p. 414). This theoretical conceptualization is developed further in Mosher's involvement theory (Mosher, 1980). Mosher and Abramson (1977) developed an affective rating scale for six adjectives; factor analysis showed it to be a cohesive measure of sexual arousal. In the original version of this instrument, the six adjectives for sexual arousal were *passionate, sensuous, excited, lustful, aroused,* and *hot*. Ratings of these adjectives

have been shown to be higher following exposure to an erotic stimulus than a neutral stimulus (Morokoff, 1980).

In order to develop multi-item scales of subjective sexual arousal, Mosher et al. (1988) developed item pools for two measures of sexual arousal: sexual arousal ratings and affective sexual arousal. This was done also to assess the discriminant and convergent validity of the scales and to examine their validity as operationalizations of the sexual arousal construct.

Eleven seven-point Likert rating scales were developed to permit ratings of sexual arousal. The 11 items to be rated were sexual arousal, genital sensations, sexual warmth, muscular tension, nongenital physical sensation, sexual absorption, sexual tension, sex drive, sexual deprivation, sexual goal value, and sexual interest. It may be noted that some of these items (especially sex drive, sexual interest, sexual deprivation, and sexual goal value) appear to tap the desire phase of sexual response more than the arousal phase. Psychometric evaluation was used to obtain the most cohesive five-item scale of rated sexual arousal. The items that resulted were ratings of sexual arousal, genital sensations, sexual warmth, nongenital physical sensations, and sexual absorption. None of the items measuring sexual desire appear in this group, and Mosher et al. indicate that two of these items (sexual deprivation and sexual goal value) were not acceptable due to low item-total correlations. Reliability coefficients for this scale range from .97 to .98 across the different fantasy arousal conditions.

Ten adjectives for sexual arousal, each rated on a five-point scale, were embedded in an adjective checklist. These constituted an expansion of the adjective checklist discussed above. The adjectives subjected to evaluation were *lustful, sexually erotic, sexually aroused, sensuous, turned on, sexually hot, horny, sexy, passionate,* and *sexually excited*. The most cohesive five-item scale included the following adjectives: *sexually aroused, sensuous, turned on, sexually hot,* and *sexually excited*.

Mosher et al. (1988) also developed an 11-item Guttman-type scale for subjective awareness of genital sensations. The scale items go from no genital sensations through multiple orgasm. (The structure of these items as a Guttman scale has not been confirmed, however.) The scale is designed to be used by either men or women. There are two problems with the structure of the scale. One is that measurement of vaginal lubrication is confounded with measurement of vasocongestion. That is, the scale assumes that vasocongestion and lubrication progress at the same pace. (For example, item #3, mild genital sensation, is defined as vasocongestion sufficient to begin penile erection or to begin vaginal lubrication; item #4, moderate genital sensations, is defined as vasocongestion sufficient to erect penis fully or to lubricate vagina fully.) These assumptions are in accord with Masters and Johnson's (1966) observations that lubrication is a response to vaginal vasocongestion. However, there is evidence that in estrogen-deficient women, lubrication is impaired despite no evidence of reduced vaginal vasocongestion (Myers & Morokoff, 1986). Such asynchrony of response suggests that further evaluation of the relation of vasocongestion to lubrication is needed. This should be done employing physiological and subjective measures of both vasocongestion and lubrication. A second problem is the assumption that orgasm follows high levels of arousal. Again, this is probably the case in the undergraduate sample utilized in the study by Mosher et al., but is not universal. It is known that orgasm and ejaculation may occur in men with a flaccid penis (Kaplan, 1989), and it is probable that a similar response pattern may occur in women, although it has not yet been documented.

The three measures of subjective sexual arousal were subjected to a multicondition-multimethod matrix to determine convergent and discriminative validity (Mosher et al., 1988). Strong evidence was found for these measures as operations for the construct of subjective sexual arousal. The three measures tended to be correlated with each other within and across types of fantasy.

Measures such as those described here are rarely, if ever, used clinically; their use has been primarily restricted to research. However, there are potential clinical applications for reliable and valid measures of subjective sexual arousal to specific experiences. Many sex therapists ask clients to keep records of their sexual activities at home, in some instances asking clients to make ratings describing their pleasure in these activities. In assessing a couple, it would be possible to ask each partner to rate arousal experienced during lovemaking using the scales described here. This would be highly desirable as a pre-post outcome measure.

Measurement of Sexual Arousal Across Situations

A single-item measure of sexual arousal during sex with one's partner is included along with single-item measures of other sexual dysfunctions in the General Information Form developed by LoPiccolo and colleagues. This instrument is described by Nowinski and LoPiccolo (1979), although the version of the survey presented in that paper does not include the item under discussion, which was added later. The question asks, "When you have sex with your mate, do you feel sexually aroused (i.e., feeling "turned on," pleasure, excitement)?" Response options are (1) nearly always, over 90%; (2) usually, about 75% of the time; (3) sometimes, about 50% of the time; (4) seldom, about 25% of the time; and (5) never. Normative data have not yet been published for this measure.

The Sexual Arousability Inventory (SAI) was developed by Hoon, Hoon, and Wincze (1976), to measure potential for sexual arousal in response to 28 erotic experiences. These include items such as "when a loved one stimulates your genitals with mouth and tongue" and "when you read suggestive or pornographic poetry." This scale demonstrated high internal consistency but a somewhat lower test-retest reliability ($r = .69$). The SAI was expanded (Hoon, 1978) to permit rating of the original situations on two additional scales—anxiety and satisfaction. The reliability, validity, and factor structure of the expanded scale were further demonstrated by Chambless and Lifshitz (1984). The relationship of the SAI to a physiological measure of sexual arousal was evaluated in two studies. Interestingly, both found a negative correlation between self-reported sexual arousability and vaginal pulse amplitude (Morokoff, 1985; Rogers et al., 1985). The asynchronous results between physiological and self-report measures suggest (as discussed earlier) that the two response modalities may not be reflecting the same underlying phenomenon. These findings highlight the importance of multimodal measures of sexual arousal.

A potential problem with the SAI is that respondents are asked to make general ratings of arousal, anxiety, and satisfaction with reference to specific sexual situations, but not to specific partners. Thus "when you dance with a loved one" or "when a loved one kisses you with an exploring tongue" may be highly arousing with one partner, but a turn-off with another partner. Variability of response depending on partner may account for the low test-retest reliability. The instrument was designed for clinical use but has not been widely adopted for this purpose—perhaps because the inventory assesses a general tendency of arousability rather than arousal within the relationship being treated. Most arousal dysfunctions are treated in a conjoint format, and therapists may find the characteristics of response in that particular relationship most relevant.

An inventory that does tap responses within a specific sexual relationship is the Sexual Interaction Inventory (SII) (LoPiccolo & Steger, 1974). This instrument is designed to be completed by both members of the couple. For each of 17 sexual activities, ranging from seeing each partner nude to having intercourse with orgasm, respondents indicate current frequency, desired frequency, pleasantness of the activity, desired pleasantness, how pleasant the partner is believed to find the activity, and how pleasant the respondent would like the partner to find the activity. Eleven scales derived from this data characterize sexual interactions between the couple. The only scale relevant to assessment of female sexual arousal is the pleasure mean (scale 6), which is simply a mean of the female partner's ratings of "pleasantness" for each of the 17 activities. The primary drawback of this instrument as a measure of sexual arousal is that a rating of pleasantness is not a straightforward way to measure sexual arousal, and it may be argued that it actually taps a different construct.

The pleasure mean scale of the SII has been found to have high internal consistency and a test-retest reliability of $r = .89$. Women in a normal sample provided an average rating of 5.11 on the six-point scale, which was significantly different from a clinical sample's mean rating of 4.69. Significant changes in this scale were reported as a result of treatment (LoPiccolo & Steger, 1974). Although this instrument has not been used to evaluate treatment of women diagnosed with sexual arousal disorder, it has been used to evaluate pre-post treatment changes for a group of women diagnosed with orgasm dysfunction. It is very likely that at least a portion of the clients would have met the criterion for female sexual arousal disorder, if it had been diagnosed. The SII pleasure mean scale showed significant improvement from pre- to post-treatment, an improvement that was maintained at follow-up three months later (Morokoff & LoPiccolo, 1986).

Evaluation of Factors Associated with Sexual Arousal

Medical Evaluation

A hormonal evaluation is the most important element of a medical evaluation to assess physical factors relevant to sexual arousal disorder in women. Determination of estrogen level will indicate whether this is a cause of vaginal dryness. Especially for women who have had their ovaries removed, evaluation of testosterone level will indicate whether testosterone deprivation may account for lack of subjective arousal.

In addition, a vaginal smear may be appropriate, especially for postmenopausal women, to determine whether thinning of the vaginal epithelium may account for vaginal irritation. For other medical factors to be assessed, see Chapters 5, 8, and 12 of this book.

The Couple's Relationship

Assessment of the quality of the couple's relationship is vital to understanding a lack of sexual arousal. Suppressed anger and associated power issues in the relationship, as well as fear of rejection, may make it very difficult for a woman to become sexually aroused. Such issues are best assessed by an experienced clinician during conjoint interviews with the couple (Kaplan, 1983).

The mutuality of the couple's relationship is so important that it seems appropriate to include it in the diagnostic criteria for sexual arousal disorder. Such a revision would add qualifications such as are required of the sexual activity in order to make a diagnosis of inhibited female orgasm (i.e., it must be judged by the clinician to be of adequate focus, intensity and duration). The new diagnosis for female sexual arousal disorder might read: "failure to attain or maintain (sexual arousal) until the completion of sexual activity in a relationship judged by the clinician to be appropriate, mutual, and noncoercive." This revision would recognize that women may be coerced into nonmutual sexual relations over an extended time, such as by an abusive partner or relative (in the case of child abuse), and that lack of sexual arousal under such circumstances should not connote a sexual dysfunction.

Family History, Sexual History, and Psychological Status

The kind of intrapsychic issues that lead to anxiety over sexual arousal must be assessed by taking a careful family history and psychological history. This is primarily accomplished through interview, although standardized measures of psychological functioning may also be employed.

Assessment of any form of sexual abuse is crucial to treatment. In an individual interview, specific questions must be asked concerning sexual experiences during childhood and adult experiences of sexual coercion or rape. The best way to assess such experiences is to ask whether the woman has experienced any unwanted sexual acts (Becker, 1989). This is because many women will not define their experience as rape. Furthermore, a wide range of experiences may have coercive elements and thus have treatment implications—for example, acquiescing to sex with a drunken partner for fear his mood will turn ugly, or agreeing to act out pornographic scenes to avoid verbal harrassment. Because the base rates of abuse in our population are so high (Alter-Reid, Gibbs, Lachenmayer, Siegal, & Massoth, 1986), questions about sexual or physical abuse should never be omitted. Discovery that the client has survived abusive experiences will have implications for treatment, since the major goal of sex therapy then becomes helping the client regain control of her body and her sexuality (Becker, 1989).

Recommendations for a Clinical Assessment Protocol

1. The interview is the most important part of the protocol, because it provides an overview of the problem and suggests areas to be followed up with further assessment using other modalities. Specific guidelines have been presented for interview assessment of female sexual arousal disorder. However, it should be clear that the interview can supply information only from the client's subjective, retrospective experience. Because it is known that subjective measures of sexual arousal do not correlate well with physiological measures in women (Morokoff, 1988a), physiological measures or prospective attempts to assess subjective awareness of physiological response are important.

2. Psychophysiological measurement of sexual arousal would be an essential component of the protocol if it were possible to measure physiological arousal experienced during lovemaking with a partner. Because our current technology

does not allow this, psychophysiological assessment is not recommended for routine clinical use. The specific situations in which psychophysiological assessment should be used are discussed in detail under the heading "Clinical uses of psychophysiological assessment." These include documentation of women's sexual arousal when she believes herself not capable of arousal, determination of arousing fantasy themes, determination of amount of vaginal lubrication, and differential diagnosis of physiological versus psychogenic arousal dysfunction.

3. Assessment should include self-report measurement of the state of sexual arousal in response to specific sexual experiences. This area of assessment is seriously neglected in the treatment of arousal dysfunction. Many clinicians ask clients to keep records of sexual activities, but measurement of arousal is not typically attempted. It would be highly desirable to use scales such as those developed by Mosher et al. (1988) for women to rate arousal experienced during sexual activity at home during an assessment phase of treatment. It would also be good if comparable ratings were made at the end of treatment, to document the extent of treatment effectiveness.

4. Inventory measurement of sexual arousal across situations should be implemented. Use of a standardized inventory to assess women's experience of arousal would be extremely beneficial clinically, both to characterize the client before treatment and to document the effectiveness of treatment. Unfortunately, all the measures currently available have drawbacks. Single-item measures such as that developed by LoPiccolo and colleagues are not psychometrically sophisticated and lack normative data. The SAI crosses partners as well as situations and therefore may not be as clinically relevant as desired. The SII does not specifically assess sexual arousal. A new instrument is called for in this area. Ideally, it would tap a variety of arousing situations, as both the SAI and SII do. It would focus on a particular sexual relationship in such a way as to take advantage of partners' responses, as the SII does. Unlike either of these scales, it would differentiate the components of sexual arousal: global perception of sexual arousal, awareness of genital vasocongestion, and awareness of vaginal lubrication. It must again be emphasized that the lack of diagnosis and treatment of arousal disorder in women is in part due to lack of conceptualization and methods of measuring the response. If we are to make accurate differential diagnoses of arousal and orgasm disorders in women, we must have a way of determining the presence and level of arousal. The need for such an instrument presents an important challenge to the community of scientists and practitioners dealing with female sexual dysfunctions.

TREATMENT

Treatment of sexual arousal disorder in women has suffered from a lack of a constituent population, due to underdiagnosis. If there are few patients, there is very little incentive for clinicians to design and evaluate treatment programs. An extensive research literature deals with the treatment of orgasmic dysfunction in women, in contrast to virtually no outcome studies of treatment of female arousal disorder. In her review of the literature, Andersen (1983) reports 28 therapy outcome studies on women diagnosed with an orgasm dysfunction. It is undoubtedly the case that many of these women were misdiagnosed and should have received a diagnosis of arousal disorder. The high degree of success in treating these cases using directed masturbation suggests that if the diagnostic assumptions presented here are correct, masturbatory treatment is effective for both arousal and orgasmic disorders. Although the treatment literature on orgasmic dysfunction may be relevant to arousal disorders, it is more appropriately discussed in Chapter 9 (Inhibited Female Orgasm), so and will not be reviewed here.

Treatment of Sexual Arousal Disorder

Many directive sex therapy approaches for treatment of sexual dysfunction in women have been used to treat arousal disorder, including

Masters and Johnson's treatment program for orgasmic dysfunction (Masters & Johnson, 1970), LoPiccolo's program of masturbation training (LoPiccolo & Lobitz, 1972), and Kaplan's (1974) program for treatment of general sexual dysfunction. Kaplan (1979) presents a treatment program specifically designed for female sexual arousal disorder. This program utilizes the following steps (quoted from Kaplan, 1979, p. 47):

1. Sensate focus I—Taking turns at pleasuring or caressing each other's bodies without genital stimulation.
2. Sensate focus II—Taking turns at pleasuring each other's bodies with gentle, nondemanding genital stimulation which does not proceed to orgasm.
3. Slow, teasing genital stimulation by partner. The vulva, clitoris and vaginal entrance and the nipples are caressed. This is interrupted if the woman feels near orgasm, and then continued a little later, when arousal has diminished somewhat.
4. Coitus is withheld until the woman is well lubricated. To avoid frustration and to reduce pressure on the woman, the partner is advised to have extracoital orgasms during this phase of treatment.
5. Slow, teasing nondemanding intromission in the female superior position under her control, for the purpose of focusing on her vaginal sensations.

Kaplan exphasizes that the aim of this program is to reduce the anxiety that is evoked when arousal begins to develop, and that flexibility to accommodate the individual client's needs is important. Unfortunately, no outcome data have been reported on this program, or any program specifically designed to treat female sexual arousal disorder.

In my clinical experience it is also important to help women become self-focused and assertive with respect to sexuality. As previously discussed, it is virtually impossible to become aroused when one has sex exclusively on someone else's timetable. Women cannot both maintain the traditional (passive) feminine role and expect to become aroused during sex. It is possible to work on this issue very effectively in therapy by giving assignments to women to initiate homework sessions such as those in Kaplan's program, or to alternate with their partners in initiating sessions. As treatment progresses, an opportunity can usually be found to discuss with the couples the conceptualization presented above and to explain the importance of saying "no" when not in the mood. Nonrejecting strategies for turning down the partner can be discussed—e.g., saying, "I'm really too stressed out right now, but I'd like to try it tomorrow." Women and their partners may be given specific assignments to decline sexual invitations in order to gain experience with feeling that they are not at the partner's beck and call.

In a case recently treated in our psychology clinic, both husband and wife reported arousal difficulties. Although treatment gains were initially made, arousal was not consistent for either partner, and the husband had not been able to maintain an erection during intercourse. It began to emerge that both were extremely reluctant to say "no" to the other in sexual and nonsexual areas. We constructed an assignment for this couple in which each had to invite the other to participate in a set number of nonsexual activities in a given day, and the other was required to decline half of them. We then extended the assignment to sexual activities. As the couple began to do these assignments, they became very concerned about technicalities, suggesting that it had struck a nerve. Following completion of the assignments, the husband remembered and revealed to his wife an event that had angered him many years earlier. The next week he was able to maintain an erection and successfully have intercourse with her for the first time in seven years. The wife also became attuned to ways in which she felt her husband had let her down. These memories, along with sharing her sexual fantasies for the first time, enabled her to begin experiencing arousal with her husband. This case may illustrate how unwillingness to appropriately decline sexual activity may passively express anger and interfere with arousal. In women, role expectations to meet the sexual needs of the male partner make it even more difficult to give up this accommodation. It is my experience that when changes can be made in this feeling of being required to service the partner's sexual needs, significant improvements in arousal occur.

For women who have been sexually abused, control over sexual activity is of paramount importance. Maltz and Holman (1987) suggest establishing a ground rule that "the couple can engage in sex only when (the) survivor really wants to and initiates it" (p. 131). In our clinic we require that partners of sexual abuse survivors be able to accept this guideline as a precondition for couples therapy. For these couples, work on sexuality often must begin with such activities as handholding and nonsexual physical affection, rather than with sensate focus. Therapists also must play a less directive role than in traditional sex therapy, so that sexual experiences can be under the survivor's control.

Research

One outcome study stands out because a group of women who probably meet the diagnostic criteria for sexual arousal disorder were evaluated using pre-post measures of sexual arousal. Treatment of "sexually unresponsive" women was evaluated by Carney, Bancroft, and Mathews (1978). Thirty-two couples were assigned to one of four treatment cells. In half the couples, women were treated with testosterone, and half were treated with diazepam. Drug treatment was factorially crossed with number of therapy sessions: Half the couples received 16 sessions of weekly therapy, half 5 monthly sessions. The diagnosis of female sexual unresponsiveness was not defined. It is specified that the problem had to have been present for at least one year and that cases of vaginismus or in which orgasmic dysfunction was the only problem were excluded. Psychological treatment was a modified version of the Masters and Johnson approach involving a ban on intercourse and

instructions to reintroduce sexual activity in a prescribed, graded sequence.

This study was unusual in that sexual arousal was assessed pre- and posttreatment. Single-item measures of sexual arousal were utilized. Results indicated in general that the testosterone group did significantly better than the diazepam group. Superiority for the testosterone group was found in the assessor's rating of the couple's sexual relationship and the female partner's rating of "interest and arousal." The latter measure unfortunately confounds sexual desire and sexual arousal. The testosterone group was also superior on the female partner's self-ratings of vaginal lubrication (a measure of sexual arousal), frequency of orgasm, genital discomfort, and pleasant sexual feelings. Two measures related to sexual arousal that failed to show group differences were self-rating on the semantic differential of "easy to arouse sexually" and assessor's rating of enjoyment during lovemaking. Thus, although testosterone administration appeared to be generally successful in improving the sexual relationship, testosterone was superior to diazepam on some measures of arousal but not on others. This could be because both treatments were successful in improving these ratings. Unfortunately, the authors do not make statistical comparisons pre- and posttreatment, so we only know whether the treatment groups differed, not whether each treatment was effective in producing improvements on the various measures. Very few differences were found between groups receiving 5 monthly sessions as against 16 weekly sessions.

The need to evaluate treatment for sexual arousal disorder is clear. As this diagnostic category is used more often and better instruments are designed to measure it, the prospect of conducting outcome studies may become more appealing to investigators. Carney et al.'s (1978) investigation stands out as a study in which approximately this diagnostic group was treated and evaluated with measures assessing sexual arousal. It is also of interest in recognizing that inhibited sexual arousal may result from a suboptimal level of testosterone, from excessive anxiety, or from other psychological causes. More studies evaluating treatment issues such as these would aid our understanding of the factors contributing to sexual arousal disorders.

CONCLUSIONS

A dysfunction associated with the arousal phase of the female sexual response cycle was not originally proposed by Masters and Johnson (1970), and the concept has undergone significant revisions in the DSM-III and DSM-III-R. Female sexual arousal disorder is a diagnostic category that is far less utilized than inhibited female orgasm, despite the much greater prevalence of arousal difficulties than orgasm difficulties in a community sample of women (Frank, Anderson, & Rubinstein, 1978). It is suggested here that the reasons for these disparities lie in (1) cultural biases, (2) an inadequate conceptualization of sexual arousal in women and men, and (3) lack of valid and reliable assessment procedures based on this conceptualization. Cultural biases suggest that sexual arousal may not be all that important in women. Conceptual and assessment issues are based on a perhaps implicit assumption that what cannot be seen also cannot be understood or measured. In men, erection can be seen, understood, and measured, but if one wishes to assess sexual arousal in men as something more than only erection, the same conceptual problems arise as exist for women. It is vital that sex researchers and clinicians reach a conceptual agreement and develop appropriate assessment procedures.

A conceptualization of sexual arousal in women is presented here. It includes physiological reactions (the two primary ones being vasocongestion and vaginal lubrication) and subjective awareness of arousal, which can be subdivided into a global sense of excitement and awareness of the physiological changes. Mosher (1980) adds a third element, affective arousal. Subjective awareness of arousal can be conceptualized as a state (and thus evaluated with respect to a specific experience) or as a trait (present across situations). Trait mea-

sures are most clinically relevant when they are conceptualized not as a global trait, but rather a tendency within a particular relationship.

A number of issues urgently require research. Determination of the reliability and validity of existing measures of sexual arousal in women is needed. With respect to interview, researchers can determine the relationship between information obtained through interviewing the client and from other sources, such as partner interview, state measures of sexual arousal, and physiological indices. A cross-situational measure of sexual arousal is clearly needed. Existing instruments do not satisfy requirements for a psychometrically sound, clinically relevant measure of sexual arousal across situations. Further work on the reliability and validity of physiological measures of sexual arousal in women is also needed. It is important to determine the extent to which low correlations between subjective and physiological measures of sexual arousal reflect the discriminative validity of separate constructs rather than just women's lack of subjective awareness of their own physiological responses. A generally accepted measure of vaginal lubrication should be developed and normative data collected with pre- and postmenopausal women. Further development of measures of nocturnal vaginal or genital response will permit assessment of the physiological causes of inhibited arousal.

When we have reliable and valid measures of female sexual arousal, clinicians and researchers will feel confident in using them to make differential diagnoses between arousal and orgasmic dysfunctions. We will then be in a better position to determine the true incidence and prevalence of these disorders, both in the general population and in the population of women seeking treatment for sexual problems. When women are correctly diagnosed with sexual arousal disorder, the need for relevant treatments that are specific to arousal deficits will be clarified. Currently, sex therapy programs include assignments specifically designed to facilitate arousal, such as sensate focus. Intrapsychic and interpersonal issues that may impede arousal in many women have not been well characterized, however. Control over sexuality is proposed here as one such important issue. Women need to have control over when they have sex and over the type of sexual activities in which they engage. Since sex involves two people, these issues must be negotiated between partners. A one-sided resolution virtually assures impairment of arousal. Treatment outcome research on sexual arousal in women is lacking, again in part because clinicians and researchers have not agreed that arousal is important and furthermore do not have good instruments with which to measure it.

In order to provide the best possible treatment for sexual arousal disorder, clinicians need a clear idea of how women's psychobiological life stages, as well as illness and dysphoria, affect their capacity for sexual arousal. Much basic research is still needed in these areas. For example, the relationship between sexual arousal and well-being needs to be established. If well-being predicts sexual arousal as it does sexual desire, we need to know whether this accounts for differences in sexual arousal across the menstrual cycle. Similarly, the predictors of sexual arousal during pregnancy and postpartum have not been established. Because these experiences involve symptoms and discomfort, it is again relevant to determine the relationship of arousal to well-being during pregnancy and postpartum. Although much important research has been done on reproductive hormones and sexuality, the role of estrogen, progesterone, and androgens in female sexuality is far from completely understood.

Assessment and treatment of sexual arousal disorder in women has advanced remarkably in the past 30 years. The state of knowledge discussed here makes it clear there is still a long way to go. A focus on sexual arousal, within the contexts of culture, psychobiological life stages, and interpersonal relationships, will aid in a more complete understanding of sexuality in women's lives. A focus on sexual arousal as an important part of the sexual response cycle will provide the opportunity for more accurate diagnosis and better treatment.

REFERENCES

Abel, G. G., Murphy, W. E., Becker, J. V., & Bitar, A. (1979). Women's vaginal responses during REM sleep. *Journal of Sex and Marital Therapy, 1,* 5–14.

Abramson, P. R., Perry, L. B., Seeley, T. T., Seeley, D. M., & Rothblatt, A. B. (1981). Thermographic measurement of sexual arousal: A discriminant validity analysis. *Archives of Sexual Behavior, 10,* 171–176.

Alter-Reid, K., Gibbs, M. S., Lachenmayer, J. R., Siegal, J., & Massoth, N. A. (1986). Sexual abuse of children: A review of empirical findings. *Clinical Psychology Review, 6,* 249–266.

American Psychiatric Association (1980). *Diagnostic and statistical manual of mental disorders* (3rd ed.). Washington, DC: Author.

American Psychiatric Association (1987). *Diagnostic and statistical manual of mental disorders* (3rd ed., rev.). Washington, DC: Author.

Andersen, B. L. (1983). Primary orgasmic dysfunction: Diagnostic considerations and review of treatment. *Psychological Bulletin, 93,* 105–136.

Annon, J. S. (1973). The therapeutic use of masturbation in the treatment of sexual disorders. In R. D. Rubin, J. P. Brady, & J. D. Henderson (Eds.), *Advances in behavior therapy* (Vol. 4). New York: Academic Press.

Armon, H., Weinman, J., & Weinstein, D. (1978). A vaginal photoplethysmographic transducer. *IEEE Transactions on Biomedical Engineering, 25,* 434–440.

Baird, D. T., McNeilly, A. S., Sawers, R. S., & Sharpe, R. M. (1979). Failure of estrogen-induced discharge of luteinizing hormone in lactating women. *Journal of Clinical Endocrinology and Metabolism, 49,* 500–506.

Bancroft, J. (1984). Hormones and human sexual behavior. *Journal of Sex and Marital Therapy, 10,* 3–21.

Bancroft, J. (1987). Hormones, sexuality and fertility in humans. *Journal of Zoology, 213,* 445–461.

Bancroft, J., & Coles, L. (1976). Three years' experience in a sexual problems clinic. *British Medical Journal, 1,* 1575–1577.

Bancroft, J., Sanders, D., Davidson, D., & Warner, P. (1983). Mood, sexuality, hormones and the menstrual cycle: III. Sexuality and the role of androgens. *Psychosomatic Medicine, 45,* 509.

Barlow, D. H. (1986). Causes of sexual dysfunction: The role of anxiety and cognitive interference.

Journal of Consulting and Clinical Psychology,
54, 140–148.

Barlow, D. H., Sakheim, D. K., & Beck, J. G. (1983).
Anxiety increases sexual arousal. *Journal of Abnormal Psychology, 92,* 49–54.

Becker, J. V. (1989). Impact of sexual abuse on sexual functioning. In S. R. Leiblum & R. C. Rosen
(Eds.), *Principles and practice of sex therapy: Update for the 1990s.* New York: Guilford.

Becker, J. V., Skinner, L., Abel, G., & Treacy, E.
(1982). Incidence and types of sexual dysfunctions
in rape and incest victims. *Journal of Sex and
Marital Therapy, 8,* 65–74.

Beggs, V. E., Calhoun, K. S., & Wolchik, S. A.
(1987). Sexual anxiety and female sexual arousal:
A comparison of arousal during sexual anxiety
stimuli and sexual pleasure stimuli. *Archives of
Sexual Behavior, 16,* 311–319.

Benoit, H. J., Borth, R., & Woolever, C. A. (1980).
Self-stabilizing system for measuring infrared light
backscattered from vaginal tissues. *Medical and
Biological Engineering and Computing, 18,* 265–
270.

Bottiglioni, F., & DeAloysio, D. (1982). Female sexual activity as a function of climacteric conditions
and age. *Maturitas, 4,* 27–32.

Bretschneider, J. G., & McCoy, N. L. (1988). Sexual
interest and behavior in healthy 80- to 102-year-olds. *Archives of Sexual Behavior, 17,* 109–129.

Briere, J. (1984). *The effects of childhood sexual
abuse on later psychological functioning: Defining
a post-sexual abuse syndrome.* Paper presented at
the Third National Conference on Sexual Victimization of Children, Children's Hospital National
Medical Center, Washington, DC.

Carney, A., Bancroft, J., & Mathews, A. (1978).
Combination of hormonal and pscyhological treatment for female sexual unresponsiveness: A comparative study. *British Journal of Psychiatry, 132,*
339–346.

Catania, J. A., Gibson, D. R., Chitwood, D. D., &
Coates, T. J. (1990). Methodological problems in
AIDS behavioral research: Influences on measurement error and participation bias in studies of sexual behavior. *Psychological Bulletin, 108,* 339–
362.

Chambless, D. L., & Lifshitz, J. L. (1984). Self-reported sexual anxiety and arousal: The expanded sexual arousability inventory. *Journal of
Sex Research, 20,* 241–254.

Chasseguet-Smirgel, J. (1970). Feminine guilt and the
oedipus complex. In J. Chasseguet-Smirgel (Ed.),

Female sexuality. Ann Arbor: University of
Michigan Press.

Chodorow, N. (1978). *The reproduction of mothering.* Los Angeles: University of California Press.

Clark, A., & Wallin, P. (1964). The accuracy of husbands' and wives' reports of the frequency of marital coitus. *Population Studies, 18,* 165–173.

Coates, R., Calzavara, L., Soskolne, C., Read, S.,
Fanning, M., Shepherd, F., Klein, M., & Johnson,
J. (1988). Validity of sexual contacts of men with
AIDS or an AIDS-related condition. *American
Journal of Epidemiology, 128,* 719–728.

Cohen, H. D., & Shapiro. A. (1970). *A method for
measuring sexual arousal in the female.* Paper
presented at the Society for Psychophysiological
Research, New Orleans.

Cowan, G., Lee, C., Levy, D., & Snyder, D. (1988).
Dominance and inequality in X-rated videocassettes. *Psychology of Women Quarterly, 12,* 199–
311.

Cutler, W. B., Garcia, C. R., & McCoy, N. (1987).
Perimenopausal sexuality. *Archives of Sexual Behavior, 16,* 225–234.

Dennerstein, L., Burrows, G. D., Wood, C., & Hyman, G. (1980). Hormones and sexuality: The effects of estrogen and progestogen. *Obstetrics and
Gynecology, 56,* 316–322.

Englander-Golden, P., Chang, H. S., Whitmore,
M. R., & Dienstbier, R. A. (1980). Female sexual
arousal and the menstrual cycle. *Journal of Human Stress, 6,* 42–48.

Falicov, C. J. (1973). Sexual adjustment during first
pregnancy and post partum. *American Journal of
Obstetrics and Gynecology, 117,* 991–1000.

Fava, G. A., Fava, M., Kellner, R., Buckman, M. T.,
Lisansky, J., Serafini, E., DeBesi, L., & Mastrogiacomo, I. (1983). Psychosomatic aspects of hyperprolactinemia. *Psychotherapy and Psychosomatics, 40,* 257–262.

Finkelhor, D. (1979a). What's wrong with sex between adults and children: Ethics and the problem
of sexual abuse. *American Journal of Orthopsychiatry, 49,* 694–695.

Finkelhor, D. (1979b). *Sexually victimized children.*
New York: Free Press.

Fischer, C., Cohen, H.,, Schiavi, R., David, D., Furman, B., Ward, K., Edwards, A., & Cunningham,
J. (1983). Patterns of female sexual arousal during
sleep and waking: Vaginal thermoconductance
studies. *Archives of Sexual Behavior, 12,* 97–122.

Frank, E., Anderson, C., & Kupfer, D. J. (1976).
Profiles of couples seeking sex therapy and marital

therapy. *American Journal of Psychiatry, 133,* 559–562.

Frank, E., Anderson, C., & Rubinstein, D. (1978). Frequency of sexual dysfunction in "normal" couples. *New England Journal of Medicine, 299,* 111–115.

Gallant, S. J., Hamilton, J. A., Popiel, D. A., Morokoff, P. J., & Chakraborty, P. K. (1991). Daily moods and symptoms: Effects of awareness of study focus, gender, menstrual cycle phase, and day of the week. *Health Psychology, 10.*

Geer, J. H., Morokoff, P. J., & Greenwood, P. (1974). Sexual arousal in women: The development of a measurement device for vaginal blood volume. *Archives of Sexual Behavior, 3,* 559–564.

Gillan, P., & Brindley, G. S. (1979). Vaginal and pelvic floor responses to sexual stimulation. *Psychophysiology, 16,* 471–481.

Gordy, P. (1983). Group work that supports victims of childhood incest. *Social Casework, 64,* 300–307.

Green, S. E., & Mosher, D. L. (1985). A causal model of sexual arousal to erotic fantasies. *Journal of Sex Research, 21,* 1–23.

Greenblatt, R. B., Oettinger, M., & Bohler, C. S. (1976). Estrogen-androgen levels in aging men and women: Therapeutic considerations. *Journal of the American Geriatric Society, 24,* 173–178.

Hallstrom, T. (1977). Sexuality in the climacteric. *Clinics in Obstetrics and Gynecology, 4,* 227–239.

Heiman, J. R. (1977). A psychophysiological exploration of sexual arousal patterns in females and males. *Psychophysiology, 14,* 266–274.

Heiman, J. R. (1980). Female sexual response patterns: Interactions of physiological, affective, and contextual cues. *Archives of General Psychiatry, 37,* 1311–1316.

Heiman, J. R., & Rowland, D. L. (1983). Affective and physiological sexual response patterns: The effects of instructions on sexually functional and dysfunctional men. *Journal of Psychosomatic Research, 27,* 105–116.

Henson, D. E., & Rubin, H. B. (1978). A comparison of two objective measures of sexual arousal of women. *Behaviour Research and Therapy, 16,* 143–151.

Henson, D. E., Rubin, H. B., & Henson, C. (1978). Consistency of the labial temperature change measure of human female eroticism. *Behaviour Research and Therapy, 16,* 125–129.

Henson, D. E., Rubin, H. B., & Henson, C. (1979). Analysis of the consistency of objective measures of sexual arousal in women. *Journal of Applied Behavior Analysis, 12,* 701–711.

Henson, D. E., Rubin, H. B., Henson, C., & Williams, J. (1977). Temperature changes of the labia minora as an objective measure of human female eroticism. *Journal of Behavior Therapy and Experimental Psychiatry, 8,* 401–410.

Hoon, E. F. (1978). *The expanded sexual arousability inventory.* Available from the author, Box j-165, JHMHC, University of Florida, Gainesville, FL 32610.

Hoon, E. F., Hoon, P. W., & Wincze, J. P. (1976). An inventory for the measurement of female sexual arousability: The SAI. *Archives of Sexual Behavior, 5,* 291–300.

Hoon, P. W., Bruce, K., & Kinchloe, G. (1982). Does the menstrual cycle affect erotic arousal? *Psychophysiology, 19,* 21.

Hoon, P. W., Wincze, J. P., & Hoon, E. F. (1976). Physiological assessment of sexual arousal in women. *Psychophysiology, 13,* 196–204.

Hoon, P. W., Wincze, J. P., & Hoon, E. F. (1977). A test of reciprocal inhibition: Are anxiety and sexual arousal in women mutually inhibitory? *Journal of Abnormal Psychology, 86,* 65–74.

Jacobson, N., & Moore, D. (1981). Spouses as observers of the events in their relationship. *Journal of Consulting and Clinical Psychology, 49,* 269–277.

Javanovic, V. J. (1971). The recording of physiological evidence of genital arousal in the human males and females. *Archives of Sexual Behavior, 1,* 309–320.

Jehu, D. (1988). *Beyond sexual abuse: Therapy with women who were childhood victims.* New York: Wiley.

Jevitch, M. J. (1983). Vascular noninvasive diagnostic techniques. In R. J. Krane, M. B. Siroky, & I. Goldstein (Eds.), *Male sexual dysfunction.* Boston: Little, Brown.

Judd, H. L. (1976). Hormonal dynamics associated with the menopause. *Clinical Obstetrics and Gynecology, 19,* 775–788.

Judd, H. L., & Yen, S. S. C. (1973). Serum androstenedione and testosterone levels during the menstrual cycle. *Journal of Clinical Endocrinology and Metabolism, 36,* 475.

Kaplan, H. S. (1974). *The new sex therapy.* New York: Brunner/Mazel.

Kaplan, H. S. (1979). *Disorders of sexual desire and other new concepts and techniques in sex therapy.* New York: Simon and Schuster.

Kaplan, H. S. (1983). *Evaluation of sexual disorders*. New York: Brunner/Mazel.

Kaplan, H. S. (1989). *How to overcome premature ejaculation*. New York: Brunner/Mazel.

Karacan, I., Rosenbloom, A., & Williams, R. (1970). The clitoral erection cycle during sleep. *Psychophysiology, 7*, 33.

Kelley, L. (1988). *Surviving sexual violence*. Minneapolis: University of Minnesota Press.

Kenney, J. A. (1973). Sexuality of pregnant and breastfeeding women. *Archives of Sexual Behavior, 2*, 215–229.

Kinsey, A. C., Pomeroy, W. B., Martin, C. E., & Gebhard, P. H. (1953). *Sexual behavior in the human female*. Philadelphia: Saunders.

Koppelman, M. C. S., Parry, B. L., Hamilton, J. A., & Alagna, S. W. (1985). *Libido and affect in hyperprolactinemic women: Effect of bromocriptine (BCPT)*. Paper presented at the meeting of the Endocrine Society.

Korff, J., & Geer, J. H. (1983). The relationship between sexual arousal experience and genital response. *Psychophysiology, 20*, 121–127.

Kumar, R., Brandt, H. A., & Robson, K. M. (1981). Childbearing and maternal sexuality: A prospective survey of 119 primiparae. *Journal of Psychosomatic Research, 25*, 373–383.

Lerner, H. G. (1988). *Women in therapy*. Northvale, NJ: Jason Aronson.

Levin, R. J., & S. Wagner, G. (1977). Haemodynamic changes of the human vagina during sexual arousal assessed by a heated oxygen electrode. *Journal of Physiology, 275*, 23P–24P.

Levine, S. B., & Yost, M. A. (1976). Frequency of sexual dysfunction in a general gynecological clinic: An epidemiological approach. *Archives of Sexual behavior, 5*, 229–238.

Lobotsky, J., Wyss, H. I., Segre, E. J., & Lloyd, C. W. (1964). Plasm testosterone in the normal woman. *Journal of Clinical Endocrinalogy, 24*, 1261–1265.

LoPiccolo, J., & Lobitz, W. C. (1972). The role of masturbation in the treatment of orgasmic dysfunction. *Archives of Sexual Behavior, 2*, 163–171.

LoPiccolo, J., & Steger, J. C. (1974). The Sexual Interaction Inventory: A new instrument for assessment of sexual dysfunction. *Archives of Sexual Behavior, 3*, 585–595.

Malinosky-Rummell, R. R., & Hoier, T. S. (1991). Validating measures of dissociation in sexually abused and nonabused children. *Behavioral Assessment, 13*, 341–357.

Maltz, W., & Holman, B. (1987). *Incest and sexuality*. Lexington, MA: Lexington Books.

Masters, W. H., & Johnson, V. E. (1966). *Human sexual response*. Boston: Little, Brown.

Masters, W. H., & Johnson, V. E. (1970). *Human sexual inadequacy*. New York: Little, Brown.

Mastrogiacomo, I., DeBesi, L., Serafini, E., Zussa, S., Zucchetta, P., Romagnoli, G. F., Saporiti, E., Dean, P., Ronco, C., & Adami, A. (1984). Hyperprolactinemia and sexual disturbances among uremic women on hemodialysis. *Nephron, 37*, 195–199.

McCoy, N., & Davidson, J. M. (1985). A longitudinal study of the effects of menopause on sexuality. *Maturitas, 7*, 203–210.

Meiselman, K. (1978). *Incest: A psychological study of causes and effects with treatment recommendations*. San Francisco: Jossey-Bass.

Meuwissen, I., & Over, R. (1991). Multidimensionality of the content of female sexual fantasy. *Behavioral Research and Therapy, 29*, 179–181.

Morokoff, P. J. (1978). Determinants of female orgasm. In J. LoPiccolo & L. LoPiccolo (Eds.), *Handbook of sex therapy*. New York: Plenum Press.

Morokoff, P. J. (1981). Female sexual arousal as a function of individual differences and exposure to erotic stimuli. *Dissertation Abstracts International, 41*, 4270-B (University Microfilms No. 8109039).

Morokoff, P. J. (1985). Effects of sex guilt, repression, sexual "arousability," and sex experience on female sexual arousal during erotica and fantasy. *Journal of Personality and Social Psychology, 49*, 177–187.

Morokoff, P. J. (1988a). Self-awareness of sexual arousal in women. In D. Smith (Chair), *Two different worlds: Women, men and emotion*. Symposium presented at the annual meeting of the American Psychological Association, Atlanta, GA.

Morokoff, P. J. (1988b). Sexuality in perimenopausal and postmenopausal women. *Psychology of Women Quarterly, 12*, 489–511.

Morokoff, P. J. (1989). Sex bias and POD. *American Psychologist, 44*, 73–75.

Morokoff, P. J. (1990). Women's sexuality: Expression of self versus social construction. In C. B. Travis (Chair), *The social construction of women's sexuality*. Symposium presented at the annual meeting of the American Psychological Association, Boston.

Morokoff, P. J., & Heiman, J. R. (1980). Effects of erotic stimuli on sexually functional and dysfunctional women: Multiple measures before and after sex therapy. *Behaviour Research and Therapy, 18,* 127–137.

Morokoff, P. J., & LoPiccolo, J. (1986). A comparative evaluation of minimal therapist contact and 15-session treatment for female orgasmic dysfunction. *Journal of Consulting and Clinical Psychology, 54,* 294–300.

Morrell, M. J., Dixen, J. M., Carter, C. S., & Davidson, J. M. (1984). The influence of age and cycling status on sexual arousability in women. *American Journal of Obstetrics and Gynecology, 148,* 66–71.

Mosher, D. L. (1966). The development and multitrait-multimethod matrix analysis of three measures of three aspects of guilt. *Journal of Consulting Psychology, 30,* 25–29.

Mosher, D. L. (1973). Sex differences, sex experience, sex guilt, and explicitly sexual films. *Journal of Social Issues, 29,* 95–112.

Mosher, D. L. (1979). The meaning and measurement of guilt. In C. E. Izard (Ed.), *Emotions in personality and psychopathology* (pp. 105–129). New York: Plenum.

Mosher, D. L. (1980). Three dimensions of depth of involvement in human sexual response. *Journal of Sex Research, 16,* 1–42.

Mosher, D. L., & Abramson, P. R. (1977). Subjective sexual arousal to films of masturbation. *Journal of Consulting and Clinical Psychology, 45,* 796–807.

Mosher, D. L., Barton-Henry, M., & Green, S. E. (1988). Subjective sexual arousal and involvement: Development of multiple indicators. *Journal of Sex Research, 25,* 412–425.

Mosher, D. L., & Greenberg, I. (1969). Females' affective responses to reading erotic literature. *Journal of Consulting and Clinical Psychology, 33,* 472–477.

Mosher, D. L., & O'Grady, K. E. (1975). Sex guilt, trait anxiety, and females' subjective sexual arousal to erotica. *Motivation and Emotion, 3,* 235–249.

Mosher, D. L., & White, B. B. (1980). Effects of committed or casual erotic guided imagery on females' subjective sexual arousal and emotional response. *Journal of Sex Research, 16,* 273–299.

Myers, L., & Morokoff, P. J. (1986). Physiological and subjective sexual arousal in pre- and postmenopausal women and postmenopausal women taking replacement therapy. *Psychophysiology, 23,* 283–292.

Noel, G. L., Suh, H. K., & Frantz, A. G. (1974). Prolactin release during nursing and breast stimulation in postpartum and non postpartum subjects. *Journal of Clinical Endocrinology and Metabolism, 38,* 413–423.

Nowinski, J. K., & LoPiccolo, J. (1979). Assessing sexual behavior in couples. *Journal of Sex and Marital Therapy, 5,* 225–241.

Palace, E. M., & Gorzalka, B. B. (1990). The enhancing effects of anxiety on arousal in sexually dysfunctional and functional women. *Journal of Abnormal Psychology, 99,* 403–411.

Perez, A., Vela, P., Masnick, G. S., & Potter, R. G. (1972). First ovulation after childbirth: The effect of breast-feeding. *American Journal of Obstetrics and Gynecology, 114,* 1041.

Persky, H., Charney, N., Lief, H. I., O'Brien, C. P., Miller, W. R. & Strauss, D. (1978). The relationship of plasma estradiol level to sexual behavior in young women. *Psychosomatic Medicine, 40,* 523–535.

Persky, H., Dreisback, L., Miller, W., O'Brien, C., Khan, M., Lief, H., Charney, N., & Strauss, D. (1982). The relation of plasma androgen levels to sexual behaviors and attitudes of women. *Psychosomatic Medicine, 44,* 305–319.

Pertot, S. (1981). Postpartum loss of sexual desire and enjoyment. *Australian Journal of Psychology, 33,* 11–18.

Pfeiffer, E., Verwoerdt, A., & Davis, G. (1972). Sexual behavior in middle life. *American Journal of Psychiatry, 128,* 1262–1267.

Pfeiffer, E., Verwoerdt, A., & Wang, H. S. (1968). Sexual behavior in aged men and women. I: Observations on 254 community volunteers. *Archives of General Psychiatry, 19,* 753–758.

Popeil, D. A., Alagna, S. W., & Morokoff, P. J. (1988, March). *The effects of mood on sexual functioning.* Paper presented at the meeting of the Association for Women in Psychology, Bethesda, MD.

Preti, G., Huggins, G. R., & Silverberg, G. D. (1979). Alterations in the organic compounds of vaginal secretions caused by sexual arousal. *Fertility and Sterility, 32,* 47–54.

Putnam, F. W., Guroff, J. J., Silberman, E. K., Barban, L., & Post, R. M. (1986). The clinical phenomenology of multiple personality disorder: A review of 100 recent cases. *Journal of Clinical Psychiatry, 47,* 285–293.

Rolland, R., Lequin, R. M., Schellekens, L. A., & De Jong, F. H. (1975). The role of prolactin in the restoration of ovarian function during the early post-partum period in the human female. *Clinical Endocrinology, 4,* 15–25.

Rogers, G. S., Van de Castle, R. L., Evans, W. S., & Critelli, J. W. (1985). Vaginal pulse amplitude response patterns during erotic conditions and sleep. *Archives of Sexual Behavior, 14.*

Rosen, R. C., & Beck, J. G. (1988). *Patterns of sexual arousal: Psychophysiological processes and clinical applications.* New York: Guilford.

Sanders, B., McRoberts, G., & Tollefson, C. (1989).Childhood stress and dissociation in a college population. *Dissociation, 2,* 17–23.

Sanders, D., Warner, P., Backstrom, T., & Bancroft, J. (1983). Mood, sexuality, hormones and the menstrual cycle. I. Changes in mood and physical state: Description of subjects and method. *Psychosomatic Medicine, 45,* 487–502.

Schmidt, G. (1975). Male-female differences in sexual arousal and behavior during and after exposure to sexually explicit stimuli. *Archives of Sexual Behavior, 4,* 353–365.

Schover, L. R., Evans, R. B., & von Eschenbach, A. C. (1987). Sexual rehabilitation in a cancer center: Diagnosis and outcome in 384 consultations. *Archives of Sexual Behavior, 16,* 445–461.

Schover, L. R., Friedman, J. M., Weiler, S. J., Heiman, J. R., & LoPiccolo, J. (1982). Multiaxial problem-oriented system for sexual dysfunctions: An alternative to DSM-III. *Archives of General Psychiatry, 39,* 614–619.

Schreiner-Engel, P., Schiavi, R. C., Smith, H., & White, D. (1981). Sexual arousability and the menstrual cycle. *Psychosomatic Medicine, 43,* 199–214.

Semlow, J. L., & Lubowsky, J. (1983). Sexual instrumentation. *IEEE Transactions on Biomedical Engineering, 30,* 309–319.

Semmens, J. P., & Wagner, G. (1982). Estrogen deprivation and vaginal function in postmenopausal women. *Journal of the American Medical Association, 248,* 445–446.

Shapiro, A., Cohen, H. D., DiBianco, P., & Rosen, G. (1968). Vaginal blood flow changes during sleep and sexual arousal. *Psychophysiology, 4,* 394 (abstract).

Sherfey, M. J. (1973). *The nature and evolution of female sexuality.* New York: Vintage.

Sherwin, B., & Gelfand, M. (1987). The role of androgen in the maintenance of sexual functioning in oophorectomized women. *Psychosomatic Medicine, 9,* 297–409.

Sherwin, B., Gelfand, M., & Brenner, W. (1985). Androgen enhances sexual motivation in females: A prospective, crossover study of sex steroid administration in the surgical menopause. *Psychosomatic Medicine, 47,* 339–351.

Sintchak, G., & Geer, J. H. (1975). A vaginal plethysmograph system. *Psychophysiology, 12,* 113–115.

Spector, I. P., & Carey, M. P. (1990). Incidence and prevalence of the sexual dysfunctions: A critical review of the empirical literature. *Archives of Sexual Behavior, 19,* 389–408.

Stoller, R. J. (1979). *Sexual excitement: Dynamics of erotic life.* Washington, DC: American Psychiatric Press.

Stoller, R. J. (1985). *Observing the erotic imagination.* New Haven, CT: Yale University Press.

Tsai, M., Feldman-Summers, S., & Edgar, M. (1979). Childhood molestation: Variables related to differential impacts on psychosexual functioning in adult women. *Journal of Abnormal Psychology, 88,* 407–417.

Tyson, J. E., Hwang, P., Guyda, H., Friesen, H. G. (1972). Studies of prolactin secretion in human pregnancy. *American Journal of Obstetrics and Gynecology, 113,* 14–20.

Vasquez, J. M., Samaras, C. A., & Nezhat, C. (1982). Endocrine studies in postmenopausal women during oral replacement therapy with unconjugated estrogens. *Reproduction, 6,* 49–59.

Vermeulen, A., & Verdonck, L. (1976). Plasma androgen levels during the menstrual cycle. *American Journal of Obstetrics and Gynecology, 125,* 491–494.

Wagner, G., & Green, R. (1981). *Impotence: Physiological, psychological, and surgical diagnosis and treatment.* New York: Plenum.

Wagner, G., & Levin, R. J. (1977). Human vaginal fluid, pH, urea, potassium and potential difference during sexual excitement. In R. Gemme & C. C. Wheelen (Eds.), *Progress in sexology.* New York: Plenum.

Wagner, G., & Levin, R. J. (1978). Oxygen tension of the vaginal surface during sexual stimulation in the human. *Fertility and Sterility, 30,* 50–53.

Wakefield, J. C. (1987). Sex bias in the diagnosis of primary orgasmic dysfunction. *American Psychologist, 42,* 464–471.

Weinman, J. (1967). Photoplethysmography. In P. Venables & I. Martin (Eds.), *A manual of psycho-*

physiological methods (pp. 283–306). New York: Wiley.

Weiss, H. D. (1972). The physiology of human erection. *Annals of Internal Medicine, 76,* 793–799.

Weizman, R., Weizman, A., Levi, J., Gura, V., Zevin, D., Maoz, B., Wijsenbeek, H., & David, M. B. (1983). Sexual dysfunction associated with hyperprolactinemia in males and females undergoing hemodialysis. *Psychosomatic Medicine, 45,* 259–269.

Wincze, J. P., Hoon, E. F., & Hoon, P. W. (1977). Sexual arousal in women: A comparison of cognitive and physiological responses by continuous measurement. *Archives of Sexual Behavior, 6,* 121–133

Wolchik, S. A., Beggs, V. E., Wincze, J. P., Sakheim, D. K., Barlow, D. H., & Mavissakalian, M. (1980). The effects of emotional arousal on subsequent sexual arousal in men. *Journal of Abnormal Psychology, 89,* 595–598.

CHAPTER 7

MALE ERECTILE DISORDER

Walter Everaerd, University of Amsterdam

DEFINITION AND DESCRIPTION OF MALE ERECTILE DISORDER

Male erectile disorder (MED) is defined in the DSM-III-R as either "(1) persistent or recurrent partial or complete failure in a male to attain or maintain erection until completion of the sexual activity, or (2) persistent or recurrent lack of a subjective sense of sexual excitement and pleasure in a male during sexual activity" (American Psychiatric Association, 1987, p. 294). The psychophysiological changes and the subjective experience that accompany sexual arousal have been specified in these criteria. In other definitions a behavioral criterion is added to the psychophysiological changes; instead of "completion of the sexual activity," the normative "sufficient for vaginal penetration" is used (Mohr and Beutler, 1990). The usage of the terms *impotence* and *frigidity* in ICD (International Classification of Diseases) classifications also makes reference to penetration or intercourse. Frigidity is the dislike of or aversion to intercourse. Impotence is the sustained inability (due to psychological causes) to maintain an erection that will allow normal heterosexual penetration and ejaculation to take place (APA, 1987).

The use of both *erectile disorder* and *impotence* (some authors use these terms interchangeably) points to some disagreements about the definition of sexual response—in particular, about the definition of erectile problems. It seems that *erectile disorder* is used, as in the DSM-III-R, when subjective experience is included in the criterion. The term *impotence* is preferred when the emphasis is given to physiological manifestations. This distinction becomes clear when browsing the urological literature. One reason for this disagreement may be different views of the principal function of sex.

Historically, the view that sex is reproductive behavior has dominated sexology. In recent decades the concept that the function of sex is recreational has been added to the reproductive view. As a consequence, the behavioral criterion of sexual performance (penetration) has been complemented with experiential and emotional criteria. Psychophysiological studies of sexual response time have been using physiological indices of sexual arousal as a crucial operationalization. However, more recent studies have made clear that subjective experience should be given a more important —perhaps even central—position in the definition of sexual response:

> Although the physiological substrate is clearly more amenable to empirical definition and measurement than are subjective components of arousal, it is clear that genital engorgement (or other autonomic changes) should not be viewed as necessary or sufficient in defining sexual response. Numerous instances have been presented in which sexual arousal may be experienced without genital responding, and vice versa (Rosen & Beck, 1988, p. 334).

In cases of erectile problems, it may also be the suffering males themselves who contribute to a more instrumental (performance-oriented) approach to the definition of sexual response.

The debate on the definition of sexual problems, especially erectile problems, is intertwined with discussions about the common causes of these disorders. In recent years important advances have been made in the assessment, and in many instances also the treatment, of the anatomical and physiological substrate of sexual response. Multiple causation of erectile disorders has lead some authors to classify the disorders according to presumed main causes, instead of the phenomenon-based description of response inhibition that has been used in the DSM-III-R. Krane, Goldstein, and Saenz de Tejada (1989) recently presented a typology based on pathophysiological mechanisms. These authors describe six types of impotence: neurogenic, endocrinologic, psychogenic, vasculogenic, drug-induced, and diabetic. Drug-induced and diabetic impotence are thought to be a consequence of neurovascular and neuroendocrine mechanisms.

The increase in knowledge of physiological mechanisms has resulted in more frequent diagnosis of biogenic causes for erectile problems (Bancroft, 1989). It also has brought a swing in the pendulum: For some time, psychological causes were favored, but now the scale leans towards the biogenic point of view. The debate is not settled, however. There is a growing awareness that sexual problems result from a complicated interplay of the anatomical and physiological substrate, psychophysiological and specifically cognitive processes, and cultural factors.

The consensus reached in the DSM-III-R specifies that defects in the anatomical and physiological substrate due to organic factors, such as a physical disorder or medication, cannot lead to a diagnosis of sexual dysfunction such as erectile disorder. Likewise, a distinction is made for the psychogenic component in the etiology of the disorder. The presence of another Axis I mental disorder, such as major depression, precludes the diagnosis of sexual dysfunction. In clinical practice, these distinctions are not made very easily. Inhibition of emotional and motivational processes (appetite) and psychophysiological changes may be attributed to psychological causes, but also to causes that result from the interaction of psychological and organic processes. In the section of the chapter on methods of assessment, this point will be elaborated.

Browsing through the literature on erectile disorders, one easily gets confused by differences in the description and definition of the disorders. The phenomenon-based definition, as it appears in the DSM-III-R, seems to meet the needs of those who do not adhere to a normative or strictly functional point of view on sexual response. When subjective experience is brought into the picture, it is left to the individual to qualify the function of sexual responding. This view is at odds with, for example, the view that sex is reproductive behavior. The situation is further complicated by the different perspectives on MED that arise from different referrals and professional interests. An endocrinologist with an interest in male fertility disorders will thus differ from a psychologist with an interest in relationship or family disorders. In this chapter I will use the perspective that is provided by the consensus as described in the DSM-III-R.

PSYCHOPATHOLOGY

Incidence and Prevalence

According to the DSM-III-R, studies in Europe and the United States indicate that in the young adult population, approximately 8% of the males have MED. Recently, Spector and Carey (1990) estimated erectile difficulty prevalence rates to be between 3% and 9%. The exact prevalence and incidence of erectile disorders is not known; there is a scarcity of data on this point. Erectile disorders are age-dependent, with an incidence of 1.9% at 40 years of age and 25% at 65 years of age (Krane et al., 1989). The prevalence is higher in certain groups of patients, such as those with diabetes, cardiovascular disorders, and chronic renal failure. In these groups, erectile disorders are estimated to be in the range of 50–60% (Segraves & Schoenberg, 1985). Krane et al. (1989) provide an estimate of 10 million men with erectile disorder in the United States. This accounts for more than 400,000 visits to physicians and more than 30,000 hospital admissions, resulting in a total cost of $146 million.

Associated Features

Numerous features are often, but not invariably, present in MED. As a further complication, it is unknown what percentage of men with erectile disorder seek to alleviate their problems. We do not know the ways in which men suffer from their erectile failure. Those who present their disorder generally are anxious, sometimes depressed, or guilty and ashamed. Most feel frustrated and helpless when confronted with erectile failure. Almost invariably, a fear of failure and self-monitoring ("spectating") has developed. Most men are very sensitive to the reactions in their social environment, especially to the reactions of the partner (Barlow, 1986). The previous section mentioned a higher prevalence for men with chronic diseases. Without being the specific (biological) cause of sexual disorders, the co-existence of chronic disease often seems to contribute to the deterioration of the relationship and sexual functioning. This is also true for other chronic conditions such as the use of medication, infertility, and the major mental disorders (e.g., schizophrenia and alcoholism). For an excellent review of sexual disorders co-existing with problems resulting from chronic illness, the reader is referred to Schover and Jensen (1988).

There is some evidence that the extent of suffering from erectile disorders is associated with hypermasculine sex-role definitions, especially in men with psychogenic erectile failure (Derogatis, 1976). However, there is no evidence that specific sex roles predispose males to sexual dysfunction.

Course and Subtypes

Erectile disorders may be subdivided into several forms according to aspects of development in time, the frequency and kind of sexual experience, and the causes of the disorder. The subdivision of erectile disorders has often been attempted retrospectively, after some form of therapy, in order to obtain prognostic indicators. An important focus of these studies has been the discrimination between biogenic and psychogenic failure (Hengeveld, 1986). The acute onset of the disorder was supposed to be a consequence of a psychogenic causes, whereas a gradual onset was attributed to biogenic causes. Advances in assessment and measurement have shown this distinction to be inadequate. Both biogenic and psychogenic disorders may arise in an acute fashion (e.g., from psychological or surgical trauma) or a more gradual way. The distinction between *primary* and *secondary* dysfunction has been introduced to indicate a difference between no history of adequate responding and a history of prior intervals of adequate response (Masters & Johnson, 1970). A slightly different distinction is made when *lifelong* and *acquired* are used as subdivisions. To indicate a specific precipitating event in cases of secondary or acquired erectile disorders, the term *situational* is sometimes used. Even when biogenic origins of the disorder are excluded, it is often difficult to decide whether a response has ever occurred. A lifelong, primary male sexual disorder is probably very rare. In a series of 157 men who presented complaints of erectile failure to a sex therapy clinic, it was found that 1.9% had never been functional in intercourse because of a continuous history of erectile failure (Wagner & Green, 1981).

Theory and Etiology

"Penile erections are elicited by local sensory stimulation of the genital organs (reflexogenic erections) and by central psychogenic stimuli received by or generated within the brain (psychogenic erections)" (Krane et al., 1989, p. 1648). According to these authors, the pathways for psychogenic erections, are less well understood. I will not dwell on the neurophysiological mechanism here; for more information, see Chapter 5. However, it is important to note that recent neurophysiological evidence points to the possibility that reflexogenic and psychogenic erectile mechanisms act synergistically in the control of penile erections. Psychogenic stimuli can facilitate or inhibit the erectile response. Two mechanisms may be involved in inhibition. First, psychogenic stimuli may inhibit reflexogenic erections and thereby the parasympathic dilator nerves to the penis. Second, excessive sympathetic outflow in anxious men may increase penile smooth-muscle tone, opposing the penile smooth-muscle relaxation necessary for erection (Krane et al., 1989).

Cognitive processing of psychological stimuli does not necessarily imply consciously controlled activity. Thus, the understanding of psychogenic mechanisms may be complicated by a subdivision into so-called automatic and controlled cognitive processing (Schneider & Shifrin, 1977). This subdivision in cognitive processing is relevant in several ways. First, the issue of voluntary control may be elucidated. Masters and Johnson (1970), in a reflexogenic spirit, considered "erections [to] develop just as involuntary and with just as little effort as breathing" (p. 196). However, a number of studies have demonstrated that inhibition of sexual responding is easily accomplished by instructing subjects to do so (e.g., Laws & Rubin, 1969). In most of these studies, to inhibit responding subjects seemed to direct their attention away from the sexual stimulus (e.g., film or slide). These experiments do not satisfy the circumstances for a demonstration of controlled or "voluntary" processing. A more relevant demonstration would require the subject to process information of the sexual stimulus in different ways, resulting in different response outcomes. A demonstration of this approach, using Lang's information-processing model, is provided in a study by Dekker and Everaerd (1988). When attention is focused on sexual responses (as contrasted with sexual stimuli) during imagery, response propositions are activated. According to Lang's prediction, activation of response propositions (as contrasted with stimulus propositions) elicits the sexual response. It was found that sexual responses of both men and women were stronger when they imagined sexual situations, actions, and feelings than when they imagined only sexual situations and actions.

The interference with controlled processing and inhibition of sexual response has been studied in a double-task paradigm, using tasks that distract from controlled attention on the sexual stimulus. The inhibitory role of distraction on sexual response in functional subjects has been demonstrated by Geer and Fuhr (1976). In dysfunctional subjects, it seems that task-irrelevant worries and fear of failure act to distract from attending to the stimulus, thereby inhibiting sexual response. The interference of this negative controlled processing with automatic processing can be alleviated when attention is directed to a task that avoids worries and fear of failure. When, while attending to erotic stimuli, dysfunctional males are instructed to attend also to a distractor (a neutral story with questioning afterwards, or sums in arithmetic), the interference with automatic processing should diminish. In a comparison of functional and dysfunctional subjects under distraction and no distraction, it was found that distraction did not result in detumescence in dysfunctional subjects, as was found for functional subjects (Barlow, 1986). Only recently have researchers begun to explore cognitive processing in sexual mechanisms from an information-processing point of view. There is some evidence of the heuristic value of such an approach, although data to support this approach is still scarce.

When reviewing the etiology and theories of erectile disorders, several sources of knowledge have to be accommodated. In this chapter the main focus will be on psychological theories that pertain to psychological factors influencing the erectile mechanism and associated aspects of subjective experience.

Psychological Theories of Erectile Dysfunction

According to the DSM-III-R, "The essential feature of sexual dysfunctions is inhibition of appetitive or psychophysiological changes that characterize the complete sexual response cycle" (APA, 1987, p. 290). Both appetitive and psychophysiological changes come about in confrontations with adequate erotic stimuli. A variety of stimuli (including visual, gustatory, auditory, imaginative, and tactile) may elicit erectile responses. A theory or model of sexual functioning should provide an explanation of how these stimuli are processed and how they are transformed into messages (in the brain) that result in neurophysiological and behavioral responses and conscious subjective experience.

The simplest model proposes a preprogrammed sexual mechanism that is activated by an "adequate" sexual stimulus (e.g., Masters & Johnson, 1970). This involuntary, reflexogenic, or conditioned mechanism accounts for the effortless and spontaneous sexual experience of many functional subjects. However, this model does not provide an explanation of the many regulatory processes related to voluntary facilitation and inhibition of the response. Nor can we understand from that simple model the many variations in subjective experience and the complicated variation in relevant stimulus and response parameters that is observed within and among subjects. To accommodate regulatory processes, most researchers adhere to models from cognitive theories of emotion, information processing, or cognitive behavior modification. The central role of cognition in these theoretical approaches has several consequences. It is implied in the model that stimuli are (cognitively) transformed into messages that eventually result in a sexual response (subjective sexual experience in particular). Thus, a stimulus is not intrinsically sexual; it becomes sexual by its transformation (Castille & Geer, 1989). We have no certainty about the existence of so-called unlearned sexual stimuli. There is ample evidence that there are stimuli (e.g., tactile) that activate arousal in the physiological component of sexual response (Bancroft, 1989). However, this arousal alone is not sufficient to produce subjective sexual experience. This experience ultimately depends on the individual's awareness and definition of the response as sexual (Rosen & Beck, 1988; Frijda, 1986).

A second important point is that a stimulus may convey several meanings, depending on the circumstances or the individual's history. Different messages, in the same or in different individuals, may thus be accessed by the same stimulus. Sexual meaning and other meanings relevant for different emotions (such as anxiety, anger, or elation) may be present at the same time. The different meanings will be processed as different messages—which, by further processing, may develop divergent physiological and behavioral responses and subjective experiences.

A simple application of this theoretical notion is to be found in the assessment of erectile disorders. One would predict that a patient with erectile disorder, when confronted with a "sexual" situation will report meaning (cognition) that predicts negative emotions, erectile failure, and avoidance of the situation. An interesting point is that functional males, as compared with females, seem to be limited in their conscious emotional experience of sexual situations. Whereas women, concurrent with sexual excitement, report many other positive and negative emotions, reports of men are almost exclusively limited to sexual excitement (Dekker, 1988).

This brings up a third point. The observed selectivity in men's sexual experience may be attributed to the contribution of sensations in the genitalia. The peripheral feedback generated by vasocongestion may act as a specific indicator of the relevant meaning to be processed ("I feel that this is sexual"). The contrast between males and females would then be that in subjective experience, females process more situational cues and males more physiological cues. However, it is not easy to decide whether males are preoccupied with genital sensations, or whether peripheral feedback dominates the quality and intensity of sexual experience. In both instances men will be vulnerable for a weakening of sensations from the penis.

In emotion research the contribution of peripheral feedback to emotions as they are subjectively experienced is still debated. For subjective sexual experience this contribution is clear when considering more intense levels of subjective experience; it is most probable in the experience of orgasm. With less intense experience the contribution of peripheral feedback to sexual experience is uncertain. There is some data to substantiate this. First, correlations between self-reported sexual excitement and penile engorgement are variable over situations, both between and within subjects. Second, in a study using a habituation paradigm, O'Donohue and Geer (1985) found low correlations between physiological and subjective responses. Physiological response seems to habituate readily, whereas subjective response does not decrease at the same rate. Further-

more, it has been observed that functional men tend to overestimate their genital arousal, while men with sexual dysfunction underestimate theirs (Barlow, 1986).

Most of the processes discussed so far seem to rely on conscious cognition. For most men this is only partly true. They know that they may consciously seek or imagine situations that will facilitate sexual excitement. In many instances excitement comes without such effort, as if it were spontaneous. At least, these men seem not to have been aware of their processing in a sexual way. This automatic processing contrasts with the threatening helplessness of men who have become dysfunctional ("It always used to come naturally, but whatever I do now, it won't work"). At this time there is no data available to determine whether automatic processing should be attributed to overlearning, conditioning, or even unlearned stimuli.

When cognitive processing is emphasized as the main psychological window on sexual excitement in males, we still have to explain how cognitive processing contributes to or interferes with neurophysiological mechanisms. Thus far, it has been demonstrated that the perception of visual stimuli results in decreased electric activity in the smooth muscles of the corpora cavernosa (Wagner et al., 1989); the resulting smooting-out is necessary for engorgement to develop. These very recent findings corroborate earlier hypotheses, derived from general theoretical ideas, that cognitive processing ultimately results in messages for motor output. Conscious cognitive interference—e.g., worries, fear of failure—are probably located in a late stage of the perceptual process. Further development of sexual responding is then inhibited, although there is some initial responding. Conceptually, this state of affairs is quite different when compared with the possibility of a very early association between a sexual stimulus and cues for nonsexual emotions (e.g., anxiety or depression). In the latter case, possibly as a result of conditioning, no initial sexual response will result.

Recent psychological theories on erectile

dysfunction have emphasized the role of conscious cognitions. Theorizing started from the observations of Masters and Johnson (1970), which are still noted in the associated features section of the DSM-III-R: "Almost invariably a fear of failure and the development of a 'spectator' attitude (self-monitoring), with extreme sensitivity to the reaction of the sexual partner, are present" (p. 292). Conscious cognitive interference has been explored in both experimental and treatment studies. These studies show that inhibition of subjective excitement and penile engorgement may be alleviated by controlling the sexually irrelevant negative conscious processing (Barlow, 1986). (These studies will be reviewed in some detail below.) There is no evidence available on the role of conditioned inhibition in erectile disorders. However, some attempts at conditioning penile tumescence have been made. Generally, conditioning effects were weak (Geer, O'Donohue, & Schorman, 1986).

Treatment of erectile disorders that are difficult to manage with available methods would possibly profit from a counterconditioning approach. This approach would not apply to the sort of inhibited sexual response that must be attributed to its defensive function. There is anecdotal evidence showing that complaints about erectile failure prevent confrontations with painful emotional experiences (Kaplan, 1974). This point is clearly illustrated by a patient who complained of erectile failure with his third sexual partner. His first and second partners had both died of genital cancer, but according to this patient, these dramatic events where unrelated to his erectile problem. In many attempts with his third partner, he had experienced no response whatsoever. His response by masturbation when alone remained intact. "There is really no way to understand why I fail with her," he concluded. Problems in the relationship often contribute considerably to the etiology and maintenance of erectile problems.

Recently, Barlow (1986) has proposed a model of erectile dysfunction that integrates much of what is known of cognitive processing in sexuality and its emotional consequences.

Empirical evidence seems to reveal five factors that differentiate between sexually functional and dysfunctional subjects.

> First, sexually dysfunctional subjects consistently evidence negative affect in the sexual context, whereas sexually functional subjects display more positive affect. Second, dysfunctional subjects consistently underreport their levels of sexual arousal and generally evidence diminished perceptions of control over their arousal. Third, dysfunctional men are not distracted by non-sexual-performance-related stimuli in that they evidence no decrease in erectile response, whereas sexually functional subjects are distracted and show decreases in sexual response. Fourth, dysfunctional men are distracted by performance-related sexual stimuli, whereas sexual arousal of sexually functional men is enhanced. Finally, anxiety inhibits sexual arousal in dysfunctional subjects but facilitates arousal in sexually functional subjects (p. 146).

In his model, Barlow suggests that a cognitive interference process interacting with anxiety is responsible for sexual dysfunction, in particular for erectile dysfunction. Barlow goes on to generalize his model as relevant also for female excitement disorders, not without observing that evidence for this generalization is only preliminary. What is felt or experienced in confrontations with sexual stimuli, according to Barlow, is specifically determined by the peripheral physiological feedback. Thus, when confronted with sexual stimuli or expectations for sexual performance, the individual may feel threatened, hurt, and rejected. The resulting perceived negative arousal will feed back on processing, eventually resulting in erectile failure and avoidance of such confrontations. In functional subjects the dominant experience is sexual excitement and positive emotions. The coexistence of autonomic arousal feeds back on and facilitates the processing of sexual cognitions, thus further enhancing sexual response. Thus, dysfunctional subjects seem to focus on or attend to task-irrelevant content, at least when they aim to become sexually aroused. It is also possible, of course, that functional subjects discard or ward off threatening aspects of the situation. Eventually they become "safe" from those threats by focusing on their sexual excitement, which obscures their emotional problems.

The literature includes long lists of possible psychological factors contributing to the etiology or maintenance of erectile disorders (Hawton et al., 1990). These proposed factors stem from different sources, such as restrictive upbringing, discord in the relationship, or reaction to illness. The common pathway resulting in erectile disorder seems to be the processing of negative emotions. The heuristic value of this approach from cognitive emotion theory has only recently been explored. Further empirical studies will be needed to establish the feasibility of this approach in advancing our knowledge of the etiology and maintenance of erectile disorders.

METHODS OF ASSESSMENT

An ideal protocol for the assessment of erectile dysfunction should be constructed in accordance with theoretical and factual knowledge of the physiological, psychophysiological, and psychological mechanisms involved. The protocol then describes the most efficient path from presentation of complaints to effective therapy. Besides financial costs, the protocol must also consider the disruption to the patient of the procedures involved. Strategy in constructing protocols also depends on what is known about the rank-order of probable causes.

Recent research on the prevalence of biogenic and psychogenic causes often begin with statements about Masters and Johnson's early findings that the psychogenic rate was 95%, then go on to present recent results showing dramatic changes in prevalence—to 50% biogenic and 50% psychogenic (e.g. Mohr & Beutler, 1990). In fact, most studies suffer from selection bias, and the clinical samples of different studies are not comparable. Furthermore, prevalence rates depend to a great ex-

tent on the development of assessment technologies. The last few years we have seen enormous progress in vascular and neural assessment techniques, but psychological and psychophysiological methods have not advanced at the same pace. In the debate on strategy, the pendulum has swung to the biological point of view. The development of vascular, pharmacological, and surgical treatments further strengthens this position. Stepping back to look at these developments, it is clear that assessment of erectile dysfunction has advanced in a rapid but unbalanced way. There is no accurate prevalence data available to help determine whether one strategy is to be prefered over the other. The literature presents different approaches, depending on selected clinical populations and assessment preferences that stem from different medical and psychological specializations (Mohr & Beutler, 1990; Meisler & Carey, 1990).

The largest differences in approach may be observed between those clinicians who consider only functional aspects of physiological mechanisms and those who start from a multivariate, or psychobiosocial, point of view. The urologic literature abounds with examples of diagnostic procedures for physiological functions. In a review of the diagnosis and treatment of erectile dysfunction, Williams (1987) described several physiological tests without even mentioning psychological explanations of erectile dysfunction. The exaggerated biogenic view results in intracavernosal injections of vasodilating drugs as the first step in assessment of erectile failure. This is a logical result when the researcher considers "the use of pharmacologically induced penile erections [to be] the most promising mode of diagnosis and treatment" (Williams, 1987, p. 2).

Assessment in a biopsychosocial context should start with a verification of the chief complaint. The aim of the initial clinical interview is to gather detailed information concerning current sexual functioning, onset of the sexual complaint, and the context in which the difficulty has occurred. This information gathering may be aided by the use of a structured interview and paper-and-pencil measures regarding sexual history and functioning. An individual and conjoint partner interview, if possible, can provide additional relationship information and can corroborate data provided by the patient. The initial clinical interview should help the clinician in formulating the problem. An important point is to seek the patient's agreement with the formulation of the problem. An agreed-upon formulation may guide further diagnostic procedures.

A man with erectile dysfunction may be wary of accepting psychological causes for his problem, since they might seem to imply that he himself is responsible for the difficulty. This may add to the threat to his male identity that he has already experienced by the inability to function sexually. Men may also be vulnerable while expecting or having encountered negative comments of the partner. Even more danger may arise when other men become aware of his problem. Furthermore, men with erectile failure often feel helpless because they fail in their own eyes, even when (or because) they put so much effort into trying to regain normal functioning.

Considering the way the man may experience his problem, it can be expected that it will not always be easy to explain to him the contribution of psychological factors. A clinician who is knowledgeable in biopsychosocial aspects of sexual functioning should be able to discuss the problem openly with the patient. Dysfunctional performance is meaningful "performance," in the sense that misinformation, emotional states, and obsessive concerns about performance give insight into the patient's "theory" of sexual functioning. When contrasting this information with what is known about variations in adequate sexual functioning, it is often clear that the patient must fail. "Whatever I do, he does not stiffen," one patient remarked. "It makes me angry to the point that I shout, 'I want an erection,' but still that will not help." In fact, contrary to the patient's expectation, it *can* help, if "I want an erection" is an effective stimulus for sexual arousal.

For the clinician, a problem arises when, even if there is adequate stimulation and adequate processing of the stimulus information (according to the clinician's judgment), no response results, either at a physiological or a psychological level. At this point a number of assessment methods, aimed at identifying different components or mechanisms of sexual functioning, may be considered. In principle two main strategies may be followed. (1) Although a psychological factor interfering with response cannot be inferred from the report of the patient, one can still suspect some psychological factor at work. Possibly the patient is not aware of this factor, so he cannot report on it. Eliminating this psychological influence may result in adequate response. (2) Perhaps, even with adequate (psychological) stimulation and processing, response is prevented by physiological dysfunction. Physiological assessment may then aid in arriving at a diagnostic conclusion. The biopsychosocial approach predicts that it is inadequate to choose one of these strategies exclusively. This is so because there may always be an unforeseen psychological or biological factor, and because sexual functioning is always psychophysiological functioning. Dysfunction in a biological system may sometimes be compensated for by psychological factors. A noncausal biological disease may become an important determinant for psychological causes.

Assessment is especially difficult in cases where psychological and biological factors interact to produce sexual dysfunction. As a consequence of this difficulty, there has emerged a classification scheme in which both clusters of factors have been accommodated (Melman, Tiefer & Pederson, 1988). The researchers present five categories: Four categories are used for decisions that assign weights to psychological and biological factors; and one category is reserved for those patients for whom no diagnostic conclusion could be established. Patients are classified as "unknown" when they did not attain maximal erections, but no psychological or biological factors were found to explain their dysfunction. Two categories allow for the classification of "pure organic" and "pure psychogenic" cases. In cases where interaction is suspected, the dysfunction is classified as either "primarily organic" or "primarily psychogenic." In an evaluation of 406 patients, Melman et al. classified 117 patients (28.8%) as having organic impotence, 161 (39.6%) as having psychogenic impotence, 62 (15.3%) as having diminished erectile capacity as a result of an organic deficit worsened by psychological factors (primarily organic), 40 (9.9%) as having psychogenic erectile dysfunction with some organic contribution (primarily psychogenic), and 26 (6.4%) as having erectile dysfunction of unknown origin.

Before elaborating on specific assessment procedures, I will review the working knowledge derived from what is stated thus far.

In assessing excitement disorders—specifically, MED—one should keep in mind that a psychophysiological mechanism is involved. When a patient reports sustained and sufficiently rigid erections in some situations (e.g., masturbation, upon waking, or with other partners), his dysfunction most probably has a psychological origin. When no response or insufficient response is reported, a psychological factor may be suspected. When the identification of a clear psychological etiology proves to be difficult, attempts at visual and tactile stimulation may be the next alternative. This may be followed by further assessment of waking (diurnal) or sleep (nocturnal) erectile capacity when one suspects that psychological factors are the most important contributing causes for erectile failure. When sustained subjective and physiological response results from this approach, one can proceed with further psychological explorations. The absence of penile response under any condition is less informative, because the clinician can conclude only that no response could be elicited or observed, or that organic factors precluded the patient's responding. At this point, methods that help to establish the differentiation and the weight of psychological and biological factors are called for. In the next few paragraphs, this difficult assessment problem will be emphasized.

Waking (Diurnal) Erectile Assessment

Before the advent of modern methods of physiological assessment, diagnostic procedures for erectile dysfunction consisted of clinical interviews and a noninvasive physical examination. Information about sexual functioning was limited to what the patient had observed and could report regarding his sexual activities. In cases of situational erectile dysfunction specifically, clinicians have always relied on information about other (nondysfunctional) sexual activities of the patient, where activation and functioning of the sexual mechanism could be observed. When a patient complains of erectile difficulties with a partner, there may be no problem when he masturbates or when he interacts with other partners. The diagnostic accuracy of this approach relies entirely on information provided by the patient. This may prove problematic because patients, specifically in cases of protracted dysfunction, are often unable to provide the relevant information. Cognitive interference with sexual responding may have become pervasive, and the patient's hope for reversal of his problem may be shattered. There may have been no occasion to observe even the slightest response, or the patient may have become biased in his observations.

Many men with erectile dysfunction strongly underestimate their sexual arousal. Noting this, Sakheim, Barlow, Abrahamson, and Beck (1985) evaluated the effectiveness of a series of explicit erotic films and self-stimulation in eliciting erectile response. Penile circumference changes were used as a response measure. (For details on the measurement of penile tumescence, see Rosen & Beck, 1988, and Geer & Orman Castille, 1989.) Results indicated that men with psychogenic erectile dysfunction could achieve tumescence in response to films or self-stimulation. In some cases erections were equal to those of functional subjects under the same conditions. Using this procedure, Sakheim et al. (1985) compared a group of organically impaired men with a group of men who had psychogenic erectile dysfunction, and with a control group of age-matched sexually functional males. They achieved 80% diagnostic accuracy, which is as accurate as typical nocturnal penile tumescence (NPT) results. Further comparisons between waking assessment and NPT will be discussed in the next section, where the NPT procedure is described.

Two factors threaten to limit the diagnostic accuracy of waking assessment. First, when no response is elicited, the deficit may be caused by cognitive interference that has not been considered in the procedure. For example, most men do not feel at ease when asked to masturbate in the laboratory, as is required in the procedure of Sakheim et al. (1985). In the diagnostic protocol at my clinic, we use vibration applied to the penis instead of self-stimulation. Vibration combined with an explicit erotic film proves to be very effective in producing erections and can to often yield unexpected ejaculations (Janssen et al., 1991).

Barlow's theory (1986) suggests a number of possible improvements that may help to minimize negative cognitive interference. Sensitivity of the waking procedure in detecting functional erectile capacity may increase when more control is achieved over inhibitory processes. The negative side of this development is that the number of false positives will also increase. In some cases of organic impairment, intense erotic stimulation will override the organic deficits (Meisler & Carey, 1990). Consistent with that suggestion, both Zuckerman et al. (1985) and Slob et al. (1990) have shown that it is difficult to distinguish between the genital responses to erotic films of diabetic and nondiabetic subjects.

There are indications that the concurrent measurement of subjective arousal obtained during waking procedures may be of some interest. It has been noted that discrepancies between subjective arousal and physiological response are different in psychogenic and organic erectile dysfunction (Rosen & Beck, 1988). Subjects with psychogenic dysfunction show low correlations between subjective and physiological response. They report weak subjective excitement and seem to be less able to track tu-

mescence. Men with vasculogenic disease also showed low correlations; they may report substantial subjective excitement while concurrently showing poor physiological response. Unfortunately, there is thus far no data available about these discrepancies to evaluate their possible contribution to assessment procedures.

Nocturnal Erectile Assessment

The occurrence of spontaneous erections during sleep was first noted in 1944 (cited in Meisler & Carey, 1990). In the intervening decades, an association has been documented between nocturnal erections and rapid eye movement (REM) cycles during sleep (Meisler & Carey, 1990). Karacan (1970) suggested that nocturnal penile tumescence changes could aid in the differentiation of organic and psychogenic erectile dysfunction. Organic pathology would supposedly lead to diminished NPT response, whereas psychogenic causes would be inoperative during sleep and result in normal NPT response. NPT assessment requires that the patient be evaluated during two or three nights in a sleep laboratory. Several nights are needed to avoid suppressed NPT response through the so-called first-night effect, in which discomfort with the clinical setting or embarrassment may preclude adequate evaluation. Many measures are recorded, to assure reliable and valid assessment. Besides penile tumescence, which implies some combination of circumference measures of the tip and base of the penis and/or a measure of rigidity, electroencephalography (EEG), electrooculography (EOG), and electromyography (EMG) are used.

In addition to these physiological measures, Karacan (1978) recommended additional direct observation of erections by a technician or by video. He also suggested that the patient be awakened at the time of maximal erection, to obtain his estimate of the percentage of full erection that was represented by the current erection. To further assure a measure of penile rigidity, a buckling pressure test is to be conducted. Since Karacan's publications, NPT assessments seem to have become standard procedure in many sexual dysfunction clinics, as a means of determining the biogenic etiology of erectile failure.

Although Karacan et al. (1977, 1978) cautioned that, in their view, erectile dysfunction should be considered as a biopsychosocial phenomenon, some have considered NPT as a gold standard for deciding between psychogenic and biogenic etiologies. Recent studies and reviews (e.g., Meisler & Carey, 1990) have questioned the diagnostic accuracy of NPT assessment and emphasized the necessity of further research to justify its use. NPT measures should therefore be compared with diagnostic groups that have been composed using NPT-independent empirical assessments. From the array of studies that have used independent assignment to diagnostic groups, the study of Wincze et al. (1988) is of special interest. In this methodologically sophisticated study, waking and sleep assessments were compared. Assignment of patients to diagnostic groups was based on clinical criteria. The following groups were described: (1) nondysfunctional subjects, (2) vasculogenic erectile dysfunction, (3) high-risk sexual dysfunction (such as diabetes or peripheral vascular disease), and (4) and (5) psychogenic erectile dysfunction. The last group was subdivided on the basis of reports of genital response in situations other than with the usual sexual partner and on the basis of penile circumference change in response to erotic film. Those who responded were assigned to group 4, the remainder to group 5. All subjects underwent psychological, vascular, endocrinological, urological, and radiological examinations in addition to NPT evaluation and daytime erotic and neutral stimulation procedures. During the daytime procedure, subjective experience of sexual arousal was continuously recorded by the use of a hand lever (Wincze et al., 1980). Statistical analysis of variance revealed that NPT penile circumference changes (in mm) were significantly smaller for groups 2 and 3 than for groups 1, 4, and 5. There were no significant differences among groups 1, 4, and 5 or between groups 2 and 3. It also was found that groups 1 and 4 had significantly greater penile responses to erotic videotapes.

There were no significant differences between groups 1 and 4 or among groups 2, 3, and 5. It is important to note that none of the groups differed significantly on the continuous measure of subjective sexual excitement. Looking at the combined nocturnal and diurnal data, it is clear that only for group 5 was there a difference between NPT response and response to the erotic video. The authors report that they were unable to assign subjects to groups on the basis of hour-long interviews. Most of the dysfunctional subjects denied having had erections under any circumstances (having masturbated or having viewed erotic movies); even nocturnal erections were denied or were thought to be irrelevant. One subject even denied an erection response after obtaining a 20 mm circumference increase while viewing an erotic video. When compared with the information provided by patients during interviews, both diurnal and nocturnal assessments provided relevant clinical information. The authors do not provide data on clinical decision analysis, so the reader is not informed about the accuracy of diagnostic classification by NPT or daytime procedure data. Data on within-group variation in response to both assessments shows considerable differences among patients. Two of the subjects in group 2 (vascular) showed stronger (> 10 mm) erections during daytime evaluation than during sleep. Furthermore, 9 out of 14 subjects in group 2 and 6 out of 14 subjects in group 3 (high risk) showed greater responses during daytime arousal than during NPT evaluation. The authors claim that NPT response is not representative of the maximum response possible. They conclude that NPT evaluation is unreliable: It may present false negative readings (no response, although response may be elicited by other means, such as film). Contrary to earlier (gold standard) expectations, it is now fair to estimate that the diagnostic accuracy of NPT evaluations is about 80% (Rosen & Beck, 1988).

Since NPT evaluations are very expensive, there have been several attempts to reduce the cost of assessment by using portable NPT devices or simpler nocturnal monitoring devices. RigiScan and SurgiTec are portable devices that electronically record tumescence and rigidity. These devices are convenient for home use, but using them does not provide other measurements and observations (EEG, REM, etc.) that are taken in standard NPT procedures. This also applies to simpler monitoring instruments. Most of these devices are low-tech and inexpensive: for example, a ring of stamps that separates at the perforations during erection (Barry et al., 1980); a snap-gauge made of layers of plastic, designed to rupture at different levels of force (Bradley, 1987); and the Erectiometer, made of felt bands with plastic sliding collars that move under prespecified strains to measure both circumference and rigidity (Slob et al., 1990). Several methodological problems are inherent in the use of portable and low-cost devices. Movement or repositioning of the device during sleep, or improper placement, may result in artifactual recordings (Rosen & Beck, 1988). In the absence of physiological sleep recording that verifies sleep stages, sleep disturbances may weaken the reliability of these measures. The usefulness of simplified NPT procedures has not been established, and the problems described certainly will not improve their diagnostic accuracy.

A Comparison of Diurnal and Nocturnal Assessments

Thus far, the diagnostic accuracy of both waking and sleep assessment procedures seems to be less than the clinical practitioner would wish. Both procedures have the advantage of informing the clinician about the erectile capacity of the patient when this remains unclear following the diagnostic interview. Earlier in this section, it was observed that when no response results from either waking or sleep procedures, the clinician is left to decide between two options: The procedure failed to elicit the response (false negative), or organic factors preclude the patient's responding (true organic). A further complication arises when the combined results of waking and sleep procedures are considered. With the introduction of NPT assessment, it is

assumed that NPT data are useful in the prediction of daytime erectile capacity. Studies on the relationship between nocturnal and daytime erections challenge this approach. Schiavi et al. (1985) found reduced NPT circumference changes in diabetic patients who were sexually functional. In aging sexually functional men, reduced NPT circumference has been found (Kahn & Fisher, 1969). Studies combining waking and sleep assessments also point to dissociation between waking and sleep erections in dysfunctions with organic involvement (Chung & Choi, 1990; Wincze et al., 1988). Waking assessments in these patients seem to be more valid; waking response may be more meaningful, since that is the context of the patient's complaints about sexual functioning. Nevertheless, we must still be concerned with the accuracy of waking procedures, because organic factors may be obscured (false positives).

It has been assumed that waking and sleep erections are based on the same biological substrate or mechanism. This provided the rationale for NPT assessments and raised the possibility that sleep might prevent cognitive interference with erectile response. The first hypothesis is questioned on the basis of data on the dissociation between waking and sleep erections. Some studies on the role of androgens in erectile response have contained speculations on different mechanisms (for a review, see Rosen & Beck, 1988). Hypogonadal men, with subphysiological levels of androgens, do show erections in response to erotic visual stimuli, but they show no response during NPT. After substitution with androgens, NPT responses do appear (Bancroft, 1989). Wincze et al. (1986) found reduced NPT but no change in waking sexual arousal in male sex offenders provided with antiandrogens.

Chung and Choi (1990) provided data that allow for the calculation of the predictive value of nocturnal assessments for waking erectile responses to audiovisual stimulation. Snap-gauge, NPT, and Rigiscan nocturnal assessments were compared with audiovisual stimulation (AVS). From Chung and Choi's data, the predictive value was calculated for both positive and negative outcomes of nocturnal evaluations. The snap-gauge is a device with three preset filaments. The response was considered positive (and normal) if all three filaments (or the blue and red ones) ruptured, or negative (and abnormal) when no filament (or only the blue one) ruptured. Positive and negative response on NPT and Rigiscan were evaluated according to the guidelines of Bradley (1987). For a positive response on the snap-gauge ($N = 49$), this results in AVS+ ($N = 15$) / AVS+ + AVS− ($N = 34$) = predictive value 15/49 = 30%. For the negative snap-gauge response, the predictive value for AVS− was 75%. For NPT the predictive values were AVS+ = 22% and AVS− = 82%; and for Rigiscan, AVS+ = 17% and AVS− = 92%. Clearly, negative nocturnal outcome is the best predictor. Chung and Choi also provided data on the relationship between diurnal and nocturnal data and their final diagnosis (organic or psychogenic). The predictive value of positive response for psychogenic as final diagnosis was 86% for combined nocturnal measures and 77% for AVS. The predictive value of negative response for the final diagnosis of organic was 75% for combined nocturnal measures and 35% for AVS. When patients with fluctuating responses during AVS ("unstables," according to Chung & Choi) are excluded, the predictive value increased to 85%. However, the available data seem to corroborate the idea that nocturnal response is not an adequate predictor of waking erections. Furthermore, independent of interactions between nocturnal and diurnal erectile capacity, the predictive values of both methods are limited to about 80%.

One would suspect that with further improvements, the waking procedure would be a cost-effective and appropriate initial screening procedure.

Psychological Measures

Several attempts have been made to establish the differentiation and weight of psychogenic and organic involvement in erectile dysfunc-

tions. Although initial reports sometimes have been promising, replications have not shown that psychological measures reliably rule out organic involvement. For example, the MMPI has been used in several studies, but, taken together, the results have shown that this approach is ineffective (Mohr & Beutler, 1990).

The Derogatis Sexual Functioning Inventory (DFSI; Derogatis, Meyer, & Dupkin, 1976) is composed of ten subscales; it is a sophisticated self-report instrument. Derogatis et al. found that with the gender role subscale alone, they were able to achieve 89% diagnostic accuracy in discriminating between organogenic and psychogenic erectile failure. Segraves et al. (1981) were unable to replicate this finding. Wincze et al. (1988), in their study on NPT and waking arousal, found that a functional group differed significantly from dysfunctional groups on the DFSI subscales of sexual fantasy and sexual experience. The groups did not differ on the subscale of accuracy of sexual information. DFSI measures are not reported to make any contribution to the differentiation between diagnostic groups.

There have been some explorations of the validity of questions, complaints, and symptoms in assessments through clinical interviews. Taken together, these studies report that the best predictive value for organic involvement in erectile disorders is found for the patient's report that no morning erections occur. Segraves, Schoenberg, & Segraves (1985) compared eight questions concerning sexual function with etiological assignment after extensive biomedical evaluation. The answers to only two of the questions proved to have appropriate predictive value: firm, lasting erections upon awakening and turgid noncoital erections predicted psychogenic etiology. Some prudence in using sexual history data is called for. Many men with erectile dysfunction report never having erections. Awareness of erections upon awakening implies that the patient awakes right after REM. It is not clear whether REM erection does not occur in men with erectile dysfunction or that they simply do not notice the occurrence. Mohr and

Beutler (1990) also point to the presence of a pelvic steal syndrome: During pelvic thrusting, blood is shunted away from the penis. These patients will report morning erections even when they are unable to perform coital penetration.

There is a scarcity of studies on the predictive value of data from clinical interviews for the differentiation and weight of psychogenic and organic etiology in MED. More information on the predictive value of symptoms and signs of MED as they appear in clinical interviews would be most helpful to the clinical practitioner. Segraves et al. (1985) propose that clinicians use history data with a certain degree of reliability to make a differential diagnosis.

> Historical data indicating the presence of decreased turgidity in noncoital activities is highly suggestive of an organic etiology to the problem. The finding that prolonged ejaculatory latency may also be predictive of organic impotence in diabetics is reflective of a peripheral neuropathy. This affects nerve pathways influencing ejaculation as well as those controlling erections in many diabetics. The complaints of decreased libido in the sexual history appears to warrant an endocrine workup (p. 169).

However, an objective assessment of the value of clinical data in this respect remains to be established.

Differentiation of Somatic Etiology

Both nocturnal and diurnal procedures have the disadvantage of not being specific regarding the differentiation of organic causes of the dysfunction. The suspicion of specific organic etiology is guided by medical history data and physical examination. A review of the medical history includes a careful review of medical conditions and pharmacotherapy associated with erectile failure. An in-depth review of these relationships is provided by Schover and Jensen (1988). Physical examination normally includes the endocrine, neurological, and vascular systems,

apart from local physical causes (e.g., plaques or fibrosis in the corpora cavernosa).

To explore vascular etiology, several methods are available. The ratio of systolic blood pressure measured at the arm and at the penile dorsal arteries (penile-brachial index, PBI) is a simple method. The predictive value for vascular etiology does not exceed 60%, resulting in a large number of false positives (Abber et al., 1986; Melman et al., 1988). Venous leakage can be detected using a radiologic cavernosography procedure (Wespes et al., 1984). Penile perfusion may be reliably assessed with the Doppler probe. "A small pneumatic cuff is positioned proximal to the Doppler probe. The cuff is inflated until arterial flow is abolished and is then allowed to slowly deflate; the point at which arterial flow returns is defined as the penile systolic pressure" (Gewertz & Zarins, 1985, p. 108). The sensitivity of Doppler seems to be less than satisfactory; known vascular involvement is detected in about 46% of the patients (Mohr & Beutler, 1990). Vascular involvement can be excluded very efficiently with smooth-muscle-relaxing drugs injected into the corpus cavernosum. With these drugs (e.g., papaverine, phenoxibenzamine), sustained erections may be produced if the vascular system is intact. Although erectile response to these drugs does not help in the differentiation of psychogenic and neurogenic erectile failure, it seems to be the most sensitive and hence the most effective method for screening vascular involvement (Bancroft, 1989).

Neurological screening is most pertinent in the evaluation of sensory and motor functioning in the perineal area and lower extremities. Elicitation of perineal reflexes, including the bulbocavernosus reflex, is routine in this screening. Any suspicion of other disorders interfering with erectile capacity leads to a more extensive neurological examination (Mancall et al., 1985).

Laboratory tests for serum testosterone and serum prolactine are often performed to assess the body's ability to use serum testosterone. Recent studies have pointed to the possibility that testosterone does not affect erectile ability

(Bancroft, 1989). However, these tests may inform the clinician about the cause of decreased sexual interest or appetite.

A Comment on Diagnostic Protocols

The formulation of diagnostic protocols rests on various considerations stemming from available assessment methods, aims in patient management, and balancing the cost of different approaches against their relative yield. Furthermore, diagnostic protocols aim at rational decision making, which requires knowledge of the prevalence rates of different etiologies and the sensitivity and specificity of symptoms, signs, and tests. Mohr and Beutler's (1990) critical comment about diagnostic approaches is to the point:

> Many diagnostic programs lose sight of the fact that the primary purpose of diagnosis is the formulation of a workable treatment plan rather than identifying which of several mutually exclusive classifications best fit the patient. For this primary purpose, the degree and nature of physiological and psychological involvement should be used together with prognostic indicators (1990, p. 130).

Several passages in this section on methods of assessment have pointed to flaws in our knowledge of erectile dysfunction. The prevalence rates of various etiological factors are not well known; estimates seem dependent on patient populations as they are studied in different clinics. Still, a rational approach to formulating a diagnostic protocol would start with data on the frequency of different etiologies. This may be done by gathering prevalence rates for the particular assessment setting where a protocol will be used. It allows for the calculation of *a priori* probabilities for different etiologies and thus for the construction of an efficient and rational assessment strategy. From available data it seems that the largest *a priori* probability of a specific etiology is psychogenic. The combined organogenic etiologies include a large number of different specific etiologies that require special diagnostic tests. It is therefore understandable that most authors plead for strategies where a thorough clinical interview and physical examination is followed by eliciting erectile response by psychological means (Segraves et al., 1985; Rosen & Beck, 1988; Bancroft, 1989; Mohr & Beutler, 1990). Most often this is done in a simple and straightforward way by exposing the patient to an explicitly erotic film or video. Concurrently, penile circumference changes and rigidity are measured, along with subjective sexual and emotional experience. The addition of vibration and tasks that help preclude negative cognitive interference may further increase the effectiveness of this approach (Janssen et al., 1991). Visual and vibrotactile stimulation may inform the clinician about erectile capacity in spite of medical disorders or pharmacotherapy that interfere with sexual response, as well as about discrepancies between self-reported excitement and erections. When no sustained response is established in this assessment, the next step is the exploration of vascular involvement. There is increased consensus that, as a first step, injection with a drug that relaxes smooth cavernosal muscle is the most efficient choice (Mohr & Beutler, 1990; Meisler & Carey, 1990). Depending on the results of that test, a further vascular and neurological workup may follow. There is less consensus about the priority of endocrinological tests. When there is a substantial probability of diabetes, glucose tolerance testing is done in relation to the physical examination. This also applies for prolactine and testosterone testing; the general use of these tests is questionable (Bancroft, 1989), as testosterone seems not to affect erectile capacity.

Thus far, proposals for diagnostic protocols have been formulated on the basis of clinical common sense, not on the basis of diagnostic accuracy of tests or on known prognostic indicators. It is worthwhile to bear in mind that many patients refuse or do not follow prescribed treatment. In the study by Melman et al. (1988), it was found that 25% of the patients did not enter any treatment. These data indicate that there is a clear need for improvement of assessment strategies to prevent costly testing with no yield for diagnostic or prognostic accuracy and no real benefit for patients.

PSYCHOLOGICAL TREATMENT

Since 1970 the psychological treatment of erectile dysfunction has been reviewed several times. A review of somatic therapies is beyond the scope of this chapter; for a summary, the reader is referred to Chapter 5 and Krane et al. (1989). Cooper's analysis (1969a, 1969b) followed the boost in sex therapy that originated with the development of behavior therapy and a little later the publication of Masters and Johnson's *Human Sexual Inadequacy* (1970). In his 1971 paper Cooper noted in a summary statement:

> On the available information there is no factual evidence that psychoanalysis or other depth psychotherapies are either effective or ineffective in these conditions; at the moment an objective evaluation is not possible. If among other qualifications, it is assumed that the natural history of the various potency disorders is that of a static process (viz., the condition would neither have worsened or improved spontaneously), a superficial behavioral approach, especially that of Masters and Johnson seems vastly superior (p. 243).

Six years later Reynolds (1977), on the basis of an extensive review, put Cooper's summary in perspective. He disagreed with Cooper on methodological grounds: "the conclusion that such approaches (superficial behavioral) provide a clear alternative to other techniques is unwarranted, given the studies available to Cooper (1971) or those conducted thereafter" (p. 1234). Mohr and Beutler (1990) drew a similar conclusion.

Cooper (1971) provided 56 references for his review; Reynolds used 63 references; and in Mohr and Beutler's review, the number increased to 124 references. There is only a small overlap of five references between Reynolds and Mohr and Beutler. One relevant controlled study of systematic desensitization (Kockott et

al., 1975) was not reviewed by Mohr and Beutler. The considerable increase in references since Reynolds' 1977 review reflects developments in diagnostic and treatment procedures for erectile dysfunction. The boost in somatic studies is indicated by 57 such references, mainly on the differentiation of psychogenic and biogenic erectile failure. Progress in psychological treatment provided 22 references on outcome studies published since 1974. Only a few of these studies have compared treatment methods. The scarcity of evidence seems to preclude a definitive statement on the superiority of one of the available methods of treatment.

Treatment of Erectile Dysfunction

Guided exposure to situations where the patient is alone or with a partner and that demand sexual interaction seems to be prevalent in psychotherapeutic endeavors to relieve MED. Guidance, in essence, is preparation for exposure, because exposure itself is experienced in private. It is not generally feasible to engage in direct observation of sexual behavior, neither for therapeutic nor for assessment purposes. Psychophysiological studies are close to direct observation, but recording of changes in penile circumference or other physiological variables on a monitoring device is still indirect. These studies generally rely on self-report to obtain data on behavior and on experience of sexual emotions. There have been some reports on the use of surrogate partners, where direct exposure was used as a treatment modality. Most of these attempts are difficult to evaluate because of the complex ethical issues involved. Surrogates are sometimes described as therapists or as sexual therapy practitioners (Bancroft, 1989). Sexual involvement of therapists is unacceptable to most practitioners and is also prohibited by professional ethical codes.

When there is no dominant somatic involvement, erectile dysfunction is caused by inadequate behavior, cognition, and affect, which prevent sustained erectile responding and the subjective sense of sexual excitement and pleasure. When confronted with what may be considered relevant stimuli for sexual response, men with erectile disorders seem to perform task-irrelevant coping, resulting in negative emotions and avoidance of the sexual aspects of the situation. Consequently, even when the man aims at sexual response, his efforts are counterproductive. For most men this contrasts sharply with earlier experiences, when erectile response occurred spontaneously.

Treatment generally aims at restoring the determinants of sexual functioning. However, there are no pertinent data to determine the crucial determinants to facilitate the choice of key ingredients for treatment. Furthermore, there is much variation in etiology among men with MED—and therefore in the weight of different determinants. For clinical practice it has become typical to use multimodal or combined treatment packages. They allow therapists to tailor treatment to the specific needs of a patient. Most studies on the treatment of erectile disorders have used multimodal interventions, thus making it difficult to evaluate the component parts of those treatments (Mohr & Beutler, 1990).

The social (relationship) function of sexual behavior stresses the importance of interaction and communication skills. Interventions aim at generating feelings of safety and positive emotions in the social context. Partners learn skills for communicating negative, aggressive, and positive feelings. They may also learn to give and receive adequate stimulation (Everaerd & Dekker, 1982; Kilmann et al., 1987; Takefman & Brender, 1984). Often these interventions are used as a first step in treatment, to ease relationship problems and improve cooperation in the couple.

There are numerous interventions directed at restoring erectile response. Some practitioners reason that the dysfunction must be attributed to intrapsychic conflicts. Thus, according to Bieber (1974), the focus in the psychoanalytic approach is on uncovering the beliefs that support the patient's fear about being free of the erectile dysfunction. Of course, there is an interaction between the patient's cognitions about sexual behavior and the resulting negative emotions (presumably consisting mainly of anxiety). Several approaches have been proposed to relieve the effects of this interaction. Systematic desensitization aims at directly reducing anxiety (Everaerd & Dekker, 1985; Kockott et al., 1975; Mathews et al., 1976). In the same vein, self-hypnosis has been studied by Araoz (1983). Rational emotive therapy has also been used, in an attempt to correct inadequate cognitions (Munjack et al., 1984; Everaerd et al., 1982).

Masters and Johnson (1970) combined the correction of relationship, emotional, and cognitive factors in a landmark approach to sexual dysfunctions. Their interventions aim at sustained positive emotions, sexual arousal, and excitement by gradually changing and shaping the interactions of the couple. In an ingenious way they create optimal conditions for couples to experience sexual arousal when coping with specific dysfunctions. The couple is instructed to perform task-relevant behaviors, and the tasks are structured to prevent or minimize the interference of negative cognitions and anxiety. The work of Masters and Johnson (1970) has been followed in several ways. Some clinicians have used some of the interventions (e.g., sensate focus, ban on sexual intercourse); others have used modifications that generally replicated Masters and Johnson's approach but changed their clinical format (Arentewics & Schmidt, 1983; Everaerd & Dekker, 1985; Mathews et al., 1976; Hawton & Catalan, 1986). Kaplan (1974) added psychodynamic and systemic interventions to Masters and Johnson's approach.

Biofeedback procedures, using feedback from penile circumference, has been reported by Reynolds (1980), who obtained disappointing results. Earlier, more optimistic reports were published by Csillag (1976) and Herman and Prewitt (1974).

Treatment Format

Masters and Johnson (1970) have put the weight of determinants of sexual dysfunction on the couple rather than on the individual patient. In their view, the unit of analysis is the couple.

They feel that patient-therapist interaction is better served when the therapists too act as a couple, matched for sex with the dysfunctional couple. As a result, most of the published studies on treatment have used therapist couples. This approach has been questioned because of cost-effectiveness considerations. However, there is no substantial data to answer these concerns. Of several possible patient-therapist formats (one or two therapists with single men or a couple as patients, or individual treatment), couple treatment has been used most frequently. Individual and group treatments have been reported, both with individuals and couples and with one or two therapists. Few differences in therapy outcome were found on the basis of the therapist's gender (LoPiccolo et al., 1985) or on the basis of single or dual therapists (Arentewics & Schmidt, 1983).

Most treatment formats use between 15 and 20 weekly sessions. There is some variation in the length and intensity of treatments (Arentewics & Schmidt, 1983). Some formats have used intensive daily sessions for two weeks, whereas others used minimal monthly contact and sometimes therapy by correspondence (Bancroft, 1989; Mathews et al., 1976; Takefman & Brender, 1984). The results of minimal contact treatment, as compared with more intensive formats, seem to be less stable and more variable among patients (Takefman & Brender, 1984).

Effects of Psychological Treatments

In *Human Sexual Inadequacy,* Masters and Johnson (1970) reported that their treatment statistics showed a failure rate of 40.6% for primary erectile dysfunction and 30.9% for secondary erectile dysfunction. Compared with statistics for other male and female dysfunctions, the outcome for erectile disorders was disappointing; Masters and Johnson considered erectile dysfunctions to be a "disaster area" for sex therapy. However, in their 1970 book, Masters and Johnson do not satisfy the curiosity of their readers by giving insight in how they arrived at their published statistics. To put their treatment

results in perspective, Masters and Johnson have stressed that their patients represented a positively biased sample. These patients were motivated, cooperative couples; they were highly educated; and they were able to stay for two weeks in Masters and Johnson's clinic. Any failure thus meant that no sexual response was observed, in spite of two weeks of intensive treatment.

No other study to be reported in this section used Masters and Johnson's two-week intensive treatment format, nor were most therapists able to restrict the availability of treatment to a selected group of patients. Reynolds (1977) still had some reservation about the effectiveness of treatment for MED. After the publication of several studies in the late '70s and in the '80s, Mohr & Beutler (1990) seem to be more optimistic. They conclude that therapy is successful, and they cite success rates between 53% and 90%. Still, this conclusion seems premature when one considers the huge differences in reported outcome measures, in most cases without direct reports of sustained erectile response.

Outcome of psychoanalysis and analytically oriented therapy has been reported in some retrospective studies. About 70% of erectile disorders were judged to have improved. However, no specific definition of improvement was provided (O'Conner & Stern, 1972). Kaplan (1974) does not provide data on outcome of her combined psychodynamic/systemic/behavioral approach.

Multimodal approaches, using a blend of communication and interaction training and some form of guided exposure (a la Masters & Johnson), seem to result in substantial improvement on self-report measures (Arentewics & Schmidt, 1983; DeAmicis et al., 1985; Dekker et al., 1985; Hawton & Catalan, 1986; Heiman & LoPiccolo, 1983). Arentewics and Schmidt found that long-term treatment (up to 40 biweekly sessions) was slightly better than 16 sessions in three weeks. However, the dropout rate was greater in long-term treatment. At 2.5 to 4.5 years follow-up, Arentewics and Schmidt found that a large number of patients judged that they had not improved at all, notwithstanding their substantial self-reported improvement at the end of therapy. The possible response shift observed in that study could have been due to the fact patients had been asked to judge their improvement retrospectively at the end of therapy. This may be a relevant point for many studies to consider, as men with erectile disorders tend to underestimate their sexual response (Barlow, 1986). Araoz (1983), using Masters and Johnson-style sex therapy, with and without self-hypnosis, found self-hypnosis to have a significant contribution to outcome.

Systematic desensitization has been studied in several controlled studies and found to result in improvements (Auerbach & Kilmann, 1977; Kockott et al., 1975). In two comparisons of systematic desensitization and a Master and Johnson approach, no differences in effectiveness emerged between these treatments (Mathews et al., 1976; Everaerd & Dekker, 1985).

Rational emotive therapy (RET) has resulted in substantial improvement (Munjack et al., 1984). RET was also effective in a group of mixed single hetero- and homosexual men (Everaerd et al., 1982). One study compared RET with Masters and Johnson-style therapy and with desensitization (Everaerd & Dekker, 1985). No differences in effect were found between treatments; RET, in contrast to the other treatments, showed improvement on relationship measures.

Earlier in this section it was mentioned that Reynolds (1980) had studied biofeedback, with disappointing results. Training in communication skills, sexual skills, dating skills, and social skills were found to be variably effective (Kilmann et al., 1987; Reynolds et al., 1981; Stravynski, 1986; Lobitz & Baker, 1979). In Lobitz and Baker's study, men with secondary erectile failure improved, while men with primary dysfunctions did not. Reynolds et al. found that dating skill training improved social anxiety and precoital erectile problems, but not coital dysfunction.

Long-term follow-up reports have shown that psychological treatment of erectile dysfunction is effective. However, several problems remain after termination of therapy (Arentewics & Schmidt, 1983; DeAmicis et al., 1985; Dekker & Everaerd, 1983; Hawton et al., 1986, Heiman & LoPiccolo, 1983). Maintenance of results over long periods seems to be uncertain and unpredictable. Recurring episodes of erectile failure are not always overcome easily. Some couples cope with these problems by using strategies learned in therapy. Everaerd and Dekker (1983) found that couples used salient aspects of the therapeutic method. Thus, couples who solved their problems with a Masters and Johnson-type approach tended to use, for example, sensate focus; when communication training had been an important therapeutic ingredient, couples tended to solve recurring problems by talking.

SUMMARY AND RECOMMENDATIONS

Diagnosis and treatment of MED have advanced since the early 1970s. Assessment methods for somatic involvement in erectile failure have boosted research on NPT procedures. The early enthusiasm about NPT's diagnostic precision has waned. Nowadays there is enthusiasm for intracavernosal injections and Doppler ultrasound, among other methods. It is fair to state that diagnostic accuracy has not increased at the same pace as newer technologies were introduced. It is to be expected that the development of neurological assessment in the near future will yield further information about the physiological mechanisms of erectile function. Thus far, the erectile mechanism has been explored peripherally, and the link with central mechanisms remains largely unknown.

Psychological assessment by self-report measures does not contribute in a substantial way to solving the diagnostic dilemma of psychogenic and organic involvement. Since the '80s there has been a growing interest in psychophysiological studies (Geer & Orman Castille, 1989; Rosen & Beck, 1988). Specifically, studies on cognitive processing, cognitive interference, and the relationship between cognition and emotion seem to provide new clues for diagnostic and therapeutic applications. Waking erectile assessment has only begun to be explored. Its face validity has already resulted in the implementation of so-called visual stimulation in most diagnostic protocols. The experimental manipulation of cognitive determinants of sexual response elucidates the complicated interplay of cognitive processing, the resulting emotions, and consequences for psychophysiological functioning (Barlow, 1986; Dekker, 1988). Barlow's proposal for a psychological model of erectile dysfunction integrates many findings of his and other research groups (Barlow, 1986). In principle his proposal reflects many conceptualizations that have been in use since Masters and Johnson (1970) formulated their therapeutic format. However, many refinements of earlier etiological hypotheses have been established. The supposedly all-important role of anxiety as an etiological factor has not been confirmed. Furthermore, in experimental studies, numerous aspects of cognitive processing (e.g., distraction, monitoring, and performance demand) seem to have differential effects on men with and without dysfunctions. This means that these factors have to be considered as playing a role in the maintenance of problems, instead of being considered as causative. A more direct approach to erectile failure will be possible when we can pin down the relevant cognitive processing factors.

Studies on the psychological treatment of erectile dysfunction, also at long-term follow-up, have shown positive outcomes from several approaches. Masters and Johnson-style ingredients seem to be incorporated in most treatment methods. Other interventions are weighted differently in the available studies. There is extensive use of training in communication and interaction skills to ensure cooperation between the partners. These interventions may also be used to foster an exchange of adequate stimulation. The task-relevant experience of sensations is aided by diverse interventions; besides Masters and Johnson's sensate focus, RET has been of some use, as well as sexual skills training and masturbation. Thus far, the available outcome data do not make it possible to specify an ideal package of interventions, nor is it possible to delineate a most efficient format.

It is fair to say that since the '70s no truly new approach to MED has been proposed. Experimental studies on emotional and cognitive factors have elucidated how task-irrelevant behaviors may interfere with the development of sexual arousal and the experience of sexual excitement (Barlow, 1986). In the near future, new applications may be expected as a result of these studies.

Methodological Issues

Is it necessary to reiterate what is written about methodological flaws in almost all diagnostic and treatment studies? What has been stressed in the literature on psychotherapy outcome in general also applies to studies on erectile dysfunction. Reynolds (1977) could not help but repeat what Cooper (1971) had said before him, and that in turn is recited by Mohr and Beutler (1990) in their review.

Few studies have applied decision analysis to assessment procedures (e.g., Schiavi, 1988), and not one study has applied this analysis to therapeutic efficacy. Decision analysis, instead of one-way ANOVAs and t-tests of between-group differences, might show progress developing at a slow rate. Despite all the recent changes, it seems very difficult to do better than a well-trained clinician who is not armed with any technology.

REFERENCES

Abber, J. C., Lue, T. F., Orvis, B. R., McClure, R. D. (1986). Diagnostic tests for impotence: A comparison of papaverine injection with penile-brachial index, and nocturnal penile tumescence monitoring. *Journal of Urology, 135,* 923–925.

American Psychiatric Association. (1987). *Diagnostic and statistical manual of mental disorders.* Washington, DC: Author.

Araoz, D. L. (1983). Hypnosex therapy. *Journal of Clinical Hypnosis, 26,* 37–41.

Arentewics, G., & Schmidt, G. (Eds.). (1983). *The treatment of sexual disorders.* New York: Basic Books.

Auerbach, R., & Kilmann, P. R. (1977). The effects of group systematic desensitization on secondary erectile failure. *Behavior Therapy, 8*(3), 330–339.

Bancroft, J. (1989). *Human sexuality and its problems.* Edinburgh, UK: Churchill Livingstone.

Barlow, D. H. (1986). Causes of sexual dysfunction:

The role of anxiety and cognitive interference. *Journal of Consulting and Clinical Psychology, 54,* 140–148.

Barry, J. M., Blank, B., & Boileau, M. (1980). Nocturnal penile tumescence monitoring with stamps. *Urology, 15,* 171–172.

Bieber, I. (1974). The psychoanalytic treatment of sexual disorders. *Journal of Sex and Marital Therapy, 1*(1), 5–15.

Bradley, W. E. (1987). New techniques in the evaluation of impotence. *Urology, 39,* 383–388.

Castille, C. O., & Geer, J. H. (1989). Sex is in the eye of the beholder. Poster presented at the meeting of the American Psychological Association, New Orleans, August.

Chung, W. S., & Choi, H. K. (1990). Erotic erection versus nocturnal erection. *Journal of Urology, 143,* 294–297.

Cooper, A. J. (1969a). Disorders of sexual potency in the male: A clinical and statistical study of some factors related to short-term prognosis. *British Journal of Psychiatry, 115,* 709–719.

Cooper, A. J. (1969b). Outpatient treatment of impotence. *Journal of Nervous and Mental Diseases, 149,* 360–371.

Cooper, A. J. (1971). Treatment of male potency disorders: The present status. *Psychosomatics, 12,* 235–244.

Csillag, E. R. (1976). Modification of penile erectile response. *Journal of Behavior Therapy and Experimental Psychiatry, 7,* 27–29.

DeAmicis, L. A., Goldberg, D. C., LoPiccolo, J., Friedman, J., & Davies, L. (1985). Clinical followup of couples treated for sexual dysfunction. *Archives of Sexual Behavior, 14,* 467–489.

Dekker, J. (1988). *Voluntary control of sexual arousal.* Dissertation, State University of Utrecht, The Netherlands.

Dekker, J., Dronkers, J., & Staffeleu, J. (1985). Treatment of sexual dysfunction in male-only groups: Predicting outcome. *Journal of Sex and Marital Therapy, 11,* 80–90.

Dekker, J., & Everaerd, W. (1983). A long-term follow-up study of couples treated for sexual dysfunctions. *Journal of Sex and Marital Therapy, 9,* 99–113.

Dekker, J., & Everaerd, W. (1988). Attentional effects on sexual arousal. *Psychophysiology, 25,* 45–54.

Derogatis, L. R. (1976). Psychological assessment of sexual disorders. In J. K. Meyer (Ed.), *Clinical management of sexual disorders* (pp. 35–73). Baltimore: Williams and Wilkins.

Derogatis, L. R., Meyer, J. K., & Dupkin, C. N. (1976). Discrimination of organic versus psychogenic impotence with the DSFI. *Journal of Sex and Marital Therapy, 2,* 229–240.

Everaerd, W., & Dekker, J. (1982). Treatment of secondary orgasmic dysfunction: A comparison of systematic desensitization and sex therapy. *Behaviour Research and Therapy, 20,* 269–274.

Everaerd, W., & Dekker, J. (1985). Treatment of male sexual dysfunction: Sex therapy compared with systematic desensitization and rational emotive therapy. *Behaviour Research and Therapy, 23,* 13–25.

Everaerd, W., Dekker, J., Dronkers, J., Rhee, K. v. d., Staffeleu, J., & Wisselius, G. (1982). Treatment of homosexual and heterosexual sexual dysfunction in male-only groups of mixed sexual orientation. *Archives of Sexual Behavior, 11,* 1–10.

Frijda, N. H. (1986). *The emotions.* Cambridge, UK: Cambridge University Press.

Geer, J. H., & Fuhr, R. (1976). Cognitive factors in sexual arousal: The role of distraction. *Journal of Consulting and Clinical Psychology, 44*(2), 238–243.

Geer, J. H., O'Donohue, W. T., & Schorman, R. H. (1986). Sexuality. In M. G. H. Coles, E. Donchin, & S. W. Porges (Eds.), *Psychophysiology: Systems, processes, and applications* (pp. 407–427). New York: Guilford.

Geer, J. H., & Orman Castille, C. (1989). Sexual disorders. In G. Turpin (Ed.), *Handbook of clinical psychophysiology.* Chichester, UK: Wiley.

Gewertz, B. L., & Zarins, C. K. (1985). Vasculogenic impotence. In R. T. Segraves & H. W. Schoenberg (Eds.), *Diagnosis and treatment of erectile disturbances* (pp. 105–113).

Hawton, K., & Catalan, J. (1986). Prognostic factors in sex therapy. *Behaviour Research and Therapy, 24,* 377–385.

Hawton, K., Salkovskis, P. M., Kirk, J. & Clark, D. M. (1990). *Cognitive behaviour therapy for psychiatric problems.* Oxford, UK: Oxford University Press.

Heiman, J. R., & LoPiccolo, J. (1983). Clinical outcome of sex therapy. *Archives of General Psychiatry, 40,* 443–449.

Hengeveld, W. M. (1986). Erectile dysfunction: Diagnosis and choice of therapy. *World Journal of Urology, 3,* 249–252.

Herman, S. H., & Prewitt, M. (1974). An experimental analysis of feedback to increase sexual arousal in a case of homo- and heterosexual impotence: A preliminary report. *Journal of Behavior Therapy and Experimental Psychiatry, 5,* 271–274.

Janssen, E., van Lunsen, R., Oerlemans, S., & Everaerd, W. (1991). The contribution of a comprehensive psychophysiological evaluation to the diagnosis of erectile disorders. Paper presented at the meeting of the Academy of Sex Research, Toronto.

Kahn, E., & Fisher, C. (1969). Some correlates of rapid eye movement sleep in the normal aged male. *Journal of Nervous and Mental Disorders, 148,* 495–505.

Kaplan, H. S., (1974). *The new sex therapy.* New York: Times Books.

Karacan, I. (1970). Clinical value of nocturnal erection in the prognosis and diagnosis of impotence. *Medical Aspects of Human Sexuality, 4,* 27–34.

Karacan, I. (1978). Advances in the psychophysiological evaluation of male erectile impotence. In J. LoPiccolo & L. LoPiccolo (Eds.), *Handbook of sex therapy* (pp. 137–146). New York: Plenum.

Karacan, I., Salis, P. J., Ware, J. C., et al. (1977). Nocturnal penile tumescence and diagnosis in diabetic impotence. *American Journal of Psychiatry, 135,* 191–197.

Karacan, I., Scott, F. B., Salis, P. J., et al. (1977). Nocturnal erections in the differential diagnosis of impotence, and diabetes. *Biological Psychiatry, 12,* 373–380.

Kilmann, P. R., Milan, R. J., Boland, J. P., Nankin, H. R., Davidson, E., West, M. O., Sabalis, R. F., Caid, C., & Devine, J. M. (1987). *Journal of Sex and Marital Therapy, 13,* 168–182.

Kockott, G., Dittmar, F., & Nusselt, L. (1975). Systematic desensitization of erectile impotence: A controlled study. *Archives of Sexual Behavior, 4,* 493–500.

Krane, R. J., Goldstein, I., & de Tejada, I. S. (1989). Impotence. *New England Journal of Medicine, 321* (24), 1648–1659.

Laws, D. R., & Rubin, H. B. (1969). Instructional control of an autonomic sexual response. *Journal of Applied Behavior Analysis, 2,* 93–99.

Lobitz, W. C., & Baker, E. L. (1979). Group treatment of single males with erectile dysfunction. *Archives of Sexual Behavior, 8,* 127–139.

LoPiccolo, J., Heiman, J. R., Hogan, D. R., & Roberts, C. W. (1985). Effectiveness of single therapists versus cotherapy teams in sex therapy. *Journal of Consulting and Clinical Psychology, 53,* 287–294.

Mancall, E. L., Alonso, R. J., & Marlowe, W. B. (1985). Sexual dysfunction in neurological disease.

In R. T. Segraves & H. W. Schoenberg (Eds.), *Diagnosis and treatment of erectile disturbances.* (pp. 65–85). New York: Plenum.

Masters, W. H., & Johnson, V. E. (1970). *Human sexual inadequacy.* New York: Little, Brown.

Mathews, A., Bancroft, J., Whitehead, A., Hackmann, A., Julier D., Bancroft, J., Gath, D., & Shaw, P. (1976). The behavioural treatment of sexual inadequacy: A comparative study. *Behaviour Research and Therapy, 14,* 427–436.

Meisler, A. W., & Carey, M. P. (1990). A critical reevaluation of nocturnal penile tumescence monitoring in the diagnosis of erectile dysfunction. *Journal of Nervous and Mental Diseases, 178,* 78–89.

Melman, A., Tiefer, L., & Pederson, R. (1988). Evaluation of first 406 patients in urology department based center for male sexual dysfunction. *Urology, 32,* 6–10.

Mohr, D. C., & Beutler, L. E. (1990). Erectile dysfunction: A review of diagnostic and treatment procedures. *Clinical Psychology Review, 10,* 123–150.

Munjack, D. J., Schlaks, A., Sanchez, V. C., Usigli, R., Zulueta, A., & Leonard, M. (1984). Rational-emotive therapy in the treatment of erectile failure. *Journal of Sex and Marital Therapy, 10,* 170–175.

O'Conner, J. F., & Stern, L. O. (1972). Results of treatment in functional sexual disorders. *New York State Journal of Medicine, 72,* 1927–1934.

O'Donohue, W. T., & Geer, J. H. (1985). The habituation of sexual arousal. *Archives of Sexual Behavior, 14,* 233–246.

Reynolds, B. S. (1977). Psychological treatment models and outcome results for erectile dysfunction: A critical review. *Psychological Bulletin, 84,* 1218–1238.

Reynolds, B. S. (1980). Biofeedback and facilitation of erection in men with erectile dysfunction. *Archives of Sexual Behavior, 9,* 101–113.

Reynolds, B. S., Cohen, B. D., Schochet, B. V., Price, S. G., & Anderson, A. (1981). Dating skills training in the group treatment of erectile dysfunction in men without partners. *Journal of Sex and Marital Therapy, 7,* 184–194.

Rosen, R. C., & Beck, J. G. (1988). *Patterns of sexual arousal.* New York: Guilford.

Sakheim, D. K., Barlow, D. H., Abrahamson, D. J., & Beck, J. G. (1985). Distinguishing between organogenic and psychogenic erectile dysfunction. *Behaviour Research and Therapy, 25,* 379–390.

Schiavi, R. C. (1988). Nocturnal penile tumescence in the evaluation of erectile disorders: A critical review. *Journal of Sex and Marital Therapy, 14,* 83–97.

Schiavi, R. C., Fischer, C., Quadland, M., & Glover, A. (1985). Nocturnal penile tumescence evaluation of erectile function in insulin-dependent diabetic men. *Diabetologia, 28,* 90–94.

Schneider, W., & Shifrin, R. M. (1977). Controlled and automatic human information processing: I. Detection, search and attention. *Psychological Review, 84,* 1–66.

Schover, L., & Jensen, S. B. (1988). *Sexuality and chronic illness: A comprehensive approach.* New York: Guilford.

Segraves, R. T., & Schoenberg, H. W. (Eds.). (1985). *Diagnosis and treatment of erectile disturbances.* New York: Plenum.

Segraves, R. T., Schoenberg, H. W., & Segraves, A. B. (1985). Evaluation of the etiology of erectile failure. In R. T. Segraves, H. W. Schoenberg (Eds.), *Diagnosis and treatment of erectile disturbances* (pp. 165–195). New York: Plenum.

Segraves, R. T., Schoenberg, H. W., Zarins, C. K., Knopf, J., & Camic, P. (1981). Discrimination of organic versus psychological impotence with the DSFI: A failure to replicate. *Journal of Sex and Marital Therapy, 7,* 230–238.

Shifrin, R. M., & Schneider, W. (1981). Controlled and automatic human information processing: II. Perceptual learning, automatic attending, and a general theory. *Psychological Review, 84,* 127–190.

Slob, A. K., Blom, J. H. M., & van der Werff ten Bosch, J. J. (1990). Erection problems in medical practice: Differential diagnosis with relatively simple method. *Journal of Urology, 143,* 46–50.

Spector, I. P., & Carey, M. P. (1990). Incidence and prevalence of sexual dysfunctions: A critical review of the empirical literature. *Archives of Sexual Behavior, 19,* 389–408.

Stravynski, A. (1986). Indirect behavioral treatment of erectile failure and premature ejaculation in a man without a partner. *Archives of Sexual Behavior, 15,* 355–361.

Takefman, J., & Brender, W. (1984). An analysis of the effectiveness of two components in the treatment of erectile dysfunction. *Archives of Sexual Behavior, 13,* 321–340.

Wagner, G., Gerstenberg, T., & Levin, R. J. (1989). Electrical activity of corpus cavernosum during flaccidity and erection of the human penis: A new diagnostic method? *Journal of Urology, 142,* 723–725.

Wagner, G., & Green, R. (1981). *Impotence—Physiological, psychological, and surgical diagnosis and treatment.* New York: Plenum.

Wespes, E., Delcour, C., Struyven, J., & Schulman, G. C. (1984). Cavernometry-cavernography: Its role in organic impotence. *European Urology, 10,* 229–232.

Williams, G. (1987). Erectile dysfunction. *British Journal of Urology, 60,* 1–5.

Wincze, J. P., Bansal, S., Malhotra, C., Balko, A., Susset, J. G., & Malamud, M. (1988). A comparison of nocturnal penile tumescence and penile response to erotic stimulation during waking states in comprehensively diagnosed groups of males experiencing erectile difficulties. *Archives of Sexual Behavior, 17,* 333–348.

Wincze, J. P., Venditti, E., Barlow, D., & Mavissakalian, M. (1980). The effects of a subjective monitoring task in the physiological measure of genital response to erotic stimulation. *Archives of Sexual Behavior, 9,* 533–545.

Zuckerman, M., Neeb, M., Ficher, M., Fishkin, R. E., Goldman, A., Fink, P. J., Cohen, S. N., Jacobs, J. A., & Weisberg, M. (1985). Nocturnal penile tumescence and penile reponses in the waking state in diabetic and nondiabetic sexual dysfunctionals. *Archives of Sexual Behavior, 14,* 109–130.

CHAPTER 8

MEDICAL ASPECTS OF ORGASM DISORDERS

R. T. Segraves, Case Western Reserve University
K. B. Segraves, Case Western Reserve University

Sexual function is the end product of complex and interactive biological and psychological factors. Thus, orgasm disorders can have their etiology in a myriad of biological, social, and psychological systems. In every case of orgasm disorder, the clinician must carefully consider whether organic factors may play a role in the genesis and maintenance of the complaint. A faulty analysis of the etiology and prescription of a psychological intervention for an organically based disorder may contribute to patient demoralization, as the symptom fails to abate in spite of sincere efforts by the clinician and the patient. Clearly, we wish to identify treatable organic etiologies. But we also wish to identify currently untreatable biogenic problems, in order to protect the patient from future exposure to unethical or uninformed providers and to help him or her adapt to organic lesions for which there is no effective treatment at present.

Although most clinicians within the field of human sexuality would agree that sexual diffi-culties have both organic and psychogenic causation and would support the concept of the necessity of biomedical evaluation of sexual disorders, (Segraves, Schoenberg, & Segraves, 1985), the actual knowledge base concerning organic factors in orgasm disorders is somewhat sparse. A number of factors contribute to the current ambiguous nature of the information available. These include (1) considerable species variation in mechanisms, rendering extrapolation from lower primates to humans risky; (2) social taboos, which until the recent past, discouraged research concerning sexual behavior; and (3) a frequent lack of cross-fertilization between the research endeavors of those in clinical medicine and those in basic sciences such as pharmacology and endocrinology (Bell, 1972). Whereas the knowledge base concerning orgasm disorders in males is merely inadequate, our knowledge concerning the basic neurophysiology of female orgasm is almost nonexistent. Presumably, this discrepancy between what we know about female orgasm and about male orgasm is related to societal taboos and will begin to be remedied in this decade. In the interim, it is important to realize that much of what is presumed to be true about female orgasm is the result of extrapolation from studies of males. The basic research concerning the neurophysiology of female orgasm has not been performed, and many clinicians who have studied the effects of disease processes on orgasm have restricted their studies to males. The purpose of this chapter will be to review the evidence concerning medical aspects of orgasm disorders. By way of orientation to the subject matter, the review will begin with a brief summary of the neurophysiology of orgasm.

NEUROPHYSIOLOGY OF MALE ORGASM

Although the neurophysiology of male orgasm is less well understood than the neurophysiology of erection, and considerable gaps remain in our knowledge base (Rivard, 1982), a review of certain basic concepts, definitions, and neuroanatomy can help us conceptualize how physical disease can interrupt this process. Most of the sexual response cycle can be conceptualized as a series of spinal reflexes in which sensory stimuli reach threshold values, triggering sexual responses. The sensory experience resulting from some of these reflex sexual responses is believed to correspond to what we call orgasm (Bell, 1972). It should be emphasized that the sexual reflexes are quite complex. For example, the stimulus of repeated tactile stimulation of the penis can evoke reflex vasodilatation of the penile vasculature, resulting in penile erection, seminal expulsion from contraction of the smooth muscle of the internal reproductive organs, glandular secretion, and rhythmic contraction of the striated musculature. All of this requires an intricate sequencing of events and is subject to inhibitory and/or excitatory influences from the brain (Reckler, 1983).

The ejaculatory reflex (seminal voiding) can be defined as consisting of three components (Siroky, 1988):

1. Emission and bladder neck closure
2. Ejaculation and
3. The experience of orgasm

Sensory impulses eliciting the ejaculatory reflex enter the sacral spinal cord via the pudendal nerve. Emission consists of the transport of the ejaculate into the pelvic urethra and is caused by contraction of the vas deferens, seminal vesicles, and smooth muscle of the prostate. As the urethral bulb is stimulated by the inflowing seminal fluid, reflex closure of the bladder neck occurs. Bladder neck closure is necessary to prevent retrograde ejaculation; it occurs over nervous pathways similar to those mediating emission (Kleeman, 1970; Stockamp & Schreiter, 1974). The motor fibers mediating emission are contained in the hypogastric nerve and consist of preganglionic fibers that arise from thoracolumbar spinal cord, segments T12–L3. These preganglionic fibers synapse with short adrenergic nerves that lie close to the innervated organ. The terminals of these short adrenergic fibers are deeply embedded in smooth muscle cells, affording them relative immunity from the action of many systematically administered drugs (Segraves, 1977). Pharmacological studies indicate that these adrenergic fibers are predominantly alpha-adrenergic (Bell, 1972). The vas deferens also receives cholinergic fibers of uncertain origin and function (Rivard, 1982). The cholinergic supply is sparse relative to the adrenergic one (Robinson, 1969).

The term *ejaculation* refers to the expulsion of the ejaculate through the external urinary meatus. Rhythmic contractions of the urethral bulb and perineal musculature propel the ejaculate along the length of the urethra. Sensory efferents from the urethra travel in the pudendal nerve to the sacral cord, where they synapse with somatic efferents that travel in the pudendal nerve, causing contraction of the ischio- and bulbocavernosus muscles.

Orgasm is a purely subjective sensory experience associated with the rhythmic contractions of ejaculation and emission. Presumably, tactile sensory impulses travel to the thalamus and then to the limbic lobe and sensory cortex to produce the sensation of orgasm.

Animal research has identified cortical and subcortical structures associated with the ejaculatory reflex (Blumer & Walker, 1975). In the monkey, ejaculation can be produced by stimulation of the anterior thalamus, along the spinothalamic pathways (MacLean, 1975) and of the preoptic area, which contains many fibers of the medial forebrain bundle (Robinson & Mishkin, 1966). Heath (1963, 1972, 1975) reported that direct stimulation of the septal region of the brain in humans produced euphoria, sexual arousal, and multiple orgasms in some patients. By the use of deep and surface electrodes, Heath (1972) demonstrated that sexual orgasm is accompanied by altered electrical discharge from the septal region. Less dramatic changes were also noted in the amygdala, thalamus, and deep cerebellar nuclei. There is limited evidence concerning the sensory representation of sexual feeling in the cerebral cortex. In their classic work on cerebral representation, Penfield and Rasmussen (1950) reported that stimulation of selected points in the posterior portion of the postcentral gyrus in the midline produced sensation in the penis. However, these sensations were not perceived as erotic. Other reports from patients with epilepsy suggests that sexual feelings have a representation in the paracentral lobule (Smith and Khatri, 1979).

Animal research has indicated that brain dopamine and serotonin levels are related to ejaculatory thresholds (Segraves, 1989). The brain has receptors to many of the reproductive hormones, and it is possible that hormones influence sexual activity by modulating neurotransmitter activity (Bancroft, 1983). While the hormones may sensitize the organs to be receptive to sensual stimuli, other psychosocial factors can inhibit or potentiate the experience of orgasm.

NEUROPHYSIOLOGY OF FEMALE ORGASM

Considerably less in known about the neurophysiology of the female orgasm than is known about male orgasm (Bancroft, 1983; Wagner & Sjostrand, 1988). Orgasm appears to be a genital reflex. A biphasic motor response depends first on intact sympathetic fibers within the lower thoracic and upper lumbar cord segments, resulting in contractions of the smooth muscles of the fallopian tubes, uterus, and paraurethral glands of Skene. The second phase consists of contractions of the striated muscles located within the pelvic floor, perineum, and anal sphincter (Griffith & Trieschmann, 1975). Theoretically, afferent impulses enter the sacral cord via the pudendal nerve (areas innervated by the pudendal nerve include the vagina, clitoris, perineum, and anus) and efferent fibers emerge from T12–L1 (Kaufman, 1983). Adrenergic terminals have been identified in the ovary, uterus, fallopian tubes, and vaginal musculature. Orgasm is probably the sensory consequence of the contraction of the internal genitalia, mediated by these fibers of the sympathetic nervous system. The female sexual organs also have a cholinergic innervation of uncertain function (Bell, 1972). The components probably involved in the orgasmic response are outlined in Table 8.1.

CLINICAL RELEVANCE

From the preceding rudimentary review of the neurophysiology of human orgasm, one can easily surmise the multiple points at which organic factors can cause orgasm disorders. Any assault to the cerebrum (e.g., stroke, tumor, trauma), spinal cord (e.g., tumor, trauma, multiple sclerosis, tabes dorsalis), or peripheral nerves (e.g., pelvic surgery, trauma, diabetes mellitus) might result in orgasm disorders. Many commonly prescribed medications (especially hypotensive agents and psychiatric drugs) alter central nervous system neurotransmission and autonomic nervous system

Table 8.1. Probable Components of the Orgasmic Reflex

A. SENSORY COMPONENT
   1. Tactile stimuli from external genitalia travel via pudendal nerve to spinal centers
   2. Threshhold values required for elicitation of the orgasmic reflex, presumably influenced by hormonal influences on brain centers that connect with spinal centers

B. MOTOR COMPONENT
   1. Motor (efferent) fibers from T12–L1 area of spinal cord travel via hypogastric nerve to genital organs (e.g., urethra, prostate, seminal vesicles, fallopian tubes, uterus, fallopian tubes) and cause rhythmic contractions of these structures
   2. Sensory fibers from these structures travel in the pudendal nerve to the sacral cord, where they synapse with motor fibers that cause contractions of the peritoneal muscles (e.g., ischiocavernosus, bulbocavernosus, and pubococcygeal muscles)

C. SENSATION OF ORGASM
   1. Sensory stimuli from the contractions of the sexual organs travel to the spinal cord, thalamus, limbic lobes, and sensory cortex
   2. The conscious recognition of these sensory impulses is believed to be the experience of orgasm

function and would be suspected to cause orgasm disturbances. As steroid hormones have powerful influences on neurotransmitter systems (Rand & Nott, 1988), certain endocrinopathies might alter orgasmic capacity.

SPINAL CORD INJURIES IN MALES

Spinal cord lesions are among the most common causes of biogenic sexual disorders. As of 1982, there were approximately 200,000 persons with spinal cord injuries in the United States, and this population is increased by between 7000 and 8000 per year (Willmuth, 1987). The sexual behavior of most of these individuals is dramatically altered postinjury.

To understand the literature on sexual function in cord-injured patients, several points need to be highlighted. Some of the seeming inconsistencies in the literature concerning preservation of function postinjury can be understood by realizing that it is easier to predict the sexual effects of a complete cord lesion than an incomplete lesion, as one is always less certain of which tracts are spared in an incom-

plete lesion (Geiger, 1979). In clinical practice, one encounters incomplete lesions more frequently than complete lesions. It is also important to note that the designation of a complete cord lesion is usually made on the basis of a neurological examination, that the term *complete* thus does not imply anatomic transection of the cord, and that the stated low percentage of patients maintaining ejaculatory function with "complete" cord lesion may indicate incorrect assignment and the presence of some communication between the partially severed cord and the brain (Bors & Comarr, 1960).

Most investigators are in agreement that spinal cord lesions are more uniformly destructive to ejaculatory function than erectile function. Also, retention of normal ejaculatory function in patients with complete cervical or complete high thoracic cord lesions is extremely rare (Yalla, 1982; Cole, 1975; Griffith et al., 1973). The largest clinical series concerning sexual function in cord-injured patients was reported by Bors and Comarr (1960). A total of 529 male patients were individually interviewed regarding their sexual function and independently examined neurologically. Neurological examination determined the level of the lesion, whether it was complete or incomplete, and whether it was an upper or lower motor neuron lesion. Patients with complete upper motor neuron lesions retained ejaculatory function less often than those with lower motor neuron lesions (5% versus 18%); a similar pattern was observed for incomplete upper and lower motor neuron lesions (32% versus 70%). There was also a tendency for patients with lesions below thoracic vertebra 9 to retain ejaculatory function better than those with higher lesions. In their conclusions, Bors and Comarr stated that the experience of orgasm required intact innervation of the internal genitalia. However, they presented no evidence that they specifically interviewed patients concerning the experience of orgasm.

Similar findings were reported by Comarr (1970). In this study 150 cord-injured patients were given an interview that specifically distinguished between ejaculation and the experience of orgasm. Patients with complete upper motor neuron lesions rarely experienced ejaculation and orgasm as compared to those with complete lower motor neuron lesions (1% versus 15%). Patients with incomplete lesions had a higher chance of experiencing ejaculation and orgasm. Dribbling ejaculate was noted to occur only in patients with lower motor neuron lesions, presumably because of paralysis of the ischio- and bulbocavernosus muscles. In no case was the perception of orgasm reported in the absence of ejaculation. He concluded that the perception of afferent impulses in the sacral elements is of crucial importance for ejaculation with orgasm.

Electro-ejaculation (induction of ejaculation by stimulating pelvic nerves through the rectal mucosa by an electrical pulse generator) (Brindley, 1980) and intense vibratory stimulation of the penis (Szasz & Carpenter, 1989; Bridley, 1981, 1984) can induce ejaculation if the thoracolumbar spinal centers are intact and connected to the lower cord. In complete lesions, of course, there is no experience of orgasm. Several investigators (Willmuth, 1987) have reported that some cord-injured men experience "orgasm" in the absence of ejaculation or emission. In other words, it is proposed that the sensory component can be experienced without the motor component and in the absence of innervation of pelvic structures. The explanation for these reports is unclear.

Figure 8.1 schematically represents the mechanism by which intense vibratory stimulation might elicit orgasm in spite of a complete midthoracic cord lesion.

Comment

Although the literature on spinal cord lesions on male orgasm appears somewhat inconsistent, the inconsistencies seem to be primarily related to the difficulty in reliably distinguishing between complete and incomplete lesions. Since most lesions are incomplete, the clinician can never be certain of which tracts are still intact. In spite of this, the literature appears consistent in demonstrating that the

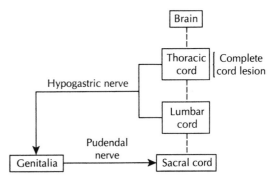

Figure 8.1. Cord lesion and intense virbratory stimulation. Above-midthoracic lesion would presumably allow lower cord to have ejaculatory reflex to intense stimulation. Separation of lower cord from brain would prevent cerebral experience of orgasm.

experience of orgasm requires communication between the sacral cord and the brain. Intense vibratory and electrical stimulation appears to be capable of inducing ejaculation if the thoracolumbar ejaculation centers of the cord are in communication with the sacral cord.

SPINAL CORD INJURIES IN FEMALES

Relatively little information in the literature on the presence or absence of orgasmic experience in women contains precise neurological description of the extent and level of cord injury. Comarr and Vigue (1978) reported on 16 women's sexual function after cord injury. The sample included 21 patients, but 4 were still in the acute stage and had not returned to sexual activity, and one other reported no sexual activity. Several patients reported orgasm after nipple manipulation. From the clinical report, it was not possible to correlate lack of orgasm with any given level of cord lesion. Berard (1989) assessed level of cord lesion and level of sexual function in 15 cord-injured females. He concluded that if the lesion is below T1, orgasm is impossible. He also noted that some patients could experience paroxysmal pleasure from stimulation of erogenous zones above the lesion and through deep mental concentration on the genital sensations, experiencing the orgasm as if it originated in the genitals. Clearly, there is a pressing need for careful investigations to delineate the preservation of various aspects of sexual function as related to level of cord lesion in female patients.

MALE ORGASM DISORDERS AFTER SURGICAL PROCEDURES

Various surgical procedures interfere with autonomic nervous system innervation of the pelvic organs and would theoretically be expected to cause orgasm difficulties. Before the advent of modern pharmacotherapy for arterial hypertensive disease, sympathectomy was a surgical procedure employed to control malignant hypertensive disease. One of the earliest attempts at systematic examination of the effects of sympathectomy on sexual behavior was reported by Whitelaw and Smithwick (1951). Questionnaries that addressed changes in sexual behavior were mailed to patients after surgery. A 69% response rate produced 161 usable questionnaires. Surgeons' reports were used to specify the sympathetic ganglia removed. They concluded that sympathectomies not removing the sympathetic chain below T-12 did not result in loss of ejaculation. Sympathectomies interfering with L1, L2, or L3 resulted in permanent loss of ejaculation in 15%, 29%, and 54% of patients, respectively.

Rose (1953) investigated sexual function in a smaller sample of patients, again using a questionnaire. His sample included 30 patients with simple bilateral ganglionectomy, 8 patients with extensive sympathetic chain removal including the splanchnic nerves, and 10 patients in a nonsympathectomy surgical control group. Of the bilateral lumbar sympathectomy group, 90% retained ejaculatory function, whereas 100% of the more extensive sympathectomy group experienced an interruption of sexual function. He concluded that the critical area for ejaculatory function is just above L1 and that variations in surgical procedures may explain why investigators concluded that the lumbar ganglia are critical to ejaculatory function.

Retroperitoneal Lymphadenectomy

Another surgical procedure that interrupts the sympathetic innervation of the sexual organs is retroperitoneal lymphadenectomy. Retroperitoneal lymph node dissection is typically performed to prevent the spread of nonseminomatous tumors of the testes. Since the lymphatic vessels and nerves are intimately interwoven, this procedure includes removal of all of the sympathetic ganglia from T12 to L3 and damage to or removal of the hypogastric plexus. Because testicular cancer is primarily a disease of young men, infertility resulting from this procedure may prove to be a serious problem for many patients.

Kedia et al. (1975) followed up 36 patients postsurgery. Thirty-five of them experienced orgasm without ejaculation. Postmasturbatory urine samples produced no evidence of retrograde ejaculation. One patient partially recovered ejaculatory function 5–7 years postsurgery. In a subsequent report (1977), the same authors presented data on 52 patients; 49 reported orgasm without ejaculation. Two patients had partial recovery of function 5–7 years postsurgery. A somewhat different result was reported by Nijman et al. (1982). After retroperitoneal lymph node dissection, 12 out of 14 patients lost antegrade ejaculation. However, 10 of these were found to have retrograde ejaculation, which responded to 50 milligrams per day of imipramine.

A number of other investigators have confirmed the occurrence of ejaculatory impairment after retroperitoneal lymphadenectomy (Bracken & Johnson, 1976; Narayan et al., 1982). Schover and Von Eschenbach (1985) reported a questionnaire study of 121 patients who had been treated for nonseminomatous testicular cancer. Reduced orgasmic intensity and difficulty reaching orgasm were rated after retroperitoneal lymphadenectomy. The percentage of men with these complaints increased if chemotherapy and/or radiotherapy was added to the treatment. Radiotherapy alone for testicular seminoma is associated with difficulty reaching orgasm and decreased orgasmic intensity. It has been speculated that radiation to the paraaortic field may be responsible for these effects (Schover, Gonzalez, & von Eschenbach, 1986).

Protocolectomy and Abdominoperitoneal Resection

Rectal excision is another surgical procedure frequently reported to cause sexual impairment (Bennett, 1982; Schoenberg, 1985). The frequency and type of sexual impairment is related to the type of surgical procedure used. A brief review of the course of the sympathetic fibers within the pelvis may clarify why certain surgical procedures are associated with a higher frequency of sexual problems. The sympathetic fibers mediating ejaculation enter the pelvis along its lateral walls as the hypogastric nerves. These nerves are joined by the parasympathetic fibers, forming the pelvic plexi, which lie lateral to the rectal ampulla. The fibers are closely applied to the lateral pelvic walls and far removed from the surgical field unless dissection is extended to the walls in removal of lymph nodes. Two major surgical procedures are employed: protocolectomy for benign disease (such as ulcerative colitis) and abdominoperitoneal resection for malignant disease. A high incidence of sexual difficulties, including ejaculatory impairment, has been reported after abdominoperitoneal resection (Aso & Yasutomi, 1974) and anterior resection of the rectum (Hellstrom, 1988). This is probably related to the wider resection necessary for malignant disease (Yeager & van Heerden, 1980).

A number of studies have reported more frequent ejaculatory impairment after abdominoperitoneal resection than after protocolectomy. Yeager and Van Heerden (1980), in a study of male patients less than 50 years old, reported that 2 out of 20 abdominoperineal resection patients were unable to ejaculate postoperatively. None of the 25 proctocolectomy patients experienced a change in ejaculation. Bernardinis et al. (1981) reported that 47 out of 84 patients undergoing colorectal resection for cancer experienced permanent loss of ejaculation, whereas none of the patients undergoing proctocolectomy for ulcerative colitis experienced permanent problems. Neal (1966) also reported a higher incidence of ejaculatory impairment in patients undergoing abdominoperineal excision than in those undergoing proctectomy. A number of other investigators have reported ejaculatory disturbance to be absent or infrequent after proctectomy for benign disease (Corman et al., 1978; Watts et al., 1966; Bauer et al., 1983; Stahlgren & Ferguson, 1958; Donovan & O'Hara, 1960).

Aortoiliac Surgery

Ejaculatory impairment has been reported after aortoiliac reconstructive surgery; it is probably related to surgical damage to the superior hypogastric plexus. A number of investigations are consistent in reporting this finding. In a questionnaire study of 35 males who had received aortoiliac surgery (thrombendarterectomy, aneurysm repair, or grafts), Hallbrook and Holmquist (1970) reported that 10 were left with permanent ejaculatory impairment (presumably retrograde ejaculation). Sabri and Cotton (1971) reported that 7 out of 9 patients undergoing a standard aortoiliac endarterectomy experienced permanent ejaculatory failure. In a second group of 10 patients undergoing endarterectomy in which special care was taken to preserve the hypogastric plexus, only one suffered ejaculatory failure. Abramovici et al. (1971) also reported three patients who retained the sensation of orgasm but lost the ability to ejaculate after aortoiliac surgery. One of the largest clinical series addressing the effect of aortoiliac surgery on sexual function was reported by May et al. (1969). Seventy patients had aortoiliac reconstructive surgery either for occlusive disease or for aneurysmal disease of the abdominal aorta; 63% of patients undergoing aneurysmectomy and 49% of patients undergoing reconstructive surgery for occlusive disease experienced change in ejaculation. Retrograde ejaculation and no ejaculation were commonly noted. Interestingly, the authors commented that only 3 out of 70 patients mentioned the sexual problem without being directly asked by the surgeon. A number of other investigators have reported ejaculatory problems after aortoiliac surgery (Weinstein & Machleder, 1976; Flanigan et al., 1982; Metz et al., 1983). Ohshiro and Kosaki (1984) also reported that the incidence of ejaculatory failure could be reduced by modifying the operative technique.

Prostatectomy

One of the most common causes of retrograde ejaculation is transurethral prostatectomy (Holtgrewe & Valk, 1964; Kaplan, 1983). In this procedure, retrograde ejaculation occurs as a consequence of ceased function of the bladder neck. Although the outcome of prostatectomy on erectile function has been studied, many investigators have been remiss in asking questions concerning ejaculatory function. In a study in which questionnaires were administered both preoperatively and six months postoperatively, Hargreave and Stephenson (1977), found that 22 out of 41 men (54%) had postoperative absence of anterograde ejaculation. Moller-Nielsen et al. (1985) conducted sex life interviews preoperatively and at 6 and 12 months postoperatively in 167 men undergoing transurethral prostatic resection. Of the men who remained sexually active postoperatively, 49% had retrograde ejaculation.

Two other operative procedures for cancer of the prostate are radical retropubic prostatectomy and transvesical prostatectomy. Hargreave and Stephenson (1977) reported that 12 out of 15 men undergoing this procedure had ejaculatory problems postoperatively. However, Walsh and Donker (1982) reported that 30 out of 31 men who received this procedure were able to achieve orgasm postoperatively. Hargreave and Stephenson (1977) also reported that 9 out of 13 men undergoing transvesical prostectomy did not have antereograde ejaculation postoperatively.

Surgical Procedure for Bladder Cancer

The frequency of orgasmic dysfunction after surgery for bladder cancer may vary according to the procedure used. Bergman et al. (1979) reported on 42 male patients with cancer of the bladder who were treated by total cystectomy, vesiculectomy, and prostatectomy. Pelvic node dissection was not performed in any patient. Although erectile impairment was common, 25 men reported masturbatory activity postoperatively. Of these, 18 reported normal orgasmic experiences. Schover et al. (1986) reported follow-up data on 73 men who had received either radiotherapy followed by cystectomy or cystectomy combined with pelvic node dissection. Of the men attempting sexual behavior after treatment, 36% reported difficulty reaching orgasm, and 100% reported failure of anterograde ejaculation.

Gunterberg and Petersen (1976) reported on a group of patients subjected to major sacral resection for extirpation of tumors, in which the sacral nerves had to be intentionally sacrificed. Ejaculation appeared unaffected unless nerves above S-3 were sacrificed, at which point ejaculation was described as less forceful and "dripping." Table 8.2 lists the effects of various surgical procedures on male orgasm.

Table 8.2. Surgical Procedures and Male Orgasmic Dysfunction

PROCEDURE	EFFECT
Sympathectomy	Loss of ejaculation with damage to T12–L3 area
Retroperitoneal lymphadenectomy	Loss of ejaculation or retrograde ejaculation common
Protocolectomy	Infrequent ejaculatory failure
Abdominoperitoneal resection	Loss of ejaculation common
Aortoiliac surgery	Ejaculatory changes related to surgical procedure
Prostatectomy	Retrograde ejaculation common with transurethral prostatectomy; failure of ejaculation common with transvesical prostectomy
Cystectomy	Ejaculatory impairment if pelvic nerves sacrificed

Summary

This review suggests that many surgical procedures can affect ejaculatory function. However, few studies asked patients about the subjective experiences of orgasm. Some investigators followed patients for longer postoperative periods and reported some return of function. This finding suggests that altering surgical techniques with preservation of sexual functioning in mind might reduce the amount of sexual impairment. Also, longer follow-up evaluation may lead to a better understanding of partial return of sexual function.

FEMALE ORGASM DISORDERS AFTER SURGICAL PROCEDURES

Surgical Procedure

Theoretically, one would expect that surgical procedures that interrupt the sympathetic innervation of the genital organs, such as sympathectomy, abdominoperitoneal resection, retroperitoneal lymphadenectomy, and aortoiliac surgery, would result in female orgasm disorders. However, there is minimal information concerning the impact of most surgical procedures on female sexuality (Schover & Jensen, 1988), and much of the available information does not directly address orgasm apart from postoperative changes in general sexual function such as lubrication and sexual desire (e.g., Brouillette et al., 1981; Gruner et al., 1977). Also, very few of the available reports define how the sexual information was obtained.

Abdominoperitoneal Resection

Cunsolo and his co-workers at the University of Bologna, Italy, reported on a series of patients with carcinoma of the rectum. This surgical series included 94 female patients; after abdominoperitoneal resection, 25% were listed as having residual changes in orgasm. Burnham et al. (1977) sent sexual questionnaires to members of the Ileostomy Association of Great

Britain. A 70% response rate yielded 175 completed forms from female patients with benign disease. For female ileostomists with intact rectum, there was no change postoperatively in orgasmic function. Metcalf et al. (1988) also reported that proctocolectomy for benign disease does not appear to be associated with an increased risk of anorgasmia.

Gynecologic Cancer

With advances in cancer treatment, there has been an increased interest in the quality of life of cancer survivors. Part of this interest has focused on complications affecting sexual functioning in women with gynecologic cancer (Andersen, 1987) and on sexual rehabilitation of cancer patients (Schover et al., 1987; Capone et al., 1980). Although this research has documented considerable psychological distress after certain surgical procedures that are disfiguring (Andersen, 1985), there is minimal evidence concerning the effect of various procedures on the biological substratum of orgasm.

A number of studies have suggested that radiation therapy produces more devastating effects on sexual life (Abitol & Davenport, 1974; Decker & Schwartzman, 1962), including orgasmic capacity, than does hysterectomy for invasive carcinoma of the cervix (e.g., Seibel et al., 1980, 1982; O'Hoy & Tang, 1985). However, this finding has not replicated by other investigators using a prospective design (Schover et al., 1989; Vincent et al., 1975; Andersen, 1987). In two of these studies, orgasmic dysfunction at follow-up was not statistically different from its frequency pretreatment (Schover et al., 1989; Andersen, 1987).

Pelvic exenteration is a life-saving and mutilating surgical procedure for recurrent pelvic malignancy. It involves surgical removal of the uterus, fallopian tubes, ovaries, urinary bladder, rectum, and vagina. Surgical reconstruction of a neovagina is often performed. As one might expect, clinical reports have indicated major difficulties in postsurgical adjustment and total cessation of sexual activity in many patients (Broun et al., 1972; Andersen & Hacker, 1983; Dempsey et al., 1975: Vera, 1981). However, based on these reports, it is difficult to document a specific influence on orgasmic capacity apart from the major medical and psychological aspects of adaptation postsurgery.

Invasive vulvar cancer is typically treated by either wide local excision or by removing the entire vulva (radical vulvectomy). In a short questionnaire study of 18 patients treated with wide local excision, it was reported that all women maintained sexual responsiveness—in contrast to two patients undergoing radical vulvectomy, who lost orgasmic ability. Andersen and Hacker (1983) reported a retrospective descriptive study of 15 women, most of whom had received radical vulvectomy. Many reported loss of orgasmic capacity, as well as blunting of genital sensitivity. Due to the small sample size, it was not possible to correlate surgically induced anorgasmia with the specific surgical procedure. In a subsequent study with a larger sample, Andersen et al. (1988) reported on 42 patients' sexual functioning postsurgery. There was a significant decrease in orgasmic capacity, and anorgasmia was related to the extent of surgical intervention. Anorgasmia postvulvectomy has also been reported by Moth et al. (1983).

Schover and Von Eschenbach (1985) reported on a series of nine sexually active women before and after radical cystectomy (removal of bladder, urethra, uterus, ovaries, fallopian tubes, and anterior vaginal wall). Of the eight women who resumed intercourse, six were coitally orgasmic, and two were orgasmic by masturbation. All had been orgasmic prior to surgery.

Gunterberg and Petersen (1976) reported on four female patients who suffered damage to the sacral nerves during major sacral surgery. Anorgasmia did not occur, although sacrifice of pelvic nerves above S3 resulted in decreased sensitivity of the labia. Information on surgical procedures and female orgasmic dysfunction is listed in Table 8.3.

Table 8.3. Surgical Procedures and Female Orgasm

PROCEDURE	EFFECT
Proctocolectomy	Minimal risk
Abdominoperitoneal resection	Risk of anorgasmia
Pelvic exenteration	Frequent cessation of sexual activity
Radical vulvectomy	Anorgasmia
Cystectomy	Minimal risk

Comment

Studies of the effects of surgical procedures on sexual function in women have varied widely in their methodological sophistication. Some comments on certain basic problems are in order here. In most situations, the ideal control group is the same group of patients prior to surgery. If this design is to be utilized, it is clearly necessary to study the patients prior to the intervention as well as after, to avoid problems in recall and faulty attribution. The study of sexual function clearly must include most aspects of sexual behavior so that the investigator can identify the specific sexual response disrupted.

In this regard, the investigator should examine libido and arousal and orgasm parameters to be certain that the procedure has had an effect on the specific sexual parameter in question rather than just leading to a general decline in sexual function. Our own preference is that the major instrument of study should be a semistructured interview by someone well acquainted with the patient and her medical condition. A good semistructured interview should avoid the problem of the patient not clearly differentiating the various phases of the sexual response cycle in the same manner as the investigator. Standardized questionnaires may need to be included to guarantee uniformity across studies.

Most patients undergoing major surgery (especially of the genital and reproductive organs) will experience psychological distress. The extent of the surgery and the degree of disfigurement can be expected to be related to the degree of distress experienced and to the time needed for adjustment. In certain situations (e.g., pelvic exenteration), it is extremely difficult to study the impact of the intervention on the biological substratum of sexual function, separate from its effect on psychological distress. Obviously, such studies require long follow-up periods to allow for adjustment postsurgery. The Andersen (1987) study illustrates this point. The frequency of patients experiencing orgasm disorders four months after treatment for cervical cancer was 23% (as compared to 12% pretreatment). After 12 months, the frequency of orgasm dysfunction returned to baseline, suggesting that the treatment did not have a lasting effect on orgasmic capacity. Similarly, the investigator must assess the degree of ongoing medical intervention and impairment. For example, if a patient with a neovagina continues to experience vaginal discharge, irritation, and recurrent infection, it will be difficult to decipher what part of her sexual impairment is due to the surgical intervention rather than to ongoing medical problems.

This area of inquiry requires close collaboration between the oncologist and the specialist in sexual medicine. Typical treatments may involve combinations of surgery, chemotherapy, and radiation—any of which may cause sexual difficulties. The particulars of the medical or surgical intervention must be specified as treatments evolve. If chemotherapy is utilized, the agents and total dosage must be specified, as must the parameters of radiation therapy. Ideally, one should review operative notes to confirm the extent of lymph node dissection, as the nerves supplying the genital organs are frequently embedded in the lymph nodes.

DIABETES AND MALE SEXUALITY

The association of diabetes mellitus with erectile dysfunction is well known (Bancroft, 1983; Mills, 1976; Karacan, 1980; McCulloch, 1984;

House & Pendleton, 1988), and the mechanism is assumed to be diabetic neuropathy (Mancall et al., 1985; Ellenberg, 1971).

Although many clinicians have reported retrograde ejaculation (Greene & Kelalis, 1968; Greene et al., 1963; Ellenberg & Weber, 1966) or ejaculatory delay (Abel et al., 1982) to be associated with diabetes mellitus, this appears to be a relatively uncommon complication of diabetes mellitus (Fairburn, 1981).

In a study of 175 male diabetic outpatients by Kolodny et al. (1974), only two were found to have retrograde ejaculation. Jensen (1981) examined sexual function in 80 diabetic men as compared to a general-medicine control group and found two cases of retarded ejaculation in diabetics. Fairburn et al. (1982a, 1982b) reported evidence that a subtle disruption of the ejaculatory process in diabetics may be more common than previously suspected. Over one-third of the men in the series noted an absence of the "pumping action" of ejaculation, and a few reported orgasm without emission.

DIABETES AND FEMALE SEXUAL FUNCTION

One of the first studies documenting an effect of diabetes mellitus on female sexuality was reported by Kolodny (1971). In this study, 125 hospitalized diabetic females and a control group of 100 hospitalized non-diabetic female patients were interviewed; 35% of the diabetic group reported total absence of the orgasmic reflex versus 6% in the control group. In all cases, the orgasmic dysfunction occurred after the onset of diabetes. In 1977, Ellenberg interviewed 100 diabetic women and found that 18% had significant orgasmic difficulty. However, no comparison group was utilized in this study. In a series of publications, Jensen (1981, 1985, 1986) compared sexual behavior in 80 Type 1 diabetic female outpatients versus 40 female controls. No significant differences in orgasmic response were found. Several other studies have failed to find a significant elevation of orgasmic dysfunction in Type 1 (Tyrer et al, 1983) or mixed diabetics (Neuman and Bertelson, 1984; Schreiner-Engel, 1985).

However, two studies have produced evidence supportive of Kolodny's original report. Zrustova et al. (1978) found anorgasmia in 33% of diabetic women and evidence of clitoral nerve neuropathy. Schreiner-Engel and coworkers (1987) examined sexual impairment in female diabetics as compared to non-diabetic medical patients. Type 1 diabetics were not significantly different from controls, but Type 2 diabetics had significantly more orgasmic impairment than control subjects.

MULTIPLE SCLEROSIS AND MALE SEXUAL FUNCTION

Multiple sclerosis is principally a disease affecting the white matter of the brain and spinal cord. Typically, it has an intermittent but progressive course with a multiplicity of symptoms (Walton, 1975). It is well established that impotence is frequently associated with this disease (Lilius et al., 1976a; Vas, 1969). However, Valleroy and Kraft (1984) reported that multiple sclerosis may also be associated with orgasmic dysfunction in male patients. Anonymous sexual questionnaires were given to 656 multiple sclerosis patients; a total of 217 usable questionnaires were returned. Of the 68 males returning questionnaires, 28 reported difficulty with ejaculation or orgasm.

MULTIPLE SCLEROSIS AND FEMALE ORGASMIC DISORDER

Lilius et al. (1976b) sent detailed questionnaires to members of the Helsinki Multiple Sclerosis Society. Orgasmic dysfunction was reported by 33% of the female patients. Lundberg (1978) studied 25 female patients with mild multiple sclerosis. Nine (36%) reported orgasmic problems. Similar findings were reported by Valleroy and Kraft (1984) in their questionnaire study of patients with multiple sclerosis.

Of the 149 females participating, 53 (37%) reported anorgasmia.

COMMENT

Although there is clear evidence of orgasmic dysfunction in both sexes with diabetes mellitus and multiple sclerosis, more information is clearly needed. The excellent work by Schneiner-Engel et al. (1987) at Mt. Sinai in New York emphasizes the critical need for researchers to document patient and treatment parameters in their investigational efforts. Failure to do this may confuse the literature rather than add to our knowledge base. The work by Fairburn et al. (1982a, 1982b) illustrates the importance of the investigator not relying solely on standard sexual diagnostic entities, but rather listening to the patient's actual descriptions of what has occurred. Most of our knowledge concerning orgasmic disturbance in patients with multiple sclerosis is based on questionnaire surveys; this must be complemented by careful, standardized interviews with patients.

PHARMACOLOGIC AGENTS AND MALE SEXUAL FUNCTION

The major classes of drugs reported to cause orgasmic dysfunction in males are the antihypertensive and the psychiatric drugs. (See Table 8.4.) Numerous clinical series have reported erectile problems (Pillay, 1976; Bulpitt & Dollern, 1973; Johnson et al., 1966; Newman & Salerno, 1974), decreased libido (Horwitz et al., 1967; Lauer, 1974), and ejaculatory impairment (Hogan et al., 1980; Brown et al., 1972; Horwitz et al., 1967; Bauer et al., 1973; Lauwers et al., 1963; Bulpitt & Dollern, 1973; Prichard et al., 1968) in patients taking methyldopa. The total number of cases in seven reports inquiring about ejaculatory function totals 264 male hypertensives; 11% (29 men) reported ejaculatory inhibition.

Table 8.4. Pharmacological Agents Association with Male Anorgasmia

Lorazepam	Chlorpromazine	Pargyline
Reserpine	Chlorprothexine	Mebanazine
Quanethidine	Mesoridazine	Imipramine
Quanoxan	Fluphenazine	Amitryptiline
Quanoclor	Thiothixine	Chlomipramine
Bethanidine	Perphenazine	Amoxapine
DeBrisoquine	Trifluoperazine	Desipramine
Phenoxybenzamine	Haloperidol	Chlordiazepoxide
Phentolamine	Phenelzine	Alprazolam
Thioridazine		

Antihypertensive Agents

Reserpine is often used as an adjunctive therapy with other drugs for the treatment of moderate to severe hypertension. This drug depletes stores of catecholamines and 5-hydroxytryptamine. Case reports have linked reserpine administration with complaints of impotence (Boyden et al., 1980), decreased libido, and the inability to ejaculate (Bulpitt & Dollern, 1973; Greenbladt & Koch-Weser, 1973; Lauer, 1974; Tuchman & Crumpton, 1955; Girgis et al., 1968).

Guanethidine is a peripheral adrenergic blocking agent used in the treatment of moderate to severe arterial hypertensive tension. In 11 separate studies of the effect of guanethidine on ejaculation, 40% of 307 hypertensives studied reported retarded ejaculation (Vejlsgaard et al., 1967; Prichard et al., 1968; Bauer et al., 1973; Reudy & Davies, 1967; Schinger & Gifford, 1962; Seedat & Pillay, 1966; Brown, 1975: Lowther & Turner, 1963; Bauer et al., 1961; Oats et al., 1965; Page et al., 1961).

Guanoxan and guanoclor, two antihypertensive agents resembling guanethidine, have been reported to be associated with ejaculatory impairment (Vejlsgaard et al., 1967; Reudy & Davies, 1967; Lawrie et al., 1964).

Bethanidine is believed to exert its hypotensive action by inhibiting the release of norepinephrine at sympathetic nerve endings. Bulpitt and Dollern (1973), in a questionnaire study of sexual side effects of antihypertensive agents,

reported that 41% of men on Bethanidine reported ejaculatory failure, as compared to 14% of men on diuretics alone. This difference was statistically significant. Debrisoquine, another agent inhibiting norepinephrine release from sympathetic fibers, has also been reported to be associated with ejaculatory failure (Lauer, 1974).

Phenoxybenzamine and phentolamine are alpha-adrenergic blocking agents with limited utility in the treatment of hypertension. Numerous case reports have indicated that these drugs cause inhibited ejaculation (Vlachakis & Mendlowitz, 1976; Lowen & Puttuck, 1953; Green & Berman, 1954; Caine et al., 1981; Kedia & Persky, 1981). Kedia and Persky (1981) examined postorgasm urine samples and concluded that retrograde ejaculation did not occur. These drugs probably inhibit ejaculation by their action of blocking alpha-adrenergic receptors in the vas deferens and seminal vesicles (Segraves, Madseu, et al., 1985).

To our knowledge, there have been no reports of ejaculatory problems in patients taking diuretics or beta blockers.

Psychiatric Medications

There have been a number of reports of failure of anterograde ejaculation in patients taking antipsychotic drugs (Freyhan, 1961; Shader, 1964; Clein, 1962; Greenberg, 1971; Boleloucky, 1965; Ditman, 1964; Shader, 1972; Blair & Simpson, 1966; Kotin et al., 1976). The antipsychotic agents implicated include thioridazine, chlorpromazine, chlorprothixine, mesoridazine, fluphenazine, thiothixine, perphenazine, trifluoperazine, and haloperidol. The usual case report is that a patient has normal erectile function, has a subjective experience of orgasm, but fails to ejaculate. In many of these cases, the problem ceased when the drug was discontinued and recurred upon readministration of the agent. One clinical series (Kotin et al., 1976) reported that 49% of male patients taking thioridazine experienced severe ejaculatory problems. This effect of the antipsychotics on ejaculation is probably secondary to their strong alpha-adrenergic blocking action (Segraves, 1989).

Although there have been case reports of anorgasmia associated with most of the antidepressants, including phenelzine (Wyatt et al., 1971; Friedman et al., 1978; Hollander & Ban, 1980; Rapp, 1979, Glass, 1981), pargyline (Kohn, 1964; Simpson et al., 1965), mebanazine (Simpson et al., 1965), imipramine (Glass, 1981; Simpson et al., 1965; Couper-Smartt & Rodham, 1973), amitryptoline (Couper-Smartt & Rodham, 1973; Nininger, 1987; Segraves, 1987a), clomipramine (Ananth et al., 1979; Eaton, 1973) amoxapine (Schwartz, 1982), and desipramine (Simpson et al., 1965), there have been relatively few controlled studies of the effects of antidepressants on ejaculatory function. Monteiro et al. (1987), in a double-blind study of the efficacy of chlomipramine in the treatment of obsessive-compulsive disease, reported that 96% of patients developed anorgasmia after two weeks on a dose of 200 mg per day. Harrison et al. (1986; 1985), in a double-blind study, reported that imipramine hydrochloride (200 to 300 mg orally for six weeks) and phenelzine sulfate (60 to 90 mg orally for six weeks) are both associated with anorgasmia. This side effect was more common with phenelzine. It should be noted that there have been no reported cases of anorgasmia caused by bupropion. Gardner and Johnson (1985) have reported that many patients experiencing anorgasmia on other antidepressants can be helped by switching them to bupropion.

There is relatively little information concerning the effects of minor tranquilizers on orgasmic function. Hughes (1964) reported one male patient with ejaculatory inhibition while taking 30 mg of chlordiazepoxide orally per day. Ejaculation returned when the drug was discontinued, and retarded ejaculation recurred upon drug readministration. There have also been reports of anorgasmia with alprazolam (Uhde et al., 1988). One clinician used the orgasm-inhibiting effects of minor tranquilizers in a successful treatment of premature ejaculation with lorazepam (Segraves, 1987b).

DRUGS AND FEMALE ANORGASMIA

Psychiatric Agents

In contrast to the relatively large literature concerning drug effects on male sexual function, that concerning drug effects on female orgasm is sparse, and most of the available work concerns psychiatric drugs (Segraves, 1985). (See Table 8.5.) A number of case reports in the clinical literature suggest that both hetereocyclic and monoamine oxidase inhibitors may cause anorgasmia (Segraves, 1988a). Wyatt et al. (1971) were the first to report female orgasmic difficulty with monoamine oxidase inhibitors. An incidental finding in their study of the usefulness of phenelzine in the treatment of intractable narcolepsy was that two out of the four female patients reported difficulty reaching orgasm on doses of 60–70 mg per day. A number of other investigators have also reported anorgasmia on this drug (Rabkin et al., 1984, 1985; Moss, 1983; Barton, 1979; Pohl, 1983, Lesko et al., 1982; Fraser, 1984; Nurnberg & Levine, 1987). Two other monoamine oxidase inhibitors (Isocarboxazid and Tranylcypromine) have also been reported to cause anorgasmia (Lesko et al., 1982; Gross, 1982). Harrison et al. (1985, 1986), in a double-blind study of the effect of imipramine and phenelzine on sexual function, reported that both drugs impaired the ability of patients to experience orgasm with masturbation. Only phenelzine significantly impaired the ability to achieve coital orgasm.

Couper-Smartt and Rodham (1973) were the first to report female anorgasmia associated

Table 8.5. Drugs Associated with Female Anorgasmia

Phenelzine	Nortriptyline
Isocarboxazid	Thioridazine
Tranylcypromine	Trifluoperazine
Imipramine	Fluphenazine
Chlomipramine	Alprazolam
Amoxapine	Diazepam

with heterocyclic antidepressants. One female patient on 100 mg daily of imipramine developed anorgasmia. There have been other reports of anorgasmia with this drug (Souner, 1983, 1984). There have been several case reports of anorgasmia induced by chlomipramine (Quirk & Einarson, 1983; Beaumont, 1973). Monteiro et al. (1987), in a double-blind study of clomipramine in obsessive-compulsive disorder, found that six out of seven previously orgasmic women became anorgasmic on this drug. Amoxapine (Gross, 1982; Shen, 1982) and nortriptyline (Souner, 1983, 1984) have also been reported to cause anorgasmia. Several lines of indirect evidence suggest that the anorgasmia induced by antidepressants may be related to their serotonergic activity. For example, anorgasmia associated with nortriptyline (Souner, 1984) and tranylcypromine (Descastro, 1985) can be relieved by the coadministration of cyproheptadine (an antiserotonergic drug). It has also been reported that patients who experience anorgasmia on imipramine have remittance of this symptom when a less serotonergic antidepressant such as desipramine is substituted (Souner, 1983). Steele and Howell reported that a 32-year-old female experienced complete anorgasmia on 150 mg per day of oral imipramine. A novel double-blind single-subject trial of cyproheptadine, diphenhydramine, or lactose was begun. Capsules were taken approximately 2 hours prior to initiating sexual activity, and afterward the patient rated ease of orgasm attainment. Cyproheptadine was considered more effective than the other two agents.

Orgasmic dysfunction has been reported with the following neuroleptics: thioridazine (Kotin et al., 1976; Shen & Park, 1982), trifluoperazine (Degen, 1982), and fluphenazine (Ghadirian et al., 1982). There have been no double-blind studies of the effect of antipsychotic drugs on orgasmic capacity.

There is some evidence that minor tranquilizers may cause anorgasmia, including alprazolam (Sangal, 1985). A controlled study by Riley and Riley (1986) demonstrated a dose response relationship between oral diazepam and difficulty of orgasm attainment.

Comment

The evidence reviewed in the preceding two sections has obviously varied widely in quality, and there are glaring gaps in our knowledge base. The deficiencies in our knowledge of drug effects on female sexuality are astounding. Surely, the cardiovascular drugs that interfere with ejaculation must have an effect on female orgasm as well. The clinician treating a female patient complaining of anorgasmia while on antihypertensive drugs does not have a database from which to evaluate this complaint.

Clearly, the preferred method for ascertaining whether or not a given drug has an effect on sexual function is a double-blind drug trial. However, large clinical series can be useful in estimating the frequency of sexual side effects if the investigator has clearly specified the method by which such information was gathered. Single case reports can be useful in drawing attention to previously overlooked side effects and may be the only method of studying rarely occurring side effects. The study by Steele and Howell (1986) is an excellent example of the contribution a case report can make.

ENDOCRINOPATHY AND MALE ORGASMIC DYSFUNCTION

Current evidence suggests that at least two endocrinopathies, hypogonadism and hyperprolactinemia, should be considered in the evaluation of male patients with a complaint with orgasmic dysfunction. Much of our knowledge concerning the effects of androgens on male sexuality comes from the study of castrates and men with severe hypogonadism. Castration (orchidectomy) eliminates the testicular sources of androgen, so the sexual behavior of castrates is a source of information concerning the role of androgens in human sexual behavior. Castration is currently used as a treatment for sex offenders in some countries (Heim, 1981; Heim & Hursch, 1979) and in the treatment of men with testicular neoplasms (Bancroft, 1984). With the removal of androgens, sexual interest and sexual activity typically show a decline in two to three weeks. Ejaculation and the capacity for orgasm also cease. With the introduction of exogenous androgens to hypogonadal men, sexual function in general (and ejaculatory function in particular) returns to normal levels (Shakkebaek et al., 1980; Luisi & Franchi, 1980). Most of the studies of the effects of androgen replacement in hypogonadal men have focused on the effects of androgen replacement on libido and arousability. From these studies, it appears that there is a certain minimal level of androgen necessary to sustain sexual function and that increases in androgen above this level have nonexistent or barely detectable effects on sexual behavior (Davidson et al., 1982). In other words, there is minimal reason to expect that exogenous androgen administration to a man with normal androgen levels and orgasmic dysfunction would be effective.

Hyperprolactinemia (elevated serum prolactin) has been recognized as a cause of diminished libido and erectile disturbances (Segraves, 1988b). This condition, which may be idiopathic, secondary to pituitary adenomas, or secondary to a number of other disease states, may also be associated with ejaculatory failure. In most cases, hyperprolactinemia is associated with low or borderline testotenone levels, but this is not invariably the case. Schwartz et al. (1982) examined prolactin levels in 136 men seeking treatment for sexual dysfunction at the Masters and Johnson Institute between 1976 and 1980. Eight patients were found to have marked hyperprolactinemia. Of these, seven reported severe difficulty with ejaculation. When the condition was effectively treated with surgery, irradiation, and/or bromocriptine, sexual function was restored. Grafeille et al. (1984) also reported a high incidence of ejaculatory difficulty in men with hyperprolactinemia. Hyperprolactinemia and ejaculatory failure have also been noted in patients undergoing hemodialysis for kidney failure. Treatment of the hyperprolactinemia restores orgasmic function (Weizman et al., 1983).

ENDOCRINOPATHIES AND FEMALE ORGASMIC DYSFUNCTION

In subprimate animals, sexual activity is strongly associated with the cyclicity or ovarian hormone production, and sexual activity is often restricted to the time around ovulation (Sanders & Bancroft, 1982). In humans, the role of hormonal factors in libido and orgasmic capacity is less clear. Certainly, there is no evidence that the surgically castrated (ovarectomized) female is incapable of orgasm in the same way as the castrated male may be unable to ejaculate. There is, however, suggestive evidence that androgen levels may be related to sexual drive. Attempts to study the effect of endocrine function on female sexuality can be grouped into three major avenues of inquiry: (1) studies of sexual behavior after menopause; (2) studies of the effects of exogenous hormones on sexual behavior; and (3) studies of the covariation between sexual behavior and cyclic endocrine changes during the menstrual cycle.

A minority of women report some decline in sexual activity associated with menopause (Bachmann et al., 1985). However, it is unclear whether endocrinological factors are responsible for this decline. Sociocultural expectations associated with menopause (Semmens & Semmens, 1984) and psychological distress associated with the symbolic meaning of menopause may be the etiological factors. Supporting this hypothesis, Myers and Morokoff (1985) found that premenopausal and postmenopausal women did not differ in their vaginal photoplethysmographic responses to erotic stimuli. The evidence concerning the effect of surgical menopause (hysterectomy and bilateral oophorectomy) on libido and orgasmic function is also unclear (Utian, 1972; Segraves, 1988b).

Studies of the effects of hormone replacement therapy for menopausal women have yielded inconclusive results concerning the effects of estrogen and suggestive evidence of a beneficial effect of androgens on libido. In a double-blind crossover study, Dennerstein and Burrows (1982) studied the effects of four different hormonal preparations on sexual responsitivity in 49 women (post hysterectomy and bilateral oophorectomy). Estrogen preparations had a significant, positive effect on libido, frequency of orgasm, and vaginal lubrication. Other studies (Studd et al, 1977; Utian, 1972) have not found an effect of estrogen replacement on libido or orgasm attainment. Any effect of estrogen on orgasm attainment may be secondary to its effects on vaginal lubrication and general well being.

There is suggestive evidence that estrogen-androgen preparations may be effective in enhancing libido in postmenopausal women (Burger et al., 1984; Shorr et al., 1938; Studd et al., 1977; Greenblatt et al., 1942). However, other investigators have not found the administration of androgens to sexually dysfunctional women to enhance orgasmic capacity (Mathews et al., 1983; Bancroft et al., 1980).

Sherwin and associates (Sherwin & Gelfant, 1984, 1985; Sherwin, Gelfant, & Brender, 1985) reported a prospective, double-blind crossover study in which surgically menopausal women were given either estrogen, androgen, placebo, or a combination of estrogen and androgen. Measures of sexual desire, arousal, and fantasy were all elevated in the groups receiving androgen. In a subsequent study, Sherwin and Gelfant (1987) investigated sexual behavior in women who had undergone total abdominal hysterectomy and bilateral salpingooophorectomy approximately four years before. One group had been receiving an estrogen-androgen preparation; another group had been receiving estrogen alone; and the third group had remained untreated. Women receiving the estrogen-androgen preparation reported higher levels of sexual desire, sexual arousal, and sexual fantasies than the other two groups. Rates of coitus and orgasm were also higher for the estrogen-androgen group than the other two groups.

A number of investigators have failed to find significant relationships between cyclic changes in estradiol and progesterone and various indices of female sexuality (Schreiner-Engel et al., 1981; Backstrom et al., 1983; Bancroft et al.,

1983; Persky et al., 1978a, 1978b, 1976). However, a number of studies have found relationships between serum androgen levels and various measures of female sexuality (Schreiner-Engel et al., 1981; Bancroft et al., 1983; Persky et al., 1978a).

There is some evidence that hyperprolactinemia may be associated with female sexual dysfunction. Grafeille et al. (1984) studied prolactin levels in 149 women with sexual complaints; 17 of them had prolactin levels higher than 30 mg/ml, and 40% of these women were diagnosed as suffering from "frigidity." Bromocriptine therapy was reported as effective in reversing sexual complaints. This report is difficult to interpret because of uncertainty regarding the authors' use of sexual diagnosis (frigidity). Riley (1984) reported that slightly less than half of female sexual dysfunction patients with plasma prolactin levels above 350 international units per liter benefited from bromocriptine therapy. There have also been reports of hyperprolactinemia being associated with anorgasmia in female patients undergoing hemodialysis (Weizman et al., 1983; Mastrogiacomo et al., 1984; Finkelstein et al., 1978; Procci et al., 1978). Weizman et al. reported that bromocriptine therapy was effective in restoring sexual function.

Comment

The available evidence suggests that ejaculatory impairment is common in severe hyperprolactinemia and severe hypogonadism in males and that routine serum prolactin and testosterone levels should be obtained in men complaining of ejaculatory failure. The evidence concerning the role of androgens and hyperprolactinemia in female anorgasmia is less clear. In premenopausal women, androgen levels are not routinely assessed, and the clinical implications of low androgen in a female with anorgasmia are unclear. In spite of the intriguing results reported by Sherwin et al. (1984, 1985a, 1985b, 1987), androgen-estrogen replacement is not standard practice for postmenopausal women with anorgasmia. It should also be noted that the doses of androgen utilized in these studies exceed physiological levels.

PREMATURE EJACULATION

Theoretically, one might expect premature ejaculation to develop as a symptom in men suffering from irritating lesions in the peripheral or central nervous system. For example, if a man had a premorbid history of normal ejaculatory function and no obvious psychosocial precipitant, one might expect the sudden onset of premature ejaculation to suggest the onset of a new disease process. We could find no data to suggest an association between any organized pathology and premature ejaculation. The one possible exception to this is the report that chomipramine may induce spontaneous orgasm in susceptible patients (McLean et al., 1983).

THE BRAIN AND ORGASMIC DYSFUNCTION

Reduction in sexual behavior and decreased libido have been recorded in association with diffuse brain disease (Mancall et al., 1985) and after cerebral vascular accident (Sadoughi et al., 1971; Fugl-Meyer & Jaasko, 1980; Kalliomaki et al., 1961; Sjogren & Fugl-Meyer, 1982; Allsup-Jackson, 1981). Decreased ejaculatory capacity (Bray et al., 1981) and anorgasmia in female (Monga et al., 1986) have also been reported in stroke patients. In these reports, it is impossible to correlate a given sexual impairment with a given focal lesion. In other words, one cannot predict the sexual symptom experienced from a knowledge of the anatomical site destroyed. Clearly, a number of psychosocial factors, as well as destruction of cerebral pathways involved in sexual behavior, may be implicated. These would obviously include fear of another cerebral vascular incident, physical limitations in movement, loss of self-esteem, and rejection by the partner.

Perhaps our only evidence of a clear relationship between a given brain site and sexual behavior comes from a few case reports of sexual behavior during well-documented temporal lobe (complex, partial, psychomotor) seizures. Erotic sensations and orgasm have been noted as part of the aura of such seizures (Van Reeth et al., 1958), and a temporal lobe seizure has been reported to end in orgasm (Bancaud, 1971).

CONCLUSION

The chapter indicates that a number of medical conditions—such as spinal cord injury, diabetes mellitus, multiple sclerosis, endocrinopathies, pharmacological agents, and surgical procedures—may cause orgasmic disturbance. A careful medical history may reveal a condition that is possibly responsible for a given patient's orgasmic dysfunction. However, most often the clinician will not be able to conclude from this history that the patient's problem is exclusively or even predominantly biologic in origin. With a few exceptions, laboratory procedures to confirm that the medical problem is responsible for the patient's difficulty are unavailable, and medical therapies (with the exception of male endocrinopathies) are also unavailable. Protocols for the medical evaluation of orgasmic disorders have not been developed. Differential diagnosis must be characterized as a combination of art and science; unfortunately, science is a relatively small part of the equation at present.

As professionals who has specialized in the field of human sexuality for over 20 years, writing this chapter has been a sobering experience for us. We were at first surprised and then appalled by how little is known about the effects of disease and medical treatment on human orgasm. We would encounter considerable uncertainty in diagnosing the contributions of medical conditions to male orgasmic dysfunction, but we have close to total ignorance in the medical evaluation of female difficulties with orgasm. We must do more. Both the clinician and the researcher must be aware of the need to ask patients about all aspects of sexual functioning if this area of study is to advance as a science. Spontaneous reports of sexual problems are rare. Physicians and health care providers should take a more aggressive stance and begin to ask the difficult questions.

REFERENCES

Abel, G. G., Becker, J. V., Cunningham-Rathner, J., Mittelman, M., & Primack, M. (1982). Differential diagnosis of impotence in diabetis—the validity of sexual symptomatology. *Neurology and Unodynamics, 1,* 57–69.

Abitol, M. M., & Davenport, J. H. (1974). Sexual dysfunction after therapy for cervical carcinoma. *American Journal of Obstetrics & Gynecology, 119,* 181–189.

Abramovici, H., Weisz, G. M., Timor-Tritsch, I., & Schramek, A. (1971). Male infertility following aortic surgery. *International Journal of Fertility, 16,* 144–146.

Allsup-Jackson, G. (1981). Sexual dysfunction of stroke patients. *Sexuality and Disability, 4,* 161–168.

Ananth, J., Pechnold, T. C., & Steern, N. U. D. (1979). Double blind comparative study of chlomipramine in obsessive neurosis. *Current Therapeutic Research, 25,* 703–709.

Andersen, B. L. (1985). Sexual functioning morbidity among cancer survivors. *Cancer, 55,* 1835–1842.

Andersen, B. L. (1987). Sexual functioning complications in women with gynecologic cancer. *Cancer, 60,* 2123–2128.

Andersen, B. L., & Hacker, N. F. (1983). Psychosexual adjustment following pelvic exenteration. *Obstetrics and Gynecology, 61,* 331–338.

Andersen, B. L., & Hacker, N. F. (1983). Psychosexual adjustment after vulvar surgery. *Obstetrics and Gynecology, 62,* 457–462.

Andersen, B. L., Lachenbruch, P. A., Anderson, B., & de Prosse, C. (1986). Sexual dysfunction and signs of gynecologic cancer. *Cancer, 57,* 1880–1886.

Andersen, B. L., Turnquist, D., LaPolla, J., & Tunner, D. (1988). Sexual functioning after treatment of in situ vulvar cancer: preliminary report. *Obstetrics and Gynecology, 71,* 15–19.

Aso, R., & Yasutomi, M. (1974). Urinary and sexual disturbances following radical surgery for rectal cancer and pudendal nerve block as a countermeasure for urinary disturbance. *American Journal of Proctology, 25,* 60–74.

Bachman, G. A., Leiblum, S. R., Sandler, B., Ainsley, W., Narcessian, R., Shelden, R., & Hymans, H. N. (1985). Correlates of sexual desire in postmenopausal women. *Maturitas, 7,* 211–216.

Backstrom, T., Sanders, D., Leask, R., Davidson, D., Warner, P., & Bancroft, J. (1983). Mood, sexuality, hormones, and the menstrual cycle. II: Hormone levels and their relationship to the premenstrual syndrome. *Psychosomatic Medicine, 45,* 503–507.

Bancaud, J. (1971). Paroxysmal sexual manifestations and temporal epilepsy. *Electroencephalograph Clinical Neurophysiology, 30,* 371–390.

Bancroft, J. (1983). *Human sexuality and its problems.* Edinburgh, UK: Churchill Livingstone.

Bancroft, J. C. (1984). Hormones and human sexual behavior. *Journal of Sex and Marital Therapy, 10,* 3–21.

Bancroft, J., Davidson, D., Warner, P., & Tyrer, G. (1980). Androgens and sexual behavior in women using oral contraceptives. *Clinical Endocrinology, 12,* 327–340.

Bancroft, J., Sanders, D., Davidson, D., & Warner, P. (1983). Mood, sexuality, hormones and the menstrual cycle. III: Sexuality and the role of androgens. *Psychosomatic Medicine, 45,* 509–516.

Barton, T. L. (1979). Orgasmic inhibition by phenelzine. *American Journal of Psychiatry, 136,* 1616–1617.

Bauer, G. E., Croll, F. J. T., & Goldrick, R. B. (1961). Guanethidine in the treatment of hypertension. *British Medical Journal, 2,* 410–415.

Bauer, G. E., Hull, R. D., & Stokes, G. S. (1973). The reversibility of side-effects of guanethidine therapy. *Medical Journal Australia, 1,* 930–933.

Bauer, J. J., Gelernt, I. M., Salky, B., & Kreel, I. (1983). Sexual dysfunction following proctocolectomy for benign disease of the colon and rectum. *Annals of Surgery, 197,* 363–367.

Beaumont, G. (1973). Sexual side-effect of clomipramine (anafranil). *International Journal of Medical Research, 1,* 469–472.

Bell, C. (1972). Autonomic nervous control of reproduction: Circulatory and other factors. *Pharmacological Reviews, 24,* 657–736.

Bennett, A. H. (1982). Organic causes of impotence: Surgical. In A. H. Bennett (Ed.), *Management of male impotence* (pp. 135–142). Baltimore: Williams and Wilkins.

Berard, E. J. J. (1989). The sexuality of spinal cord injured women: Physiology and pathophysiology: A review. *Paraplegia, 27,* 99–112.

Bergman, B., Nilsson, S., & Petersen, I. (1979). The effect on erection and orgasm of cystectomy, prostatectomy, and vesiculectomy for cancer of the bladder: A clinical and electromyographic study. *British Journal of Urology, 51,* 114–120.

Bernardinis, G. D., Tuscano, D., Negro, P., Flati, G., Flati, D., Bianchini, A., & Carboni, M. (1981).

Sexual dysfunction in males following extensive colonectal surgery. *International Surgery, 66,* 133–135.

Blair, J. H., Simpson, G. M. (1966). Effects of antipsychotic drugs on reproductive function. *Diseases of the Nervous System, 27,* 645–647.

Blumer, D., & Walker, E. A. (1975). The neural basis of sexual behavior. In D. F. Benson, & D. Blumer (Eds.), *Psychiatric aspects of neurologic disease* (199–217). New York: Grume & Stratton.

Boleloucky, Z. (1965). Chlorpromazine inhibition of ejaculation. *Activitas Nervosa Superior* (Praha). 7, 145.

Bors, E., & Comarr, A. E. (1960). Neurological disturbances of sexual function with special reference to 529 patients with spinal cord injury. *Urological Review, 10,* 191–222.

Boyden, T. W., Nugent, C. A., & Ogihara, T. (1980). Reserpine hydrochorothiazide and pituitary gonadal hormones in hypertensive patients. *European Journal of Clinical Pharmacology, 17,* 329–332.

Bracken, R. B., & Johnson, D. E. (1976). Sexual function and fecundity after treatment for testicular tumors. *Urology, 7,* 35–38.

Bray, G. P., DeFrank, R. S., Wolfe, T. L. (1981). Sexual functioning in stroke survivors. *Archives Physical Medical Rehabilitation, 62,* 286–288.

Brindley, G. S. (1980). Electroejaculation and fertility of paraplegic men. *Sexuality and Disability, 3,* 3. 223–229.

Brindley, G. S. (1981). Reflex ejaculation under vibratory stimulation in paraplegic men. *Paraplegia, 19,* 299–302.

Brindley, G. S. (1984). The fertility of men with spinal injuries. *Paraplegia, 22,* 337–348.

Brouillette, J. N., Pryor, E., & Fox, T. A. (1981). Evaluation of sexual dysfunction in the female following rectal resection and intestinal stoma. *Diseases of the Colon and Rectum, 24,* 96–102.

Broun, R. S., Haddox, J., Posada, A., & Rubio, A. (1972). Social and psychological adjustment following pelvic exenteration. *American Journal of Obstetrics & Gynecology, 114,* 162–171.

Brown, W. J. (1975). The use of guanethidine and hydrochlorothiazide in the long term treatment of essential hypertension. *Current Therapy and Research, 17,* 544–554.

Brown, J., Davies, D. L., & Ferriss, J. B. (1972). Comparison of surgery and prolonged spironlactone therapy in patients with hypertension, aldosterone excess, and low plasma renin. *British Medical Journal, 1,* 729–734.

Bulpitt, C. J., Dollern, C. T. (1973). Side-effect of hypotensive agents evaluated by a self-administered questionnaire. *British Medical Journal, 3,* 485–490.

Burger, H. G., Hailes, J., Menelaus, M., Nelson, J., Hudson, B., & Balazs, N. (1984). The management of persistent menopausal symptoms with oestradiol-testosterone implants—clinical, lipid, and hormonal results. *Maturitas, 6,* 351–358.

Burnham, W. R., Lennard-Jones, J. E., & Brooke, B. N. (1977). Sexual problems among married ileostomists. *Gut, 18,* 673–677.

Caine, M., Perlman, S., & Shapiro, A. (1981). Phenoxyhenzamine for benign prostatic obstruction. *Urology, 17,* 542–546.

Capone, M. A., Good, R. S., Westie, K. S., & Jacobson, A. F. (1980). Psychosocial rehabilitation of gynecologic oncology patients. *Archives of Physical Medicine and Rehabilitation, 61,* 128–132.

Clein, L. (1962). Thioridazine and ejaculation. *British Medical Journal, 2,* 548–549.

Cole, T. M. (1975). Sexuality and physical disabilities. *Archives of Sexual Behavior, 4,* 4, 389–403.

Comarr, A. E. (1970). Sexual function among patients with spinal cord injury. *Urology Internationalis, 25,* 134–168.

Comarr, A. E., Vigue, M. (1978). Sexual counseling among male and female patients with spinal cord and/or cauda equina injury. *American Journal of Physical Medicine, 57,* 5, 215–227.

Corman, M. L., Veidenheimer, M. C., & Coller, J. A. (1978). Impotence after proctectomy for inflammatory disease of the bowel. *Disease of the Colon and Rectum, 21,* 418–419.

Couper-Smartt, T. D., & Rodham, R. (1973). A technique for surveying side-effects of tricyclic drugs with reference to reported sexual effects. *Journal International Medicine Research, 1,* 473–476.

Cunsolo, A., Bragaglia, R. B., Petrucci, C., Poggioli, G., & Gozzetti, G. (1989). Survival and complications after radical surgery for carcinoma of the rectum. *Journal of Surgical Oncology. 41,* 27–32.

Davidson, J. M., Kwan, M., & Greenleaf, W. (1982). Hormonal replacement and sexuality in men. *Clinics in Endocrinology and Metabolism, 11,* 599–623.

Decker, W. H., & Schwartzman, E. (1962). Sexual function following treatment for carcinoma of the cervix. *American Journal of Obstetrics & Gynecology, 83,* 401–405.

Degen, K. (1982). Sexual dysfunction in women using major tranquilizers. *Psychosomatics, 23,* 959–961.

Dempsey, G. M., Buchsbaum, H. J., & Morrison, J. (1975). Psychosocial adjustment to pelvic exenteration. *Gynecological Oncology, 3,* 325–334.

Dennerstein, L., Burrows, G. D. (1982). Hormone replacement therapy and sexuality in women. *Clinics in Endocrinology and Metabolism, 11,* 661–679.

Decastro, R. M. (1985). Reversal of MAOI-induced anorgasmia with cyproheptadine. *American Journal of Psychiatry, 147,* 783.

DiSala, P. J., Creasman, W. T., & Rich, W. M. (1979). An alternative approach to early cancer of the vulva. *American Journal of Obstetrics and Gynecology, 133,* 825–829.

Ditman, K. S. (1964). Inhibition of ejaculation by chloroprothixine. *American Journal of Psychiatry, 120,* 1004–1005.

Donovan, M. J., & O'Hara, E. T. (1960). Sexual function following surgery for ulcerative colitis. *New England Journal of Medicine, 262,* 719–720.

Eaton, H. (1973). Chlomipramine (Anafranil) in the treatment of premature ejaculation. *Journal of Clinical Medical Research, 1,* 432–434.

Ellenberg, M. (1971). Impotence in diabetes: The neurologic factor. *Annals of Internal Medicine, 75,* 213–229.

Ellenberg, M. (1977). Sexual aspects of the female diabetic. *Mt. Sinai Journal of Medicine, 44,* 495–500.

Ellenberg, M., & Weber, H. (1966). Retrograde ejaculation in diabetic neuropathy. *Annals of Internal Medicine, 65,* 1237–1246.

Fairburn, C. (1981). The sexual problems of diabetic men. *British Journal of Hospital Medicine, 12,* 484–491.

Fairburn, C. G., McCulloch, D. K., & Wu, F. U. (1982a). The effects of diabetes on male sexual function. *Clinics in Endocrinology and Metabolism, 11,* 749–767.

Fairburn, C. G., Wu, F. C. W., McCulloch, D. K., Borsay, D. Q., Ewing, D. J., Clarke, B. F., & Bancroft, J. H. J. (1982b). The clinical features of diabetic impotence: A preliminary study. *British Journal of Psychiatry, 140,* 447–452.

Finkelstein, F. O., & Steele, T. E. (1978). Sexual dysfunction and chronic renal failure. A psychosocial study of 77 patients. *Dialysis and Transplantation, 7,* 877–878.

Flanigan, D. P., Schuler, J. J., Keifer, T., Schwartz, J. A., & Lim, L. T. (1982). Elimination of iatrogenic impotence and improvement of sexual function after aortoiliac revascularization. *Archives of Surgery, 117,* 544–550.

Fraser, A. R. (1984). Sexual dysfunction following antidepressant drug therapy. *Journal of Clinical Psychopharmacology, 3,* 62–63.

Freyhan, F. A. (1961). Loss of ejaculation during mellaril treatment. *American Journal of Psychiatry, 118,* 171–172.

Friedman, S., Kantor, J., & Sobel, S. (1978). A follow-up study on the chemotherapy of neurodenmatitis with a monoamine oxidase inhibitor. *Journal of Nervous and Mental Diseases, 166,* 349–357.

Fugl-Meyer, A. R., & Jaasko, L. (1980). Post-stroke hemiplegia and sexual intercourse. *Scandinavian Journal of Rehabilitation Medicine, 7,* 158–166.

Gardner, E. A., & Johnson, A. (1985). Bupropion—an antidepressant without sexual pathophysiological action. *Journal of Clinical Psychopharmacology, 5,* 24–29.

Geiger, R. C. (1979). Neurophysiology of sexual response in spinal cord injury. *Sexuality and Disability, 2, 4,* 257–266.

Ghadirian, A. M., Chouinard, G., & Annable, L. (1982). Sexual dysfunction and plasma prolactin levels in neuroleptic-treated schizophrenic outpatients. *Journal of Nervous Mental Diseases, 170,* 463–467.

Girgis, S. M., Etriby, A., & El-Hefnawy, H. (1968). Aspermia: A survey of 49 cases. *Fertility and Sterility, 19,* 580–588.

Glass, R. M. (1981). Ejaculatory impairment from both phenelzine and imipramine with tinnitus from phenelzine. *Journal of Clinical Psychopharmacology, 1,* 152–164.

Grafeille, N., Joutard, J. C., & Ruffie, A. (1984). Plasma prolactin levels in 300 cases of sexual disorders. In R. T. Segraves & E. J. Haeberle (Eds.), *Emerging dimensions of sexology.* New York: Praeger.

Green, M., & Berman, S. (1954). Failure of ejaculation produced by dibenzyline. *Connecticut State Medical Journal, 18,* 30–34.

Greenberg, H. R. (1971). Inhibition of ejaculation by chlorpromazine. *Journal of Nervous and Mental Diseases, 152,* 364–366.

Greenbıadt, D. J., & Koch-Weser, J. (1973). Gynecomastia and impotence complications of spironolactone therapy. *Journal of the American Medical Association, 233,* 82.

Greenblatt, R. B., Mortara, F., & Torpin, R. (1942). Sexual libido in the female. *American Journal of Obstetrics and Gynecology, 44,* 658–663.

Greene, L. F., & Kelalis, P. P. (1968). Retrograde

ejaculation of semen due to diabetic neuropathy. *Journal of Urology, 98,* 693–696.

Greene, L. F., Kelalis, P. P., & Weeks, R. E. (1963). Retrograde ejaculation of semen due to diabetic neuropathy. *Fertility and Sterility, 14,* 617–625.

Griffith, E. R., Tomko, M. A., & Timms, R. J. (1973). Sexual function in spinal cord-injured patients: A review. *Archives of Physical Medicine and Rehabilitation, 54,* 539–543.

Griffith, E. R., & Trieschmann, R. B. (1975). Sexual functioning in women with spinal cord injury, *Archives of Physical Medicine and Rehabilitation, 56,* 25—40.

Gross, M. D. (1982). Reversal by bethanechol of sexual dysfunction caused by anticholinergic antidepressants. *American Journal of Psychiatry, 139,* 1193–1194.

Gruner, O. P. N., Naas, R., Fretheim, B., & Gjone, E. (1977). Marital status and sexual adjustment after colectomy. *Scandinavian Journal of Gastroenterology, 12,* 193–197.

Gunterberg, B., & Petersen, I. (1976). Sexual function after major resection of the sacrum with bilateral or unilateral sacrifice of sacral nerves. *Fertility and Sterility, 27,* 1146–1153.

Hallbrook, T., & Holmquist, B. (1970). Sexual disturbances following dissection of the aorta and the common iliac arteries. *Journal of Cardiovascular Surgery, 11,* 255–260.

Hargreave, T. B., & Stephenson, T. P. (1977). Potency and prostatectomy. *British Journal of Urology, 49,* 683–688.

Harrison, W. M., Rabkin, J. G., Ehrhardt, A. A., Stewart, J. W., McGrath, P. J., Ross, D., & Quitkin, F. M. (1986). Effects of antidepressant medication on sexual function: A controlled study. *Journal of Clinical Psychopharmacology, 6,* 144–149.

Harrison, W. M., Stewart, J., Ehrhardt, A. A., Rabkin, J., McGrath, P., Liebowitz, M., & Quitkin, F. M. (1985). A controlled study of the effects of antidepressants on sexual function. *Psychopharmacology Bulletin, 21,* 85–88.

Heath, R. G. (1963). Electrical self-stimulation of the brain in man. *American Journal of Psychiatry, 120,* 571–577.

Heath, R. G. (1972). Pleasure and brain activity in man: Deep and surface electroenaephalograms during orgasm. *Journal of Nervous and Mental Diseases, 154,* 3–18.

Heath, R. G. (1975). Brain function and behavior. *Journal of Nervous and Mental Diseases, 160,* 159–175.

Heim, N. (1981). Sex behavior of castrated sex offenders. *Archives of Sexual Behavior, 10,* 11–19.

Heim, N., & Hursch, C. J. (1979). Castration for sex offenders: Treatment or punishment? A review and critique of recent European literature. *Archives of Sexual Behavior, 8,* 281–305.

Hellstrom, P. (1988). Urinary and sexual dysfunction after rectosigmoid surgery. *Annales Chirurgiae et Gynaecologiae, 77,* 51–56.

Hogan, M. J., Wallin, J. D., & Baer, R. M. (1980). Antihypertensive therapy and male sexual dysfunction. *Psychosomatics, 12,* 234–237.

Hollander, M. H., & Ban, T. A. (1980). Ejaculatio retarda due to phenelzine. *Psychiatry Journal of the University of Ottawa, 4,* 233–234.

Holtgrewe, H. L., & Valk, W. L. (1964). Late results of transurethral prostatectomy. *Journal of Urology, 92,* 51–55.

Horwitz, D., Pettinger, W. A., & Gruis, H. (1967). Effects of methyldopa in fifty hypertensive patients. *Clinical Pharmacology and Therapeutics, 8,* 224–234.

House, W. C., & Pendleton, L. (1988). Sexual functioning in male diabetics with impotence problems. *Sexual and Marital Therapy, 3,* 205–212.

Hughes, J. M. (1964). Failure to ejaculate with chlordiazepoxide. *American Journal of Psychiatry, 121,* 610–611.

Jensen, S. B. (1981). Diabetic sexual dysfunction: A comparative study of 160 insulin treated diabetic men and women and an age-matched control group. *Archives of Sexual Behavior, 10,* 493–504.

Jensen, S. B. (1985). Sexual dysfunction in younger insulin-treated diabetic females. *Diabetes and Metabolism (Paris) 11,* 278–282.

Jensen, S. B. (1986). The natural history of sexual dysfunction in diabetic women. *Acta Medica Scandinavica, 219,* 73–78.

Johnson, P., Kitchin, A. H., & Lowther, C. P. (1966). Treatment of hypertension with methyldopa. *British Medical Journal, 1,* 133–137.

Kalliomaki, J. L., Markkanen, T. K., & Mustonen, V. A. (1961). Sexual behavior after cerebral vascular accident: Study on patients below age 60 years. *Fertility and Sterility, 12,* 156–158.

Kaplan, H. S. (1983). The comprehensive evaluation. In H. S. Kaplan (Ed.), *The evaluation of sexual disorders* (pp. 199–272). New York: Brunner/Mazel.

Karacan, I. (1980). Diagnosis of erectile impotence in diabetes mellitus. *Annals of Internal Medicine, 92* (part 2), 334–337.

Kaufman, S. A. (1983). The gynecological evaluation

of female orgasm disorders. In H. S. Kaplan (Ed.), *The evaluation of sexual disorders: Psychological and medical aspects* (pp. 117–121). New York: Brunner/Mazel.

Kedia, K. R., Markland, C., & Fraley, E. E. (1975). Sexual function following high retroperitoneal lymphadenectomy. *Journal of Urology, 114,* 237–239.

Kedia, K. R., Markland, C., & Fraley, E. E. (1977). Sexual function after high retroperitoneal lymphadenectomy. *Urologic Clinics of North America, 4,* 523–528.

Kedia, K. R., & Perskly, L. (1981). Effect of phenoxybenzamine (Dibenzyline) on sexual function in man. *Urology, 18,* 620–622.

Kleeman, F. J. (1970). The physiology of the internal urinary sphincter. *Journal of Urology, 104,* 549–554.

Kohn, R. M. (1964). Nocturnal orthostatic syncope in pargyline therapy. *Journal of the American Medical Association, 187,* 229.

Kolodny, R. C. (1971). Sexual dysfunction in diabetic females. *Diabetes, 20,* 557–559.

Kolodny, R. C., Kahn, C. B., Goldstein, H. H., & Barnett, D. M. (1974). Sexual dysfunction in diabetic men. *Diabetes, 23,* 306–309.

Kotin, J., Wilber, D. E., & Verburg, D. (1976). Thioridazine and sexual dysfunction. *American Journal of Psychiatry, 133,* 82–85.

Lauer, M. C. (1974). Sexual behavior patterns in male hypertensives. *Australian–New Zealand Journal of Medicine, 4,* 29–31.

Lauwers, P., Verstraete, M., & Joossen, J. V. (1963). Methyldopa in the treatment of hypertensives. *British Medical Journal, 1,* 295–300.

Lawrie, T. D. V., Lorimer, A. R., & McAlpine, D. S. G. (1964). Clinical trial and pharmacological study of compound 1029 ("vatensol"). *British Medical Journal, 1,* 402–406.

Lesko, L. M., Stotland, N. L., & Segraves, R. T. (1982). Three cases of female anorgasmia associated with MAOIs. *American Journal of Psychiatry, 139,* 1353–1354.

Lilius, H. G., Valtonen, E., & Wikstrom, J. (1976a). Sexual problems in patients suffering from multiple sclerosis. *Scandinavian Journal of Social Medicine, 4,* 41–44.

Lilius, H. G., Valtonen, E. J., & Wikstrom, J. (1976b). Sexual problems in patients suffering from multiple sclerosis. *Journal of Chronic Diseases, 29,* 643–647.

Lowen, S., & Puttuck, S. L. (1953). Anti-ejaculatory effect of sympatholytic ganglionytic and spasmo-

lytic drugs. *Journal of Pharmacology and Experimental Therapeutics, 107,* 379–384.

Lowther, C. P., & Turner, R. W. (1963). Guanethidine in the treatment of hypertension. *British Medical Journal, 2,* 776–781.

Luisi, M., & Franchi, F. (1980). Double-blind group comparitive study of testosterone undeconoate and mesterolone in hypogonadal male patients. *Journal of Endocrinologic Investigation, 3,* 305–308.

Lundberg, P. O. (1978). Sexual dysfunction in patients with multiple sclerosis. *Sexuality and Disability, 1,* 218–222.

Luttge, W. B. (1971). The role of gonadal hormones in the sexual behavior of the rhesus monkey and human: A literature survey. *Archives of Sexual Behavior, 1,* 61–68.

Maclean, J. D., Sorsythe, R. G., & Kapkin, I. A. (1983). Unusual side-effects of domipramine associated with yawning. *Canadian Journal of Psychiatry, 28,* 569–570.

MacLean, P. D. (1975). Brain mechanisms of primal sexual functions and related behavior. In M. Sandler & G. L. Gessa (Eds.), *Sexual behavior: Pharmacology and biochemistry* (pp. 1–11). New York: Raven Press.

Mancall, E. L., Alonso, R. J., & Marlowe, W. B. (1985). Sexual dysfunction in neurological disease. In R. T. Segraves & H. W. Schoenberg (Eds.), *Diagnosis and treatment of erectile disturbances* (pp. 65–85). New York: Plenum.

Mastrogiacomo, I., DeBesi, L., Serafini, E. Zussa, S., Zucchetta, P., Romagnoli, G. F., Sadoriti, E., Dean, P., Ronco, C., & Adami, A. (1984). Hyperprolactinemia and sexual disturbances among uremic women on hemodialysis. *Nephron, 37,* 195–199.

Mathews, A., Whitehead, A., & Kellet, J. (1983). Psychological and hormonal factors in the treatment of female sexual dysfunctions. *Psychological Medicine, 13,* 83–92.

May, A. G., DeWeese, J., & Rob, C. G. (1969). Changes in sexual function following operation of the abdominal aorta. *Surgery, 65,* 41–47.

McCulloch, D. K., Young, R. J., Prescott, R. J., Campbell, I. W., & Clarke, B. F. (1984). The natural history of impotence in diabetic men. *Diabetologia, 26,* 437–440.

Metcalf, A. M., Dozois, R. R., & Kelly, K. A. (1988). Sexual function in women after proctocolectomy. *Annals of Surgery, 204,* 624–627.

Metz, P., Frimodt-Moller, C., & Mathiesen, F. R. (1983). Erectile function before and after reconstructive arterial surgery in men with occlusive arterial leg disease. *Scandinavian Journal of Thoracic and Cardiovascular Surgery, 17*, 45–50.

Mills, L. C. (1976). Sexual disorders in the diabetic patient. In W. W. Oaks, G. A. Melchiode, & I. Ficher (Eds.), *Sex and the life cycle* (pp. 163–174). New York: Grune & Stratton.

Moller-Nielsen, C., Lundhus, E., Moller-Madsen, B., Norgaard, J. P., Simonsen, O. H., Hansen, S. L., & Birkler, N. (1985). Sexual life following minimal and total transurethral prostatic resection. *Urologia Internationalis, 40*, 3–4.

Monga, T. N., Lawson, J. S., & Inglis, J. (1986). Sexual dysfunction in stroke patients. *Archives of Physical Medicine and Rehabilitation, 67*, 19–22.

Monteiro, W. O., Noshirvani, H. F., Marks, I. M., & Lelliott, P. T. (1987). Anorgasmia from chlomipramine in obsessive-compulsive disorder: A controlled trial. *British Journal of Psychiatry, 151*, 107–112.

Moss, H. B. (1983). More cases of anorgasmia after MAOI treatment. *American Journal of Psychiatry, 140*, 266.

Moth, I., Andreasson, B., Jensen, S. B., & Bock, J. E. (1983). Sexual function and somatopsychic reactions after vulvectomy. *Danish Medical Bulletin, 30*, 27–30.

Myers, L., & Morokoff, P. (1985). Physiological and subjective sexual arousal in pre and post menopausal women. Poster presented at the meeting of the American Psychological Association, Los Angeles.

Narayan, P., Lange, P. H., & Fraley, E. E. (1982). Ejaculation and fertility after extended retropeutoneal lymph node dissection for testicular cancer. *Journal of Urology, 127*, 685–687.

Neal, D. E. (1966). The effects on pelvic visceral function of anal sphincter ablating and anal sphincter preserving operations for cancer of the lower part of the rectum and for benign colo-rectal disease. *Annals of the Royal College of Surgeons of England, 66*, 7–13.

Neuman, A. S., & Bertelson, A. D. (1986). Sexual dysfunction in diabetic women. *Journal of Behavioral Medicine, 9*, 261–270.

Newman, R. J., & Salerno, H. R. (1974). Sexual dysfunction due to methyldopa. *British Medical Journal, 4*, 106.

Nijman, J. M., Jager, S., Boer, P. W., Kremer, J., Oldhoff, J., & Kopps, H. S. (1982). The treatment of ejaculation disorders after retroperitoneal lymph node dissection. *Cancer, 50*, 2967–2971.

Nininger, T. E. (1987). Inhibition of ejaculation by amitryptiline. *American Journal of Psychiatry, 135*, 750–751.

Nurnberg, H. G., & Levine, P. E. (1987). Spontaneous remission of MAO-I-induced anorgasmia. *American Journal of Psychiatry, 144*, 805–807.

Oats, J. A., Seligmann, A. W., & Clark, M. A. (1965). The relative efficacy of guanethidine, methyldopa, and pargyline as antihypertensive agents. *New England Journal of Medicine, 273*, 729–734.

O'Hoy, K. M., & Tang, G. W. K. (1985). Sexual function following treatment for carcinoma of the cervix. *Journal of Psychosomatic Obstetrics and Gynecology, 4*, 51–58.

Ohshiro, T., & Kosaki, G. (1984). Sexual function after aorto-iliac vascular reconstruction. *Journal of Cardiovascular Surgery, 25*, 47–50.

Page, I. H., Hurley, R. E., & Dustan, H. P. (1961). The prolonged treatment of hypertension with guanethidine. *Journal of the American Medical Association, 175*, 543–549.

Penfield, W., & Rasmussen, T. (1950). *The cerebral cortex of man.* New York: Macmillan.

Persky, H., Channey, N., Lief, H. I., O'Brien, C. P., Miller, W. R., & Strauss, D. (1978a). The relationship of plasma estradiol level to sexual behavior in young women. *Psychosomatic Medicine, 40*, 523–535.

Persky, H., Lief, H. I., Strauss, D., Miller, W. R., & O'Brien, C. P. (1978b). Plasma testosterone level and sexual behavior of couples. *Archives of Sexual Behavior, 7*, 157–173.

Persky, H., O'Brien, C. P., & Kahn, M. A. (1976). Reproductive hormone levels, sexual activity and moods during the menstrual cycle. *Psychosomatic Medicine, 38*, 62–63.

Pillay, V. K. G. (1976). Some side-effects of alpha-methyldopa. *South African Medical Journal, 50*, 625–626.

Pohl, R. (1983). Anorgasmia caused by MAOIs. *American Journal of Psychiatry, 140*, 310.

Prichard, B. N. C., Johnston, A. W., & Hill, I. D. (1968). Bethanidine, guanethidine, and methyldopa in treatment of hypertension: A written patient comparison. *British Medical Journal, 1*, 135–144.

Procci, W. R., Hoffman, K. I., & Chatterjee, S. N. (1978). Persistent sexual dysfunction following renal transplantation. *Dialysis and Transplantation, 7*, 981–984.

Quirk, K. C., & Einarson, T. R. (1983). Sexual dysfunction and clomipramine. *Canadian Journal of Psychiatry, 27,* 228–231.

Rabkin, J., Quitkin, F., Harrison, W., Tricamo, E., & McGrath, P. (1984). Adverse reactions to meonoamine oxidase inhibitors. Part I. A comparative study. *Journal of Clinical Psychopharmacology, 4,* 270–278.

Rabkin, J., Quitkin, F., McGrath, P., Harrison, W., & Tricamo, E. (1985). Adverse reactions to monoamine oxidase inhibitors. Part II. Treatment correlates and clinical management. *Journal of Clinical Psychopharmacology, 5,* 2–9.

Rand, M. J., & Nott, M. W. (1988). Basic neuropharmacology in sexology. In JMA Sitsen (Ed.), *Handbook of sexology* (Vol. 6): *The pharmacology and endocrinology of sexual function* (pp. 1–31). Amsterdam: Elsevier.

Rapp, M. S. (1979). Two cases of ejaculatory impairment related to phenelzine. *American Journal of Psychiatry, 136,* 1200–1201.

Reckler, J. M. (1983). The urologic evaluation of ejaculatory disorders (male orgasm disorders, RE and PE). In H. S. Kaplan (Ed.), *The evaluation of sexual disorders: Psychological and medical aspects.* (pp. 139–149). New York: Brunner/Mazel.

Reudy, J., & Davies, R. O. (1967). A comparative clinical trial of guanoxan and guanethidine in essential hypertension. *Clinical Pharmacology and Therapeutics, 8,* 38–47.

Riley, A. J. (1984). Prolactin and female sexual function. *British Journal of Sexual Medicine, 11,* 14–17.

Riley, A. J., & Riley, E. J. (1986). The effect of single dose diazepam on female sexual response induced by masturbation. *Sexual and Marital Therapy, 1,* 49–53.

Rivard, D. J. (1982). Anatomy, physiology, and neurophysiology of male sexual function. In A. H. Bennett (Ed.), *Management of male Impotence* (pp. 1–25). Baltimore: Williams and Wilkins.

Robinson, B. W., & Mishkin, M. (1966). Ejaculation evoked by stimulation of the preoptic area in monkey. *Physiology and Behavior, 1,* 264–272.

Robinson, P. M. (1969). A cholinergic component in the innervation of the longitudinal smooth muscle of the guinea pig vas deferens. *Journal of Cell Biology, 41,* 462–476.

Rose, S. S. (1953). An investigation into sterility after lumbar ganglionectomy. *British Medical Journal, 1,* 247–250.

Sabri, S., & Cotton, L. T. (1971). Sexual function following aortoiliac reconstruction. *Lancet, 2,* 1218–1219.

Sadoughi, W., Leshner, M., & Fine, H. L. (1971). Sexual adjustment in chronically ill and physically disabled population: Pilot study. *Archives of Physical Medicine and Rehabilitation, 52,* 311–317.

Sanders, D., & Bancroft, J. (1982). Hormones and the sexuality of women—the menstrual cycle. *Clinics in Endocrinology and Metabolism, 11,* 639–659.

Sangal, R. (1985). Inhibited female orgasm as a side-effect of alprazolam. *American Journal of Psychiatry, 142,* 1223–1224.

Schinger, A., & Gifford, R. W. (1962). Guanethidine, a new antihypertensive agent: Experience in the treatment of patients with severe hypertension. *Mayo Clinic Proceedings, 37,* 100–108.

Schoenberg, H. W. (1985). Other causes of erectile impotence. In R. T. Segraves & H. H. Schoenberg (Eds.), *Diagnosis and treatment of erectile disturbances* (pp. 159–164). New York: Plenum.

Schover, L. R., Evans, R., & von Eschenbach, A. C. (1986). Sexual rehabilitation and male radical cystectomy. *Journal of Urology, 136,* 1015–1017.

Schover, L. R., Evans, R. B., & von Eschenbach, A. C. (1987). Sexual rehabilitation in a cancer center: Diagnosis and outcome in 384 consultations. *Archives of Sexual Behavior, 16,* 445–461.

Schover, L. R., Fife, M., & Gershenson, D. M. (1989). Sexual dysfunction and treatment for early stage cervical cancer. *Cancer, 63,* 204–212.

Schover, L. R., Gonzales, M., & von Eschenbach, A. C. (1986). Sexual and marital relationships after radiotherapy for seminoma. *Urology, 17,* 117–123.

Schover, L. R., & Jensen, S. B. (1988). *Sexuality and chronic illness.* New York: Guilford.

Schover, L. R., & von Eschenbach, A. C. (1985). Sexual and marital relationships after treatment for nonseminomatous testicular cancer. *Urology, 25,* 251–255.

Schover, L. R., & von Eschenbach, A. C. (1985). Sexual function and female radical cystectomy: A case series. *Journal of Urology, 134,* 465–468.

Schreiner-Engel, P., Schiavi, R. C., Smith, H., & White, D. (1981). Sexual arousability and the menstrual cycle. *Psychosomatic Medicine, 43,* 199–214.

Schreiner-Engel, P. Schiavi, R. C., Vietorisz, D., Eichel, J., & Smith, H. (1985). Diabetes and female sexuality: A comparative study of women in relationships. *Journal of Sex and Marital Therapy, 11,* 165–175.

Schreiner-Engel, P., Schiavi, R. C., Vietorisz, D., &

Smith, H. (1987). The differential impact of diabetes type on female sexuality. *Journal of Psychosomatic Research, 31*, 23–33.

Schwartz, G. (1982). Case report of inhibition of ejaculation and retrograde ejaculation as a side-effect of amoxapine. *American Journal of Psychiatry, 139*, 233–234.

Schwartz, M. F., Bauman, J. E., & Masters, W. H. (1982). Hyperprolactinemia and sexual disorders in men. *Biological Psychiatry, 17*, 861–876.

Seedat, Y. K., & Pillay, V. K. G. (1966). Further experience with guanethidine—a clinical assessment of 103 patients. *South African Medical Journal, 40*, 140–143.

Segraves, R. T. (1977). Pharmacological agents causing sexual dysfunction. *Journal of Sex and Marital Therapy, 3*,3, 157–176.

Segraves, R. T. (1985). Psychiatric drugs and orgasm in the human female. *Journal of Psychosomatic Obstetrics and Gynaecology, 4*, 125–128.

Segraves, R. T. (1987a). Reversal of amitryptoline induced anorgasmia by bethanechol. *American Journal of Psychiatry, 144*, 1243.

Segraves, R. T. (1987b). Treatment of premature ejaculation with lorazepam. *American Journal of Psychiatry, 144*, 1240.

Segraves, R. T. (1988a). Psychiatric drugs and inhibited female orgasm. *Journal of Sex Education and Marital Therapy, 14*, 202–207.

Segraves, R. T. (1988b). Hormones and libido. In S. R. Leiblum & R. C. Rosen (Eds.), *Sexual desire disorders* (pp. 271–312). New York: Guilford.

Segraves, R. T. (1989). Effects of psychotrophic drugs on human erection and ejaculation. *Archives of General Psychiatry, 46*, 275–284.

Segraves, R. T., Madsen, R., Carter, S. C., & Davis, J. M. (1985). Erectile dysfunction associated with pharmacological agents. In R. T. Segraves & H. W. Schoenberg (Eds.), *Diagnosis and treatment of erectile disturbances* (pp. 23–63). New York: Plenum.

Segraves, R. T., Schoenberg, H. W., & Segraves, K. A. B. (1985). Evaluation of the etiology of erectile failure. In R. T. Segraves & H. W. Schoenberg (Eds.), *Diagnosis and treatment of erectile disturbances* (pp. 165–195). New York: Plenum.

Seibel, M. M., Freeman, M. G., & Graves, W. L. (1980). Carcinoma of the cervix and sexual function. *Obstetrics Gynecology, 55*, 484–487.

Seibel, M., Freeman, M. G., & Graves, W. L. (1982). Sexual function after surgical and radiation therapy for cervical carcinoma. *Southern Medical Journal, 85*, 1195–1197.

Semmens, J. P., & Semmens, E. C. (1984). Sexual function and the menopause. *Clinical Obstetrics and Gynecoloy, 27*, 717–722.

Shader, R. I. (1964). Sexual dysfunction associated with thioridazine hydrochloride. *Journal of the American Medical Association, 188*, 1007–1009.

Shader, R. I. (1972). Sexual dysfunction associated with mesoridazine besylate (Serentil). *Psychopharmacologia, 27*, 193–194.

Shakkebaek, N. E., Bancroft, L., Davidson, D. W., & Warner, P. (1980). Androgen replacement with oral testosterone undecanoate in hypogonadal men: A double-blind controlled study. *Clinical Endocrinology, 14*, 49–61.

Shen, W. W. (1982). Female orgasmic inhibition by amoxapine. *American Journal of Psychiatry, 139*, 1221.

Shen, W. W., & Park, S. (1982). Thioridazine-induced inhibition of female orgasm. *Psychiatry Journal of the University of Ottawa, 7*, 249–251.

Sherwin, B. B., & Gelfant, M. M. (1984). Effects of parenteral administration of estrogen and androgen on plasma hormone levels and hot flashes in the surgical menopause. *American Journal of Obstetrics and Gynecology, 148*, 552–557.

Sherwin, B. B., & Gelfant, M. M. (1985). Differential symptom response to parenteral estrogen and/or androgen administration in the surgical menopause. *American Journal of Obstetrics and Gynecology, 151*, 153–160.

Sherwin, B. B., Gelfant, M. M., & Brender, W. (1985). Androgen enhances sexual motivation in females. A prospective, crossover study of sex steroid administration in the surgical menopause. *Psychosomatic Medicine, 47*, 339–351.

Sherwin, B. B., & Gelfant, M. M. (1987). The role of androgen in the maintenance of sexual functioning in oophorectomized women. *Psychosomatic Medicine, 49*, 397–409.

Shorr, E., Papanicolaou, G. N., & Stimmel, B. F. (1938). Neutralization of ovarian follicular hormone in women by simultaneous administration of male sex hormone. *Proceedings of the Society for Experimental Biology and Medicine, 38*, 759–767.

Simpson, G. M., Blair, J. H., & Amuso, D. (1965). Effects of antidepressants on genitourinary function. *Diseases of the Nervous System, 26,* 787–789.

Siroky, M. B. (1988). Neurophysiology of male sexual dysfunction in neurologic disorders. *Seminars in Neurology, 8,* 2, 137–140.

Sjogren, K., & Fugl-Meyer, A. R. (1982). Adjustment to life after stroke with special reference to sexual intercourse and leisure. *Journal of Psychosomatic Research, 26,* 409–417.

Smith, B. H., & Khatri, A. M. (1979). Cortical localization of sexual feeling. *Psychosomatics, 20,* 771–776.

Souner, R. C. (1983). Anorgasmia associated with imipramine but not desepramine. A case report. *Journal of Clinical Psychiatry, 44,* 345–346.

Souner, R. C. (1984). Treatment of tricyclic antidepressant induced orgasmic dysfunction with cyproheptadine. *Journal of Clinical Psychopharmacology, 4,* 169.

Stahlgren, L. H., & Ferguson, L. K. (1958). Influence on sexual function of abdominoperitoneal resection for ulcerative colitis. *New England Journal of Medicine, 259,* 873–875.

Steele, T. E., & Howell, E. F. (1986). Cyproheptadine for imipramine-induced anorgasmia. *Journal of Clinical Psychopharmacology, 6,* 326–327.

Stockamp, K., & Schreiter, F. (1974). Function of the posterior urethra in ejaculation and its importance for urine control. *Urology International, 29,* 226–230.

Studd, J. W., Collins, W. P., Charkrauarti, S., Newton, J. R., Oram, D., & Parsons, A. (1977). Oestradiol and testosterone implants in the treatment of psychosexual problems in the postmenopausal woman. *British Journal of Obstetrics and Gynecology, 84,* 314–316.

Szasz, G., & Carpenter, C. (1989). Clinical observations in vibratory stimulation of the penis of men with spinal cord injury. *Archives of Sexual Behavior, 18,* 461–474.

Tuchman, H., & Crumpton, C. W. (1955). A comparison of Rauvolfia serpentia compounds cruderout, alseroxylon derivatives and single alkaloid in the treatment of hypertension. *American Heart Journal, 49,* 742–750.

Tyrer, G., Steel, J. M., Ewing, D. J., Bancroft, J., Warner, P., & Clarke, B. F. (1983). Sexual responsiveness in diabetic women. *Diabetologia, 24,* 166–171.

Uhde, T. W., Tancer, M. E., & Shea, C. A. (1988). Sexual dysfunction related to alprazolam treatment of social phobia. *American Journal of Psychiatry, 145,* 531–532.

Utian, W. H. (1972). The true clinical features of postmenopause and oophorectomy, and their response to estrogen therapy. *South African Medical Journal, 46,* 732–737.

Valleroy, M. I., & Kraft, G. H. (1984). Sexual dysfunction in multiple sclerosis. *Archives of Physical Medicine and Rehabilitation, 65,* 125–128.

Van Reeth, P. C., Olericens, J., & Luminet, D. (1958). Hypersexuality in epilepsy and temporal lobe tumors. *Acta Neurology Psychiatry, 58,* 194–203.

Vas, C. J. (1969). Sexual impotence and some autonomic disturbances in men with multiple sclerosis. *Acta Neurologica Scandinavica, 45,* 166–182.

Vejlsgaard, V., Christensen, M., & Classen, E. (1967). Double-blind trial of four hypotensive drugs (methyldopa and three synpatholytic agents). *British Medical Journal, 2,* 598–600.

Vera, M. I. (1981). Quality of life following pelvic exenteration. *Gynecologic Oncology, 12,* 355–366.

Vincent, C. E., Vincent, B., Greiss, F. C., & Linton, E. B. (1975). Some marital sexual concomitants of carcinoma of the cervix. *Southern Medical Journal, 68,* 552–558.

Vlachakis, N. D., & Mendlowitz, M. (1976). Alpha and beta-adrenergic receptor blocking agents combined with a diuretic in the treatment of essential hypertension. *Journal of Clinical Pharmacology, 111,* 352–360.

Wagner, G., & Sjostrand, N. O. (1988). Autonomic pharmacology and sexual function. In JMA Sitsen (Ed.), *Handbook of sexology* (Vol. 6): *The pharmacology and endocrinology of sexual function* (pp. 32–43). Amsterdam, Elsevier.

Walsh, P. C., & Donker, P. J. (1982). Impotence following radical prostatectomy: Insight into etiology and prevention. *Journal of Urology, 128,* 492–497.

Walton, J. N. (1975). *Essentials of neurology.* London: J. P. Lippincott.

Watts, J. M., deDomibal, F. T., & Goligher, J. C. (1966). Long-term complications and prognosis following major surgery for ulcerative colitis. *British Journal of Surgery, 53,* 1014–1019.

Weinstein, M. H., & Machleder, H. I. (1976). Sexual function after aorto-iliac surgery. *Annals of Surgery, 181,* 787–790.

Weizman, R., Weizman, A., Levi, J., Gura, V.,

Zevin, D., Maoz, B., Wijsenbeek, H., & David, M. B. (1983). Sexual dysfunction associated with hyperprolactinemia inmales and females undergoing hemodialysis. *Psychosomatic Medicine, 45,* 259–269.

Whitelaw, G. P., & Smithwick, R. H. (1951). Some secondary effects of sympathectomy. *New England Journal of Medicine, 245,* 121–130.

Willmuth, M. E. (1987). Sexuality after spinal cord injury: A critical review. *Clinical Psychology Review, 7,* 389–412.

Wyatt, R. J., Fram, D. H., & Buchbinder, R. (1971). Treatment of intractable narcolepsy with a monoamine oxidase inhibitor. *New England Journal of Medicine, 285,* 987–991.

Yalla, S. V. (1982). Sexual dysfunction in the paraplegic and quadriplegic. In A. H. Bennett (Ed.), *Management of male impotence* (pp. 181–191). Baltimore: Williams and Wilkins.

Yeager, E. S., & Von Heerden, J. A. (1980). Sexual dysfunction following proctocolectomy and abdominoperineal resection. *Annals of Surgery, 191,* 169–170.

Zrustova, M., Rostlapid, J., & Kabshelova, A. (1978). Sexual disorders in diabetic women. *Cesk Gynekol, 43,* 277–281.

CHAPTER 9

INHIBITED FEMALE ORGASM

Wendy Stock, Texas A&M University

INTRODUCTION

It is impossible to separate the subject of inhibited female orgasm from the social context in which women learn about and experience their sexuality. Thus, this chapter will critically examine the current diagnostic concept of inhibited female orgasm, its socially constructed limitations, omissions, and the resulting implications for assessment and treatment. This critical analysis is intended to enhance the reader's awareness in applying the current diagnostic system, the better to identify, diagnose, and treat women who experience difficulty attaining orgasm.

Definition

The DSM-III-R (American Psychiatric Association, 1987), the diagnostic system according to which this book is organized, defines inhibited female orgasm (302.73) as follows:

A. Persistent or recurrent delay in, or absence of, orgasm in a female following a

normal sexual excitement phase during sexual activity that the clinician judges to be adequate in focus, intensity, and duration. Some females are able to experience orgasm during noncoital clitoral stimulation, but are unable to experience it during coitus in the absence of manual clitoral stimulation. In most of these females, this represents a normal variation of the female sexual response and does not justify the diagnosis of Inhibited Female Orgasm. However, in some of these females, this does represent a psychological inhibition that justifies the diagnosis. This difficult judgment is assisted by a thorough sexual evaluation, which may even require a trial of treatment.

B. Occurrence not exclusively during the course of another Axis I disorder (other than a sexual dysfunction), such as Major Depression (p. 294).

Subtypes

Many variations of inhibited female orgasm are possible within this diagnosis. Among these subtypes are women who may experience a global inability to achieve orgasm through any means; women who are inorgasmic except for either masturbation, partner manipulation, or both; women who never or infrequently experience coital orgasm; and women who are anorgasmic except for vibrator or other mechanical stimulation (Schover et al., 1982). Contained within this diagnosis are numerous subtypes with dramatically different characteristics and etiologies.

Clitoral vs. Vaginal Orgasm

The long-standing confusion regarding coital orgasm continues to haunt the current diagnostic system. On one hand, the DSM-III-R correctly acknowledges that some females are unable to experience orgasm during coitus in the absence of manual clitoral stimulation and that this usually represents a "normal variation" of the female sexual response, which does not justify a diagnosis of inhibited female orgasm. At this point, the DSM opens a veritable Pandora's box of confusion by indicating that in some cases, lack of unassisted coital orgasm "does represent a psychological inhibition that justifies the diagnosis" (p. 294). This nosological fence-sitting may represent an attempt to satisfy both sides of the debate over clitoral vs. vaginal orgasm (the latter being rooted in Freudian theory).

Freud (1961) regarded coitus as the only legitimate means to sexual pleasure. An adult woman who had failed to transfer her locus of sexual sensation from the clitoris to the vagina was considered to be neurotic, immature, and masculine-identified. Freud's ideas were theoretical, not based on any controlled empirical data. Recent research has challenged the theory that it is pathologic for a woman to prefer or require clitoral stimulation to attain orgasm. Kinsey et al. (1953) noted the relative insensitivity of the vagina, reporting that 84% of their sample of 2480 women relied primarily on labial and clitoral stimulation to attain masturbatory orgasm. Masters and Johnson (1966) reported that the site of effective stimulation for orgasm is the clitoris, refuting the notion that there was such a thing as a clitoral orgasm distinct from a vaginal orgasm. Physiologic recordings of responses at the outer portion of the vagina indicated that the same orgasmic response occurred regardless of the site of stimulation. Hite (1976) found, on the basis of voluntary questionnaire responses of approximately 3000 women, that intercourse was generally considered peripheral to sexual pleasure, and that only 30% of her orgasmic respondents were able to experience coitally induced orgasms most or nearly all of the time (75–100%). Kinsey's, Masters and Johnson's, and Hite's research represented an effective and empirically based challenge to the tyranny of the Freudian-based and purely theoretical primacy of the vaginal orgasm.

However, more recent research has suggested that female orgasm is more complex than a solely clitoral model can account for. The installation of the clitoral model carried with it a danger of imposing another restrictive standard of normality of female sexual functioning, failing to allow for the wide range of individual variability that exists among women (Ellison, 1980; Warner, 1982). Critics of the clitoral model argue that Kinsey was in error by assuming that a light touch from a probe in an *unaroused* vagina is analogous to a penis thrusting in the vagina of a woman who is highly subjectively and physiologically aroused. Ellison (1980) found that a significant portion (49%) of her sample of 145 women reported having experienced vaginal orgasms and that 25% of the women mentioned deep internal sensations as one of their triggers to orgasm. Alzate (1985) notes the ample evidence indicating that coitus is an inefficient method of eliciting female orgasm but points out that orgasmic response by vaginal stimulation generally requires strong frictional pressure applied at an angle to the vaginal wall. This is impossible via penile stimulation, since the penis usually moves parallel to the vaginal walls, exerting only light friction at the erogenous zone(s). When a woman reaches an advanced stage of sexual arousal, a ballooning of the upper part of the vagina may occur, precluding any further contact between the glans penis and any intravaginal erogenous zones. Alzate proposes that there may be an optimal coital position for each woman, according to her idiosyncratic areas of vaginal sensitivity. In addition, the orgasmic latency of many women is relatively longer than that of their male sexual partners. Given these considerations, it is not surprising that the vagina has been undervalued in terms of its potential for erotic responsivity. It may be the case that many women have never received effective vaginal stimulation, which could result in orgasmic responsiveness.

Several studies report that women make subjective distinctions between masturbatory and coital orgasms (Robertiello, 1970; Singer & Singer, 1972). Allgeier and Allgeier (1984, p. 235) summarize Singer and Singer's typology of three types of orgasms, which is closely paraphrased below.

1. A *vulval orgasm* is induced by coital or noncoital stimulation and does not have a refractory period following it. At high levels of sexual arousal, the outer third of the vagina becomes constricted through blood engorgement. This constriction forms a narrow tube, referred to as the *orgasmic platform* by Masters and Johnson (1966). Vulval orgasm is characterized by involuntary rhythmic contractions of the orgasmic platform; this is the type measured by Masters and Johnson (1966).

2. The *uterine orgasm,* in contrast, is characterized by a gasping type of breathing that culminates in involuntary breath holding. At orgasm the breath is explosively exhaled, and a feeling of relaxation and sexual satiation follows. This response seems to occur upon repeated deep stimulation of the cervix, which displaces the uterus and causes stimulation of the membrane lining the abdominal cavity (peritoneum). This type of orgasm is followed by a refractory period.

3. The *blended orgasm* combines elements of the other two types. It is experienced as deeper than a vulval orgasm and includes breath holding and contractions of the orgasmic platform. This model would account for the great individual variability in emotional

satisfaction and physiologic response to orgasm in women.

With respect to diagnosis and treatment of inhibited female orgasm, it should be made clear to female patients that there is no single correct or "normal" way to experience an orgasm. Women can achieve orgasm through various types of stimulation, not limited to penile and vaginal contact. Although the physiologic and subjective processes that constitute female orgasm are not fully understood, research seems to indicate that many different physical, psychological, and subjective factors are involved; any one-dimensional view of normality is outdated and limiting. The current DSM-III-R diagnosis implies, unfortunately, that some women may have a "psychological inhibition" preventing them from experiencing coital orgasm. This inclusion implies psychopathology where none exists. Some women may be able to learn certain techniques that allow them to experience coital orgasm, but others may be physiologically unable to attain orgasm in this manner, regardless of the amount of practice. To diagnose this as psychopathology is equivalent to diagnosing all runners as psychopathological who cannot learn to run a four-minute mile. Based on the available data, it is simply not possible for the clinician to differentiate "psychological inhibition" from normal variation in the area of female coital orgasm. Utilizing this diagnosis only in the case of lack of coital orgasm is to risk pathologizing normal individuals. Treatment approaches that enhance and expand female orgasmic capability, without using pathologizing diagnoses, are discussed below.

PREVALENCE

As Kaplan (1974) noted, there is much conceptual ambiguity and confusion regarding the nosology of "frigidity" in women. According to the DSM-III-R, approximately 30% of the female population has inhibited female orgasm. In our culture, it appears that a significant number of women do not achieve orgasm during sexual relations. Kinsey et al. (1953) found that 30% of the women in their large sample of 2480 women did not have orgasms when they were first married and that 10% remained anorgasmic after ten years of marriage. It is Kaplan's (1974) estimate, 20 years after Kinsey reported his findings, that currently 8–10% of the female population has never experienced an orgasm, as compared to less than 1% of the male population. Other estimates range from 7% (Hunt, 1974) to 15% of the adult female population (Andersen, 1983), with a standard figure of about 10% (Hite, 1976). Approximately 90% of women seem able to achieve orgasm by some means. There are methodological limitations to these studies: They generally do not include a demographically representative population sample that is balanced for race, ethnic, and socioeconomic status. Volunteer bias may also affect the representativeness of the samples, in terms of the percentage of individuals willing to report sexual dysfunction. However, in spite of interpretive difficulties in survey data, Andersen (1983) maintains that the convergent evidence from such research indicates that a considerable number of women do not experience orgasm.

In the past, global, lifelong inability to have an orgasm (Masters & Johnson's (1970) diagnostic category of primary orgasmic dysfunction) was a common presenting complaint (LoPiccolo & Stock, 1986). In the first 100 successive admissions to LoPiccolo's Sex Therapy Center between 1974 and 1975, there were 29 cases of global, lifelong lack of female orgasm. During the period 1983–1984, there were only two such cases. This change in incidence may reflect an increase in the amount of information available to women, particularly information concerning masturbation. Until the late 1970s, women presenting with global anorgasmia often lacked basic information about the anatomy and physiology of their sexual response and were more influenced by cultural negativity toward female sexuality (LoPiccolo & Stock, 1986). Women now have greater access to such information, and some are more likely to have experienced their first orgasm during masturbation, sometimes with a mechanical aid such as a vibrator. Often, these women have been unable to experi-

ence the necessary conditions to have orgasm with a partner—including factors such as partner willingness to devote time to noncoital stimulation (foreplay), poor sexual communication between partners, or difficulty generalizing orgasm from masturbatory stimulation to that provided by a partner. Regarding the latter, certain masturbatory patterns that produce orgasm for women are incompatible with having coitus or receiving partner stimulation. For example, certain women may attain orgasm only by lying face down with their ankles crossed and pressing their thighs together while rhythmically rocking (LoPiccolo & Stock, 1986).

Thus, the fact that a woman is able to achieve orgasm does not mean that she will do so on a dependable basis during sexual activity with a partner. The average married woman may not necessarily attain orgasm often, even if she is orgasmic. In a study of the frequency of sexual dysfunction in 100 white, well-educated, middle-class couples who were recruited for a study of marriages that were "happy," Frank et al. (1978) found that 48% of the women reported difficulty getting excited, 33% had difficulty maintaining interest, and 46% had difficulty reaching orgasm. Significantly, only 15% reported an inability to have orgasm. These figures suggest that inhibited female orgasm is extremely common; something is preventing women who are otherwise sexually functional from actualizing this potential. Frank et al. (1978) also asked respondents to indicate sexual "difficulties" that do not fall under the current diagnostic nomenclature. The most commonly listed difficulties for women were:

1. Inability to relax (47%)
2. Partner choosing inconvenient time (31%)
3. Too little foreplay (38%)
4. Disinterest (35%)
5. Feeling "turned off" (28%)
6. Too little "tenderness" after intercourse (25%)

As Frank et al. (1978) emphasized, "In general, the women's reports of sexual *difficulties,* both in themselves and in their husbands, showed a stronger relation with ratings of sexual dissatisfaction than their reports of sexual *dysfunctions.*"

DIAGNOSTIC ISSUES

The Social Construction of DSM Diagnoses: Pathologizing the Normative

As Tiefer (1990) notes, the DSM carries incredible political influence, as it creates nomenclature and conceptualizations used by researchers, teachers, mental health professionals, physicians, the judicial system, and insurance companies. Tiefer notes that classification creates and enforces norms, creates culturally dominant language and imagery, and determines gender meanings and relations. In the DSM-III-R, sexual dysfunction is defined as follows (APA, 1987, pp. 290–291):

> The essential feature of this subclass is inhibition in the appetitive or psychophysiologic changes that characterize the complete sexual response cycle. . . . The complete sexual response cycle can be divided into the following phases: 1) appetitive, 2) excitement, 3) orgasm, 4) resolution.

The orgasm phase is described in more detail:

> This consists of a peaking of sexual pleasure, with release of sexual tension and rhythmic contraction of the perineal muscles and pelvic reproductive organs. . . . In the female there are contractions, not always subjectively experienced as such, of the wall of the outer third of the vagina. In both the male and the female there is often generalized muscular tension or contractions, such as involuntary pelvic thrusting (p. 291).

As Tiefer (1990) points out, "sexual abnormality is defined as deviation from a fixed sequence of physical changes." The act of reducing sexual dysfunction to a deficit in following a physiological response sequence is accomplished at the expense of decontextualizing sexuality from social reality, and this is only possible by making many assumptions about sexuality. Tiefer (1990) identifies these assumptions as follows:

1. Sexuality is apparently universal, unlearned, and innate;
2. Sexuality has to do with reactions of fragmented body parts;
3. Sexuality is obsessively genitally focused;
4. Heterosexual intercourse is the normative sexual activity, with sexual dysfunctions described as performance failures in coitus.

How do these assumptions shape and narrow our view of sexual dysfunction? (1) The effects of learning and sexual experience are overlooked, with the assumption that adequate physical stimulation will release an encoded biological reaction. (2) The body becomes a fragmented collection of disconnected physical parts in a performance sequence, leading to a view of sexual problems as "machines in disrepair." (3) The nomenclature implies that when genitals perform correctly, there is no sexual problem. (4) Dysfunctions are repeatedly described as performance failures in coitus. (5) Heterosexual intercourse is the "default" mode of sexual activity; other forms of sexual activity are qualified by the adjective *noncoital.* For example, in the description of female orgasm, a group of women are identified as not having orgasm during intercourse unaccompanied by clitoral stimulation, but also having orgasm during noncoital clitoral stimulation. Women who have orgasm only during noncoital clitoral stimulation are never mentioned (Tiefer, 1990).

To what extent does the current diagnostic system address women's experience of inhibited orgasm? The study by Frank et al. (1978) indicates that a number of nonphysiological, nongenital factors determine whether women experience orgasm—more significantly than ability to respond genitally. Tiefer (1990) lists areas that should be included in the classification, description, and assessment of women's sexual dysfunctions. Inclusion of "women's actual sexual voices," as heard in popular surveys, questionnaire studies, and writings, would address such concerns as emotion and communication, whole-body experience, commitment, attraction, sexual knowledge, safety, respect, body image, effects of menstrual cycle, menopause, and aging. Second, the DSM implies gender equity through its equally detailed description of genital response and denies women's social reality. Tiefer (1990) calls this *gender inequality*. Specifically, women lack equal opportunity for sexual freedom and social permission to experiment, are burdened with poorer physical self-image, have weaker status and economic bargaining position in intimate relationships with men, are frequently traumatized by past sexual exploitation, are concerned about unwanted pregnancy due to the unavailability of safe contraception and threats to reproductive choices, and are devalued by a "limited window of sexual attractiveness" (Tiefer, 1990, p. 10). Thus, women enter the sexual arena at a great disadvantage compared to men. As Tiefer argues, to speak of "a normal sexual excitement phase" as being determined by "activity that the clinician judges to be adequate in focus, intensity and duration" (APA, p. 294) trivializes and ignores women's sociosexual reality. The current diagnostic system is woefully inadequate in providing accurate descriptive and clinically relevant information. It obscures the contextual background that is necessary to understand and treat inhibited female orgasm.

Alternative Diagnostic Approaches

Originally, one diagnostic term—*frigidity*—was used to describe all female inhibitions and dysfunctions. Although the DSM classification system is a vast improvement over simply describing a woman as frigid, which is pejorative and imprecise, the current diagnostic system leaves much to be desired in terms of specifity and precision. If we diagnose a woman as having inhibited female orgasm, this could include a woman who has never had an orgasm in any way in her whole life, a woman who previously had

orgasms but has not had them for some time, a woman who can have orgasm with some men but not with her current partner, a woman who can have orgasm in her own masturbation but not with a partner, a woman who can have orgasm in many ways but not during intercourse, and a woman who can have orgasm only with the use of an electric vibrator—among other possibilities.

A more precise diagnostic system was developed by Schover et al. (1982). This multiaxial system has separate axes for desire, arousal, orgasm, coital pain, frequency disagreement, and additional information. The nature of the problem is further delineated by describing the problem as either lifelong or not lifelong in history of occurrence, and as global (present across situations) or situational. The orgasm phase axis contains seven categories, shown below, which must also be described in historical and situational terms:

- Anhedonic orgasm
- Anorgasmic (total)
- Anorgasmic except for masturbation
- Anorgasmic except for partner manipulation
- Anorgasmic except for masturbation or partner manipulation
- Infrequent coital orgasms
- Anorgasmic except for vibrator or mechanical stimulation

The addition of historical and situational information clears up some confusion from other diagnostic systems, such as Kaplan's (1974) and Masters and Johnson's (1970). In these systems, disorders are described as either primary or secondary. However, these terms contain elements both of the history of the disorder and its current global or situational nature. For example, a woman who had been orgasmic across situations but experienced a brutal rape and was then no longer orgasmic at all would have been diagnosed as primary anorgasmic, whereas in the above system she would be diagnosed as anorgasmic, not lifelong and global, alerting the clinician of the need to seek further historical information.

A recent controversy has emerged regarding the diagnostic category of primary orgasmic dysfunction (POD) in the clinical literature. Wakefield (1987b) argues that this term overpathologizes women by including those who simply have not experienced genital stimulation sufficient to have an orgasm. For cultural reasons, many women do not masturbate, a behavior that is generally acknowledged to be the most reliable method of producing orgasm in women (Kinsey, Pomeroy, & Martin, 1953; Masters & Johnson, 1966). In addition, it is well known that many women cannot easily have orgasms from coitus alone, without additional stimulation (Hite, 1976; Kaplan, 1974). Wakefield criticizes the POD diagnosis for including women who may never have achieved an orgasm for many reasons that do not indicate a true inability to have an orgasm and do not imply an orgasmic disorder. For example, a woman might lack knowledge about masturbation, or she might have religious convictions or fears that prevent her from masturbating. Wakefield argues that it does a disservice to women to assign a pathological condition to what may be merely a behavioral deficit. He argues that the DSM avoids the confusion between insufficient stimulation and orgasmic inhibition by requiring *adequate stimulation* as a precondition for diagnosis of primary anorgasmia. In the DSM-III-R, the diagnostic category of inhibited female orgasm specifies that the female has experienced "persistent or recurrent delay in, or absence of, orgasm in a female following a normal sexual excitement phase during sexual activity that the clinician judges to be adequate in focus, intensity, and duration" (p. 294). This requires that the clinician be able to judge accurately what constitutes adequate stimulation for an individual woman, in order to assign this diagnosis.

In the case of inhibited female orgasm, the DSM-III-R has moved from a decriptive diagnostic category (requiring few assumptions) to a diagnosis requiring assumptions and clinical intuition regarding what constitutes adequate sexual stimulation for another person. Although the intent of the authors of the DSM-III-R is commendable—a desire not to misdiagnose women who have not experienced adequate sexual stimulation—this assumes that there is a clinical pathological condition in which a woman would be anorgasmic *with* sufficient stimulation. This diagnosis cannot be assigned in coexistence with another severe Axis I disorder (e.g., major depression or schizophrenia). The current diagnosis, as worded, reveals the assumption that some people with sexual dysfunctions suffer from a truly pathological condition, and that those with learning or behavioral deficits do not qualify. Wakefield's (1989) examples of women with "no pathology" include "those who have never masturbated due to religious beliefs and who are married to prematurely ejaculating husbands" (p. 77). Does this mean that women who have masturbated and/or received "adequate" sexual stimulation, but who do not experience orgasm because they fear the loss of control which occurs (perhaps because of a sexually or psychologically abusive or damaging experience) are more pathological? Both types are based on having had certain learning experiences. Barbach (1980) points out that Kinsey et al.'s (1953) data "laid the foundation for the important assumption that orgasm could be considered a learned response for some women and that failure to achieve it was therefore not necessarily a sign of neurosis, but rather due to faulty learning" (Barbach, 1980, p. 110).

A number of researchers and clinicians suggest that a pattern of sexual response that includes arousal and pleasure but excludes orgasm may represent a normal variation on the continuum of female sexual response (Ford & Beach, 1951; Kaplan, 1974; Newcomb & Bentler, 1983). Medical conditions that create or contribute to an inability to experience orgasm, including the use of certain antihypertensive medications, substance abuse, or an atypically high threshold for sensory stimulation, should not be confused with psychopathology (see Chapter 8). There is no empirical documentation of a psychopathological condition that would substantiate Wakefield's argument or correspond to the DSM-III-R category.

Morokoff (1989), in her reply to Wakefield (1987a), addresses another mistaken assumption required by the inhibited female orgasm diagnosis in the DSM-III-R. Women who are capable of having intercourse may be assumed to be sexually aroused, as the male equivalent for intercourse is having an erection, which requires sexual arousal. However, Morokoff points out that many women are socialized to engage in intercourse as an obligation, based on the definition of a "good wife," even in the absence of any significant sexual arousal. Morokoff argues that female sexual arousal disorder, if appropriately utilized, would increase in prevalence, with a resultant decrease in diagnosis of inhibited female orgasm. Morokoff contends that the DSM-III-R diagnostic criteria are consistent with women's experiences. However, a clinical judgment of adequate sexual stimulation is still required to differentiate inhibited arousal from inhibited orgasm, since they are mutually exclusive diagnoses. In addition, clinical judgment as to the presence or absence of sexual arousal is required—a judgment that even Morokoff argues is difficult for women themselves to make reliably, let alone another party. Among the implications of this position are to acknowledge the inherent limitations of clinical judgment in making this diagnosis and to place more importance on lack of orgasm as a diagnostic criterion.

The above controversy highlights a major flaw inherent in the DSM-III-R, a diagnostic system based on the medical model. To pathologize or medicalize what Szasz (1961) called *problems in living* is to force social reality into a Procrustean bed. The sexual dysfunctions, when medical etiology is exempt, are not inherently pathological or necessarily indicative of other psychopathology. A frankly descriptive system would avoid assumptions regarding lack of sufficient stimulation, behavioral deficits, or attempts to distinguish these from "true" psychopathology. For this reason, a diagnosis of inhibited orgasm should not preclude an inhibited arousal diagnosis, or vice versa. Regardless of etiology, roughly 10% of the female population does not experience orgasm. A diagnostic system that recognizes this population without pathologiz-

ing it and that includes temporal, situational, and behavioral qualifiers and subcategories (e.g., Schover et al., 1982) would best serve this population.

Finally, researchers, diagnosticians, and clinicians would do well to consider developing a normative model of women-defined sexual problems based on "women's experience and women-generated goals, established by women of diverse experiences and backgrounds" (Tiefer, 1988, p. 11). To this end, Tiefer suggests utilizing a qualitative approach such as Hite's (1976) survey of women's sexual practices. Hite rejected traditional standards and norms, instead asking women to describe, in open-ended answers, their practices, experiences, preferences, dissatisfactions, etc. Tiefer urges the development of a system of classification of women's sexual dysfunctions based on Hite's data—which would be very different from the current diagnostic system.

Assessment Implications

The diagnostic system used determines what information is sought during assessment. This information may be pertinent not only for a correct and reliable diagnosis, but also for conceptualization and treatment. The inadequacies of the current DSM-III-R, discussed above, should inspire the development of a broader, detailed assessment procedure for women presenting with inhibited female orgasm. Ideally, assessment should include the following:

1. Detailed information on current specific sexual behaviors, including frequency and method of masturbation; sexual behaviors engaged in with a partner; degree of physiological and subjective sexual arousal; relative effectiveness of various types of sexual stimulation; and focus, intensity, and duration of sexual activity
2. History of presenting problem (lifelong vs. not lifelong) and situational factors (global vs. situational)
3. Medical factors relating to sexual functioning

(ruling out medical etiology or major Axis I disorder)

4. Relational context in which sexual behavior takes place: under what circumstances sexual behavior is engaged in; the meaning of sexual interaction within the relationship; perceptions about partner's involvement in the sexual relationship and relationship quality (Frank, Downard, & Lang, 1986); to what degree other nonsexual needs are addressed within the relationship (the need for shared home responsibilities, emotional support and nurturance, woman's perceived choice to engage in or refuse sexual activity)—Frank et al. (1978) may serve as guide, since 46% of women in this survey reported difficulty reaching orgasm, and only 15% reported inability to have orgasm, which suggests assessment of other sexual problems such as fatigue, lack of foreplay, inconvenient time, disinterest, inability to relax, or too little tenderness after intercourse

The above framework represents the minimum information necessary to make an accurate DSM diagnosis. Prior to treatment, of course, a much more detailed assessment, including historical and current information, is needed; an excellent outline for taking a sex history is included in Heiman and LoPiccolo's self-treatment book, *Becoming Orgasmic: A Sexual Growth Program for Women* (1986). This outline includes early learning experiences about sexuality; parental attitudes; religious influences; experiences during childhood, puberty, and adulthood; body image; use and content of sexual fantasy; and additional items.

FEMALE ORGASMIC FUNCTION AND DYSFUNCTION

Although much of the research on determinants of sexual functioning in women uses orgasm as the criterion of sexual functioning and satisfaction, it should be emphasized that orgasm represents only one aspect of female sexuality. As Jayne (1981) points out, many women persist in a sexual activity that, in Kinsey's terms, provides no "outlet." Masters and Johnson (1966) found that the most physiologically intense orgasms occur as a result of masturbation, and the lowest-intensity orgasms were found during intercourse (intensity being defined by both objective recording and subjective report). It appears that women persist in and prefer sexual activities that may not produce orgasm consistently and that the intensity of orgasmic contraction is not related to the subjective satisfaction (Jayne, 1981). Not surprisingly, those activities most preferred and rated as most satisfying were those that included a partner, independent of the occurrence of orgasm. It appears that factors other than orgasmic outlet must be evaluated to understand what constitutes sexual satisfaction for women. Hite (1976), for example, asked women what gave them the greatest pleasure in sex. The most frequent response was "emotional intimacy, tenderness, closeness, sharing deep feelings with a loved one."

Physiologic Factors in Female Orgasm

Hormonal Factors

Hormones play a complex role with regard to sexual drive, arousal, and perhaps orgasmic capacity in women. The only hormone that has been positively associated with increased capacity for orgasm is testosterone (Bancroft, 1984). When women have been administered large amounts of testosterone for medical reasons, the clitoris becomes enlarged, and orgasm is reached more easily. It has been reported that women who had never experienced sexual desire in the past reported their first strong sexual urges while undergoing treatment with testosterone (Bancroft, 1984). However, the hormonal system in females is so complex that much research will be necessary to determine the interactions of hormonal influences on sexual behavior, arousal, drive, and orgasm in women.

Pubococcygeal Muscle Strength

In the 1950s, Arnold Kegel (1952) proposed that orgasmic dysfunction in women could be attributed, in large part, to the poor tone of the vaginal musculature, or damage to it. A treatment program developed by Kegel for urinary stress incontinence had the inadvertent effect of increasing orgasmic responsiveness in female patients. These exercises were developed to strengthen the pubococcygeal (PC) muscle, which surrounds the vagina, urethra, and anus and corresponds to that area of the vagina labeled the "orgasmic platform" by Masters and Johnson (1966). In a retrospective survey of 281 female patients, Graber and Kline-Graber (1979) found that PC strength varied in the predicted direction, with women having the weakest muscle strength being completely anorgasmic, women with a moderate amount of muscle tone being orgasmic but not during coitus, and women with the most highly developed muscles being orgasmic during coitus. The statistically significant differences were between anorgasmic and orgasmic women—not within the two orgasmic groups.

Recently, a number of studies have failed to demonstrate a relationship between PC muscle strength and orgasmic ability. Sultan et al. (1980) found that PC strength was not related to frequency of orgasm in coitus or due to clitoral stimulation. Only 19% of the subjects reported orgasmic frequency during coitus on 60–100% of occasions, while 75% reported this orgasmic frequency on occasions involving clitoral stimulation.

Another study on PC muscle strength and the effect of PC exercise on coital orgasm in women (Chambless et al. 1984) found that although Kegel exercises improved PC muscle strength, women practicing Kegel exercises did not show greater improvement on coital orgasmic frequency compared to two control groups.

To summarize findings on the PC muscle, research does not conclusively demonstrate that PC muscle strength is related to orgasmic frequency or intensity. Women with a global, lifelong lack of orgasm do tend to have weaker PC musculature, but there is no evidence that increasing PC muscle strength results in greater orgasmic ability.

The Grafenberg Spot and Female Ejaculation

Another area of research on the relationship of female anatomy to orgasmic functioning concerns the Grafenberg spot, or G spot, and the phenomenon that has been labeled *female ejaculation* (Ladas et al., 1982). The Grafenberg spot is described as a small, erotically sensitive structure located within the anterior wall of the vagina. In some women it has been found that orgasm can be produced through stimulation of this spot, without any concurrent clitoral stimulation. In addition to the G spot being a sensitive area in the vagina for some women, it has been suggested that following its stimulation, a small percentage of women emit during orgasm a fluid that is described as "unlike urine" (Belzer, 1981). Addiego et al. (1981) made chemical comparisons of urine with samples of this fluid from one subject. The ejaculate was found to differ from her urine in that it contained prostatic acid phosphatase, a chemical secreted primarily by the prostate and periurethral gland. This finding has led to the speculation that the female ejaculate comes from a vestigal prostate gland that some women have located at the G spot. A later study by Goldberg et al. (1983), comparing the fluid emitted at orgasm by six female ejaculators and six orgasmic women, found that the "ejaculate fluid" was indistinguishable from urine. However, as the PC muscle strength of female ejaculators is very high (Perry & Whipple, 1981), it should not be assumed that women who emit fluid at orgasm have urinary stress incontinence. It may be that women with very high PC muscle strength emit a fluid at orgasm as a function of these very strong muscles milking residual urine from the bladder and bladder neck.

A recent survey study (Darling et al., 1991) examined a number of variables thought to be associated with female ejaculation in a sample of 1172 professional women. Of these respondents, 40% reported having a fluid release (ejaculation) at the moment of orgasm, and 82% of the women who reported the sensitive area (Grafenberg spot) also reported ejaculation with their orgasms. Interestingly, 40% of the women who reported ejaculation believed that urination had occurred. The authors note that anecdotal data suggested that the physiological sensations associated with this expulsion of fluid are similar to those associated with the voiding of urine, which could explain this perception of urination at the moment of orgasm. Importantly, a greater number of reported ejaculators inhibited their orgasm due to the fear of accidental urination. This fact is of clinical significance in understanding contributing factors of inhibited orgasm in women.

To summarize, although the existence of the G spot and the chemical content of the fluid expelled at orgasm are controversial at present, the expulsion of fluid at orgasm can be a nonpathologic variation of the female sexual response.

Cognitive Factors in Female Orgasm

A significant clinical literature exists on the effects of distraction and attention on sexual arousal processes (Abel et al., 1975, 1981; Cerny, 1978; Geer & Fuhr, 1976; Laws & Rubin, 1969). A frequent clinical observation is that anorgasmic women have difficulty attending to and positively evaluating physiologic changes during sexual arousal (Heiman, 1978; Kaplan, 1974; Masters & Johnson, 1970). Lifshitz and Adams (1980) tested this hypothesis with orgasmic and anorgasmic female subjects. The orgasmic group reported that during sexual activity they cognitively focused on their own physical responses as well as on pleasing their partner. The anorgasmic group reported a similar cognitive pattern initially, then shifted at the point of advanced foreplay and/or intercourse to excessive focus on achieving orgasm and increased awareness of external stimuli. The effect of distraction on genital arousal in the laboratory was increased vaginal blood volume pulse (BVP) for the orgasmic females, but a decrease in BVP for the anorgasmic females. This study indicated

that anorgasmic women were able to achieve high levels of physiologic sexual arousal but were easily distracted from arousal by competing external stimuli and cognitive events.

Adams, Haynes, and Brayer (1985) examined the role of cognitive distraction in female sexual arousal, finding significant decreases in subjective measures and physiological measures (vaginal pulse amplitude) of sexual arousal during the distraction task. Women participants were also divided into "frequently" and "infrequently" orgasmic groups. Correlations between the two measures of sexual arousal were significant during both the erotic stimulus presentation and the distraction task. The results of this study did not support the idea that infrequently orgasmic women, compared to frequently orgasmic women, are physiologically or subjectively less sexually responsive during erotic stimulation, nor for the differential effect of cognitive distraction on these two groups. However, it appears that the "infrequently" orgasmic women did show a differential tendency to respond to distracting stimuli, with decreased ability to monitor physiological changes that accompany sexual arousal.

Another study on cognitive determinants of sexual arousal (Smith et al., 1983) found support for the negative effect of "spectating" on female sexual arousal (focusing on how one appears to others). Female subjects listening to an erotic stimulus were given one of three instructional sets preceding exposure: (1) focus on stimulus material; (2) focus on one's bodily sensations; (3) focus on how one appears to others in a spectator role. Vaginal blood volume amplitude in response to erotic material was highest for the stimulus-focus condition and lowest for the spectator condition. These researchers concluded that women with sexual arousal dysfunctions might be treated more effectively by giving them instruction and practice exercises in focusing their attention primarily on their partner as a sexual stimulus, with an emphasis on reducing "spectating."

Several psychophysiological studies have examined demographic, cognitive, and behavioral variables related to forms of sexual expression.

In a sample of 370 respondents, Hoon and Hoon (1978) delineated three styles of sexual expression in women. Women who were most highly satisfied with their sexual responsivity also experienced orgasm consistently, and they enjoyed gently seductive erotic activities and breast stimulation. It was also found that women who achieved orgasm most consistently were older, were more aware of physiologic changes during arousal, reported higher frequencies of masturbation and intercourse, and were less likely to be aroused by erotic preliminaries. Since the most consistently orgasmic subjects were found to be more aware of physiologic changes during sexual activity, it was suggested that treatment strategies for lack of orgasm should teach patients to focus on sensations that occur prior to orgasm. An earlier laboratory study on the effects of biofeedback and cognitive mediation on vaginal blood volume also found that when subjects were directed to use fantasy in combination with vaginal blood volume biofeedback, with knowledge of the target response, they were more effective at producing increases in VBV. These results are somewhat inconsistent with those of Smith et al. (1983) in the recommendation of focus on the self, rather than the partner. Any attentional focus that breaks the pattern of overconcern with one's sexual performance is likely to have positive effects. When performance anxiety is not present, focus on pleasurable physiological cues of sexual arousal may be most effective.

A cognitive means of augmenting sexual arousal is the use of sexual fantasy, which has been documented in the research literature as normative in women (Hariton & Singer, 1974) and as effective in generating sexual arousal (Stock & Geer, 1982). Heiman (1977) found that ability to visualize a sexual fantasy was highly correlated with ability to perceive arousal to it. Lentz and Zeiss (1984) examined the use of sexual fantasy during masturbation and its relationship to responsiveness. They found that women who reported a high percentage of intercourse-related fantasies during masturbation were more likely to experience orgasm during intercourse. This study suggests specific clinical applications of cognitive techniques that may enhance orgasmic ability.

A study by Bridges et al. (1985) examined a cognitive stylistic pattern (fear of losing control) and its relationship to orgasm during intercourse. Fear of losing control has been hypothesized by both psychoanalytic and social learning theorists (Adams, 1966; Fisher, 1973) as a determinant of orgasmic difficulty in women. Bridges et al. found a higher frequency of coital orgasms reported by women who rated high in hypnotic susceptibility, who enjoy the feeling of getting "carried away" while drinking alcoholic beverages, and who reported less ability to control thoughts or movements near the end of coitus. Conversely, this study would suggest that women who feel that they must remain in control, who perhaps have learned to fear the loss of control, are less likely to experience coital orgasm. Survivors of rape and childhood sexual abuse frequently present with experience-based fears of letting their guard down, of losing control of their awareness of the environment or control of their physical boundary, particularly in a sexual interaction. It is possible that the stylistic cognitive variable of loss of control may be an important determinant of orgasm in women.

Individual Factors in Female Orgasm

In general, investigations relating background and personality variables to orgasmic functioning have been characterized by few significant associations (Morokoff, 1978). As orgasm rate tends to be related to happiness in general, many correlations between sexual functioning and personality variables are spurious, reflecting the underlying influence of this "happiness" variable. Fisher's (1973) comprehensive investigation of background and personality variables found few significant associations. One group of variables that did discriminate between consistently orgasmic and rarely orgasmic women concerned the quality of the father/daughter relationship. Fisher found low orgasmic experience to be consistently related to actual childhood loss or separation from the father, fathers who had been emotionally unavailable to their daughters (i.e., uncommunicative, casual, or uninterested), or father figures with whom the women did not have a positive childhood relationship. Fisher's theory holds that the experience of high sexual arousal creates a more vulnerable emotional state, in which the dependability of the love object becomes particularly salient. A state of high sexual arousal entails a "fade-out" of other love objects, which may be particularly threatening to a woman who, because of a poor child/father relationship, is especially concerned with object loss. The result might be a tendency for these women to inhibit a fading out and consequently to fail to reach orgasm.

Derogatis et al. (1986) have developed profiles for two types of anorgasmic women, suggesting the existence of at least two psychologically distinct subtypes. Earlier research on anorgasmic women by Derogatis et al. (1979, 1981) found this population to suffer from high levels of psychological symptomatic distress and dysphoria. However, a significant degree of heterogeneity existed, with a considerable number of subjects displaying low levels of symptomatic distress. Whether these symptoms were primary or secondary to the sexual dysfunction is impossible to establish—and therefore without etiological import. In the more recent study, two subtypes emerged: (1) a high-drive/high-fantasy subgroup with a greater variety of sexual experiences and relatively low levels of psychological distress and (2) a low-drive/low-fantasy subgroup with some constriction of sexual fantasies and experiences and high levels of psychological distress. Derogatis et al. (1986) speculate that the first subtype would reveal a higher prevalence of constitutional or interpersonal etiologies, while the second subtype would more likely have psychogenic etiology, manifesting higher levels of psychological distress, negative self-concepts, poorer body image, and much lower levels of investment in sexuality. Derogatis contends that the failure of therapeutic approaches to treat more anorgasmic women successfully is due to the lack of a nosology of anorgasmic conditions.

Fear and anxiety based on a traumatic sexual incident, such as rape or incest, may prevent women who have been victims of such assaults from responding sexually to their partners. A number of studies have shown a high rate of sexual dysfunction (generally 50%) among rape survivors, as well as anxiety, depression, and general disruption of life (Becker et al., 1982; Ellis et al., 1980; Kilpatrick et al., 1981; Miller et al., 1982). Consistent with Fisher's (1973) hypothesis, rape and incest survivors may have difficulty attaining orgasm, because the "letting go" response requires a relinquishing of control that these women find extremely threatening. In addition, Miller et al. (1982) found that the serious relationship dysfunctions may continue for years following a rape. Becker et al. (1982) found that for many victims the passage of time following the assault does not appear to heal sexual fears and dysfunctions. It has also been suggested (Riger & Gordon, 1981) that even women who have not been victimized may feel constrained sexually by the high frequency of sexual aggression tolerated as normal interaction in this society.

A recent study on attitudinal and experiential correlates of anorgasmia (Kelly et al., 1990) compared 24 orgasmic women to 10 anorgasmic women on laboratory sexual arousal and sexual attitudes, knowledge, and guilt. As compared to the orgasmic women, the anorgasmic women reported (1) greater discomfort in communicating with a partner regarding only those sexual activities involving direct clitoral stimulation (cunnilingus and manual stimulation by partner); (2) more negative attitudes toward masturbation; (3) greater endorsement of sex myths; and (4) greater sex guilt. (These findings overlap with most areas within this section on female orgasm, but they are discussed here as individual difference variables.) As the authors note, the ability to communicate clearly regarding sexual preferences and other intimate issues has been implicated in the etiology and maintenance of anorgasmia and other sexual dysfunctions. A woman's success at achieving orgasm during coitus or any other sexual interaction requires that she be able to indicate what type of stimulation, timing, and touch is most stimulating at the moment. The discomfort indicated regarding both partner stimulation and masturbation is precisely centered on the sexual activities most likely to result in female orgasm. The latter two findings (regarding endorsement of sex myths and greater sex guilt in anorgasmic women) are consistent with recent research on the effects of distraction, which suggests that even low levels of cognitive interference during sex may inhibit orgasm (Kelly et al., 1990).

Social/Cultural Factors in Female Orgasm

More than any other variable, cultural factors seem to account for the diversity and range of women's orgasmic experiences. In her cross-cultural exploration of the influences of sex roles, Margaret Mead (1949) emphasized the ability of human societies "to build cultural systems that are extraordinarily detached from any biological base" (p. 217). Mead contrasted two primitive South Seas societies. One society expected women to derive the same satisfaction from sex that men do, and the other society did not recognize the existence of female orgasm. Mead concluded that the potential for orgasm in the human female is determined by cultural values. In societies that consider the orgasmic release of the female important, the lovemaking techniques that facilitate women's orgasm will be valued and practiced. When the female orgasm is considered unimportant or nonexistent, the members of a culture will not practice the techniques essential for women's orgasmic release—and women in these cultures are likely to be anorgasmic. Mead (1949) concludes that "there seems to be a reasonable basis for assuming that the human female's capacity for orgasm is to be viewed much more as a potentiality that may or may not be developed by a given culture" (p. 217).

Barbach (1980) reviewed many of the possible causes of lack of orgasm and concluded that a number of "nonpathological" factors are in-

volved: (1) lack of information; (2) belief in vaginal orgasm and belief that clitoral orgasm is somehow immature and infantile; (3) belief in a standard, normal, or "one right" type of sexual response; (4) adherence to a female role or "script" dictating that women are passive and unassertive; and (5) a fear of losing control, based on cultural indoctrination that women should be ladylike and restrained.

One means through which culture influences our sexual behavior is by teaching us "sexual scripts." Stock (1984) reviewed several female sexual scripts that have been found to influence sexual functioning. The "good girl" script (Moulton, 1976) is associated with passivity, obedience, docility, and "niceness." O'Connor (1979) found that difficulty in achieving orgasm is correlated with the "good girl" script. Six hundred women presenting for sex therapy were classified as nonorgasmic or orgasmic. Of the nonorgasmic group, 88% described themselves as having been "good girls" as children and teenagers. They were obedient, did well in school, and never had major conflicts with their patients. Only 30% of the orgasmic women fell into this "good girl" category. This study suggests a possible correlation with the ability to experience orgasm. Barbach (1975) points out that in early dating experiences, boys are expected to "get away" with anything they can, whereas girls are expected to stop them from doing so. A "good girl" restrains her sexuality, whereas "loose girls" participate in and enjoy sex (at the cost of losing respect and reducing their marital potential). In this script, the girl who acts on her sexual feelings would get a bad reputation, and a boy's social status would rise with each sexual conquest. After ignoring and repressing sexual feelings during adolescence, many women have difficulty becoming responsive and "letting go" in the context of a "legitimate" sexual relationship. Indeed, some men may be uncomfortable with their wives' being too responsive, since they have internalized the script that "nice girls" do not fully desire or enjoy sex.

Similar to the "good girl" script is the "madonna/whore" script. Many women have difficulty reconciling their sexuality with other aspects of the female role (mother, daughter, wife). Often these women have received strict religious training that denies enjoyment of sexuality separate from procreation and particularly negates the possibility of being both sexual and religious. This dichotomy places such women in a painful contradiction, the resolution of which involves either denying their sexuality or else risking being viewed by themselves and others as ''whores.''

''Sleeping beauty'' is a cultural script emphasizing sexual passivity, in which the woman remains totally passive, waiting for the male partner to engineer her arousal and orgasm. Typically, women who adhere to this script are uncomfortable with initiating sex, giving feedback to partners, masturbating, knowing their own sexual needs, being sexually assertive, or taking an active role in achieving their own orgasms.

Recently, our culture has come to view female orgasm as a required ability. This new cultural demand concerning female sexuality can cause women painfully ambivalent conflict about their own sexual needs. Darling and Davidson (1986) suggest that ''as individuals become increasingly aware of their sexuality and orgasmic responsiveness, concomitantly, the phenomenon of pretending orgasm is becoming a greater part of the sexual relationship for many couples'' (p. 182). These researchers found that almost 95% of a sample of 805 professional nurses had experienced sexual intercourse, 97% of the sample had experienced orgasm, and 58% had at some time pretended to achieve orgasm through sexual intercourse. Reasons cited by Darling and Davidson (1986) for pretending orgasm are the female's desire to please her partner and to avoid disappointing or hurting him, and the women's fears that her inability to fulfill this expectation will injure her partner's sense of masculinity. This pretense may protect the egos of both partners; it may also disguise a variety of sexual problems in both partners. Other reasons cited for pretending to have an orgasm include fear (of inadequacy as a female and of inability ever to achieve orgasm), desire

to prevent the current partner from seeking another sex partner, and wishing to conclude boring or painful sexual intercourse (Darling & Davidson, 1986). These researchers obtained responses from 805 profesional women, indicating that 58% had pretended orgams: 4.5% frequently pretend, 95.4% occasionally pretend, and 8.5% no longer pretend. Approximately 97% of the pretenders and nonpretenders had experienced orgasm. Variables that differentiated pretenders from nonpretenders were primarily relational: conflicts with partner, partner's lack of interest in foreplay and/or lack of tenderness, difficulty in becoming sexually aroused with current sex partner, desire to perform well, premature ejaculation, and fear of not satisfying partner. Another important aspect of this study was the inclusion of a checklist ascertaining what changes respondents desired in their sex lives. The desired changes that differentiated pretenders from nonpretenders included more frequent orgasms, more manual stimulation of the clitoral area, a more assertive role for themselves during intercourse, sexual intercourse with mutual love, petting with mutual love, and finding a new sex partner. The authors note that while relational factors are present, women who pretend orgasm desire greater self-determination in their sexual interactions.

Women who have been taught to repress and control their sexuality but who are nowadays also ''required'' to respond orgasmically (but only in the appropriate situation) find themselves confused and resentful about these competing expectations. The cultural confusion about the acceptability of female sexual response reflects a societal ambivalence about the expression and control of female sexuality. Such qualities as adventurousness, self-confidence, assertiveness, and premarital sexual experimentation are in direct opposition to the qualities considered feminine (passivity, timidity, virginity, and naivete). Kirkpatrick (1980) presents evidence suggesting an inverse relationship between identification with the feminine sex role and sexual satisfaction, noting that the more effectively women are socialized into the feminine role, the more likely they are to repress sexual feelings and interests. Thus, diagnosing women as pathological when they are actually conforming to a social role for which they have been rewarded is placing women in a no-win situation. Kirkpatrick's (1980) research suggests that sexual satisfaction in women is more likely to be related to the adoption of a single standard of equality than adherence to traditional "double standard" rules. It is clear that acceptance of the wide range of variability in female sexual functioning (including the experience of different types of orgasms, the need for different types of sexual stimulation, and an end to dogmatic insistence on the correctness of one type of stimulation or one type of orgasm over another) will help women move in the direction of greater sexual satisfaction and a higher level of sexual functioning.

Relationship Factors in Female Orgasm

For women, satisfaction with the marital relationship seems to be an important factor in sexual functioning. Kaplan (1974) noted that a woman's sexual response is highly contingent on having positive and loving feelings toward her partner and on her acceptance of him. Gebhard (1966) observed that wives who reach orgasm 90–100% of the time during marital coitus are found more often in very happy marriages, whereas wives who never reach orgasm in marital coitus are found most often in very unhappy marriages. Seidler-Feller (1985) has argued that women's sexual dysfunctions are often forms of resistance to inequality and exploitation in a relationship—positive expressions of self-ownership and the right to privacy. Women have been found to view their personal efforts, their partners' efforts, and the quality of their relationships as major influences on whether sexual experiences are satisfying or unsatisfying (Frank, Downard, & Lang, 1986). These authors suggest that the assessment of a woman's sexual health should elicit information about her level of satisfaction with both her own and her partner's sexual participation and involvement. In

addition, the expectations for the desired level of intimacy within a given sexual interaction should be explored in the context of the couple's view of the overall relationship.

TREATMENT

Global (Primary) Anorgasmia

Arousal and orgasm problems in women are the most common sexual problems presenting for treatment (LoPiccolo & Stock, 1986). Most often, inhibited sexual desire in women is secondary to lack of arousal and orgasm. The term *primary orgasmic dysfunction* will apply here to women who have never experienced orgasm through any means. The most effective treatment at present for lifelong lack of orgasm in women is a program of directed masturbation designed by LoPiccolo and Lobitz (1972). Masturbation has proved to be the most reliable method of producing an orgasm, as well as producing the most intense orgasm (Masters & Johnson, 1966). Masturbation enables the woman to experience proprioceptive feedback directly linked to her own self-stimulation, allowing identification of effective stimulation to occur more easily than in the case of partner stimulation. Other positive cognitive and physiological effects associated with increased rate of orgasm are increased psychological anticipation of pleasure in sex (Bardwick, 1971), and increased vascularity of the pubococcygeal muscle, which may increase orgasmic potential (Kegel, 1952). The masturbation program developed by LoPiccolo and Lobitz (1972) is based on a sexual skills learning model; it has been used effectively in a time-limited behavioral treatment program involving both partners in a couple. The basic elements of treatment for lack of orgasm include education, self-exploration and body awareness, and directed masturbation. Because some women and their partners have little knowledge of the anatomy and physiology of the female sexual response cycle, bibliotherapy is used as an adjunct to treatment. Among the excellent books on the subject are

Becoming Orgasmic: A Sexual Growth Program for Women (Heiman & LoPiccolo, 1986); *For Yourself: The Fulfillment of Female Sexuality* (Barbach, 1975). In a study by Morokoff and LoPiccolo (1986), use of *Becoming Orgasmic* together with a film of the same title was found to be equally effective in helping women attain orgasm in a minimal therapist contact format when compared to weekly therapy (four sessions during a 15-week period, as compared to 15 sessions.) Both treatment formats produced gains in overall marital and sexual satisfaction, demonstrating the utility of a self-help program in the treatment of orgasmic dysfunction. This study indicates that for clients who have no other major clinical presenting complaints, an approach that relies on education, information, and systematic progress through a program of directed masturbation will be effective in treating inorgasmia (LoPiccolo & Stock, 1986).

A second component in treatment of orgasmic dysfunction involves self-exploration, body awareness, and directed masturbation (LoPiccolo & Lobitz, 1972; Heiman & LoPiccolo, 1986). The program developed by LoPiccolo and Lobitz, which forms the basis of the *Becoming Orgasmic* self-help book, involves nine steps, as summarized in LoPiccolo and Stock (1987; pp 345–346; reprinted with permission of McGraw-Hill, Inc.).

> In step 1, the woman is supplied with the *Becoming Orgasmic* book, which contains diagrams and drawings of the female genitals. She learns to identify the various parts of her genitals and is encouraged to do some attitudinal work on body acceptance and acceptance of female sexuality as a legitimate expression for a decent woman, and to examine her own sexual history in terms of pathogenic influences.
>
> In step 2, the woman is encouraged to repeat this visual exploration, this time adding exploration of her body and genitals by touching. Again, considerable attitude change work is done in this stage of the program as well.
>
> In step 3, the woman attempts to locate areas of her body and genitals that produce pleasure when touched. Not surprisingly,

most women identify the obvious erogenous zones, including the clitoris, as the focus for their sexual pleasure.

> In step 4, the woman is directly instructed in techniques of masturbation. She is encouraged to explore varieties of pressures and speeds in stimulating her own genitals.
>
> In step 5, an attempt is made to make this procedure more erotic and sexual. The woman is encouraged to develop sexual fantasies and imagery; to read sexual books, including one of the many popular anthologies of women's sexual fantasies (Friday, 1973); and to use this visual, written, and fantasy material as an aid to facilitate her arousal.
>
> In step 6, if the woman has not yet reached orgasm, the use of the electric vibrator is introduced. When introducing the vibrator at this late stage in treatment, the risk is less that the woman will remain orgasmic only with the vibrator at the end of treatment, because she will have already learned to generate her own sexual arousal via other methods, i.e., touch, fantasy. Women who do have their first orgasm with a vibrator while in treatment routinely go on to have orgasms in other forms of sexual stimulation, but the vibrator is a useful means of obtaining the first orgasm.
>
> As the woman has been progressing through the first six steps in the sex therapy program, she and her partner have been typically assigned to do the standard Masters & Johnson (1970) "sensate focus," or body awareness, exercises, involving mutual caressing, touching, and communication. At this point, the woman's masturbation program and the couple exercises converge.
>
> In step 7, the woman demonstrates to her partner the technique she has learned that produces arousal and orgasm for her. In sex therapy, the partner is routinely encouraged to demonstrate his masturbation techniques for the woman, so this is a reciprocal learning process.
>
> In step 8, the woman instructs her male partner in his caressing and touching of her genitals to produce orgasm through his direct stimulation of her genitals.
>
> In step 9, the couple resumes penile-vaginal intercourse with the woman and/or the partner continuing direct manual stimulation of the clitoris to facilitate orgasm during penetration. Positions that facilitate

this continued clitoral stimulation include coitus with the man supine and the woman kneeling above him, the Masters & Johnson (1970) lateral-coital position, and rear entry intercourse during which the man can reach around the woman's body and have easy access to her clitoris. Although female orgasm during intercourse should not be emphasized as a goal for all couples, as this is not always a realistic expectation, concurrent clitoral stimulation may maximize this occurrence, if so desired by a couple in treatment (LoPiccolo & Stock, 1986).

Results based on approximately 150 women treated in a clinic directed by LoPiccolo indicate about 95% success in terms of the woman being able to reach orgasm in her own masturbation. About 85% of these women are also able to have orgasm during direct genital stimulation by the male partner. Around 40% of these women are able to have orgasm during penile-vaginal intercourse following this treatment program. This frequency may be comparable to the incidence for coital orgasm in the general population (Hunt, 1974).

Although this program has been found to be highly effective in treating global, lifelong lack of orgasm, and may require relatively small amounts of therapeutic time in the self-help format, there can be problems in clients' acceptance of the treatment package (LoPiccolo & Stock, 1987). Older women who have been raised very restrictively with regard to sex will often balk at the idea of masturbation. The most effective manner of dealing with this seems to be simply supplying the woman with the self-help book and allowing her to make a decision, without the therapist attempting to impose it as "required" treatment.

Another element in the treatment of women's orgasmic difficulties is a training program for increasing strength in the PC muscle, which is often low in women with global, lifelong lack of orgasm. A program of Kegel exercises is a standard treatment element for this problem.

For the woman who may become highly aroused but is just not able to reach orgasm, several other sex therapy techniques can be used. One technique involves the use of "orgasm triggers" (Heiman & LoPiccolo, 1986)—behaviors that are involuntary and occur spontaneously during orgasm. When performed voluntarily during high sexual arousal, these activities may imitate or trigger the orgasm. These behaviors include holding the breath, displacing the diaphragm downward, "bearing down" with the pelvic muscles, contracting the vaginal muscles, pointing the toes and tensing the leg and thigh muscles, throwing the head back and displacing the glottis, and pelvic thrusting. The actual mechanism by which these procedures work is not known. It may involve providing the woman with arousing proprioceptive feedback, disinhibiting her response by permission-giving, or cognitive distraction (eliminating excessive focus on having an orgasm). Although these triggers will not initiate an orgasm in a person who is not highly aroused, they are of some use in triggering orgasm for women who otherwise have difficulty reaching the threshold.

Another effective technique for women who can have orgasm alone in masturbation but cannot do so with their partner is the "role play" orgasm. Many women experience inhibition, modesty, or fear of displaying to a male the relatively uncontrolled, "unladylike" aspect of orgasm. The "role play orgasm" is a grossly exaggerated orgasm—conducted alone first, if the woman is inhibited in her own masturbation, and in the presence of a partner, if this is where inhibition is experienced. This technique works for women already experiencing a high level of arousal but a specific inhibition about having an orgasm (Heiman & LoPiccolo, 1986).

Situational (Secondary) Anorgasmia

This diagnosis, as noted above, has been applied to women with a wide range of sexual functioning, including those who attain orgasm only with masturbation and/or vibratory stimulation, those who are capable of multiple orgasms through partner stimulation but not with sexual intercourse, and those who are infrequently orgasmic with a partner.

Secondary anorgasmia is a conceptually nonspecific term. This diagnosis has been applied pejoratively to women who may in fact be functioning in a completely adequate and normal manner (LoPiccolo & Stock, 1986). In addition, due to sexual performance demands by partners and cultural myths about sexual functioning, some patients may identify unrealistic goals for therapeutic intervention (e.g., orgasm during intercourse without clitoral stimulation). A more realistic goal to adopt in this case is enabling a woman to experience orgasm through some means of partner stimulation if she has previously experienced orgasm only through masturbation. Heiman and Rowland (1981) have stressed the importance of ensuring that the woman is receiving adequate stimulation and that the couple enjoy sex, and determining why coital orgasm is important to them. They suggest that teaching the male to delay his ejaculation by pause or squeeze techniques may be helpful.

Heiman and Rowland (1981) have noted that there is no major treatment strategy for secondary orgasmic dysfunction. Because this dysfunction covers such a broad range of problems, different approaches are necessary. For women who are orgasmic during masturbation but not in the presence of a partner, various desensitization, disinhibition, and role play strategies may be helpful if self-consciousness or performance pressure are clinical issues. Other components of treatment packages have included assertiveness training, modeling, behavior rehearsal, and education (Munjack et al., 1976). Providing couples with accurate information in a solely educational intervention (Kilman et al., 1983) resulted in a reduction in sexual anxiety, increased orgasmic frequency, and increased female perceptions of foreplay activities and manual clitoral stimulation. Couple sexual communication is often necessary if the woman is to become able to indicate precisely what type, duration, and intensity of sexual stimulation she requires during sexual activity. Heiman and Rowland (1981) note that when the woman's inhibitions, performance anxiety, and reluctance to take responsibility for her sexual pleasure are factors, the man's encouragement, re-

spect and cooperation are required—and he must not require his partner to have an orgasm as proof of his own sexual adequacy.

One factor that appears to contribute to treatment success, particularly for secondary anorgasmia, is marital happiness prior to therapy. McGovern, Stewart, and LoPiccolo (1975) found that secondary anorgasmic females did not report increased frequency of orgasm from genital caressing by partner or during intercourse. It was hypothesized that a combination treatment approach—marital therapy and sex treatment—might be most effective in these cases.

A more recent study (Fichen et al., 1986) of 23 couples, in which the presenting problem was secondary orgasmic dysfunction in the wife, found that cognitive-affective changes (enjoyment, satisfaction) were twice as likely to occur as changes in behaviors (reported frequency, orgasmic response). The authors consider these results to indicate that sex therapy for secondary orgasmic dysfunction produces important gains, the recognition of which hinges on the selection of relevant dependent measures.

One modality that has demonstrated effectiveness in treatment of both primary and secondary orgasmic dysfunction in women is group treatment (LoPiccolo & Stock, 1986). Dimensions on which group treatment has varied include inclusion of male partners, number of treatment sessions, inclusion of primary versus secondary anorgasmic women, and selection of treatment techniques (LoPiccolo & Stock, 1986). In general, the literature indicates that group treatment can provide an affordable and supportive intervention that is most effective for clients who have no severe psychopathology, relationship distress, or other major psychological disturbance. Although evidence indicates that behavioral group treatment approaches are quite effective, research has not determined the reasons for the success (Bogat et al., 1987). Kuriansky and Sharpe (1981) propose four components of group treatment that may be crucial to its success: (1) disclosure and support in a group; (2) focus on arousal and pleasure rather than orgasm; (3) responsibility for sexual satisfaction and increased assertiveness; and (4) the empowerment of women by fulfilling their personal sexual needs through masturbation. Barbach (1974) reported a 100% success rate in attainment of orgasm through masturbation, and over 87% of the women were orgasmic in partner-related activities.

Schneidman and McGuire (1976) included male partners in several group sessions, finding that for most couples the sexual relationship continued to improve after therapy. During treatment some women reported that this therapy was perceived as threatening to their male partners. As they became more assertive sexually, the men became uneasy in response to their new behaviors. Prior to therapy, these male partners had been the sole initiators of intercourse, and the women had been passive recipients who participated out of obligation. When the women were instructed to initiate sexual activity as home assignments in therapy, male partners reacted either by being supportive or (in a smaller number of cases) by becoming resistant and refusing to cooperate fully. This development necessitated a separate meeting for all male partners in one group, to discuss their anxieties and treatment goals. Most couples found that the sexual relationship continued to improve after therapy; orgasm had become generalized from masturbation to partner-related activities in most cases by eight-month follow-up.

Ersner-Hershfield and Kopel (1979) evaluated the effects of partner participation on group treatment. Although partner presence did not seem to enhance orgasmic capacity, enhanced marital and sexual satisfaction occurred more in groups that included partners. In this study, the percentage of women who experienced orgasm in couple activities was 73% posttreatment and 82% at ten-week follow-up. The authors caution against generalizing their results to couples in which the male partner is unwilling *or* extremely willing to participate, as the average rating by males on their willingness to participate in their study was "slightly positive."

Leiblum and Ersner-Hershfield (1977) questioned whether orgasm during intercourse is a reasonable goal for all women in therapy. These authors stress consideration of the extent to which the male partner has negative sexual attitudes, or is himself sexually dysfunctional, in assessing treatment effectiveness.

Wakefield (1987a) has criticized the use of masturbation exercises assigned in preorgasmic women's groups. He considers the success rates reported by Barbach (1975) and Ersner-Hershfield and Kopel (1979) to be inflated and based on a semantic distortion of orgasmic success. Wakefield criticizes the criterion of partner orgasm as including any orgasm experienced while a partner is present—however, it may be accomplished. He proposes that a woman's orgasm during partner sex include only orgasm resulting from the direct stimulation of her genitals by her partner's penis, hand, or mouth. Wakefield refers to his definition as the "folk concept" of partner orgasm. He criticizes preorgasmic women's groups for a concept of orgasm that emphasizes the importance of the personal orgasmic pleasure of the woman, irrespective of relationship issues, and that encourages the woman to take responsibility for her own pleasure and to focus initially on self-sexuality. Wakefield may not have conceived of the possibility of intercourse with concurrent vibrator stimulation, or manual stimulation of the vagina or breasts concurrent with vibrator stimulation. Wakefield emphasizes that the woman should achieve orgasm only through direct stimulation by the male partner, not by herself and certainly not with the aid of a vibrator. One concern that others have raised repeatedly is that women in treatment should not be dependent on a narrow range or type of erotic stimulation. The therapist should employ treatment that maximizes women's ability to respond to the broadest range of sexual stimulation desired, and the pleasure and satisfaction of a woman's orgasm is not necessarily lessened by the means by which it is obtained. It should go without saying that individual sex therapy with one member of a couple will not necessarily have directly positive effects for both partners, and that partners should ideally be included at appropriate times during sex therapy.

Techniques for Facilitating Coital Orgasm

Leiblum and Ersner-Hershfield (1977) questioned whether orgasm during intercourse for all women is a necessary goal—or even a reasonable one. However, many couples present with a wish to have the female experience coital orgasm, not out of a feeling that it is pathologic not to do so, but simply as an experience they would like to have. Given the strong cultural bias toward coital orgasm, it is impossible to make a complete separation between functional and dysfunctional desire for coital orgasm. In couples who have good sexual communication, whose repertoire already includes other stimulation techniques, where the female is already orgasmic, and where there is no undue pressure on the woman by herself or by her partner, certain techniques can be tried. First, the woman can be advised to continue doing during coitus whatever behavior produces orgasm for her (e.g., clitoral stimulation by self or partner, or vibrator stimulation). If the type of extracoital stimulation does not lend itself to simultaneous intercourse (for example, oral sex), the woman is encouraged to engage in this behavior until highly sexually aroused, at which point the couple can shift to intercourse. Should she lose her arousal during intercourse, the couple can shift back to oral sex until high arousal is reestablished, then switch back to coitus.

A second type of situational orgasmic dysfunction that does not respond to pairing coitus with direct genital stimulation involves women who do not find coitus arousing, or who find concurrent clitoral stimulation during intercourse ineffective or irritating. Zeiss et al. (1977) developed a successful approach in which gradual changes are made in stimulation. Initially, the woman may be instructed to masturbate as she always has, but to insert a finger in the vagina without moving it. This enables her to learn to experience orgasm with something contained in the vagina. Once this has been accomplished, she can be instructed to masturbate while thrusting the finger in the vagina. Following success with this activity, the partner can then ma-

nipulate her clitoris, first with nothing in the vagina, then with either her or his finger inserted. If this is successful, the progression can then be made to having his penis passively contained in the vagina while she masturbates to orgasm. The next step involves passive penile containment while *he* stimulates her to orgasm manually. The final step, thrusting of the penis in the vagina with direct manual stimulation, may now be effective in producing orgasm. By breaking down the differences between masturbation and coitus into a series of small, discrete changes, Zeiss et al. have reported greater success in broadening the women's range of orgasmic responsivity (LoPiccolo & Stock, 1987). It is important, however, for researchers and therapists to take care not to overemphasize coital orgasm. It is apparent from the preceding fairly involved description of the treatment program that coital orgasm is not an easy goal for many women to attain—nor inherently a necessary one.

Eichel, Eichel, and Kule (1988) have developed a controversial treatment to facilitate coital orgasm. It consists of teaching couples the "coital alignment" technique, which combines the "riding high" variation of the "missionary" coital posture with genitally focused pressure-counterpressure stimulus applied by both partners during intercourse. In their study, a questionnaire was given, *post hoc,* to 21 males and 22 females who had learned the alignment technique, and to a volunteer group (22 females, 21 males) who had had no knowledge of the alignment technique. Of the 43 experimental participants, 39 had learned the alignment technique while participating in a two-year group therapy program for couples. Experimental females showed higher ratings of orgasm during coitus, simultaneous orgasm, and satisfaction criteria. Eichel et al. claim on the basis of this study that the coital alignment technique provides direct clitoral contact in coitus, facilitates female orgasm, and synchronizes the timing of male and female sexual responses. Although the technique is not yet well accepted in the discipline of sex therapy and research, it suggests the possibility that close partner communication may facilitate coital positions and movements that increase the likelihood of coital orgasm.

Therapeutic Issues

Kilmann (1978) and Andersen (1983) both performed comprehensive reviews of a large number of studies on the treatment of primary and secondary orgasmic dysfunction. In addition to directed masturbation for treatment of primary orgasmic dysfunction, other treatment approaches included sexual technique training, systematic desensitization, communication training, and reeducation procedures, presented in different treatment modalities (individual, couple, and group therapy). A number of interventions included in treatment have never been systematically evaluated: for example, inclusion of the partner in treatment and directed homework assignments. The efficacy of different assignments has not been studied. Another unknown is whether continued intercourse during treatment, on the one hand, and abstinence, on the other, have differential effects on treatment outcome, or whether identification of specific characteristics of women would help determine this. It has been argued by some (Madsen & Ullmann, 1967) that permitting sexual activity during treatment provides a direct means for couples to assess progress in their sexual functioning. Others have contended that continued intercourse without arousal or orgasm may constitute repeated failure experiences for the woman, undermining treatment gains in other areas (Masters & Johnson, 1970).

The most common criterion for treatment success has been self-report of orgasm (Kilmann, 1978; Andersen, 1983). Only a few researchers have reported on measures of satisfaction with sexual functioning, regardless of changes in orgasmic responsivity. Jayne (1981) raised the issue of whether orgasmic ability can be equated with sexual satisfaction in women, finding that women prefer the emotional closeness and intimacy associated with intercourse to masturbation, although orgasmic reliability is superior with masturbation. Assessment of sexual satisfaction, independent of outcome regard-

ing orgasm, is an important aspect of therapy and research outcome measures.

REFERENCES

Abel, G., Barlow, D., Blanchard, E., & Mavissakalian, M. (1975). Measurement of sexual arousal in male homosexuals: Effects of instructions and stimulus modality. *Archives of Sexual Behavior, 4,* 623–629.

Abel, G., Blanchard, E., & Barlow, D. (1981). Measurement of sexual arousal in several paraphiliacs: The effects of stimulus modality, instructional set and stimulus content. *Behavior Research and Therapy, 19,* 25–33.

Adams, A., Haynes, S., & Brayer, M. (1985). Cognitive distraction in female sexual arousal. *Psychophysiology, 22,* 689–696.

Adams, C. (1966). An informal preliminary report on some factors relating to sexual responsiveness of certain college wives. In M. De Martino (Ed.), *Sexual behavior and personality characteristics.* New York: Grove Press.

Addiego, F., Gelzer, E., Conolli, J., et al. (1981). Female ejaculation: A case study. *Journal of Sex Research, 17,* 13–21.

Allgeier, E., & Allgeier, R. (1984). *Sexual interactions.* Lexington, MA: D.C. Heath.

Alzate, H. (1985). Vaginal eroticism and female orgasm: A current appraisal. *Journal of Sex and Marital Therapy, 11,* 271–284.

American Psychiatric Association (1987). *Diagnostic and statistical manual of mental disorders* (3rd ed., rev.). Washington, DC: Author.

Andersen, B. (1983). Primary orgasmic dysfunction. *Psychological Bulletin, 43,* 105–136.

Bancroft, J. (1984). Hormones and human sexual behavior. *Journal of Sex and Marital Therapy, 10,* 3–22.

Barbach, J. (1974). Group treatment of preorgasmic women. *Journal of Sex and Marital Therapy, 1,* 139–145.

Barbach, J. (1975). *For yourself: The fulfilment of female sexuality.* Garden City, New York: Doubleday.

Barbach, J. (1980). Group treatment of anorgasmic women. In S. Leiblum & L. Pervin (Eds.), *Principles and practice of sex therapy.* New York: Guilford.

Bardwick, J. (1971). *Psychology of women: A study of biocultural conflicts.* New York: Harper & Row.

Becker, J., Skinner, L., Abel, G., & Trecy, E. (1982). Incidence and types of sexual dysfunctions in rape and incest survivors. *Journal of Sex and Marital Therapy, 8*, 65–74.

Belzer, E. (1981). Orgasmic expulsions of women: A review and heuristic inquiry. *Journal of Sex Research, 17*, 1–12.

Bogat, G., Hamernik, K., & Brooks, L. (1987). The influence of self-efficacy expectations on the treatment of preorgasmic women. *Journal of Sex and Marital Therapy, 13*, 128–136.

Bridges, C., Critelli, J., & Loos, V. (1985). Hypnotic susceptibility, inhibitory control, and orgasmic consistency. *Archives of Sexual Behavior, 14*, 373–376.

Butler, C. (1976). New data about female sexual response. *Journal of Sex and Marital Therapy, 2*, 40–46.

Cerny, J. (1978). Biofeedback and the voluntary control of sexual arousal in women. *Behavior Therapy, 9*, 847–855.

Chambless, D., Sultan, F., Stern, T., et al. (1984). The pubococcygeous and female orgasm: A correlational study with normal subjects. *Archives of Sexual Behavior, 11*, 479–490.

Darling, C., & Davidson, J. (1986). Enhancing relationships: Understanding the feminine mystique of pretending orgasm. *Journal of Sex and Marital Therapy, 12*, 182–196.

Darling, C., Davidson, J., & Cox, R. (1991). Female sexual response and the timing of partner orgasm. *Journal of Sex and Marital Therapy, 17*, 3–21.

Derogatis, L. (1981). Psychopathology in individuals with sexual dysfunction. *American Journal of Psychiatry, 6*, 1378.

Derogatis, L., Fagan, P., Schmidt, C., Wise, T., & Gilden, K. (1986). Psychological subtypes of anorgasmia: A marker variable approach. *Journal of Sex and Marital Therapy, 12*, 197–210.

Derogatis, L., & Meyer, J. (1979). A psychological profile of the sexual dysfunctions. *Archives of Sexual Behavior, 8*, 201–223.

Eichel, E., Eichel, J., & Kule, S. (1988). The technique of coital alignment and its relation to female orgasmic response and simultaneous orgasm. *Journal of Sex and Marital Therapy, 14*, 129–141.

Ellis, E., Calhoun, K., & Atkeson, B. (1980). Sexual dysfunction in victims of rape: Victims may experience a loss of sexual arousal and frightening flashbacks even one year after the assault. *Women and Health, 5*, 39–47.

Ellison, C. (1980). *A critique of the clitoral model of female sexuality*. Paper presented at the meeting of the American Psychological Association, Montreal, September 4.

Ersner-Hershfield, R., & Kopel, S. (1979). Group treatment of preorgasmic women: Evaluation of partner involvement and spacing of sessions. *Journal of Consulting and Clinical Psychology, 47*, 750–759.

Fichen, C., Libman, E., & Brender, W. (1986). Measurement of therapy outcome and maintenance of gains in the behavioral treatment of secondary orgasmic dysfunction. *Journal of Sex and Marital Therapy, 12*, 22–34.

Fisher, S. (1973). *The female orgasm*. New York: Basic Books.

Ford, C., & Beach, F. (1951). *Patterns of sexual behavior*. New York: Paul Hoeber.

Frank, D., Downard, E., & Lang, A. (1986). Androgyny, sexual satisfaction, and women. *Journal of Psychosocial Nursing, 24*, 10–15.

Frank, E., Anderson, D., & Rubenstein, D. (1978). Frequency of sexual dysfunction in "normal" couples. *New England Journal of Medicine, 299*, 111–115.

Friday, N. (1973). *My secret garden*. New York: Pocket Books.

Freud, S. (1961). Some psychical consequences of the anatomical distinction between the sexes. *Collected works of Sigmund Freud* (standard edition, vol. 19, pp. 248–260). London: Hogarth Press.

Gebhard, P. (1966). Factors in marital orgasm. *Journal of Social Issues, 22*, 88–95.

Geer, J., & Fuhr, R. (1976). Cognitive factors in sexual arousal: The role of distraction. *Journal of Consulting and Clinical Psychology, 44*, 238–243.

Goldberg, D., Whipple, B., Fishkin, R., et al. (1983). The Grafenberg spot and female ejaculation: A review of initial hypotheses. *Journal of Sex and Marital Therapy, 9*, 27–37.

Graber, B., & Kline-Graber, G. (1979). Female orgasm: Role of pubococcygeous muscle. *Journal of Clinical Psychiatry, 40*, 348–351.

Hariton, E., & Singer, J. (1974). Women's fantasies during sexual intercourse. *Journal of Consulting and Clinical Psychology, 42*, 313–322.

Heiman, J. (1977). A psychophysiological exploration of sexual arousal patterns in females and males. *Psychophysiology, 14*, 266–274.

Heiman, J. (1978). Uses of psychophysiology in the assessment and treatment of sexual dysfunction.

In J. LoPiccolo & L. LoPiccolo (Eds.), *Handbook of sex therapy*. New York: Plenum Press.

Heiman, J., & LoPiccolo, J. (1986). *Becoming orgasmic: A sexual growth program for women*. Englewood Cliffs, NJ: Prentice-Hall.

Heiman, J., & Rowland, D. (1981). Sexual dysfunction from a psychophysiological perspective. *International Journal of Mental Health, 10*, 134–147.

Hite, S. (1976). *The Hite report*. New York: Macmillan.

Hoon, E., & Hoon, P. (1978). Styles of sexual expression in women: clinical implications of multivariate analysis. *Archives of Sexual Behavior, 1*, 105–116.

Hunt, M. (1974). *Sexual behavior in the 1970's*. Chicago: Playboy Press.

Jayne, J. (1981). A two-dimensional model of female sexual response. *Journal of Sex and Marital Therapy, 7*, 3–30.

Kaplan, H. (1974). *The new sex therapy*. New York: Brunner/Mazel.

Kegel, A. (1952). Sexual functions of the pubococcygeus muscle. *Western Journal of Surgery, 60*, 521–524.

Kelly, M., Strassberg, D., & Kircher, J. (1990). Attitudinal and experiential correlates of anorgasmia. *Archives of Sexual Behavior, 19*, 165–177.

Kilman, P. (1978). The treatment of primary and secondary orgasmic dysfunction: A methodological review of the literature since 1970. *Journal of Sex and Marital Therapy, 4*, 155–175.

Kilman, P., Mills, K., Bella, B., Caid, C., Davidson, E., Drose, G., & Wanlass, R. (1983). The effects of sex education on women with secondary orgasmic dysfunction. *Journal of Sex and Marital Therapy, 9*, 79–87.

Kilpatrick, D., Resick, P., & Veronan, L. (1981). Effects of rape experience: A longitudinal study. *Journal of Social Issues, 37*, 105–122.

Kinsey, A., Pomeroy, W., & Martin, C. (1953). *Sexual behavior in the human female*. Philadelphia: W.B. Saunders.

Kirkpatrick, C. (1980). Sex roles and sexual satisfaction in women. *Psychology of Women Quarterly, 4*, 444–459.

Kuriansky, J., & Sharpe, I. (1981). Clinical and research implications of the evaluation of women's group therapy for anorgasmia: A review. *Journal of Sex and Marital Therapy, 7*, 268–277.

Ladas, A., Whipple, B., & Perry, J. (1982). *The G-spot and other recent discoveries about human sexuality*. New York: Holt.

Laws, D., & Rubin, H. (1969). Instructional control of autonomic sexual response. *Journal of Nervous and Mental Diseases, 136*, 272–278.

Lentz, S., & Zeiss, A. (1984). Fantasy and sexual arousal in college women: An empirical investigation. *Imagination, Cognition and Personality, 3*, 185–202.

Lieblum, S., & Ersner-Hershfield, R. (1977). Sexual enhancement groups for dysfunctional women: An evaluation. *Journal of Sex and Marital Therapy, 2*, 139–152.

Lifshitz, J., & Adams, H. (1980). *Female sexual arousal: Distraction and attention in orgasmic and nonorgasmic women*. Paper presented to the annual convention of the Association for the Advancement of Behavior Therapy, New York.

LoPiccolo, J., & Lobitz, C. (1972). The role of masturbation in the treatment of orgasmic dysfunction. *Archives of Sexual Behavior, 2*, 163–172.

LoPiccolo, J., & Stock, W. (1986). Sexual counseling in gynecological practice. In Z. Rosenwaks, F. Benjamin, & M. Stone (Eds.), *Gynecology: Principles and practice*. New York: Macmillan.

LoPiccolo, J., & Stock, W. (1987). Treatment of sexual dysfunction. *Journal of Consulting and Clinical Psychology, 54*, 158–167.

Madsen, C., & Ullmann, L. (1967). Case histories and short communications. *Behaviour Research and Therapy, 5*, 67–68.

Masters, W., & Johnson, V. (1966). *Human sexual response*. Boston: Little, Brown.

Masters, W., & Johnson, V. (1970). *Human sexual inadequacy*. Boston: Little, Brown.

McGovern, K., Stewart, R., & LoPiccolo, J. (1975). Secondary orgasmic dysfunction: Analysis and strategies for treatment. *Archives of Sexual Behavior, 4*, 265.

Mead, M. (1949). *Male and female: A study of the sexes in a changing world*. New York: Dell.

Miller, W., Williams, A., & Bernstein, M. (1982). The effects of rape on marital and sexual adjustment. *American Journal of Family Therapy, 10*, 51–58.

Morokoff, P. (1978). Determinants of female orgasm. In J. LoPiccolo & L. LoPiccolo (Eds.), *Handbook of sex therapy*. New York: Plenum.

Morokoff, P. (1989). Sex bias and POD. *American Psychologist, 44*, 73–75.

Morokoff, P., & LoPiccolo, J. (1986). A comparative evaluation of minimal therapist contact and fifteen session treatment for female orgasmic dysfunction. *Journal of Consulting and Clinical Psychology, 54,* 294–300.

Moulton, R. (1976). *Some effects of the new feminism.* Paper presented to the joint meeting of the American Academy of Psychoanalysis and the American Psychiatric Association.

Munjack, D., Cristol, A., Goldstein, A., Phillips, D., Goldberg, A., Whipple, K., Staples, F., & Kanno, P. (1976). Behavioral treatment of orgasmic dysfunction: A controlled study. *British Journal of Psychiatry, 129,* 497–502.

Newcomb, M., & Bentler, D. (1983). Dimensions of subjective female orgasmic responsiveness. *Journal of Personality and Social Psychology, 44,* 862–873.

O'Connor, D. (1979). Good girls and orgasms. *Newsweek* (October 22).

Perry, J., & Whipple, B. (1981). Pelvic muscle strength of female ejaculators: Evidence in support of a new theory or orgasm. *Journal of Sex Research, 17,* 22–39.

Riger, S., & Gordon, M. (1981). The fear of rape: A study in social control. *Journal of Social Issues, 37,* 71–92.

Robertiello, R. (1970). The "clitoral versus vaginal orgasm" controversy, and some of its ramifications. *Journal of Sex Research, 6,* 307–11.

Schneidman, B., & McGuire, L. (1976). Group therapy for nonorgasmic women: Two age levels. *Archives of Sexual Behavior, 5,* 239–248.

Schover, L., Friedman, J., Weiler, S., Heiman, J., & LoPiccolo, J. (1982). Multiaxial problem-oriented system for sexual dysfunctions: An alternative to DSM-III. *Archives of General Psychiatry, 39,* 614–19.

Seidler-Feller, D. (1985). A feminist critique of sex therapy. In L. Rosewater & L. Walker (Eds.), *Feminist therapy: A coming of age.* New York: Springer.

Singer, J., & Singer, J. (1972). Types of female orgasm. *Journal of Sex Research, 8,* 255–267.

Smith, A., Calhoun, K., & Chambless, D. (1983). Stimulus focus, sensate focus, and spectatoring: Effects on female arousal. Presented at the annual meeting of the American Psychological Association, Anaheim, CA.

Stock, W. (1984). Sex roles and sexual dysfunction. In C. Widom (Ed.), *Sex roles and psychopathology.* New York: Plenum.

Stock, W., Geer, J. (1982). A study of fantasy-based sexual arousal in women. *Archives of Sexual Behavior, 11,* 33–47.

Sultan, F., Chambless, D., Stem, T., et al. (1980). The relationship of pubococcygeal condition to female sexual responsiveness in a normal population. Paper presented at a meeting of the Association of the Advancement of Behavior Therapy, New York.

Szasz, T. (1961). *The myth of mental illness: Foundations of a theory of personal conduct.* New York: Hober-Harper.

Tiefer, L. (1988). A feminist critique of the sexual dysfunction nomenclature. *Women and Therapy, 7,* 5–21.

Tiefer, L. (1990). *Gender and meaning in DSM-III (& III-R) sexual dysfunctions.* Panel: Postmodern Gender Issues, annual meeting of the American Psychological Association, August 10, Boston.

Wakefield, J. (1987a). The semantics of success: Do masturbation exercises lead to partner orgasm? *Journal of Sex and Marital Therapy, 8,* 135–150.

Wakefield, J. (1987b). Sex bias in the diagnosis of primary orgasmic dysfunction. *American Psychologist, 42,* 464–471.

Wakefield, J. (1989). Manufacturing female dysfunction: A reply to Morokoff. *American Psychologist, 44,* 75–77.

Warner, J. (1982). *The rebirth of the vaginal orgasm blues: Old and new myths and confusion about female orgasm.* Paper presented at the annual meeting of the American Psychological Association, Division 35, Open Symposium of Research in Psychology and Women, Washington, DC.

Zeiss, A., Rosen, G., & Zeiss, R. (1977). Orgasm during intercourse: A treatment strategy for women. *Journal of Consulting and Clinical Psychology, 45,* 891–895.

CHAPTER 10

INHIBITED MALE ORGASM

Joost Dekker, Netherlands Institute of Primary Health Care

Research on inhibited male orgasm is rather scarce. There are some studies on psychopathology and treatment of this disorder, but the greater part of the literature consists of clinically derived hypotheses and opinions. Several factors may have contributed to this state of affairs. Inhibited male orgasm is a relatively rare condition. Both in the general population and in clinical practice, the prevalence of this disorder is rather low (Nathan, 1986). Furthermore, inhibited male orgasm is known as a disorder that is relatively difficult to treat. Although controlled studies do not exist, clinical experience suggests that the outcome is rather poor. These features make inhibited male orgasm a less than inviting topic of research, which may explain the paucity of research in this area.

The understanding of inhibited male orgasm is also hampered by our limited knowledge of the physiological and psychological mechanisms of normal orgasm. Research concerning mechanisms of orgasm has only recently begun, and the body of knowledge on orgasm is not very

impressive as yet. However, knowledge about normal orgasm is necessary in order to understand the inhibition of orgasm. Understanding of the inhibition of orgasm means that one knows how certain etiological factors interfere with the mechanisms that normally produce orgasm. It will be argued in this chapter that research on variations in normal orgasm should have a high priority. Better knowledge of normal orgasm can be expected to facilitate research into etiological factors in inhibited orgasm.

DEFINITION AND DESCRIPTION OF THE DISORDER

Definition

Inhibited male orgasm is defined in the DSM-III-R (American Psychiatric Association, 1987) as follows:

> Persistent or recurrent delay in, or absence of, orgasm in a male following a normal

sexual excitement phase during sexual activity that the clinician, taking into account the person's age, judges to be adequate in focus, intensity, and duration. This failure to achieve orgasm is usually restricted to an inability to reach orgasm in the vagina, with orgasm possible with other types of stimulation, such as masturbation (p. 295).

The DSM-III-R requires three specifications of this (and other) sexual dysfunctions. First, it should be specified whether the dysfunction is "psychogenic only" or psychogenic and biogenic. If the disorder is biogenic only—due to a physical disorder or to medication—a physical disorder or condition should be diagnosed. In addition, if another mental disorder is the primary cause of the sexual difficulties, a sexual dysfunction should not be diagnosed; in that case the other mental disorder should be diagnosed. However, personality disorders and other problems may coexist with sexual dysfunctions. Second, it should be specified whether the disorder is lifelong or acquired. The disorder is listed as acquired if the patient has previously functioned well but then develops symptoms. If the disorder has always been present, the disorder is listed as lifelong. Third, it should be specified whether the disorder is generalized or situational. If the disorder is present in all situations and with all partners, it is generalized. On the other hand, the disorder is situational if it is limited to certain situations or with certain partners. In this respect, the distinction between sexual interaction with a partner and masturbation is particularly important: In many patients, orgasm is inhibited during sexual interaction with a partner, but not during masturbation.

Many authors have made a distinction between primary and secondary sexual disorders. It appears that in the DSM-III-R, the distinction between primary and secondary disorders has been replaced by a distinction on two axes: lifelong vs. acquired and generalized vs. situational. This is an improvement, because in the primary-secondary distinction, the time frame and the situation frame are confounded. For example, in the primary-secondary system it is not

clear how to diagnose a patient who has a lifelong disorder during interaction with a partner but has no problems during masturbation; in the DSM-III-R system this patient is diagnosed as lifelong-situational.

In the DSM-III-R, no other subclassifications or subtypes are mentioned. However, a number of subtypes have been described in the literature (Vandereycken, 1986; Kothari, 1984). Traditionally, a distinction has been made between delayed and absent orgasm. Other names for these disorders are *retarded* and *deficient* orgasm, respectively. In the DSM-III-R, both disorders are mentioned in the definition of inhibited male orgasm, but no formal distinction is made.

Another set of subtypes may be characterized as cases of incomplete orgasmic response. One of these subtypes comprises patients who seem to have a normal ejaculation (including both emission and expulsion of ejaculate), but who complain of loss of or a marked decrease in their orgasmic sensation. This disorder has been labeled *anaesthetic ejaculation* (Williams, 1985). The experience of orgasm and ejaculation are presumably two separate entities. In this disorder the experience of orgasm is selectively impaired, while ejaculation is not affected.

The latter disorder should be distinguished from a disorder called *partial ejaculatory incompetence* (Kaplan, 1974) or *squirtless seminal dribble* (Kothari, 1984). In this condition, semen seeps out of the penis instead of being propelled. The associated orgasmic experience is weak or absent. Normally, ejaculation starts with the emission of ejaculate from various vesicles. Within seconds the emission phase is followed by the expulsion phase: Muscle contractions expel the ejaculate through the penis. The experience of orgasm is associated in time with the expulsion phase. In partial ejaculatory incompetence there is a normal emission of ejaculate, but the expulsion of ejaculate and the orgasmic experience are impaired.

In association with the expulsion of ejaculate by means of muscle contractions, there is a contraction of the bladder neck. If this contraction is impaired, the ejaculate ends up in the bladder.

This disorder is called *retrograde ejaculation*. These individuals do experience emission, expulsion (without the transportation of semen), and orgasm.

The emission phase of the ejaculation may be selectively impaired (Kothari, 1984). These patients have a normal expulsion phase and orgasmic experience, but they lack the emission of semen.

Kothari (1984) has given a classification of the various orgasmic dysfunctions in men:

1. Early orgasmic response (or premature ejaculation)
2. Delayed orgasmic response
3. Absent orgasmic response
4. Incomplete orgasmic response (subdivided as follows)
   a. Emission phase disorders
   b. Contractile (or expulsion) phase disorders:
      (1) squirtless seminal dribble
      (2) retrograde ejaculation (or *seminal reflux,* as Kothari calls this disorder)
   c. Anaesthetic ejaculation (in Kothari's classification this category is lacking, but it seems logical to include it here)

To specify some of these disorders, Kothari makes a distinction between primary and secondary disorders and between partial and total disorders. These specifications do not seem entirely satisfactory; I prefer the DSM-III-R specifications: lifelong vs. acquired and generalized vs. situational. The combination of Kothari's classification and the DSM-III-R specifications seems to offer an adequate classification of the various manifestations of inhibited male orgasm.

Diagnostic Problems

In applying the DSM-III-R diagnostic criteria, the clinician has to judge whether the inhibition of orgasm occurs despite a normal sexual excitement phase during adequate sexual activity. Thus, it is assumed that one knows which events cause an orgasm. However, these events are not known. Various authors have hypothesized that pelvic muscle contractions trigger orgasm (see Rosen & Beck, 1988). But other peripheral and/or central processes may also function as orgasm triggers. There exist only theoretical accounts of how orgasm is caused; specific, empirical evidence does not exist. This leaves the clinician with only a rather vague idea of "normal sexual excitement" and "adequate sexual activity." A certain level of sexual arousal in combination with continuing genital stimulation will be regarded as adequate conditions in most cases, but this is far from a precise definition of adequate sexual arousal and activity.

There is also a problem with the definition of delay of orgasm. The range of orgasmic latency is very wide (Kinsey et al., 1948; Fisher et al., 1986). Fisher et al. reported a latency of 495 seconds (a little more than eight minutes), with a standard deviation of 219 seconds (almost four minutes) in men masturbating to orgasm in the laboratory while viewing a movie of "average" arousal quality. The wide range of orgasmic latency precludes an objective definition of delay of orgasm. In the absence of objective standards on orgasmic latency, the clinician must rely on the subjective judgment of the patient. Generally, if the patient feels that it takes too long to reach orgasm, the diagnosis of inhibited orgasm will be considered. Therefore, the patient's subjective judgment is an important element in the diagnosis. This conclusion also pertains to the diagnosis of absent orgasm. In the case of an older man, who does not have an orgasm in every sexual encounter, it may not be easy to decide whether this is abnormal or not. Probably, the clinician will be more inclined to make the diagnosis if the patient is very dissatisfied and concerned. Thus, in the case of both delayed and absent orgasm, the subjective judgment of the patient plays an important role in the decision to make the diagnosis. However, in some cases the patient's standards may be unrealistic and may themselves need to be targeted in treatment.

Finally, there may be a semantic problem between the patient and the clinician. It is not uncommon for patients to complain of the absence of orgasm when erectile difficulties are the actual problem. Erectile difficulties often lead to the absence of orgasm. Presumably, the absence of orgasm is the cardinal condition for some patients, so they complain of that rather than erectile difficulties. Of course, this semantic problem can be solved by a careful questioning of the patient. A careful history taking will indicate whether the actual problem is inhibition of orgasm, erectile dysfunction, or a combination of both. The latter possibility should also be kept in mind, since erectile difficulties may precede or follow orgasmic problems.

Reaction of the Patient and His Partner

There is a myth that the patient and his female partner actually enjoy inhibited male orgasm, since it enables the man "to go on forever." This surely is a mistake. The male patient is often very frustrated about his problem. One aspect of this frustration is the absence of orgasmic release. Another, more important aspect is the loss of lust and pleasure. These men often describe sexual activity as "hard work." To reach an orgasm becomes an overriding goal. The man obsessively works to reach this goal, but sexual activity is no longer pleasurable.

Frequently, the female partner does not appreciate the inhibition of her partner's orgasm either; prolonged sexual activity is not very enjoyable for her. If coitus goes on too long, it may become painful. Stimulating her partner's genitals in another way (e.g., with her hand) becomes "work" for her too. Also, the partner often complains that her partner is "untouchable"; these men seem to avoid extensive touching and caressing. This avoidance—which may be a manifestation of the way these patients cope with sexual feelings, as discussed in the next section—frustrates their partners.

Both the man and his partner may interpret the absence of orgasm as a rejection of the partner. The inhibition of orgasm is taken as evidence of a lack of love for or interest in the partner. According to Kaplan (1974), some pa-

tients fake an orgasm. This enables them to keep their partners from feeling rejected.

Finally, patients may bring inhibited male orgasm to the attention of a clinician because it causes infertility. Couples who are infertile because of inbited male orgasm usually do not seek treatment for the loss of orgasmic release or sexual lust. The infertility due to the lack of ejaculation is the primary reason for seeking treatment.

The statements above apply to heterosexual patients. Homosexual patients and their partners react in similar ways. Inhibited orgasm may possibly even more aversive for some homosexual men because of a higher value is placed on short orgasmic latency in certain homosexual encounters. Wilensky and Myers (1986) have described nine cases of inhibited orgasm in homosexual men. Three of these men simulated orgasm to hide their orgasmic inhibition from their partners.

PSYCHOPATHOLOGY

Prevalence

Inhibited male orgasm is a relatively uncommon condition in clinical practice. Several studies have described the distribution of diagnoses in male patients presenting a sexual dysfunction. The distribution of diagnoses in several studies describing relatively large samples has been summarized in Table 10.1. The distribution varies between studies, probably reflecting differences in patterns of referral to the various clinics and/or differences in diagnostic criteria. But in all studies, inhibited male orgasm is the least frequently diagnosed disorder; the frequency ranges from 0% to 12.5%. A survey of sex therapy providers shows a similar result: Inhibited male orgasm was among the least commonly treated dysfunctions (Kilmann et al., 1986).

As Table 10.1 indicates, Masters and Johnson (1970) reported a relatively low percentage (3.8%) of patients with inhibited male orgasm. In five studies, a higher percentage has been

Table 10.1. Distribution of Diagnoses (Percentages) in Male Patients Presenting a Sexual Dysfunction

		DIAGNOSIS				
	N	INHIBITED MALE ORGASM	PREMATURE EJACULATION	ERECTILE DYSFUNCTION	OTHER*	
Masters & Johnson, 1970	448	3.8	41.5	54.7	-	100%
Bancroft & Coles, 1976	73	12.3	31.5	56.2	-	100%
Arentewicz & Schmidt, 1980	88	0.0	35.2	64.8	-	100%
Dekker & Everaerd, 1983	46	10.9	17.4	71.7	-	100%
De Amicis et al., 1984	40	5.0	40.0	35.0	20.0	100%
De Amicis et al., 1985	44	2.3	45.5	34.1	18.1	100%
Dekker et al., 1985	46	13.0	19.6	54.3	13.0	100%
Wilensky & Myers, 1987	72	12.5	—————	87.5	—————	100%

* Desire phase disorders probably have been underestimated.

reported. Thus, the prevalence in clinical practice may be somewhat higher than Masters and Johnson's often cited figure.

The prevalence of inhibited male orgasm in the general population is also rather low. Nathan (1986) has reanalyzed the data of general population sex surveys. The results indicate that lifelong inhibition is a very rare condition: the prevalence is probably around 1.5 in 1000. Acquired inhibition has a higher prevalence, but according to Nathan, even including these cases, inhibited orgasm affects not more than 3–4% of the nongeriatric male population.

There are two general population studies that have not been reviewed by Nathan. Frenken (1980) has reported on frequency of orgasm during coitus in a sample of 250 men. These were heterosexual men, with a steady partner, ranging in age from 18 to 55. In answering questions, the men referred to their sexual experience in the past half year. For every ten coital encounters, 1% indicated that they had an orgasm once or twice; 3% had an orgasm three to five times; and 4% had an orgasm six times. All these men (8% in total) were dissatisfied with the frequency of orgasm. Based on further data, Frenken estimated that 2% had a serious inhibition of orgasm, and 6% had a mild inhibition. Bancroft (1989) cites research by Sanders, who reported that 1% of men responding to a questionnaire in a women's magazine had difficulty with orgasm (other than premature ejaculation). This figure is

less than the 3–4% estimated by Nathan, but men who respond to a questionnaire in a women's magazine are probably not very representative of the general population. The Frenken data (2% serious and 6% mild inhibition or orgasm) are rather consistent with Nathan's estimate of 3–4% of the nongeriatric male population.

Nathan has discussed the methodological deficiencies that characterize epidemiological studies in the field of sex research. These deficiencies can be summarized as follows. Diagnostic criteria are often not explicitly stated, which seriously impedes interpretation of the findings. In addition, the DSM-III-R does not consider a sexual problem to be a dysfunction if it is exclusively biogenic or if it is caused by another mental disorder, but in the surveys this differentiation is not made. In many cases, the samples studied are not representative or are rather small. Finally, many studies fail to give a specific time frame for the respondent to consider when giving an answer. This may introduce error in the data. For these reasons, one should be very cautious in interpreting these studies. This warning also applies to the findings on inhibited male orgasm.

Associated Features

An erectile disorder may be associated with inhibited male orgasm. In some patients the erectile disorder develops after (and probably as the result of) the orgasmic disorder. In other patients the erectile disorder precedes the orgasmic problem. Desire-phase disorders are seldom associated with inhibited male orgasm (see, e.g., Dekker et al., 1985). Some men with inhibited orgasm tend to avoid sexual activity. This kind of avoidance should not be confused with hypoactive sexual desire; in extreme cases the extent of avoidance may justify the diagnosis of sexual aversion disorder.

Marital difficulties may coexist with inhibited male orgasm. An ongoing power struggle, hostility towards the partner, and a lack of commitment to the relationship have been mentioned in particular (Munjack & Kanno, 1979; Schull & Sprenkle, 1980). Marital difficulties have been conceptualized both as an etiological factor and as a result of the orgasmic disorder (Munjack & Kanno, 1979).

Finally, intrapersonal disorders may be associated with inhibited male orgasm. Fear (in many different manifestations), anxiety, and hostility have been observed in these patients. Also, some patients are rather depressed. Depressed feelings may precede the inhibition of orgasm, or they may develop in reaction to the disorder.

Course and Subtypes

Various subtypes of orgasmic disorders were described in the first section of this chapter. These include delayed orgasmic response, absent orgasmic response, and incomplete orgasmic response. In the latter category, a further distinction has been made between emission phase disorders, contractile or expulsion disorders (squirtless seminal dribble and retrograde ejaculation), and anaesthetic ejaculation (see Table 10.2). Emission phase disorders and retrograde ejaculation most probably are completely biogenic (Kothari, 1984). These disorders would therefore not belong to the diagnostic category inhibited male orgasm, as defined by the DSM-III-R. The other disorders do belong to that category. The disorders can be specified on two dimensions: first, lifelong vs. acquired; second, generalized vs. situational.

Clinical experience seems to suggest that life-

Table 10.2. Subtypes of Inhibited Male Orgasm

SUBTYPES OF INHIBITED MALE ORGASM
1. Delayed orgasmic response
2. Absent orgasmic response
3. Incomplete orgasmic response
   a. Emission phase disorders
   b. Contractile or expulsion phase disorders:
      (1) Squirtless seminal dribble
      (2) Retrograde ejaculation
   c. Anaesthetic ejaculation
SPECIFICATIONS
1. Lifelong versus acquired
2. Generalized versus situational

long disorders are much more resistant to therapy than acquired disorders. Similarly, it is thought that in a generalized disorder the prognosis is worse than in a situational disorder (Kaplan, 1974). However, there is no empirical evidence to support these views. The prognostic value of these dimensions is therefore uncertain.

It is also thought that the prognosis is better in patients whose disorder is relatively independent of deeper psychopathology or sexual trauma (Masters & Johnson, 1970; Kaplan, 1974). In a report on nine homosexual men with inhibited orgasm, Wilensky and Myers (1986) indeed found that as the level of general psychopathology increased, the prognosis deteriorated. Further evidence is required to substantiate this view.

Finally, the natural course of inhibited male orgasm varies considerably. Some patients report a very long duration of their disorder—15 to 20 years (Dekker et al., 1985). At the other extreme are men who occasionally experience a modest difficulty in reaching orgasm (Kaplan, 1974). Evidently, the range of the natural course is very wide. In the absence of further data, the distribution of men over this range is unknown.

Theories and Etiology

There are quite a number of theories on the causes of inhibited male orgasm. They describe etiological factors at levels ranging from spinal reflexes to the relationship between partners. A common deficiency of these theories is the lack of an understanding of *how* the indicated etiological factors interfere with orgasm. This is mainly due to limited knowledge of normal orgasm, which is essential for an understanding of inhibited orgasm. Once normal orgasm and the mechanisms that lead to it are understood, it will be possible to study how etiological factors interfere with orgasm. Unfortunately, orgasm and its determinants constitute a relatively neglected area of research. In the last decade, however, researchers seem to have realized the importance of understanding orgasm. Some empirical and theoretical studies have been published (Szasz & Carpenter, 1989; Davidson, 1980; Bancroft, 1989). This could be the beginning of a better grasp of normal orgasm (and thus of the etiology of inhibited orgasm as well).

This section starts with a discussion of research on normal orgasm; then theories and research on the etiology of inhibited male orgasm are reviewed.

Orgasm

Orgasm is a complex response involving the whole body. During orgasm there are changes in the genitalia, other peripheral physiological systems, and subjective experience. Bancroft (1989) has classified these changes into five categories:

- Genital changes
- Changes in skeletal muscle tone and semi-voluntary movements
- General cardiovascular and respiratory changes
- Somatic sensory experiences
- Altered consciousness

Contractions of facial musculature are only superficially mentioned by Bancroft, and he fails to mention vocal reactions. Thus, it seems that a sixth category should be added to this list:

- Vocal and facial expressive reactions

The *genital response* during orgasm in men consists of ejaculation. Masters and Johnson (1966) have divided ejaculation into two distinct phases, known as the *emission phase* and the

expulsion (or *contractile*) *phase*. During the emission phase, sperm and seminal fluids are collected by means of smooth muscle contractions of internal reproductive organs (the seminal vesicles, vas deferens, and prostate). These fluids—the semen—are deposited in the prostatic urethra. At the same time, the internal sphincter of the urinary bladder is closed, thereby preventing retrograde passage of the semen into the bladder. This also prevents urine from mixing with the semen. During the expulsion phase, the semen is forcefully transported outward. This phase starts with the relaxation of the external sphincter of the bladder, which allows the semen to arrive in the penile urethra. Through forceful contractions of striated muscles (perineal musculature, bulbospongiosus and ischiocavernosus muscles, and urethral sphincter), the semen is propelled through the penis.

As the excitement increases, changes occur in general *skeletal muscle activity*. Most of these changes depend on the kind of sexual activity the subject is involved in, but some changes are stereotyped and are more or less involuntary. During orgasm, characteristic spastic contractions of muscle groups (such as rectus abdominus, sternomastoid, and striated muscles of the hand and feet) are often present (Masters & Johnson, 1966). Using an anal probe, Bohlen et al. (1980) assessed pelvic muscle contractions. At orgasm, subjects produced a characteristic series of about 10 to 15 contractions. In most subjects the pattern of contractions was a simple series of regular contractions, but in a number of men irregular contractions preceded or followed a regular series.

During orgasm *cardiovascular responses* increase. Masters and Johnson (1966) recorded heart rates ranging from 110 to 180 bpm. They also recorded elevation in systolic (40/100 mm Hg) and diastolic (20/50 mm Hg) blood pressure. The *respiratory rate* increases during orgasm: Masters and Johnson reported respiratory rates as high as 40 per min.

Somatic sensory experiences during orgasm relate to ejaculation and other peripheral responses. Masters and Johnson (1966) have divided the ejaculatory experience into two phases: (1) the sensation of ejaculatory inevitability, which parallels the emission phase of ejaculation; and (2) contractile sensations and the feeling of a buildup of fluid volume, which parallels the expulsion phase of ejaculation. Apart from the ejaculation, subjects may be aware of various peripheral responses, such as increased heart rate and muscle tension.

At orgasm, subjects experience *altered consciousness*. With an intense orgasm, awareness of the environment (including the partner) seems to be considerably reduced (Bancroft, 1989; Everaerd & Dekker, 1981). Instead, the subject is primarily aware of his private experience. This experience varies considerably from subject to subject (see Vance & Wagner, 1976; Hite, 1978). However, an intense feeling of pleasure or lust seems to be a common aspect of these experiences. Despite the intensity of the experience of orgasm, attempts to demonstrate EEG changes during orgasm have not been very successful (Graber et al., 1985).

In addition to an increased breathing rate, subjects often produce *vocal expressive reactions* such as moaning or sighing (Pomeroy, 1967; Kinsey et al., 1948). These vocal reactions seem to increase as orgasm approaches. During orgasm, subjects often show a distorted *facial expression*. Possibly this is a stereotyped expression, characteristic of orgasm.

Mechanisms of Orgasm

The mechanism underlying orgasm has been conceptualized as a *spinal reflex*. In an article on women's orgasm, Mould (1980) gave a critical discussion of the then existing spinal models. Mould also proposed an alternative spinal model that incorporates essential features of previous models into one more consistent with the neurological functioning of skeletal muscles. According to Mould, a high level of vasocongestion leads to a biasing of muscle spindles and to elevated levels of tension in the pelvic muscles. These effects set the stage for clitoral stimulation to produce rhythmic, orgasmic contractions. Clitoral stimulation elicits these contractions via a spinal effect on the biased muscle

spindles, which produces rhythmic contractions in the highly tensed pelvic muscles. Thus, processes in the pelvic muscles are hypothesized to trigger orgasm. Mould hypothesizes that this model also applies to men: ". . . other than changing a word or two the model could be applied almost equally to men—'almost' because the model does not account for the emission stage of orgasm in men . . ." (p. 200).

Human evidence for the existence of a spinal mechanism of orgasm has been produced by Szasz and Carpenter (1989). Vibratory stimulation of the glans penis triggered a series of body reactions in most men with spinal cord lesions above T11. These reactions were very similar to the physical manifestations of sexual arousal and orgasm in men with intact nervous systems. A typical series of events ran as follows: abdominal spasms; loss of erection (in subjects normally capable of touch-reflex reactions); toe and leg spasms; a drop of pulse rate; a purplish color in the glans penis; the sensation of inevitability of ejaculation; further strengthening of muscle spasms; a purple and swollen glans, increase of pulse rate, perspiration on forehead and face; ejaculation, accompanied by vocalizations and high blood pressure and pulse rate; lessening and stopping of spasms; and tired but elated feeling, with reduction of blood pressure and pulse rate. In men with lesions at the T11 or below, no ejaculation could be elicited, and only one subject showed other peripheral responses to vibration.

The results of this study suggest that a spinal mechanism exists in the segments below T11. This mechanism functions in response to stimulation of the glans penis in the absence of higher-level control. Several subjects also reported subjective reactions (e.g., muscle tension, ejaculatory inevitability, feeling of elation), but it is not clear how these sensations come about when the spinal cord is injured. The report of Szasz and Carpenter does not clearly mention the intense feelings of pleasure and lust that accompany orgasm in men with intact nervous systems, but it seems that these feelings were absent in the men with spinal cord injuries. Thus, these feelings seem to require input from the segments T11 and below into higher neural levels.

In addition to spinal mechanisms there may exist *central mechanisms* of orgasm. Bancroft (1989) has argued that the altered state of consciousness during orgasm suggests a central neurophysiological event. Indeed, if my interpretation of the Szasz and Carpenter study is correct, that study seems to indicate that intense feelings of pleasure and lust require input to higher spinal and/or brain levels. Of course, this does not prove the existence of a separate central mechanism of orgasm or orgasmic experience. Orgasmic experience may simply be a reflection of lower-level neural input. But— especially because of the intenseness of the experience—a central mechanism of orgasm and/ or orgasmic experience is a possibility.

In addition there are at least two phenomena that suggest separate mechanisms for ejaculation and the subjective experience of orgasm. In research on spinal cord-injured men, Money (1960) described "phantom orgasms." These subjects experienced orgasm in the absence of ejaculation. The reverse event also exists; ejaculation without the experience of orgasm has been described by Williams (1985), who called this phenomenon *anaesthetic ejaculation*. In these patients both the emission phase and the expulsion (or contractile) phase of ejaculation seem to be present. Thus there is a full ejaculation, but no orgasmic experience. Finally, men may have multiple orgasms (Robbins & Jensen, 1978; Dunn & Trost, 1989). But multiple orgasms in men seem to consist of a selective inhibition of the emission phase of ejaculation, while the expulsion phase is present (Robbins & Jensen, 1978). Therefore, this phenomenon is probably not an example of a complete dissociation of ejaculation and orgasmic experience.

In summary, phantom orgasms, anesthaetic ejaculation, and the data of Szasz and Carpenter suggest that ejaculation and orgasmic experience are seperate events. Ejaculation appears to be based on a spinal mechanism. It can be speculated that orgasmic experience is based on spinal input to a central mechanism.

However direct evidence for such a central mechanism is lacking (Graber et al., 1985; Bancroft, 1989).

Davidson (1980) has suggested a division of orgasmic mechanisms that is different from the division into ejaculation and orgasmic experience discussed above. On the one side, according to Davidson, there is a neural mechanism that causes the emission of semen *and* loss of arousal (causing the refractory period). On the other side, there is a neural mechanism causing contractions of striated muscles *and* an altered state of consciousness. Davidson argues that this *bipolar model* gives the most adequate explanation of orgasm, but there are some problems with it. First, as pointed out by Rosen and Beck (1988), the phenomena of phantom orgasm and of anaesthetic ejaculation are contrary to a direct linking of an altered state of consciousness and contraction of striated muscles. Second, men who are capable of multiple orgasms may still have an erection and orgasm after they have had an orgasm with ejaculation (Dunn & Trost, 1989). This is contrary to a direct link between emission and loss of arousal.

Arguments in favor of and against Davidson's model lack a sound body of physiological data. The same applies to arguments concerning a model that assumes mechanisms in the spinal cord and at the brain level. Reports on phantom orgasms, anaesthetic ejaculation, and multiple orgasms in men all lack data on muscle contractions, penile tumescence, etc. These reports are based solely on subjective reports. More sophisticated data on physiological events would be very informative.

So far, the discussion has focused exclusively on neural mechanisms of orgasm. *Psychological effects* of orgasm have not yet been mentioned; indeed, psychological theories of orgasm are almost completely absent. Genital reactions and other peripheral physiological changes are the primary focus of recent theorizing on orgasm. To a lesser extent, central neural mechanisms have been considered, but psychological theories do not seem to exist. This is a conspicious deficiency, since most theories on inhibited male orgasm hypothesize psychological causes. A psychological theory of inhibited male orgasm must explain how psychological processes inhibit orgasm—which requires a theory of how psychological factors affect orgasm. Only a few attempts at a psychological theory have been made. There is general acceptance of orgasm as a primary reinforcer. On the basis of classical or operant conditioning processes, it is thought that orgasm comes under the control of certain stimuli. Although he did not state a general theory of orgasm, Dow (1981) used this model as an explanation of inhibited male orgasm (see the next section). In a study on inhibited female orgasm Everaerd (Everaerd & Schacht, 1978; Everaerd & Dekker, 1981) discussed the idea that orgasm requires a subject to divert her (or his) attention away from the sexual interaction. Instead, the subject must focus on internal arousal and sensations. If such a shift of attention does not occur, orgasm is inhibited. If a subject keeps monitoring the sexual interaction, the necessary shift of attention (and thus orgasm) does not occur. In descriptions of orgasm, subjects frequently mention such a shift of attention (Vance & Wagner, 1976; Davidson, 1980), but further evidence in support of this theory does not seem to exist. Nevertheless, it is quite possible that—just as in sexual arousal (cf. Dekker & Everaerd, 1989)—cognitive processes play an important role in orgasm.

This discussion of the mechanisms of orgasm can be summarized as follows. (1) There is evidence in support of a spinal mechanism of ejaculation located at T11 or below. This spinal mechanisms leads to ejaculation, muscle spasms, and cardiovascular responses. (2) Orgasmic experience, however, seems to require input from the spinal mechanism to higher spinal and/or brain levels. Whether there exists a separate central mechanism of orgasm and/or orgasmic experience is not known. The few existing data do not allow a firm conclusion. (3) There is a conspicious lack of psychological theories of orgasm. There seem to exist only a few attempts at identification of psychological effects on orgasm.

Etiology of Inhibited Male Orgasm

There is a wide range of etiological theories of inhibited male orgasm. The causes of inhibited orgasm proposed by these theories lie at various levels of biobehavioral functioning, ranging from spinal mechanisms to the relationship of the patient with his partner. Each of these theories will be discussed, along with the empirical evidence, which is mostly weak.

It has been argued that *organic abnormalities* in the spinal cord contribute to causing inhibited orgasm in men (as well as women) (Brindley & Gillan, 1982). This theory is based on the authors' finding that a spinal reflex (the glandipudendal or bulbocavernosus reflex) is deficient in a proportion of cases of primary inhibited orgasm in both sexes. In women, it was also found that the absence of this reflex strongly correlated with failure of sex therapy. Brindley and Gillan concluded from these findings that a structural defect in the spinal cord is a possible etiological factor in inhibited orgasm in both sexes, at least in patients who lack the glandipudendal reflex. Although this theory can be rather easily tested, there seems to be no independent evidence in support of it.

A *learning theory* formulation of the etiology of inhibited male orgasm was proposed by Dow (1981). According to this theory, for some individuals orgasm becomes a much more likely occurrence under the discrete stimulus conditions associated with masturbation than under the contrasting conditions of sexual intercourse. This is due to the fact that orgasm follows masturbation for these men, thus providing the reinforcing event for conditioning the complex of stimuli accompanying and preceding masturbation. Dow presented some evidence derived from case studies to support his hypothesis, but firm evidence is lacking. Because most men seem to have masturbated before they have ever had intercourse, this theory would predict a much higher prevalence of inhibited coital orgasm than is actually present. It is not clear how this theory can account for the very low prevalence of inhibited male orgasm.

Inhibited male orgasm has been conceptualized as the result of a masculine tendency to avoid strong feelings or emotions (Everaerd, 1982; Everaerd et al., 1982). The *stereotyped masculine role* conditions a man not to show strong feelings. As a result, some men are also unable to focus on the internal sensations that precede or accompany orgasm. Because such a shift of attention toward internal sensations is supposed to be a necessary condition of orgasm, the inability to focus on internal sensations causes inhibition of orgasm. This theory predicts that men with inhibited male orgasm have a heightened masculinity score on a sex-role inventory. Some evidence in support of this prediction has been found (Munjack et al., 1978; Everaerd et al., 1982), but this theory clearly requires further investigation.

Apfelbaum (1980) has postulated that men with inhibited orgasm have an *"autosexual" orientation.* For these men, self-stimulation is hypothesized to be much more sexually arousing than stimulation by a partner. According to this theory, inhibited male orgasm during interpersonal sexual interaction is the result of a deviant sexual orientation, which causes these men to prefer self-stimulation. This conceptualization differs from Dow's (1981) model in that inhibited orgasm is attributed to a generalized autosexual preference rather than to a conditioning of orgasm to stimuli accompanying or preceding masturbation. Another theory, which also draws upon the concept of sexual orientation, postulates that inhibited orgasm during coitus is due to a *nonheterosexual preference.* This preference would cause inhibition of orgasm during sexual interaction with a woman (Cooper, 1968a; Munjack & Kanno, 1979). Adequate empirical evidence in support of both the autosexual and the nonheterosexual theory is lacking, however.

Many theories attribute the disorder to *anxiety, fear, or hostility.* These theories have been reviewed by Munjack and Kanno (1979) and Schull and Sprenkle (1980). Many different manifestations of anxiety and fear have been hypothesized. As enumerated by Munjack and Kanno, these manifestations of anxiety and fear include fears of death and castration, fear of loss of self and death resulting from loss of semen, fear of castration by the female genitals, fear that ejaculation would hurt the female, fear of being hurt by the female, fear of retaliation by other males for ejaculating, performance anxiety, fear of exposure and shame about the dysfunction, unwillingness to give of oneself as an expression of love, fear of impregnating the female, and guilt secondary to a strict religious upbringing. Anxiety and fear may also stem from disease of the patient or his partner. After myocardial infarction, men often fear that orgasm is too strenuous for the heart. If the female partner has (or has had) cancer, the man may fear an infection. In both cases, fear may inhibit orgasm. Finally, hostility is also frequently mentioned as a etiological factor in inhibited male orgasm. This involves hostility and hate toward women. Alternatively, hostile rivalry toward other men may also be involved—with intercourse as a symbolic extension of competition between men.

Evidence in support of these hypotheses on the etiological role of anxiety, fear, and hostility comes from studies that used standardized questionnaires or clinical interviews to assess the emotional state of patients with inhibited orgasm. Elevated levels of hostility (Cooper, 1968c), coital anxiety (Cooper, 1969), and anxiety (Munjack et al., 1978) have been demonstrated in men with inhibited orgasm. Studies on neuroticism and other personality characteristics show inconsistent results (Munjack et al., 1978; Cooper, 1968b; Razani, 1972). Thus, it seems that men with inhibited orgasm have elevated levels of hostility and anxiety. The interpretation of this finding is ambiguous, however. Hostility and anxiety may be causes as well as effects of inhibited orgasm. Because these studies lack an experimental or prospective design, the causal connections of these emotional states and the inhibition of orgasm is not known. Just as in the area of sexual arousal (see Rosen & Beck, 1988; Dekker & Everaerd, 1989) psychophysiological studies on the effect of emotional states on orgasm might be helpful in this area.

Finally, it has been hypothesized that difficulties in the *relationship* between partners play a role in the etiology of inhibited male orgasm. A power struggle or ambivalence towards the partner (Kaplan, 1974) or hostility and resentment (Masters & Johnson, 1970) may contribute to inhibition of orgasm. Conceivably, these relationship difficulties are related to the hostility that was mentioned above as a possible etiological factor. Controlled empirical studies on the relationship of men with inhibited orgasm do not seem to be available. In addition, the formulations on the etiological significance of relationship difficulties are very general, rather than being specific to inhibited male orgasm. For example, ambivalence toward the partner has been regarded as an etiological factor in many sexual (and nonsexual) problems. A more specific theory on the relationship as a cause of inhibited orgasm seems to be required.

The conclusion of this section is that quite a variety of hypotheses on the causes of inhibited male orgasm exist, but the empirical evidence in support of these theories is very weak. There is an urgent need for further research in this area. It can be suggested that studies examining variables that affect the duration of the interval before orgasm and the control of orgasm in "normal" subjects would be an expedient way to gain an insight into the determinants of orgasm. Such studies would not be hampered by the problem of low prevalence that hinders research into inhibited male orgasm. Once an insight into the determinants of male orgasm has been gained, specific etiological hypotheses can be tested in studies on patients. This strategy might be more fruitful than a continuation of the rather long series of descriptive studies on limited numbers of patients with inhibited orgasm.

METHODS OF ASSESSMENT

A general strategy that applies to all sexual dysfunctions can be followed to assess inhibited male orgasm. This strategy has been ex-

plicitly stated by Kaplan (1983). In this section, this strategy as applied to inhibited male orgasm will be discussed first. Then follows a description of the instruments available to assess this disorder.

Strategy

The general strategy for assessing sexual dysfunctions can be described as a number of hierarchical questions and related decisions in a decision tree. Each of these decisions gives rise to a certain therapeutic approach. As modified after Kaplan (1983) and applied to inhibited male orgasm, the following questions should be answered:

1. Does the patient really have inhibited male orgasm?
2. Is the inhibition of orgasm biogenic, psychogenic, or a mixture of the two?
3. Is the inhibition of orgasm secondary to another psychiatric disorder?
4. What are the immediate and underlying psychological causes of the inhibition of orgasm?

1. Does the Patient Really Have Inhibited Male Orgasm?

Patients may present with concerns about orgasm that do not justify the diagnosis of inhibited male orgasm. The patient's expectations about orgasm and the time it takes to reach it may be unrealistic. For example, with increasing age it takes many men longer to reach an orgasm. This may give rise to concerns. But as long as the time to reach an orgasm remains within "normal" limits, there is no need for a diagnosis of inhibited orgasm. Similarly, the patient's concerns may be based on general uncertainties or anxieties ("neuroticism"), when in fact there is no real delay of orgasm. These uncertainties may give rise to unrealistic expectations concerning the time it takes to reach an orgasm. Unrealistic expectations may also be due to relationship difficulties. A woman who is dissatisfied with her partner may complain that it takes her partner too long to reach an orgasm. This may lead an adequately functioning man to complain of inhibited orgasm, but the diagnosis is not justified in this case either. In these cases treatment is primarily aimed at reassurance and correction of the unrealistic expectations; treatment aimed at improvement of orgasmic functioning is not indicated. As discussed earlier in this chapter, it may not be easy to decide whether or not the patient really has inhibited male orgasm. Lacking clearly defined criteria for the inhibition of orgasm, the clinician must rely on his or her experience.

Finally, some patients complain of an inability to reach on orgasm when in fact erectile difficulties are the real problem. Erectile dysfunction frequently results in an absence of orgasm, which evidently leads some patients to complain of orgasmic instead of erectile problems. In these cases the diagnosis should be male erectile disorder.

2. Is the Inhibition of Orgasm Biogenic, Psychogenic, or a Mixture of the Two?

Once it is established that the diagnosis of inhibited orgasm is justified, it should be determined whether the causes of the disorder are biological and/or psychological. Two strategies can be used to reach a decision. First, it can be determined whether the disorder is situational or generalized. If the disorder is situational, a biological cause is less likely. For example, a biological cause is not very likely in a patient who is orgasmic during masturbation but not during partner interaction. In such cases the disorder is likely to be psychogenic. However, in situational disorders, biological causes may exist. If there exists a biological impairment of the sexual system, this may give rise to a disorder under stressful conditions. Thus, one should be careful not to equate situational disorders with psychogenic disorders. The second strategy for deciding the question of biological or psychological causes of inhibited orgasm aims directly at the identification of biological causes. It can be determined whether certain biological conditions are present that are known to cause inhibited orgasm. Various drugs and illnesses may cause inhibited orgasm (see Chapter 8). If such a drug or illness is present, it is a possible cause of the disorder. However, it is not always certain that the drug or illness is the actual or only cause. Psychological causes may contribute to the disorder, even if there is a biological cause.

The clinician should be aware of the fact that certain conditions almost always have a biological cause. This applies to retrograde ejaculation and to emission-phase disorders.

If biological factors contribute to the inhibition of orgasm, appropriate treatment is indicated. This applies both to cases that are entirely biogenic and to cases that have a mixture of bio- and psychogenic etiologies. If psychological factors seem to contribute to the inhibition of orgasm, further evaluation of these factors is necessary.

3. Is the Inhibition of Orgasm Secondary to Another Psychiatric Disorder?

In some cases the inhibition of orgasm is secondary to another major psychiatric disorder. These cases should be screened out, because sex therapy may not be appropriate. Also, the psychiatric disorder may constitute a contraindication for sex therapy (Kaplan, 1983). Among the psychiatric disorders that cause inhibited orgasm are depression, anxiety disorders, and major pathology such as schizophrenia. These examples are based on clinical experience; systematic studies do not seem to be available in this area. Thus, although it is assumed that psychiatric disorder is a contraindication for sex therapy, empirical evidence for that assertion is lacking.

4. What Are the Immediate and Underlying Psychological Causes of the Inhibition of Orgasm?

In this step, the nature of the psychological causes should be determined. Just as with the biological causes, two strategies may be used to identify psychological causes. First, it can be determined whether the inhibition of orgasm occurs in certain conditions. For example, if the disorder occurs with one partner and not with another, the relationship or the man's attitude towards that partner would seem to be etiologically implicated. The other strategy consists of identifying the presence of psychological conditions that are "known" to cause inhibition of orgasm. In such a case one must rely on clinical experience and the scarce knowledge about factors that contribute to inhibited male orgasm, since no firm body of empirical evidence on psychological causes is available.

Kaplan (1974, 1983) has divided the causes of sexual dysfunctions into two categories: the immediate causes and the deeper or underlying causes (including the partner relationship). Immediate causes are defined as follows: "The immediate psychological causes or antecedents of the sexual symptom are comprised of the patient's current ineffective sexual behavior and destructive interactions with his sexual partner and the obsessive thoughts and fearful and angry emotions which he experiences just prior to the experience of the sexual impairment" (Kaplan, 1983, p. 42). Thus, immediate causes include anxiety, hostility, spectating, etc. In addition to immediate causes, there may exist deeper or underlying causes. These are defined as "neurotic needs to avoid sexual pleasure and adequacy" (p. 44). Apart from general neurotic needs, these deeper causes include difficulties due to cultural indoctrination and traumatic sexual experiences. Kaplan discusses relationship difficulties as a seperate category, but it seems that these causes can also be included in the category of deeper or underlying causes.

Assessment Instruments

Presently, the clinical interview is the major instrument for the assessment of inhibited male orgasm. Apart from tests to identify biological causes and screening instruments to identify other psychiatric pathology, no specific instrument seems to be available to assess inhibited male orgasm (see also Conte, 1986).

Potentially, the measurement of anal contractions (Bohlen et al., 1986) can be developed into a specific test on the functioning of orgasm. But this is mere speculation, since this approach has not been developed yet. In questionnaires on sexual functioning, some questions on orgasm are usually asked (e.g., LoPicolo & Steger, 1974; Frenken & Vennix, 1981). In Frenken and Vennix's questionnaire there is a subscale that specifically concerns orgasm. The frequency of orgasm and the evaluation of orgasm are the main items of this subscale. Potentially, this and other questionnaires are useful instruments in the assessment of inhibited male orgasm, but no studies seem to have been done to validate this scale.

This leaves the clinical interview as the major assessment tool. The general approach in a clinical interview on sexual functioning has been described by others (e.g., Kaplan, 1983). There is no need to reiterate this general approach here. The specific goals of this interview were described above, in the section on assessment strategy: identifying patients who do not really suffer from inhibited orgasm; evaluating the likelihood of biological causes of the disorder; screening for other major psychiatric disorders; and identifying immediate and deeper psychological causes of the disorder. No studies on the reliability and validity of the clinical interview applied to inhibited male orgasm seem to be available.

So far, the discussion has focused on issues in the diagnosis of inhibited male orgasm. Methods to assess the outcome of therapeutic efforts have not been discussed yet, but, in keeping with the diagnostic assessment, the clinical interview seems to be the major instrument in assessing outcome. In most outcome studies (see next section), the therapeutic result has been determined by means of a clinical interview. In some studies, standardized questionnaires have been used, but these do not provide specific information on orgasm; they reflect only the general level of sexual functioning. (Although Frenken and Vennix's questionnaire (1981) contains a subscale on orgasm, separate results of this subscale have not been reported in studies using this scale.)

TREATMENT

Quite a number of interventions have been used to treat men with inhibited orgasm: vibratory and electrical stimulation, a variety of sexual exercises, and a range of general psychotherapeutic techniques. These interventions have been used separately or in combination with one or more others. Research on the effectiveness of these therapeutic interventions is limited to uncontrolled studies on individual patients or short series of patients. Controlled outcome studies do not seem to be available. Thus, the choice of a certain intervention is necessarily based on clinical experience and uncontrolled studies rather than on a firm body of empirical knowledge.

In this section the major therapeutic interventions and their rationale will be described first. Then follows a discussion of empirical studies on the outcome of therapeutic interventions.

Therapeutic Interventions

Vibratory and Electrical Stimulation

Vibratory stimulation to the penis has been used to induce ejaculation. The primary goal of this intervention has been to collect semen, which is used to inseminate the female partner. This procedure has been used both in men with intact nervous systems (Schellen, 1968) and in paraplegic men (Comarr, 1970). In Schellen's study it was not reported whether this procedure had any influence on the inhibition of orgasm during sexual interaction with a partner. However, Newell (1976) reported a case study on a man with an intact nervous system who suffered from inhibited orgasm. Vibratory stimulation of the penis induced ejaculation. The patient subsequently reported that he was able to ejaculate during intercourse with his wife. Ejaculation was accompanied by "a pleasant sensation."

Electrical stimulation of the internal ejaculatory organs by a transrectal electrical probe has been used to obtain semen in paraplegic men (see Bennett et al., 1988). This procedure has been called electro-ejaculation. Stewart and Ohl (1989) used the procedure to induce ejaculation in a man with inhibited orgasm and to inseminate his wife. However, because electrical stimulation is extremely painful in men with normal sensation, the patient required general anaesthesia for the procedure. This requirement seems to preclude regular use of this procedure in cases of inhibited orgasm. In addition, the only goal of this intervention has been to obtain semen for an insemination; orgasm during sexual interaction with a partner has not been its object.

Thus, vibratory stimulation can be used for ejaculation and insemination. It seems that the experience of ejaculation and orgasm is also helpful in enabling men to reach an orgasm during sexual interaction. The application of electro-ejaculation seems to be limited to obtaining an ejacaluation for insemination in very special cases.

Sexual Exercises

Sexual exercises have been extensively used in the treatment of inhibited male orgasm. Many therapists have used a series of exercises that successively approximate orgasm during intercourse (e.g., Masters & Johnson, 1970; Kaplan, 1974; Oziel, 1978; Schull & Sprenkle, 1980; Libman et al., 1984; Campden-Main & Sara, 1985). Following a period of undemanding sensate focus exercises, the patient is instructed to masturbate to orgasm in the presence of his partner. Of course, this presupposes that the man is able to have an orgasm during masturbation. If not, any other technique that is effective can be used. For example, if a man can reach an orgasm only when he is alone, he is instructed to masturbate to orgasm outside the room; in a subsequent encounter he tries to masturbate to orgasm inside the room (Kaplan, 1974). Once the patient has had an orgasm in the presence of his partner, a number of steps are implemented, which successively approximate vaginal intercourse. These steps may include moving the penis closer to the vagina during masturbation. Subsequently he enters the vagina. Combined coital and manual stimulation is then used to induce orgasm, and finally he uses only coital stimulation to reach an orgasm. Other methods of stimulation can be incorporated into these exercises: manual or oral stimulation by the partner can be incorporated at any point in the series of exercises.

Various theoretical explanations for the efficacy of this procedure have been offered. The procedure has been conceptualized as a variant of *in vivo* systematic desensitization (Kaplan, 1974). It is assumed that sexual arousal—instead of the usual muscle relaxation—prevents the occurrence of sexual anxiety; when anxiety is eliminated, the patient is able to experience orgasm. Evidently, this explanation assumes that anxiety is an important etiological factor in inhibited male orgasm. It should be noted that—rather than inhibition of anxiety—extinction of anxiety due to exposure to the anxiety eliciting stimuli may also be the effective ingredient of successively approximating coital orgasm. According to the latter explanation, anxiety reduction is also the essential feature of this procedure. The difference between the former and the latter explanation consists of the way anxiety reduction is thought to occur: by means of inhibition of anxiety through sexual arousal or by means of extinction of anxiety through exposure, respectively.

Other authors have conceptualized this procedure as involving stimulus generalization (Libman et al., 1984). It is assumed that orgasm in patients can be elicited only by stimuli accompanying masturbation (Dow, 1981; Libman et al., 1984). Effective therapy requires broadening the range of stimuli that elicit orgasm. This is achieved by successively approximating the masturbatory pattern to the interpersonal context. Reduction of anxiety does not play a role in this explanation.

Masturbation exercises have also been used in the treatment of inhibited male orgasm (Everaerd et al., 1982; Dekker el al., 1985). These exercises are meant to teach the patient how to focus on his own internal sensations. Patients with inhibited orgasm have been hypothesized to focus selectively on the sexual interaction. It is thought that they fail to shift attention towards their own arousal and body sensations.

This failure leads to the inhibition of orgasm, and the masturbation exercises are meant to remedy this situation. Patients are instructed to focus gradually on their own arousal and sensation during self-stimulation. They start with modified sensate focus exercises (masturbatory exercises instead of the usual couple exercises), and step by step they move on to higher levels of sexual arousal. This gradual approach is thought to enable men to overcome their fear of high levels of arousal and body sensations. It should be noted that this treatment approach is more or less contrary to the hypothesis that inhibited male orgasm is due to a preference for self-stimulation (Dow, 1981; Apfelbaum, 1980). Instead of moving the patient away from self-stimulation, the clinician actively encourages him to explore self-stimulation. Different conceptualizations of the etiology of inhibited male orgasm thus lead to opposing approaches to its treatment.

In addition to the exercises mentioned above, other exercise approaches have been described. Razani (1972) described a treatment approach called *systematic desensitization*. The couple was taught the Semans technique, according to which the female stimulated the erect penis to the point premonitory of ejaculation. She then stopped stimulation. It was expected that the sexual arousal would inhibit fear of ejaculation. In addition, systematic desensitization was applied in one session to the image of intravaginal ejaculation. Pryde and Woods (1980) described a cognitive approach to the treatment of inhibited orgasm. The patient was instructed to imagine a short series of items relating to ejaculation (and urination, which appeared to be linked to ejaculation for the patient). The items were arranged in order of anxiety-evoking potential. The man was instructed to imagine himself successfully performing the behavior. The couple also did sensate focus exercises and had intercourse.

Hypnotherapy

Hypnotic techniques for the treatment of sexual dysfunctions have been described by Araoz (1982). For inhibited male orgasm, a specific technique is described. Once the patient has entered hypnosis, it is suggested that one of his fingers, which represents his penis, is hypersensitive. By means of posthypnotic suggestion, the transfer of hypersensitivity to the penis is effected.

General Psychotherapeutic Techniques

Various therapeutic techniques that are not specificly designed for sexual problems have been used with inhibited male orgasm:

- Individual psychotherapy, with a psychodynamic orientation (e.g., Kaplan, 1974; Friedman, 1973; Wilensky & Myers, 1986)
- Marital therapy (e.g., Kaplan, 1974; Hartman, 1983; Hawton, 1982)
- Rational emotive therapy (e.g., Everaerd et al., 1982; Everaerd & Dekker, 1985)
- Social skills training (Everaerd et al., 1982)

These techniques have been applied seperately or in combination with sexual exercises. Issues that are more or less directly linked to the inhibition of orgasm are addressed using these techniques. Examples include oedipal problems, success phobia, feelings of inadequacy, sexual anxiety, and attitudes toward and expectations about the partner. These issues correspond to the various psychological causes that have been hypothesized in inhibited male orgasm (see the Psychopathology section of this chapter). Assuming certain psychological causes, a particular psychotherapeutic intervention aims at elimination of these causes. An illustration can be found in the application of rational emotive therapy (Everaerd & Dekker, 1985). It was hypothesized that (because of a stereotyped masculine role) the patient is unable to focus on internal sensations that precede or accompany orgasm. Instead, the patient seems to monitor the sexual interaction, which is thought to cause the inhibition of orgasm. Rational emotive therapy (RET) is used to analyze and modify the patient's cognitions, emotions, and behavior. First, the patient uses RET to identify disruptive cognitions: "My partner will ridicule me if I let myself go";

"During orgasm I will loose control of my body"; etc. Because of these and similar thoughts the patient avoids focusing on his internal sensations and keeps monitoring the interaction. Once the disruptive cognitions have been identified, the second step consists of modifying them. Using various RET techniques, the patient is encouraged to replace the disruptive cognitions by more adaptive ones. This is thought to enable the patient to "let himself go"—to focus on and indulge in his own bodily sensations. In accordance with the hypothesized psychological model of orgasm, this is expected to lead to the experience of orgasm.

Therapeutic Outcome

Munjack and Kanno (1979) have summarized the outcome of a number of studies on single patients or short series of patients. A favorable outcome was reported after application of psychodynamically oriented psychotherapy; after sexual exercises that succesively approximated coitus, alone or in combination with brief psychotherapy; and after vibrator therapy. However, because the design of these studies was very weak, it is not possible to make any statements about the effectiveness of these treatments.

Studies published after Munjack and Kanno's review are also limited to case histories and short series of patients. These studies have been summarized in Table 10.3. Pryde and Woods (1980) successfully applied to a single subject a cognitive approach (covert self-modeling) in combination with sensate focus and coital exercises. Hawton (1982) reported on a series of patients, three of whom complained of inhibited orgasm. Patients were treated with various sexual exercises (including sensate focus and masturbation exercises), counseling, education, and marital therapy. One patient with inhibited orgasm improved somewhat; two others did not change. Libman et al. (1984) reported on a successfully treated man; treatment consisted of sensate focus exercises and successive approximation of orgasm during intercourse. Dekker et al. (1985) reported on a series of men with various sexual dysfunctions, ten of whom com-

Table 10.3. Studies on the Treatment of Inhibited Male Orgasm Published in 1980 and After

AUTHORS	N	PATIENT CHARACTERISTICS	DESIGN	TREATMENT MODALITIES	FORMAT	OUTCOME
Pryde & Woods (1980)	1	Couple "in their late twenties"	Case study; pre- and posttest, 7-month follow-up	Nongenital and genital exercises; covert self-modelling	Couple therapy by dual-sex co-therapists; 10 sessions in a period of 5 months	Ejaculation during intercourse at the end of treatment and also after 7 months of follow-up
Hawton (1982)	3*	-	Series of patients; pre- and posttest, 3-month follow-up	Sex therapy; counseling; education; marital therapy	Couple therapy by single therapist; weekly sessions	At the end of treatment, one patient had improved somewhat, and two patients had not changed
Libman et al. (1984)	1	Couple, male 28 and female 26 years	Case study; pre- and posttest, 1-year follow-up	Nongenital and genital exercises; approximation of orgasm during intercourse by means of shaping and fading	Couple therapy by single therapist	At the end of treatment, intravaginal orgasm occurred in every coitus, and at one year follow-up "almost always"
Dekker et al. (1985)	10*	-	Series of patients; pre- and posttest	Rational emotive therapy; masturbation exercises and social skills training	Male-only groups with two male co-therapists; 15 to 21 weekly sessions	Significant improvement on measures of sexual and social functioning at the end of treatment

| De Amicis et al. (1985) | 5* | - | Series of patients; pre- and posttest, 3-month and 3-year follow-up | Nongenital and genital exercises; communication skills building; developing social awareness | Couple therapy; weekly sessions for 15 to 20 weeks | At the end of treatment, four patients had not changed, and one had improved. At 3-year follow-up, one patient was worse, one had not changed, and three had improved |
| Wilensky & Myers (1986) | 9 | Homosexual men, age 21 to 50 years | Series of patients; pre- and posttest | Individual psychotherapy; sex therapy; masturbatory training | On average 23 sessions (range: 9–50) | At the end of treatment, three patients were unchanged, three had a few orgasms with their partner, and three had orgasms with their partners regularly |

* A number of patients with other dysfunctions were also included in this study. Patient characteristics were not separately reported for patients with inhibited orgasm.

plained of inhibited orgasm. Treatment consisted of rational emotive therapy, masturbation exercises, and social skills training. Patients were treated in male-only groups. Outcome was assessed in a pretest-posttest design, using questionnaires on sexual and social functioning. Both sexual and social functioning improved in the group as whole. There were no significant differences between patients with inhibited orgasm and patients with erectile dysfunction or premature ejaculation, indicating that these three diagnostic groups improved to the same extent. De Amicis et al. (1985) treated a series of patients, five of whom complained of inhibited orgasm. Treatment consisted of training in sensual awareness, successive approximation of coitus, communication skills building, and developing awareness of affective states and consequences of behavior. Outcome was assessed in a design that included a pretest, a posttest, and three-month and three-year follow-up. At the end of therapy, four patients had not changed, and one patient had improved. At three-year follow-up (in comparison to pretreatment) one patient was worse, one patient had not changed and three patients were improved. Wilensky and Myers (1986) reported on nine homosexual men with inhibited orgasm. Treatment consisted of either psychodynamically oriented psychotherapy, couple therapy, or sex therapy. At the end of treatment, three patients were unchanged, three had had a few orgasms with their partner, and three had regular orgasms with their partner. Finally, in some studies men with inhibited orgasm were included, but the results for these men were not reported seperately (Hartman & Daly, 1983; Everaerd & Dekker, 1985).

This review indicates that the treatment of inhibited male orgasm has met with both success and failure. Because controlled studies are not available, it is very difficult to evaluate results: It is not known how treatment compares to no treatment. Nevertheless, in reviewing these studies, one gets the impression that the outcome is rather poor. The overall impression is that some patients are really cured after treatment, but that most patients are "somewhat improved" or unchanged.

In the absence of comparative studies, it is not possible to compare the effectiveness of different treatments. In addition, there are other methodological deficiencies. In most studies, outcome is assessed only by means of a single statement ("improved," "cured," or "unchanged"). More refined instruments such as questionnaires on sexual functioning, marital relationship, or social functioning have not been extensively used. In the cases where they have been used, the questionnaire reflects only general sexual functioning; more specific information on orgasmic functioning is lacking. Also, in quite a number of studies there is no follow-up. Finally, treatment has not been standardized in most studies. Thus, it is not clear exactly which treatment modalities have been applied.

Because of these methodological deficiencies, no firm conclusion or recommendation on the optimal treatment approach can be given. Apparently, various therapeutic techniques are associated with a favorable outcome. At the present state of knowledge, the best recommendation seems to be to use a combination of sexual exercises and general therapeutic interventions. The selection of the sexual exercises and the therapeutic interventions is up to the clinician who is treating the man with inhibited orgasm.

CONCLUSIONS

The major conclusions of this chapter can be summarized as follows:

1. The category of inhibited male orgasm consists of a number of diagnostic subtypes. Various classifications of these orgasmic disorders have been proposed. An adaptation of Kothari's (1984) scheme seems to offer the best classification of the subtypes of inhibited male orgasm.
2. The prevalence of inhibited male orgasm is rather low, both in the general population and in clinical samples. Nevertheless, the prevalence in clinical samples seems to be somewhat higher than the often quoted figure of 3.8% reported by Masters and Johnson (1970).

3. At present, the clinical interview is the major tool for the assessment of inhibited male orgasm. However, measurement of anal contractions and questionnaires on orgasm may prove to be useful instruments in the future.

4. Inhibited male orgasm is often considered rather difficult to treat. In the literature, both success and failure have been described as the outcome of therapy. Vibratory and electrical stimulation, sexual exercises, hypnotherapy, and general psychotherapeutic interventions have been applied in these cases. But because of methodological deficiencies, it is not possible to draw conclusions on treatment outcome.

5. Both the epidemiological and the clinical research on inhibited male orgasm is methodologically rather weak. Consequently, our knowledge of the assessment and treatment of inhibited male orgasm is limited. One way to improve this state of affairs is to design methodologically sound studies on assessment and treatment of the disorder. However, because of the rather low prevalence of the disorder, this will probably prove a very difficult approach. An alternative approach has been described in this chapter. It is suggested that research should focus on mechanisms of normal orgasm in "normal" samples. Knowledge of normal orgasm is essential for an understanding of inhibited orgasm. Once orgasm and the mechanisms that lead to it are understood, it should prove much easier to identify factors that interfere with orgasm and to develop rational treatment strategies for inhibited orgasm.

In this chapter, the existing biological and psychological theories of orgasm, together with the empirical support for these theories, have been reviewed. Possibly, this review will contribute to future research into the mechanisms of orgasm.

REFERENCES

American Psychiatric Association. (1987). *Diagnostic and statistical manual of mental disorders* (3rd ed., rev.). Washington, DC: Author.

Apfelbaum, B. (1980). The diagnosis and treatment of retarded ejaculation. In S. R. Leiblum & L. A. Pervin (Eds.), *Principles and practice of sex therapy*. London: Tavistock.

Araoz, D. L. (1982). *Hypnosis and sex therapy*. New York: Brunner/Mazel.

Arentewicz, G., & Schmidt, G. (1980). *Sexuell gestorte Beziehungen*. Berlin: Springer.

Bancroft, J. (1989). *Human sexuality and its problems* (2nd ed.). Edinburgh, UK: Churchill Livingstone.

Bancroft, J., & Coles, L., (1976). Three years' experience in a sexual problems clinic. *British Medical Journal, 1,* 1575–1577.

Bennett, C. J., Seager, S. W., Vasher, E. A., & McGuire, E. J. (1988). Sexual dysfunction and electroejaculation in men with spinal cord injury: A review. *Journal of Urology, 139,* 453–457.

Bohlen, J. G., Held, J. P., & Sanderson, M. O. (1980). The male orgasm: Pelvic contractions measured by anal probe. *Archives of Sexual Behavior, 9,* 503–521.

Brindley, G. S., & Gillan, P. (1982). Men and women who do not have orgasms. *British Journal of Psychiatry, 140,* 351–356.

Campden-Main, B. C., & Sara, M. L. (1985). Retarded ejaculation. *Medical Aspects of Human Sexuality, 19,* 21–29.

Comarr, A. E. (1970). Sexual function among patients with spinal cord injury. *Urologia Internationalis, 25,* 134.

Conte, H. R. (1986). Multivariate assessment of sexual dysfunction. *Journal of Consulting and Clinical Psychology, 54,* 149–157.

Cooper, A. J. (1968a). A factual study of male potency disorders. *British Journal of Psychiatry, 114,* 719–731.

Cooper, A. J. (1968b). Neurosis and disorders of sexual potency in the male. *Journal of Psychosomatic Research, 12,* 141–144.

Cooper, A. J. (1968c). Hostility and male potency disorders. *Comprehensive Psychiatry, 9,* 621–626.

Cooper, A. J. (1969). A clinical study of coital anxiety in male potency disorders. *Journal of Psychosomatic Research, 13,* 143–147.

Davidson, J. M. (1980). The psychobiology of sexual experience. In J. M. Davidson & R. J. Davidson (Eds.), *The psychobiology of consciousness*. New York: Plenum.

De Amicis, L. A., Goldberg, D. C., LoPicollo, J., Friedman, J., & Davies, L. (1984). Three-year follow-up of couples evaluated for sexual dysfunction. *Journal of Sex and Marital Therapy, 10,* 215–228.

De Amicis, L. A., Goldberg, D. C., LoPicollo, J., Friedman, J., & Davies, L. (1985). Clinical follow-up of couples treated for sexual dysfunction. *Archives of Sexual Behavior, 14,* 467–489.

Dekker, J., Dronkers, J., & Staffeleu, J. (1985). Treatment of sexual dysfunctions in male-only groups: Predicting outcome. *Journal of Sex and Marital Therapy, 11,* 80–90.

Dekker, J., & Everaerd, W. (1983). A long-term follow-up study of couples treated for sexual dysfunctions. *Journal of Sex and Marital Therapy, 9,* 99–113.

Dekker, J., & Everaerd, W. (1989). Psychological determinants of sexual arousal: A review. *Behaviour Research and Therapy, 27,* 353–364.

Dow, M. G. T. (1981). Retarded ejaculation as a function of nonaversive conditioning and discrimination: A hypothesis. *Journal of Sex and Marital Therapy, 7,* 49–53.

Dunn, M. E., & Trost, J. E. (1989). Male multiple orgasms: A descriptive study. *Archives of Sexual Behavior, 18,* 377–387.

Everaerd, W. (1982). Current research on sexual dysfunction. In J. Boulougouris (Ed.), *Learning theory approaches to psychiatry.* New York: Wiley.

Everaerd, W., & Dekker, J. (1981). A comparison of sex therapy and communication therapy: Couples complaining of orgasmic dysfunction. *Journal of Sex and Marital Therapy, 7,* 278–289.

Everaerd, W., & Dekker, J. (1985). Treatment of male sexual dysfunction: Sex therapy compared with systematic desensitization and rational emotive therapy. *Behaviour Research and Therapy, 23,* 13–25.

Everaerd, W., Dekker, J., Dronkers, J., Rhee, K., van der Staffeleu, J., & Wiselius, G. (1982). Treatment of homosexual and heterosexual sexual dysfunction in male-only groups of mixed sexual orientation. *Archives of Sexual Behavior, 11,* 1–10.

Everaerd, W., & Schacht, H. (1973). Man en vrouw: Stoornissen in hun seksuele relatie. *Intermediair, 34,* 9.

Fisher, T. D., Pollack, R. H., & Malatesta, V. J. (1986). Orgasmic latency and subjective ratings of erotic stimuli in male and female subjects. *Journal of Sex Research, 22,* 85–93.

Frenken, J. (1980). Het voorkomen van seksuele problemen in man-vrouw relaties. In J. Frenken (Ed.), *Seksuologie.* Deventer, Netherlands: Van Loghum Slaterus.

Frenken, J., & Vennix, P. (1981). *Sexuality Experience Scales—Manual.* Lisse: Swets and Zeitlinger.

Friedman, M. (1973). Success phobia and retarded ejaculation. *American Journal of Psychotherapy, 27,* 78–84.

Graber, B., Rohrbaugh, J. W., Newlin, D. B., Varner, J. L., & Ellingson, R. J. (1985). EEG during masturbation and ejaculation. *Archives of Sexual Behavior, 14,* 491–503.

Hartman, L. M. (1983). Effects of sex and marital therapy on sexual interaction and marital happiness. *Journal of Sex and Marital Therapy, 9,* 137–151.

Hartman, L.N., & Daly, E. M. (1983). Relationship factors in the treatment of sexual dysfunctions. *Behaviour Research and Therapy, 21,* 153–160.

Hawton, K. (1982). The behavioral treatment of sexual dysfunction. *British Journal of Psychiatry, 140,* 94–101.

Hite, S. (1978). *The Hite report on male sexuality.* New York: Knopf.

Kaplan, H. S. (1974). *The new sex therapy.* New York: Brunner/Mazel.

Kaplan, H. S. (1983). *The evaluation of sexual disorders.* New York: Brunner/Mazel.

Kilman, P. R., Boland, J. P., Norton, S. P., Davidson, E., & Caid, C. (1986). Perspective of sex therapy outcome: A survey of AASECT providers. *Journal of Sex and Marital Therapy, 12,* 116–138.

Kinsey, A. C., Pomeroy, W. B., & Martin, C. E. (1948). *Sexual behavior in the human male.* Philadelphia: Saunders.

Kothari, P. (1984). For discussion: Ejaculatory disorders—a new dimension. *British Journal of Sexual Medicine, 11,* 205–209.

Libman, E., Brender, W., Burstein, R., & Hodgins, S. (1984). Ejaculatory imcompetence: A theoretical formulation and case illustration. *Journal of Behavior Therapy and Experimental Psychiatry, 15,* 127–131.

LoPicollo, J., & Steger, J. (1974). The sexual interaction inventory: A new instrument for the assessment of sexual dysfunction. *Archives of Sexual Behavior, 3,* 585–595.

Masters, W. H., & Johnson, V. E. (1966). *Human sexual response.* Boston: Little, Brown.

Masters, W. H., & Johnson, V. E. (1970). *Human sexual inadequacy.* Boston: Liitle, Brown.

Money, J. (1960). Phantom orgasm in the dreams of paraplegic men and women. *Archives of General Psychiatry, 3,* 373–382.

Mould, D. E. (1980). Neuromuscular aspects of women's orgasms. *Journal of Sex Research, 16*, 193–201.

Munjack, D. J., & Kanno, P. H. (1979). Retarded ejaculation: A review. *Archives of Sexual Behavior, 8*, 139–150.

Munjack, D. J., Kanno, P. H., & Oziel, L. (1978). Ejaculatory disorders: Some psychometric data. *Psychological Reports, 43*, 783–787.

Nathan, S. G. (1986). The epidemiology of the DSM-III psychosexual dysfunctions. *Journal of Sex and Marital Therapy, 12*, 267–281.

Newell, A. G. (1976). A case of ejaculatory incompetence treated with a mechanical aid. *Journal of Behavior Therapy and Experimental Psychiatry, 7*, 193–194.

Oziel, L. J. (1978). Treating retarded ejaculation in the male. *Medical Aspects of Human Sexuality, 12*, 111–112.

Pomeroy, W. B. (1967). The Masters-Johnson report and the Kinsey tradition. In R. Brecher & E. Brecher (Eds.), *An analysis of human sexual response*. London: Deutsch.

Pryde, N., & Woods, B. (1980). A case of absolute ejaculatory incompetence treated without extravaginal ejaculation. *Journal of Behavior Therapy and Experimental Psychiatry, 11*, 219–222.

Razani, J. (1972). Ejaculatory incompetence treated by deconditioning anxiety. *Journal of Behavior Therapy and Experimental Psychiatry, 3*, 65–67.

Robbins, M. B., & Jensen, G. D. (1978). Multiple orgasm in males. *Journal of Sex Research, 14*, 21–26.

Rosen, R. C., & Beck, J. G. (1988). *Patterns of sexual arousal*. New York: Guilford.

Schellen, T. M. C. M. (1968). Induction of ejaculation by electrovibration. *Fertility and Sterility, 19*, 566–569.

Schull, G. R., & Sprenkle, D. H. (1980). Retarded ejaculation: Reconceptualization and implications for treatment. *Journal of Sex and Marital Therapy, 6*, 234–246.

Stewart, D. E., & Ohl, D. A. (1989). Idiopathic anejaculation treated by electroejaculation. *International Journal of Psychiatry in Medicine, 19*, 263–268.

Szasz, G., & Carpenter, C. (1989). Clinical observations in vibratory stimulation of the penis of men with spinal cord injury. *Archives of Sexual Behavior, 18*, 461–474.

Vance, E. B., & Wagner, N. N. (1976). Written descriptions of orgasm: A study of sex differences. *Archives of Sexual Behavior, 5*, 87–98.

Vandereycken, W. (1986) Towards a better delineation of ejaculatory disorders. *Acta Psychiatrica Belgica, 86*, 57–63.

Wilensky, M., & Myers, M. F. (1987). Retarded ejaculation in homosexual patients: A report of nine cases. *Journal of Sex Research, 13*, 85–91.

Williams, W. (1985). Anaesthetic ejaculation. *Journal of Sex and Marital Therapy, 11*, 19–29.

CHAPTER 11

PREMATURE EJACULATION

William O'Donohue, Northern Illinois University
Elizabeth Letourneau, Northern Illinois University
James H. Geer, Louisiana State University

The DSM-III-R defines premature ejaculation as follows:

> Persistent or recurrent ejaculation with minimal sexual stimulation or before, upon, or shortly after penetration and before the person wishes it. The clinician must take into account factors that affect duration of the excitement phase, such as age, novelty of the sexual partner or situation, and the frequency of sexual activity (American Psychiatric Association, 1987, p. 295).

Given the small subject size of sexual disorder studies in the DSM field trials (see Chapter 1), the taxonomic adequacy of this diagnostic category appears to be an unresolved question. Thus, the extent to which this definition allows consistent diagnoses from clinicians has yet to be determined. There is considerable looseness in this definition, which may give rise to poor reliability. The terms *persistent, recurrent, minimal,* and *shortly after* are obviously quite vague. Moreover, individuals' "wishes" may be quite variable on different occasions. Finally, there is no indication of precisely what factors to take into account—or what roles they should be assigned. For example, what is the relationship between age and the duration of the excitement phase? What data are there that bear on this question? Is the relationship a monotonic one, such that the excitement phase systematically increases after adolescence, for all individuals in all situations?

There is no generally accepted definition of *premature ejaculation* (Kaplan, Kohl, Pomeroy, Offit, & Hogan, 1974; Kilman & Auerbach, 1979; Ruff & St. Lawrence, 1985). In fact, LoPiccolo indicates that it may be easier to define what is *not* premature ejaculation: when "both the husband and wife agree that the quality of their sexual encounters is not influenced by efforts to delay ejaculation" (as recounted in Kolodny, Masters, & Johnson, 1979, p. 524).

We will not dwell on the worrisome aspects of the definition of premature ejaculation contained in the DSM-III-R, but simply make two additional points. First, our criticism must be tempered with the admission that premature ejaculation is extremely difficult to define, probably for three reasons. (1) There is a lack of clear information on normative ejaculatory latency. (2) It seems likely that the range of normal, unproblematic ejaculatory latency is quite broad. In part, this arises from the interpersonal dimension that must be taken into account in any definition of premature ejaculation; what is considered "premature" depends to some extent on the partners' needs and wishes, which can be quite variable. Where male premature ejaculation ends and female orgasmic deficiency begins is a difficult but essential question. The complex nature of sexual functioning suggests that many variables can affect ejaculatory latency; presumably, premature ejaculators are qualitatively different from normal ejaculators. However, we do not have a clear idea of the all the variables that affect ejaculatory latency, their additive and interactive effects, and the proper way to delimit deviation from the "normal." (3) Finally, to the extent that an individual's wishes are taken into account in the definition, the category becomes somewhat capricious. "Wishes" might be construed as idiosyncratic preferences, which may not be entirely in accord with normative statistical indices. Individuals' wishes concerning ejaculatory latency are especially problematic in a cultural climate that emphasizes sexual athleticism for males.

More research is needed to identify the psychometric properties of any definition of premature ejaculation. Reliability sets an upper limit on validity, so attention must be given to possible ambiguities in any proposed definition. Moreover, the definition must be evaluated on the extent to which it picks out the essential features without adding any "noise." However, if the phenomenon is fairly plastic itself (varying by partner characteristics and wishes), then any definition would necessarily be ambiguous, so as to track this looseness in the phenomenon.

EPIDEMIOLOGY

Epidemiological studies suggest that premature ejaculation may be one of the most common sexual dysfunctions (Spector & Carey, 1990). Kinsey, Pomeroy, and Martin (1948) reported that, in a sample of 12,000 North American caucasian males, 75% ejaculate within two minutes of intromission. However, Gebhard and Johnson (1979), with a sample of 5460 white males and 177 black males, found that only 26% of men ejaculate within the first two minutes after intromission. Frank, Anderson, and Rubenstein (1978), using a sample of 100 mostly middle-class couples whose marriages were "working out," found that 36% reported problems with premature ejaculation. Nettelbladt and Uddenberg (1979) interviewed 58 randomly selected males from Swedish families and found that 38% complained of premature ejaculation. Finally, Bell and Weinberg (1978) found premature ejaculation in 27% of homosexual men.

The vast range of results in these studies is difficult to interpret. Of particular concern is the vast difference between Kinsey's results and those of his colleague Gebhard (Gebhard & Johnson, 1979). It does not seem likely that the inclusion of more recent interviews and a few minority subjects would result in such a dramatic decline in prevalence. Nonetheless, it appears that anywhere from 26% to 75% of individuals not presenting to clinics have experienced problems with premature ejaculation at some point in their lives. If Kinsey's data are to be believed, premature ejaculation is the "normal" state of affairs.

Studies utilizing clinic samples reveal that premature ejaculation is often a presenting problem in sex clinics. In a clinical sample of 790 cases over six years, Masters and Johnson (1970) found that 186 (approximately 24%) experienced problems with premature ejaculation. Similarly, in a sample of 98 males and 102 females presenting to a sexual problems clinic, Bancroft and Coles (1976) found that approximately 25% of the cases involved premature ejaculation. Hawton (1982) evaluated 289 consecutive cases over a four-year period in a sexual problems clinic and found that 15% of males presented with premature ejaculation. Renshaw (1988) evaluated 1071 married couples seeking sex therapy between 1972 and 1987 and found that 21% presented with complaints concerning premature ejaculation.

All of these studies suffer from methodological problems (Nathan, 1986; Spector & Carey, 1990), so conclusions from these must be drawn with caution. Even though there may be no wholly accurate estimates of the relevant population parameters, it does seem that premature ejaculation is a prevalent problem and one that is frequently seen in sex therapy clinics. Further epidemiological research—of increased methodological sophistication—is needed.

ETIOLOGICAL HYPOTHESES

Certain etiological hypotheses have been proffered regarding premature ejaculation. For example, Kaplan (1974) hypothesizes that premature ejaculation occurs in individuals who have excessive sensitivity to erotic stimulation, which causes them to become aroused faster than normal males. Kaplan further hypothesizes that "premature ejaculators do not perceive the sensations premonitory to orgasm, which in turn deprives them of the regulatory power of the higher nervous influences" (p. 301). Semans (1956) attributes premature ejaculation to the abnormal rapidity of the ejaculatory reflex in some males. Kinsey et al. (1948), Tuthill (1955), and Hastings (1966) each assert that ejaculation occurs more rapidly after a period of sexual abstinence—which leads to the hypothesis that premature ejaculators experience longer periods of abstinence.

These theories are relatively straightforward: Since they are not predicated upon references to underlying psychological constructs, they are open to empirical testing. Spiess, Geer, and O'Donohue (1984) addressed each of these hypotheses in an investigation of differences between premature ejaculators and normal males. In this study, objective (penile plethysmo-graphic) and subjective (self-report) measures were gathered in response to erotic stimuli for 10 premature ejaculators and 14 normal males. Premature ejaculation was defined as two minutes or less of ejaculatory latency upon vaginal intromission. Males in the control group indicated latencies of three minutes or longer. Spiess et al. reported no significant differences between the groups in rate of arousal, latency to maximum erection, or maximum penile response to erotic audiotapes or fantasy. Moreover, premature ejaculators did not show greater arousal in identical situations, nor did they show more arousal across potentially erotic situations. Thus, Kaplan's hypothesis regarding excessive sensitivity was not supported. In addition, Spiess et al. examined the distribution of correlation coefficients between penile and subjective measures of sexual arousal. They again found no differences between the groups; in fact, the trend was toward premature ejaculators showing higher correlation coefficients. Thus, premature ejaculators were not shown to be worse at perceiving sensations indicative of arousal, so doubt was cast on Kaplan's (1974) other hypothesis (stated above).

Data from this study did corroborate three etiological hypotheses. (1) Seman's (1956) hypothesis regarding rapid ejaculatory reflex was supported by self-report of subjects to the question, "Do you feel fully aroused when you ejaculate through intercourse?" Premature ejaculators were more likely to report being fully aroused "sometimes," whereas control subjects were more likely to report being "always" fully aroused when ejaculating. (2) It was found that the latency of ejaculation was inversely related to both the subjects' period of abstinence from intercourse and the length of time since the previous ejaculation—supporting the theory that ejaculation occurs more quickly after longer periods of abstinence. (3) In addition, premature ejaculators reported having had a longer period of abstinence from intercourse and from ejaculation than did normal ejaculators. The picture that emerges from this study is that the premature ejaculators ejaculate at lower levels of sexual arousal and have relatively infrequent sexual activity. Spiess et al. point out that their study was correlational and based on a small sample. Nonetheless, they indicate that the results suggest a therapeutic strategy in which premature ejaculators are instructed to ejaculate more frequently and to learn to ejaculate at higher levels of arousal.

Strassberg, Kelly, Carroll, and Kircher (1987) also provide data refuting Kaplan's hypothesis that premature ejaculators are less able to evaluate their level of sexual arousal accurately. Thirteen premature ejaculators and 13 nonpremature ejaculators viewed sexually explicit videotapes while their physiological arousal was measured through penile plethysmography; self-report of subjective arousal was simultaneously recorded. No differences were found between these two groups in the correlations between subjective and physiological arousal. However, unlike Spiess et al. (1984), Strassberg et al. did not find that premature ejaculators gave different responses regarding frequency of intercourse and masturbation.

Anxiety plays a prominent role in many theories of sexual dysfunction (Barlow, Sakheim & Beck, 1983; Beck, Barlow, Sakheim, & Abrahamson, 1987; Masters and Johnson, 1970). For example, Wolpe (1969) has suggested that ejaculation and anxiety are both activities of the sympathetic nervous system. Thus, sympathetic activity elicited by anxiety might aid in meeting the threshold for ejaculation, resulting in a decreased latency to ejaculation.

Strassberg, Mahoney, Schaugaard, and Hale (1990) attempted to evaluate the relationship of anxiety to premature ejaculation. They asked 15 premature ejaculators and 17 normal controls to engage in self-stimulation in the laboratory and at home and had the subjects fill out a questionnaire regarding sexual cognitions. The results indicated that anxiety experienced during intercourse, as measured by questionnaire responses, was not significantly different between the two groups. These authors also found no significant improvement in the length of ejaculatory latency during masturbation. Thus, when

the interpersonal source of anxiety is (presumably) removed, ejaculatory latency failed to improve significantly. Strassberg et al. (1990) concluded that these results were inconsistent with the theory that interpersonal subjective distress (such as performance anxiety) plays an etiologic role in premature ejaculation. They went on to suggest an etiological model in which an individual's somatic tendency toward a lower orgasmic threshold interacts with stress to produce premature ejaculation. However, these authors neglect to specify possible somatic pathways. Also, the results of their study are vitiated by the pitfalls of self-reporting and the use of a questionnaire (designed to measure anxiety) that has unknown psychometric properties.

One such pathway, suggested by Damrav (1963) is that premature ejaculation may result from a hypersensitivity of the glans penis. He suggestion that the source of this hypersensitivity is an abnormally extensive covering of the glans penis by the prepuce. One testable prediction from this conjecture is that uncircumcised males whose erections expose the glans should be predisposed toward premature ejaculation. However, this has not been evaluated to date. Moreover, Shapiro (1943) in a review of 1130 cases over a 20-year period, concluded that physiological explanations could account for only 4% of the cases of premature ejaculation.

Cooper and Magnus (1984) provided additional data casting doubt on the role of anxiety in the etiology of premature ejaculation. In a double-blind study, 12 premature ejaculators and their partners were randomly assigned to placebo and Propranolol conditions for four weeks and then crossed over to the other condition. Couples were required to engage in intercourse twice a week and to record the time from intromission to ejaculation with a stopwatch. The results indicated that the drug had the expected effect on anxiety, but there were no differences in the latency times or subjective ratings of anxiety compared to the placebo and drug washout periods. Other possible interpretations of these results include inadequate drug dosage and variations in reactivity in using a stopwatch.

Masters and Johnson (1970) suggest a learning account of the role of anxiety in the etiology of premature ejaculation. Although they provide no well-controlled data for their assertion, Masters and Johnson suggest that premature ejaculators have backgrounds of having engaged in sexual intercourse in situations that encouraged short ejaculatory latencies (e.g., in the back seats of cars, in semiprivate locations where detection was possible, in intercourse with prostitutes who encouraged quick performance, and so on). They also suggest that the use of "withdrawal" for contraceptive purposes might be a factor involved in conditioning premature ejaculation. However, these possibilities await further systematic scrutiny.

Finally, Hong (1984) provides an evolutionary account of premature ejaculation—although Kinsey et al. (1948) and Symons (1987), among others, have also alluded to this. The evolutionary focus in not on proximate causes but rather on what circumstances in the ancestral populations probably led to selection of the particular trait (Symons, 1987). Hong proposes that rapid ejaculation was selected for (perhaps along with a highly sensitive glans) because faster ejaculators were less likely to be repelled by females or higher-ranking males—and thus likely to impregnate larger numbers of females. Hong hypothesizes that "this once superior trait" (p. 109) is currently overrepresented in the species. The reproductively advantageous strategy of premature ejaculation has been regarded by humans as a problem only in very recent times, since the recreational aspect of sex and female sexual satisfaction have come to receive a higher priority.

Hong addresses evidence that is consistent with his account. (1) Many primates ejaculate almost immediately after intromission. (2) There is an inverse correlation between speedy intercourse and male-male aggression in species. Speedy intercourse decreases male aggression because it increases the likelihood that many males will have an opportunity to mate. Any-thing that decreases such aggression has survival value. (3) Speedy intercourse has been observed to decrease the likelihood of damage to the female in primate copulation, which is often relatively rough.

However, Bixler (1986) criticizes Hong's account on the following grounds. (1) Some primates who live in multimale groups (e.g., chacmo and olive baboons and the rhesus) are not quick ejaculators. (2) Speedy ejaculation can be disadvantageous because it allows other males more opportunity to mate with an ovulating female. (3) Speedy ejaculation may be inconsistent with bonding, which is an important factor in producing successful progeny. (4) There is evidence that "sneak" copulations from subordinate males rarely lead to impregnation. Thus, the notion of evolutionary mechanisms being responsible for premature ejaculation, although fascinating, is quite controversial.

ASSESSMENT

Reliable and valid measurement of sexual dysfunction and its underlying variables are necessary for the development of empirically sound diagnostic and treatment protocols in this area (see Chapter 1; Malatesta & Adams, 1986; Ruff & St. Lawrence, 1985). Assessment is also vital in tailoring treatment to the specific needs of clients. For example, of ten couples treated with instruction manuals modeled after the Masters and Johnson protocol, only one considered sensate focus to be useful, whereas the other nine couples considered this component of treatment to be a hindrance (Lowe & Mitculas, 1985). The investigators hypothesize that either the sensate focus section of the instruction manual was poorly written, or those particular clients did not have deficits in the area in question.

When assessing the sexually dysfunctional client, information should be gathered from the three response systems (verbal, motoric, and physiological) in each of several areas pertaining to sexuality: sexual desire, arousal, and orgasm and heterosocial and heterosexual skills (Malatesta and Adams, 1986). Assessment devices within these areas will be reviewed in the remainder of this section.

Interview Assessment

Assessment of sexual dysfunction involves many steps, the first of which is usually the clinical interview. There are several reasons for employing an initial clinical interview, not the least of which is the building of good rapport. In areas as sensitive as sexual functioning and dysfunction, the importance of trust and rapport cannot be overemphasized. Other goals of the clinical interview include (1) provision of information regarding the etiology and maintenance of the problem; (2) assessment for contraindications to sex therapy (e.g., other psychopathology, relationship difficulties beyond difficulty with sexual activities, and medical problems); (3) development of tentative case formulations; and (4) provision of direction for more formal assessment to follow the initial interview (Malatesta & Adams, 1986). Several authors offer guidelines and formats specific to interviewing clients with sexual dysfunctions (Kaplan, 1983; Masters & Johnson, 1970; Ruff & St. Lawrence, 1985; Tollison & Adams, 1979). By and large, these interview protocols are similar in the kinds of information they assess: demographics, historical information (e.g., dating behavior, sex education, sexual experiences), sexual attitudes and behaviors, gender identity, gender preferences, communication skills, current relationship satisfaction, extrarelationship sexual activities, and information about specific sexual dysfunctions.

In Vivo Assessment

Motoric, or behavioral, assessment has been largely avoided, because of the private nature of the behaviors under study. Although some individuals advocate the occasional use of *in vivo* observation or surrogate partners for the purpose of assessment and treatment (Dauw, 1988; Masters & Johnson, 1970), these activities have profound ethical and legal implications and are therefore generally avoided (Malatesta &

Adams, 1986; Ruff & St. Lawrence, 1985). Furthermore, reactivity must be assumed to affect any findings gathered via these methods (Ruff & St. Lawrence, 1985). Nonetheless, accurate, objective information is useful to determine whether treatment is having a positive effect on ejaculatory latency. Zeiss has partially overcome the problems of *in vivo* assessment by having couples use a stopwatch to time ejaculatory latency (Zeiss, 1978). Of course, reactivity may still influence the sexual behavior, but Zeiss had couples take more than one reading and then averaged the times. Another way to address the issue of reactivity is to discount initial recordings. Another, more common way to gather *in vivo* data is to question the sexual partners of clients. However, the partners may be no less susceptible to social influences than the clients themselves, or they may be less than completely accurate informants for other reasons.

Physiological Assessment

Physiological measurements have been introduced in the assessment, treatment, and research of premature ejaculation (Ruff & St. Lawrence, 1985; Spiess et al., 1984). For example, Earls, Morales and Marshall (1988) reported a study in which penile plethysmography was used to evaluate the sexual arousal of 19 normal males. While their tumescence was being monitored, subjects were asked to signal when they had attained an erection that they judged sufficient for penetration, and also when a full erection had been reached. The results indicated that subjective assessment of tumescence was insensitive to penile changes between these two points. The experimenters also reported that 37% of the subjects were unable to achieve a full erection during presentation of visual sexual cues under these laboratory conditions. The authors suggested that penile plethysmography may therefore be insensitive for measuring some of the variables (or their magnitude) that are of interest in assessing premature ejaculation. However, there are other possible explanations for these findings. For example, all subjects viewed the same erotic film. Perhaps pretesting stimuli for erotic value or interviewing subjects to obtain their idiosyncratic preferences would decrease the high nonresponse rate of the subjects, which could lead to different results. The authors used a mercury-in-rubber strain gauge, whereas other experimenters have suggested that the volumetric penile measurement device is more sensitive to changes in tumescence occurring at the extreme levels of arousal (Freund & Blanchard, 1981). Thus, the methodological characteristics of this study might have contributed to these results; it is too early to make any conclusions about the usefulness of penile tumescence measurements in this area. (See Hatch (1981) and Rosen & Beck (1988) for reviews of physiological measurement of sexual arousal.)

Medical Assessment

If the clinical interview reveals that a sexual dysfunction is indicated, the next step in the assessment process should involve a medical evaluation (Malatesta & Adams, 1986). Thorough medical history, physical examination, and laboratory evaluation should all be conducted by a physician knowledgeable in the area of urology. However, little is known about the pathophysiology of premature ejaculation, and research in this area is quite sparse (see Chapter 8 and LoPiccolo & Stock, 1986). Some authors feel that the intrusiveness of this type of examination is not necessarily offset by the possibility that organic causes of premature ejaculation may soon be uncovered (Hawton, 1985). In general, however, the therapist is urged to have patients medically examined.

Assessment of Sexual Functioning

Although premature ejaculation is considered a disorder of orgasmic functioning, it is useful to assess overall sexual functioning patterns, as problems in other areas of sexual functioning (e.g., arousal or desire) may undermine or contraindicate therapy for premature ejaculation. Furthermore, measurement of overall sexual functioning may provide evidence for or against hypotheses regarding the etiology and maintenance of the dysfunction (see Spiess et al., 1984). An inventory designed to provide information for such hypotheses is the Sexual Interaction Inventory (SII), developed by LoPiccolo and Steger (1974). This paper-and-pencil inventory is given to both the client and his partner, to assess several dimensions of 17 heterosexual activities (e.g., frequency of the activity, pleasure from the activity, estimated partner pleasure from the activity). The responses are combined to form 11 scale scores, although the individual responses must be reviewed in order to determine the nature of any difficulties indicated by the scaled scores. The scaled scores include frequency of dissatisfaction—male; self-acceptance—male; pleasure mean—male; perceptual accuracy—male of female; mate acceptance—male of female; the female equivalents of these five scales; and a total disagreement score.

The reliability of the SII was assessed by administering it to a sample of normal couples ($N = 15$) twice over a two-week period. Correlations for the 11 scales were significant at the 0.05 level or better, ranging from 0.533 to 0.902. The experimenters argued that the reactive nature of this device caused the absolute values of the correlations to be less than optimal. Results from a different sample of married couples ($N = 79$) were used to calculate Cronbach's alpha coefficient to measure internal consistency. These coefficients ranged from 0.795 to 0.933, indicating good internal consistency for all scales. Convergent validity was assessed by comparing the single rating of overall sexual satisfaction (1, indicating extremely unsatisfactory, to 6, indicating extremely satisfactory) of sexually functional couples ($N = 70$) with the scaled scores. Although all correlations were in the expected direction, their absolute magnitudes were relatively low (except for scale 11), and the authors hypothesize that a global rating of sexual satisfaction does not correspond to the individual components measured by the SII scales. Discriminant validity was determined by comparing the results of a dysfunctional group

($N = 28$) and a "normal" group ($N = 63$). Nine of the 11 scales discriminated between these two groups.

Another sex inventory is the Golombok-Rust Inventory of Sexual Satisfaction (GRISS) (Rust & Golombok, 1985). This 28-item questionnaire may be given to both partners or to individual clients who are in heterosexual relationships. The GRISS measures sexual dysfunction and satisfaction and yields main scale scores of the overall quality of current sexual functioning, as well as 12 subscale scores: impotence, premature ejaculation, anorgasmia, vaginismus, infrequency, noncommunication, male and female dissatisfaction, male and female nonsensuality, and male and female avoidance.

Standardization of the GRISS was carried out on a sample of 88 sex therapy clients, and transformed scores were found to give good indications of the existence and severity of sexual problems (Rust & Golombok, 1985). The main scales had split-half reliabilities of 0.94 and 0.87 for the female and male scales, respectively. The reliabilities of subscales ranged between 0.61 and 0.83, with a mean of 0.74. Regarding validity, the overall female and male scores were found to discriminate between clinical ($N = 99$) and nonclinical ($N = 59$) groups ($p < 0.001$ for female score and $p < 0.005$ for male score). The overall scores were also found to correlate with therapists' ratings of severity ($p < 0.001$ for males and females). Specific dysfunctional groups were differentiated from the control group by the various subscales, with the differentiation of the premature ejaculators ($N = 19$) from "normal" subjects reaching significance at $p < 0.001$. Lastly, the overall scores were found to correlate with therapists' estimates of clients' improvement at five weeks of therapy ($p < 0.005$ for males and $p < 0.01$ for females).

The Derogatis Sexual Functioning Inventory (DSFI; Derogatis & Melisaratos, 1979) was designed to measure the current sexual functioning of an individual (p. 247). Originally constructed to gather information in eight areas related to sexual functioning, the DSFI currently measures functioning in ten areas: sexual knowledge, sexual experience, sexual drive, sexual

attitudes (liberal/conservative), psychological symptoms, emotional affect (positive/negative), gender-role definition (masculinity/femininity), sexual fantasies, body image, and sexual satisfaction. In addition, there are two global scores, the Sexual Functioning Score (SFI) and the Global Sexual Satisfaction Index (GSSI). The latter is measured by a nine-point scale, ranging from 0 "could not be worse" to 8 "could not be better." The SFI is simply a summation of all ten subtest scores.

Test-retest reliability coefficients were reported for all DSFI domains except body image and satisfaction, which were the two domains added after initial psychometric testing was completed with 60 sexually dysfunctional clients (Derogatis & Melisaratos, 1979). These coefficients ranged from 0.42 for the negative affect subscale to 0.96 for the attitude subscale. According to the authors, the low coefficients for the affect components (positive and negative) are due to expected fluctuations in mood. The reliabilities for information and the two component scores under gender role (masculinity and femininity) were also rather low (0.61, 0.60, and 0.58, respectively). Derogatis and Melisaratos hypothesized that some of the questions regarding sexual knowledge may be too difficult, thus resulting in guessing, which decreases reliability. They do not offer any hypotheses as to the low correlations of the gender-role definition components. Reliability scores were not reported for the two global scores.

Internal consistency scores were also reported, based on a sample size of 325 subjects. These ranged from 0.56 for the information domain to 0.97 for the experience domain. Internal consistency reliabilities were not reported for those domains that have scores base on differences between two dimensions (i.e., attitude, affect, gender role), nor for the psychological symptoms subtest, which comprises nine subtests.

Validation of the DSFI was carried out on four subject samples, normal males ($N = 76$), sexually dysfunctional males ($N = 91$), normal females ($N = 154$), and sexually dysfunctional females ($N = 59$). The SFI scores of the sexually dysfunctional subjects were significantly lower than those of the normals ($p < 0.001$). Thus, the dysfunctional males had a mean SFI score of 434 (s.d. = 35), compared to the mean score of 513 (s.d. = 44) for normal males. For the females, the dysfunctional subjects had a mean score of 456 (s.d. = 42), and the normals had a mean of 503 (s.d. = 29). GSSI scores were also significantly different between the normal and dysfunctional groups ($p < 0.001$). On this measure, normal males had a mean of 5 (s.d. = 1.5), while dysfunctional males had a mean of only 2.5 (s.d. = 1.6). Normal females had a GSSI mean of 4.8 (s.d. = 2), and dysfunctional females had a mean of 2.3 (s.d. = 1.5). Most subtests also discriminated between the two male groups, at the 0.01 level. However, gender-role and attitude differences both fell below this level. Several subtests were not significantly different between the female groups. The experience, drive, attitude, gender role, and fantasy subtests all fell below an alpha level of 0.01. The authors offer possible explanations for each instance of nonsignificance but fail to address the poorer overall performance of the DSFI when utilized with females.

Discriminative functional analyses were also conducted with the DSFI, although only on the original eight-subtest version (Derogatis & Melisaratos, 1979). The classification matrices employed led to 77% correct classification of males and 75% correct classification of females as either normal or dysfunctional. Although this represents an increase of approximately 25% over chance, the classification of individuals into such broad categories as sexually dysfunctional and nondysfunctional does not seem to add "unique predictive information" to the clinical fund of knowledge. Nonetheless, the DSFI does gather information in several areas of relevance to the clinician and does appear to possess adequate reliability and validity in several of its subtests. However, further testing is indicated, as is possible revision of the subtests that have not proven to distinguish between normal and dysfunctional samples.

The Sex History Form (SHF) is another self-report questionnaire that assesses the quality,

quantity, and nature of the sexual functioning of couples (Nowinski & LoPiccolo, 1979). In addition, overall sexual satisfaction for both the client and the partner is measured. This 19-item questionnaire is designed to serve as a measure of treatment effects, in terms of reversal of symptoms, as well as an assessment measure of sexual dysfunction and dissatisfaction (LoPiccolo, Heiman, Hogan, & Roberts, 1985). However, psychometric testing does not appear to have been reported for this instrument.

All of the inventories reviewed above are relatively inexpensive and quick, with the exception of the DSFI, which takes between 45 and 50 minutes. Other modes of measuring of sexual functioning include self-monitoring, behavioral observation, and physiological assessment. The objectivity of these measures may allow them the potential benefit of increased validity. However, as discussed earlier, there are numerous difficulties with the first two of these modalities, and the use of physiological devices to gather data on sexually dysfunctional males has not been thoroughly researched.

Assessment of Relationship Variables

A brief review of some devices that measure relationship variables will now be given, as these variables are often hypothesized to affect the etiology and maintenance of sexual dysfunctions and treatment outcome.

The Marital Adjustment Scale (Locke & Wallace, 1959) is a relatively well-known and well-researched questionnaire that yields two factor scores: sexual congeniality and compatibility. Research on a revision of this questionnaire, the Dyadic Adjustment Scale (DAS; Spanier, 1976) indicated that overall factor scores differentiate between satisfied (happily) and dissatisfied (unhappily) married men and women. Normative testing on the DAS indicates a mean adjustment score of approximately 71 for divorced couples and 115 for happily married couples. Couples known to be maladjusted (unhappy) had a mean of 71.7. In a study involving only nondysfunctional couples ($N = 44$), Kimmel and Van der Veen (1974) tested the short form of this marriage inventory. Test-retest was conducted, with a twenty-seven-month break between testing. Correlations ranged between 0.65 and 0.78 for the factor scores. Given the substantial length of time between testing and the relatively adequate correlations, Kimmel and Van der Veen concluded that "factors appear to tap enduring characteristics of marital relationships" (p. 62).

Another measure of relationship was developed by Mathews, Whitehead, and Kellett (1983). Their Relationship Questionnaire is composed of 30 items rated on a five-point scale. Part (i) assesses primarily cognitive/affective aspects of relationships (e.g., commitment, contentment, tension, communication, enjoyment of sexual activity, frequency of sexual thoughts, and communication of needs and feelings). Part (ii) assesses primarily behavioral aspects of relationships (e.g., frequency of social and spare time, frequency of communication and sexual activities over the past month, desired future frequencies, and estimation of partner's desired future frequencies). This questionnaire is reported as being sensitive to changes in marital adjustment following sex therapy (Hawton & Catalan, 1986).

One difficulty with these self-report indices of relationship is that they are susceptible to the influences of social desirability. A stronger argument is that, to the extent that various feelings, cognitions, and other nonobservable dimensions are used in assessment and therapy, the validity may be untestable (Margolin & Fernandez, 1983). However, at least one device that assesses relationships, the Marital Satisfaction Inventory, includes a validity scale measuring social desirability and thus provides a way in which invalid protocols may be recognized (Weiss & Margolin, 1986). This instrument is composed of 280 items, yielding one global affective score and 11 subscale scores: affective communication, problem-solving communication, quality and quantity of leisure time together, finances, sexual dissatisfaction,

sex-role orientation, family and marital disruption, dissatisfaction with children, and conflict over childbearing (Weiss & Margolin, 1986). Disharmony and disaffection are two scales found in a more recent item analysis (Snyder & Regts, 1982). Excellent concurrent and discriminant validity of each scale has been demonstrated (Weiss & Margolin, 1986).

Assessment of Heterosocial Skills

Malatesta and Adams (1986) list heterosocial skills as those falling between social competence and heterosexual functioning, including (1) sensitivity and discrimination of heterosocial cues; (2) evaluation and processing of these cues; (3) selection and effective execution of appropriate responses in heterosocial situations; and (4) processing and responding to feedback (Malatesta & Adams, 1986). These skills are important because, as Zilbergeld (1975) notes, satisfactory sexual encounters can take place only if the individual possesses the skills necessary to bring about opportunities for such encounters. Thus, the treatment of premature ejaculation may be clinically irrelevant if the client cannot convince others to engage in sexual activities with him.

Two measures of heterosocial dysfunction are the Social Anxiety and Distress Scale (SAD) and the Fear of Negative Evaluation Scale (FNE) (both by Watson & Friend, 1969). The SAD is a 28-item true-false questionnaire that measures avoidance of social situations due to anxiety, fear, and distress. The FNE assesses social avoidance caused by anticipatory fears of loss of approval and negative evaluation. Both measures have been found to have good reliability and internal consistency (Malatesta & Adams, 1986).

Another measure of heterosocial interaction is the Survey of Heterosocial Interactions (SHI; Twentyman & McFall, 1975). This measure includes questions regarding dating and self-perception of heterosocial dexterity, as well as 20 realistic depictions of heterosocial encounters, to which the client is to respond.

Psychometric development is extensive but limited to college males.

In addition to self-report inventories, self-monitoring and behavioral observation may provide useful information. Given the limitations of self-reporting and the time-consuming nature of behavioral observation, therapists may wish to use role-playing techniques to gather analogue information on clients' heterosocial skills. Using opposite-sex confederates can help make role-play scenarios as realistic as possible (see Zilbergeld, 1975).

Assessment of Heterosexual Skills

Heterosexual skills are those necessary for the initiation and maintenance of mutually satisfying sexual relationships. They include knowledge of human sexuality, intimacy skills, skills in affectional touching and reciprocity of sexual needs, ability to express positive emotions, and, of course, specific sexual functioning skills such as coitus and cunnilingus (Malatesta & Adams, 1986).

As mentioned earlier, the private nature of sexual behavior dictates an almost exclusive reliance on self-report measures for the gathering of information on heterosexual skills. As a partial control for the biases of subjectivity, it is recommended that partners of clients (if available) be involved in the assessment procedures. Areas to focus on include (1) sexual history, (2) sexual knowledge and experiences, (3) specific sexual responses and affectional behaviors employed by the client, and (4) current status of the sexual relationship (Malatesta & Adams, 1986). In addition, extrarelationship activities, if acknowledged by the client, should be assessed. Questionnaires have been developed to assess sexual knowledge, attitudes, and experiences. These include the Miller-Fisk Sexual Knowledge Questionnaire (Gough, 1974); the Sexual Knowledge and Attitude Test (Lief & Reed, 1972); the Sexual Knowledge Inventory (Casselman & Durham, 1979); and the Heterosexual Behavior Assessment (Bentler, 1968). More novel ap-

proaches to assessment include the development of computer programs designed specifically for the assessment of sexual dysfunctions (Binik, Servan-Schreiber, Freiwald, & Hall, 1988). These computer programs have not yet undergone psychometric evaluation, so they must be considered preliminary at this point. However, these and similar programs are likely to be available to the clinician before too long.

TREATMENT

By and large, the treatment of premature ejaculation has undergone relatively little change since it was first systematized by Semans in the mid-1950s (Semans, 1956). However, there have been some variations on the standard techniques. This section will recount the standard treatments for premature ejaculation and also review variations thereof. In addition, factors that have often been assumed to affect treatment (e.g., number of therapists) and outcome studies will be reviewed.

Traditional Therapies

There is reason to believe that premature ejaculation has plagued men (and indirectly, women) for quite some time; written accounts of the problem are found in Greek mythology (Ruff & St. Lawrence, 1985). However, treatments for the problem did not appear in the literature until relatively recently, and these were developed not in the laboratory or therapy room of the psychologist but in the clinic of the medical doctor (Tuthill, 1955; Semans, 1956; Hastings, 1966; Masters & Johnson, 1970). Tuthill (1955) conceptualized premature ejaculation as the almost inevitable outcome of a man's early experiences with intercourse. It is the individual's reaction to these initial experiences that leads either to the development of a sexual problem or to eventual satisfactory control of ejaculation, according to Tuthill. Those men who remain nonplussed by their too-quick response and are "eager to repeat intercourse" will gain control of their response (p. 125). On the other hand, men who decrease the frequency with which they engage in intercourse will continue to have difficulty. Tuthill's treatment, therefore, is simply to "abandon all restraint and have more frequent intercourse" (p. 126). In support of this hypothesis, Tuthill reported that 51 of 60 couples given this advice indicated significant improvement after only one office visit. In the other nine cases, only two to six additional sessions were required before improvement was reported by the couples. This technique is also supported by Spiess et al.'s (1984) finding that premature ejaculators tended to have less frequent intercourse than "normal" males. Of course, a decrease in frequency of intercourse may have resulted from the dysfunction, rather than vice versa. However, regardless of etiology, a simple increase in frequency of intercourse may be a valid form of intervention for some premature ejaculators.

Despite Tuthill's reported 100% rate of effectiveness and the high face validity of his "treatment," some rather obvious problems with this account must be noted. First of all, it is not clear what criteria Tuthill used to assess progress. Secondly, Tuthill does not supply information as to how the initial problem and changes in this problem were assessed. In addition, several other methodological errors are evident, including lack of a control group and lack of information about the couples. However, considering the cost-effectiveness and simplicity of this treatment plan, more methodologically adequate studies are warranted.

Hastings (1966) reports on various techniques for treating premature ejaculation. These are similar to that of Tuthill in that they might best be construed as recommendations rather than actual treatments. These techniques are divided into two categories: those that will reduce the effects of stimulus (both psychic and tactile) input and those that allow the male to lower his ejaculatory threshold (Hastings, 1966). In the first category Hastings

includes (1) distraction with nonsexual fantasies (e.g., of a hunting trip or multiplication tables); (2) tightening the anal sphincter muscles and concentrating on keeping the anus closed, (3) activities that cause some pain (e.g., biting the inside of one's cheek, pinching the skin of one's arm); (4) the "judicious" use of alcohol (p. 132); (5) use of a condom, perhaps with gauze inside, wrapped around the head of the penis; (6) deeper insertion of the penis into the vagina coupled with fewer, shorter strokes; and (7) a change in coital position (to be determined on an individual basis).

In order to increase the amount of stimulus the male can withstand before ejaculating, Hastings refers to the stop-start treatment described by Semans (discussed below). In addition, he presents information from a single case in which a client reported gaining control of ejaculation by practicing light stroking of the penis in non-interactional situations. This allowed the client to postpone ejaculation during masturbation, and after four or five such episodes, to postpone ejaculation during intercourse.

Although the techniques of distraction recommended by Hastings may work to a limited degree (Geer & Fuhr, 1976), it is likely that many men who reach a level of distress severe enough to warrant a visit to a professional have already attempted to employ at least one of these, with limited success. In addition, most of Hastings' techniques involve some level of discomfort. Certainly the goal of sexual intercourse is neither to be distracted nor in pain but quite the opposite. In fact, McCarthy (1989) suggested that "do-it-yourself" techniques such as those reported above have iatrogenic effects. He proposed that such techniques may cause erection difficulty by reducing arousal and may contribute to the deterioration of the bond between a couple, because the man is not participating fully in the act of lovemaking. Additionally, Hastings' report suffers from inadequacies similar to those in the Tuthill study.

Semans (1956) developed what is now known as the *stop-start* technique for treating premature ejaculation. It has been suggested that this technique is rather mechanical in nature (McCarthy, 1989), but it was not recommended in a vacuum but rather embedded within a framework of therapy that involved the partner as well as the individual client. The first step of Semans' treatment is to interview each partner separately, with the aim of modifying any misconceptions the partners may have about therapy. Also, the partners are instructed to rest, if either is fatigued, before beginning the therapy. Once they are rested, "loveplay" is begun, with the partners instructed to touch each other and to progress towards genital stimulation. During this initial stage, partners are to inform one another about their level of sexual excitement in response to the stimulation of being touched. When the man experiences sensations indicative of forthcoming ejaculation, he informs the partner and stops the partner from stimulating him. Once the subjective sensation of high arousal disappears, stimulation is reintroduced, and again interrupted when similar sensations reappear. This cycle is repeated until the male is able to postpone ejaculation indefinitely (clinicians often use 15–20 minutes as indicative of reasonable ejaculatory control). In the event of accidental ejaculation, the male is instructed to bring the female to orgasm via clitoral stimulation, and the session is then postponed. Postponement is also indicated if the erection subsides without returning immediately.

Upon successful postponement of ejaculation with the above instructions, the partners are again interviewed—separately and then together—with the aim of introducing the next step, which is stimulation of the penis with the aid of lubrication. Semans's reasoning behind this is that the "dry" stimulation of the penis initially used has not adequately mimicked the sensations that will be felt once vaginal penetration is reintroduced. Once indefinite postponement of ejaculation is reached using the lubricant, intercourse without premature ejaculation should be possible (Semans, 1956). After a few weeks, separate follow-up interviews are held with the wife and husband, to ensure that instructions have been understood and followed correctly and that treatment gains have been maintained.

Semans (1956) presented the results of this treatment for eight out of an initial 14 couples. (the remaining 6 were dropped from treatment or could not be followed up.) In seven of these cases, couples reported that premature ejaculation had disappeared and that treatment gains were maintained (follow-up intervals ranged from five weeks to one year). In the couple that did not report consistent improvement in ejaculatory control, the husband was diagnosed as having "depressive psychoneurosis" (p. 356). Some control was learned initially but was then lost during a return of the depression. In general, however, couples reported that ejaculatory control was readily learned.

As with the studies cited earlier, there are several methodological weaknesses in Semans' study. For example, there was no control group, and assessment of change relied solely upon the self-report of the husband and the wife, with more weight given to the veracity of the wife's account. Follow-up times were occasionally too short to be considered adequate. Although Semans does not address this issue specifically, he does demonstrate awareness of the role of social pressures (e.g., to report sexual satisfaction rather than dissatisfaction) by recommending the separate assessment of both partners.

Masters and Johnson (1970) present the most comprehensive theoretical framework, within which is outlined a treatment plan for premature ejaculation (reviewed below). Their treatment is similar to Semans' in that it involves inclusion of a partner, manual stimulation of the penis prior to vaginal stimulation, and the use of a modified stop-start technique (where, in addition to cessation of movement, the penis is squeezed by the female to reduce tumescence). These researchers also emphasize the benefits of first explaining to the couple that their problem is readily amenable to treatment (as did Semans). A major departure in the treatment approach of Masters and Johnson is their advocacy of intense, daily therapy sessions and, when possible, the social seclusion of the treatment couple.

The initial component of the Masters and Johnson therapy involves "sensate focus," in which the partners are instructed to touch each other in a nondemanding manner (that is, without focusing on the end goals of orgasm or ejaculation). Thus, for the first few days, there is a ban on contact with genitalia between the partners. Later, as such contact is included in the sensate-focus sessions, the female is instructed to stimulate the penis until full erection occurs. At this point, the squeeze technique is employed: The female places her thumb on the frenulum and two fingers on the dorsal side of the penis (above and below the coronal ridge) and then puts pressure on the penis for 3–4 seconds. This is to cause the male to lose his urge to ejaculate. The female then waits 15–30 seconds after the urge subsides and begins again to stimulate the male. The entire process is repeated for 15–20 minutes without ejaculation (Masters & Johnson, 1970). This type of stimulation is carried out for two or three days, so that the male can obtain satisfactory control over manually stimulated erections. After this has occurred, the partners progress to "nondemanding intromission" (p. 106). Here, after first manually stimulating the male and employing the squeeze technique two or three times, the couple assumes the female-superior position, in which the female is sitting atop the male, who is lying flat. The female inserts the penis into her vagina and remains motionless, to allow the male to concentrate on the sensations created by this positioning. If the male develops the urge to ejaculate, the female is to elevate off of the penis, employ the squeeze technique, and then reinsert the penis. This process is carried out over the next couple of days, with the male gradually beginning to add pelvic thrusting in order to maintain erection. Again, the goal is approximately 15–20 minutes of ejaculatory control. Once this criterion has been reached, the female may initiate pelvic thrusting, slowly at first but eventually with full intensity, with the goal of both partners reaching orgasm. Lastly, the couple is instructed to change from the female-superior position to the lateral-coital position. This position permits the male to have maximum control over erections while still allowing the female unhindered pelvic movement and thus sexual satisfaction (Masters & Johnson, 1970).

At this point the formal treatment of the couple is over. However, they are warned that ejaculatory control problems may occasionally arise over the course of the ensuing year. Consequently, they are instructed to maintain a pattern of regular intercourse, to continue to employ the squeeze technique at least once a week, and to take one 15–20 minute session per month, going back to the sensate focus and manual stimulation of the penis and using the squeeze technique. Separations of a few weeks or more are seen as high-risk situations, and the couple is encouraged to employ the techniques they have learned whenever a separation of sufficient length has taken place. Before therapy is terminated, one last word of caution is given regarding treatment-related complications. Masters and Johnson found that a small but substantial percentage of males (approximately 12%) developed secondary impotence just prior to or just after termination of treatment. They reasoned that this was a result of increased frequency of intercourse relative to pretreatment rates. Masters and Johnson hypothesized that the reaction of the couple to this failure determines whether or not a more serious problem will ensue. Couples who are able to shrug off this problem will be less likely to develop problems than those who, due to lack of warning, experience a return of performance fears (Masters & Johnson, 1970).

Utilizing the procedure outlined above, Masters and Johnson reported having significantly helped 182 out of 186 men who presented with premature ejaculation over a span of 11 years. This represents a failure rate of only 2.2% (Masters & Johnson, 1970). The criterion on which they based treatment evaluation was the ability of the male to maintain ejaculatory control enough to satisfy his partner in 50% or more of their coital encounters. Thus, four men are reported not to have attained this criterion.

The explanation given for two of these failures was that the men were not motivated to learn ejaculatory control. In the other two cases, the researchers could offer no explanation. Although it would no doubt be instructional to know why these two men failed to achieve adequate control, the success rate reported by Masters and Johnson is nonetheless astonishing.

Unfortunately, Masters and Johnson's report suffers from some severe methodological flaws (Zilbergeld & Evans, 1980). First, the authors do not describe their treatment group, except to indicate that couples who present with premature ejaculation as the primary concern tend to be more highly educated and of upper socioeconomic status. There is no information regarding couples who were turned away from treatment (if any). Thus, generalization of findings is consequently diminished. (This problem is given cursory acknowledgment in the the preface to Master and Johnson's 1970 text.) There were no control or placebo groups with which to compare outcome results, so one cannot rule out placebo effects or the possibility that experimenter expectations account for the results. There is also a problem with Masters and Johnson's choice of the criterion variable for judging success and failure rates. Masters and Johnson are to be commended for explicitly stating and defining their criterion, but the subjectivity and vagueness of "satisfying the female partner on at least 50% of all coital engagements" must be noted. What constitutes "satisfaction" for the female? Is coital orgasm the goal? What of the woman who is satisfied with less than 60 seconds of penetration? What of the woman who requires 25–30 minutes of intercourse before she is "satisfied?" Obviously, different women will have different criteria by which they judge their partners' abilities. The same man could, therefore, be considered a premature ejaculator with one partner and a retarded ejaculator with another. It is not unheard of for men and women to change their partners, and even spouses. Is a man cured of premature ejaculation simply because he changes partners? Obviously, a less subjective criterion should be employed in order to determine treatment effectiveness.

Lastly, the follow-up data present a problem. There is only indirect indication of the length of follow-up, given in the preface (p. v), where the authors claim that "imperfect five-year patient follow-up" has been carried out. No data are reported indicating any degree of attrition during follow-up. Masters and Johnson did not conduct a valid experiment, nor do they indicate that this was their goal. However, their presentation of results implies a certain scientific rigor, which was not in fact upheld (Zilbergeld & Evans, 1980). The fact that several other researchers have not found "cure rates" anywhere near those reported by Masters and Johnson gives weight to the idea that Masters and Johnson's success rates were artificially inflated, possibly due to vague treatment criteria and a general lack of precise scientific methodology.

McCarthy (1989) presents a cognitive-behavioral approach for the treatment of premature ejaculation. This approach emphasizes the formation of new attitudes that may affect not only the problem of premature ejaculation but also the entire sexual relationship, as well as making the task of learning ejaculatory control the responsibility of both partners rather than solely that of the man. Behavioral techniques are employed for the strict purpose of developing ejaculatory control; they are quite similar to those of Semans (1956) and Masters and Johnson (1970). Specifically, McCarthy recommends that the couple participate in two or more "nongenital sensuality exercises" and "nondemand pleasuring exercises" (p. 149). Manual (and/or oral) stimulation of the penis is then introduced, coupled with the stop-start technique developed by Semans (1956). However, McCarthy notes that some males may wish to practice the stop-start technique on their own in order to gain some ejaculatory control in a more private setting.

Once ejaculatory control has been acquired during manual (and/or oral) stimulation, the stop-start technique is employed during intercourse. As in Masters and Johnson's treatment, the female-superior position with minimal movement is employed, allowing the male to focus on ''containment'' sensations without the distractions of pelvic movements. This ''nondemand'' intercourse is carried out for 10–15 minutes. Positions and types of pelvic thrusting are varied and added as the male acquires more ejaculatory control. The final goal of McCarthy's therapy is for the couple to develop intimacy. McCarthy hypothesizes that sexual functioning is facilitated by a more cooperative and intimate relationship.

McCarthy indicates that he believes his approach to be unique, but this is to distinguish between his cognitive-behavioral approach and that presented by Masters and Johnson. McCarthy borrows heavily from Masters and Johnson's terminology (e.g., *pleasuring*) and seems to mimic their and Semans' treatment protocols. The underlying treatment rationales are also quite similar: For example, female partners should be intimately involved in the treatment procedure; intimacy is a primary factor in positive sexual experiences; and men should not always bear the onus of demand in the sexual context.

Cognitive and Behavioral Treatments

The reported successes of Semans' (1956) and Masters and Johnson's (1970) programs seems to have curtailed research into this area of behavior (LoPiccolo, 1985). Consequently, many studies involving the treatment of premature ejaculation employ the primary components of these treatments. However, variations have occasionally been introduced into the standard approach, frequently in an attempt to tease out the necessary (as against the gratuitous) components of therapy for premature ejaculation (LoPiccolo et al., 1985; Lowe & Mikulas, 1975; Mathews, Bancroft, Whitehead, Hackmann, Julier, Bancroft, Gath, & Shaw, 1976; McCarthy, 1989; Zeiss, 1978). Occasionally, completely different treatment components have been added to the standard package with the goal of improving on it (Hartman & Daly, 1983;

Mathews et al., 1976; Yulis, 1976). Those studies that include behavioral and/or cognitive treatment components are reviewed in this section.

Mathews and colleagues (1976) reported a comparison study of three different treatment methods used with sexually dysfunctional couples ($N = 36$). The three treatment protocols were (1) systematic desensitization plus counseling, (2) directed practice with counseling, and (3) directed practice with minimal counseling. Other variables manipulated in this study were gender and number of therapists. Couples were seen by a dual-sex team or by a therapist of the same gender as the person with the presenting problem. Thus, the 12 couples for whom premature ejaculation was the primary dysfunction were treated by either teams or by male therapists. In this protocol, couples were initially interviewed and their primary problem determined by two psychiatrists. They were then randomly allocated to one of the three treatment programs. During a baseline pretreatment period (four weeks), couples completed self-report diaries for the purpose of gathering baseline information on frequency and satisfaction with sexual contacts. All therapies began with a history-gathering session and a feedback session, in which the therapy to be used with that couple was explained.

In systematic desensitization treatment, weekly sessions were held. The couple developed a hierarchy of sexual situations and learned relaxation and desensitization skills. Subjects were encouraged to practice relaxation and desensitization at home; toward the end of therapy, treatment sessions were used mainly for general sexual counseling. The program of directed practice with counseling treatment was similar to Master and Johnson's, but it was carried out in weekly rather than daily treatment sessions. In the group treated with directed practice with minimal contact, couples were seen for the initial sessions, where it was emphasized that only occasional clinic visits would be necessary. Thereafter, instructions for directed practice (again based on Masters and Johnson's techniques) were mailed to couples on a weekly basis, along with therapists' comments. Mid-treatment and end-of-treatment sessions were the only other direct contact sessions scheduled in this treatment protocol.

Between-group comparisons yielded nonsignificant results, due primarily to the heterogeneity of the within-group results (especially the directed practice groups) (Mathews et al., 1976). No significant differences were found in between-group ratings of general and sexual relationship status made by therapists, patients, and independent assessors. There was, however, a nonsignificant trend for the group that received directed practice with counseling to show the most gains. Number of therapists, gender of the partner presenting the problem, and interactions between these two variables were also analyzed, and no significant between-groups differences were reported. Again, however, a nonsignificant trend was reported: Couples who were seen by two therapists and given the directed practice with counseling showed the most gains. The minimal-contact group was reported to be most likely to experience relapse to or below initial levels of sexual relationship and frequency of sexual contact. The desensitization group showed less variability overall and fewer gains than the group that received directed practice with counseling. Mathews et al. concluded that directed practice with counseling was superior to the other two treatments. However, they also hypothesized, due to variability within the groups, that some couples may respond more to behavioral direction (as in the minimal-treatment group), while others require more counseling. The use of systematic desensitization was not supported for the treatment of sexual dysfunction, as this group showed only minimal changes. The small number of couples in each group and the lack of statistically significant findings preclude any firm conclusions about treatment differences. Unfortunately, the findings were not broken down by type of dysfunction, so the usefulness of the various treatment procedures specifically with premature ejaculation cannot be directly assessed from this study.

Yulis (1976) treated 37 couples in which the males were premature ejaculators, as assessed by diagnostic interviews by cotherapists (patterned after the assessment protocol of Masters and Johnson, 1970). Therapy involved a synthesis of sensate focus (Masters & Johnson, 1970), squeeze techniques (Semans, 1956), and controlled intromission and pelvic thrusting (Wolpe, 1969). However, assertiveness training was also given to those males who were assessed as possessing deficiencies in the areas of social interaction, dating, and sexual contact. Couples were seen by cotherapist teams three times per week for up to 18 weeks. The criterion used for assessment of treatment effect was the attainment of ejaculatory control in 80–100% of all sexual encounters at six-month follow-up. Based on this criterion, 89% of the subjects were considered treatment successes at six-month follow-up (Yulis, 1976). Since the goal of this study was to provide information on the generalization of therapy to new partners, Yulis did not go into significant detail about the treatment outcome. However, this high level of success at six-months after treatment indicates the usefulness of these techniques. Unfortunately, Yulis did not provide differential information for subjects treated with and without assertiveness training. The primary interest of the author was in the generalization of treatment effects to new sexual partners. At six-month follow-up, 23 subjects reported having had sexual encounters with partners other than those with whom they had gone through the treatment process. Thirteen of these subjects had received sex therapy with assertive therapy, and 11 of these reported adequate generalization. Of the ten subjects who had not received assertiveness training and who had new sexual partners, only three reported adequate generalization. Fisher's Exact Probability Test was performed, indicating a statistically significant ($p = .011$) gain in generalization effect for the assertive group. The author concluded that inclusion of assertive training when treating premature ejaculation is strongly indicated for generalization of positive results to new sexual partners.

Zilbergeld (1975) developed a therapy program targeting attitudes and beliefs that are hypothesized to contribute to clients' sexual dysfunctions. These include "myths" that (1) Performance is more important than enjoyment; (2) performance is valued more by women than expression of affection and caring; (3) the male must be the initiator and director of sexual encounters; (4) sex is the logical conclusion of all physical contact; (5) sex and intercourse are the same thing; (6) to have sex, one must have an erection; and (7) males can have sex on demand. Zilbergeld attempted to counter the notion that men are "sex machines" by emphasizing that certain individually determined conditions must exist in order for men to respond sexually. In the treatment of sexual dysfunction, the client determines what conditions he requires for successful sexual encounters, and the therapist assesses whether the client has the necessary skills to achieve those conditions. Social skills training in the areas of assertiveness, communication, relaxation, and coping with interpersonal encounters is offered to clients deficient in any of these areas. If, after the client develops the appropriate skills, the sexual dysfunction persists, exercises are taught to help him gain voluntary control over his erection. These focus on thrusting (slower and in different directions) and movement of pelvic muscles (constricting and relaxing) (Zilbergeld, 1975).

Ince (1973) presented a case study in which premature ejaculation (as defined by ejaculation immediately upon vaginal intromission) was treated with several behavioral techniques. Systematic desensitization was employed at the outset of therapy, as the patient was determined to have developed anxiety regarding intercourse secondary to his sexual problems. A hierarchy was created, with the different scenarios involving kissing, mutual petting, and intercourse. After relaxation training, the therapist verbally presented the items to the patient, with the usual backtracking whenever the patient indicated he was becoming anxious. As with the study by Mathews et al. (1976), systematic desensitization did not have a significant effect on premature ejaculation, although the patient did report feeling less anxious about engaging in

intercourse. After two sessions of systematic desensitization, thought-stopping training was given to the patient. The patient was instructed to visualize sexual encounters, and when he indicated he was at the point where premature ejaculation was likely to occur, the therapist shouted "stop." After three such trials, the patient was instructed to mentally shout "stop" while visualizing the same scenes. He was to continue this practice during actual intercourse until his partner reached orgasm. As a result, the patient became able to postpone ejaculation for approximately one minute after intromission. In the third and last week of treatment, the patient was instructed to masturbate for 30–40 minutes before intercourse. The patient reported that masturbation, coupled with the thought-stopping technique, resulted in sufficient delay of ejaculation for his partner to reach orgasm. Results at follow-up, conducted five weeks posttreatment, indicated that the patient was able to delay ejaculation without the use of any behavioral techniques. The author concluded that this was a successful example of short-term behavior therapy for premature ejaculation. However, the very short follow-up period is inadequate for measuring long-term treatment effects. Also, baseline information was not collected, so it is unknown whether the results were due to one or a combination of the behavioral manipulations, to a placebo effect, or to the increased frequency with which the patient and his partner engaged in intercourse. Lastly, outcome was based on a criterion potentially unrelated to ejaculatory control (the sexual partner's orgasmic latency). Thus, the absolute magnitude of change in the client's control is unknown.

Stravynski (1986) reported a case study in which social skills training and *in vivo* exposure were used to modify an individual client's sexual disorder indirectly. Stravynski hypothesized that patients who present with sexual dysfunction but without a cooperating partner (as had this patient) may have more general difficulties in heterosocial functioning. Stravynski therefore treated his client with a combination of behavioral techniques aimed at improving the client's poor social and heterosexual skills and decreasing his interpersonal anxiety. Sexual functioning was discussed when the patient brought it up, but treatments were not aimed at sexual dysfunction per se. A single-subject, multiple-baseline design was used. Frequency of successful intercourse experiences was assessed, as were the targeted behaviors of initiating conversation, expressing interest, expressing positive emotions, and expressing empathy. In addition, anxiety during targeted behaviors was rated on a five-point scale, where 0 indicated "perfect calm" and 5 indicated "terrified." A three week baseline prior to treatment showed no instances of successful intercourse or the targeted behaviors (except expression of interest, which occurred once).

Anxiety surrounding interpersonal situations was targeted through prolonged exposure with female acquaintances of the client in pubs and cafes. Sexual overtures were prohibited at this stage of therapy. Prosocial behaviors such as initiating conversations, showing interest, and expressing positive emotions were taught through modeling, instructions, and role rehearsal. Throughout treatment, therapist feedback and client self-monitoring of the frequencies of targeted behaviors and subjective anxiety were used to provide reinforcement and correction when needed.

The results indicated that anxiety decreased, and frequency of targeted behaviors increased, immediately following treatment onset. However, the client had difficulty expressing empathy and felt anxious around women even after these areas were targeted. An increase in successful intercourse experiences was reported after six weeks of treatment. All results were maintained at six-month follow-up, indicating the usefulness of skills training with this client. Unfortunately, in this otherwise well-designed study, Stravynski fails to provide an operational definition of "successful" intercourse—the patient made this determination. Also, as noted by Stravynski, it is impossible to distinguish necessary from unnecessary treatment components in this design. Of course, generalization is limited by the single-subject focus. Nonetheless, it is intriguing that a client experienced improvement in ejaculatory control without this ever being targeted in treatment.

Other Treatments

Gentry (1978) presented a variation of "brief therapy" in the treatment of premature ejaculation. Brief therapy is defined as a communication and systems approach in which behaviors assumed to maintain symptoms are targeted for change. In this study, Gentry discussed a client with premature ejaculation (not operationally defined). Over the span of eight treatment sessions, the client was placed in several different "therapeutic paradoxes" (p. 33)—situations in which the client may perceive any result as positive. The first paradox occurred when the client was told that he and the therapist would proceed slowly toward improving his condition—even though the treatment contract was for only ten sessions. The goal of contracting for such a short time was that the client would develop positive expectations regarding quick behavioral changes. The admonition to proceed slowly was designed to create in the client the desire to prove to the therapist that he was able to work quickly toward problem resolution.

The second paradox was created by telling the client to have a premature ejaculation during his next sexual interaction. This enabled the client to feel in control of the situation, regardless of whether he did or did not ejaculate prematurely. The final paradox was created by telling the client that he would have a relapse. Thus, relapse was placed in the paradoxical context of "a step forward in therapy" rather than its usual context of an instance of regression. The client's knowledge of the impending relapse presumably allowed him to feel in control of the situation. According to Gentry, a client may feel apprehensive regarding therapeutic change (presumably because he or she has become accustomed to the symptomatic behaviors) and a relapse helps the client control this apprehension.

After six weeks of treatment, the client was

no longer experiencing difficulties with ejaculation and was having positive sexual encounters more frequently, so treatment was terminated after only the eighth week. A 12-month follow-up indicated no return of the sexual dysfunction. Gentry concluded that the second paradox (to continue the symptomatic behavior) resulted in increased control of ejaculation. The motivation to attain this control was created by the first paradox, and the third paradox allowed the client to maintain his gains by decreasing apprehension regarding his newfound control. Although Gentry may be correct in his hypotheses, there are other possible explanations for the results he reported. For example, it is possible that the client was already highly motivated for change before the initial paradox was introduced, thus making this manipulation unnecessary. Secondly, an overall increase in sexual encounters may have influenced the client's increase in positive experiences with intercourse, rather than the paradox of instructing the client to try to have an instance of premature ejaculation (the second paradox). Lastly, Gentry assumed that the client would experience apprehension regarding his newly formed ejaculatory control—hence the necessity of the last paradox. However, informing the client of the possibility of relapse may have served a function other than to decrease fear of success—such as helping the client to accept such an occurrence as normal rather than as a complete relapse. Nonetheless, Gentry presents an intriguing and novel approach to the treatment of premature ejaculation.

Dauw (1988) reported the use of an eclectic therapy program for the treatment of male sexual dysfunctions. Client-centered, behavioral, insight-oriented and cognitive techniques were all used on an "as needed" basis for each client. Additionally, all clients were instructed to (1) study at least five self-help books, (2) listen to two audiotape series concerning self-esteem and intimacy, (3) view at least one of twelve videotapes (regarding sexual functioning and dysfunctions), (4) complete homework assignments (regarding masturbatory practice and, when necessary, assertion skills), and (5) visit a sur-rogate sex therapist if no other partner was available.

Over a ten-year period, 127 clients who were treated with surrogate sex therapy had a primary diagnosis of premature ejaculation, as assessed through self-report measures and two separate interviews conducted by different clinical psychologists. The average number of treatment sessions for all subjects was one session per week for ten weeks. Treatment success was defined as ability to maintain an erection for ten minutes of continual thrusting during intercourse, as reported by the surrogate at the end of treatment and as reported by the client at three-month follow-up (Dauw, 1988). Of the premature ejaculators, 122 (96%) were considered successes according to the above criteria. However, various difficulties with this study were noted by the author. For example, the reliability of the surrogates' and clients' reports of ejaculatory control are unknown. However, this is the case with most studies. Given that the surrogates were masters-level professionals in the helping fields who had undergone a 100-hour training program and who were closely supervised by both the director of clinical services and the surrogate supervisor, their assessment of ejaculatory control was probably more than adequate. A more serious complication is that it is unclear which treatment manipulation(s) actually had an impact on positive effect. Clients' programs were all individually tailored and involved several different treatment components. However, Dauw reported that a larger percentage of clients benefited from this therapy program than from non-surrogate-assisted programs and concluded that the use of surrogates in addition to the other components is a successful component in the treatment of sexual dysfunction. Unfortunately, there was a general lack of detail reported about this therapy program. This was a provocative study, and certainly the use of such a controversial treatment component as surrogates is worthy of a more detailed report. There are, of course, several ethical dilemmas involved in the use of sexual surrogates, and this remains a controversial area (Zilbergeld, 1975)

VARIATIONS OF
TREATMENT PROCEDURES

As noted in some of the reviews of studies above, the confounding of several different treatment components makes it difficult if not impossible to determine which are necessary and/or sufficient in the effective treatment of premature ejaculation. Yet much has be written on the "necessity" of various conditions for the optimal treatment of sexual dysfunctions (e.g., Masters & Johnson, 1970). Some researchers have attempted to determine the relative efficacy of various treatment conditions, such as type of therapist contact, degree of therapist professionalism, number of therapists, sex of therapists, and availability of cooperative partners. Studies relevant to these treatment variables are reviewed below.

Therapist Contact and Level of Professional Training

There is controversy regarding the optimal amount of therapist contact for treatment of premature ejaculation. A related controversy involves what level of professional training individuals treating these types of clients should have attained. For example, McCarthy (1989) argues that "sex therapy for early ejaculation is not simply a mechanical procedure that can be easily performed by an unsophisticated and uninterested paraprofessional technician" (p. 159). Marks (1986), makes the opposite argument. He states that "most behavioral psychotherapy can probably by given by non-specialists" and specifically includes treatment of premature ejaculation in his argument for minimal clinician contact. In support of this position, Marks relates a case study where, after only three half-hour therapy sessions, his client was able to gain ejaculatory control. This brief therapy was modeled after the Masters and Johnson treatment protocol and included banning of coitus, instruction in mutual caressing, gradual inclusion of genital caressing, and instruction regarding the squeeze technique. Given these tools, the client and his wife were able to prolong coitus to 30 minutes,

and this was maintained at one-month follow-up. Marks points out that some cases may require additional help, in which case the use of specialists may be indicated. However, his position is clearly that nonspecialists (e.g., general psychiatrists and nurses) can, after only brief instruction, effectively and with minimal contact treat various psychological disorders, including premature ejaculation.

In further support of the argument for minimal contact are several studies, published over the past two decades, which look at the use of bibliotherapy in the treatment of premature ejaculation (Lowe & Mikulas, 1975; Mathews et al., 1976; Zeiss, 1978; Trudel & Proulx, 1987). In each of these studies the basis of the text or manual was similar to Masters and Johnson's protocol. Lowe and Mikulas (1975) reported the results of therapy using an 80-page program covering the following areas: (1) conceptualization of premature ejaculation; (2) sensate focus; (3) the "squeeze" procedure; (4) the female-superior position and related intravaginal control; and (5) the lateral-coital position. Quizzes were available at the end of each section to assess subjects' understanding of chapter content, and advancement through treatment levels was based on the subjects' individual experiences at the previous level.

Ten couples, four who were referred and six who answered a newspaper advertisement, met the following prerequisites: (1) The male partner experienced premature ejaculation (defined as ejaculation before penetration, upon penile-vaginal contact, or within three minutes of penetration), (2) the female partner was willing to be involved in the program, and (3) there were no interpersonal problems that were considered to require primary attention. Five couples were randomly assigned to a control group and five to the experimental group. All ten couples were contacted by phone two times per week for encouragement and were allowed to contact their therapist at any time. All males were given a questionnaire on ejaculatory experiences, including an estimation of the time between sexual stimulation and ejaculation. Couples in the experimental group were given the treatment manuals. Progression through each section of the manual depended on the male's experiences with the previous section. Treatment averaged three weeks, although couples progressed at their own pace (no range of treatment duration is given). After three weeks, the control group couples were given copies of the manual and became a second experimental group. At the end of treatment, all males again estimated the time between sexual stimulation and ejaculation.

The results indicated that the mean time of ejaculatory control for the first experimental group increased from approximately two minutes pretreatment to 37 minutes posttreatment. For the control group, the posttreatment mean (taken three weeks after initial contact) did not change from a pretreatment mean of approximately one minute of ejaculatory control. This mean did change after the control group became another experimental group, increasing to approximately 19 minutes. Although the posttreatment ejaculatory control mean of the second experimental group was significantly lower than that of the first experimental group, both groups evidenced statistically significant changes from pre- to posttreatment. The lower posttreatment mean of the second group appeared to be due to one subject whose ejaculatory control increased only 4.5 minutes, as compared to the other subjects' increases of 14 to 29 minutes.

This short-term bibliotherapy was determined to have a clinically significant effect on nine of the ten clients. The authors concluded that some cases of premature ejaculation may be conceptualized as behavioral deficits without recourse to theories of underlying interpersonal problems; for these cases, psychotherapy or Masters and Johnson's intensive sex therapy program may be unnecessary (Lowe & Mikulas, 1975). However, as noted by Zeiss (1978), the length of phone contact between clients and therapists was not reported, although it is assumed to be substantially less than the amount of time spent in more traditional therapy. Interestingly, only one couple in this study indicated that sensate focus was useful. Thus, the authors hypothe-

sized that this may be an unnecessary component in the treatment of such clients (i.e., volunteers, who may be more highly motivated and thus more likely to benefit from bibliotherapy than clients who are referred for treatment). Unfortunately, follow-up of results was not reported. Moreover, some of the extreme ejaculatory latency results (e.g., 58 minutes) may be indicative of inhibited orgasm rather than a treatment success.

One problem with lack of follow-up is that maintenance of treatment effects is impossible to assess. Zeiss (1978) carried out a study that addressed the question of maintenance as well as several other fundamental concerns about minimal-contact therapy. This study involved 18 couples who complained of premature ejaculation and met four prerequisite conditions: (1) mean latency of ejaculation of less than 5 minutes, (2) both partners willing to participate, (3) no serious gynecological problems in the female, and (4) persistence of premature ejaculation for at least six months. These couples were randomly assigned to one of three treatment groups; two couples dropped out before posttreatment data were collected, leaving six couples in each group. One was a traditional sex therapy group in which couples saw a therapist once per week for no more than 20 weeks. Couples in this group ($N = 6$) were seen by an individual paraprofessional or a graduate student therapist. The second group ($N = 5$) was a self-administered treatment group, using a manual and having minimal phone contact with therapists. Contact averaged six minutes per week and was primarily supportive rather than treatment-oriented. Lastly, there was a self-administered treatment group, with no therapist contact after an initial two sessions (during which various measures and histories were taken). Although subjects in this last group ($N = 7$) were told they could call their therapists in the event of insurmountable difficulties, none did. The manual used in the two self-administration groups (developed by Zeiss and Zeiss (1978)) is divided into 12 weekly sessions, which describe the techniques of Masters and

Johnson (1970) and Semans (1956). Approximately three hours of sexual and talking activities are assigned each week, and discussions of commonly encountered difficulties are provided in each manual section.

Three assessment measures were used during this study. On two occasions before treatment, the couple timed ejaculatory latency from intromission to ejaculation during intercourse. Couples also filled out the Marital Adjustment Test (Locke & Wallace, 1959), and a sex history inventory. At posttreatment, couples timed ejaculatory latency while employing pauses and "squeezes" and twice while not using these techniques. They also filled out the marital and sex history questionnaires. At three-month follow-up, couples were mailed the two questionnaires.

Results indicated that 11 of the 18 couples completed treatment successfully—defined as (1) a mean timed latency using treatment techniques of greater than five minutes, or at least three minutes over pretreatment means, and (2) both partners reporting improved satisfaction with the male's ejaculatory control. One couple in the phone-contact group was unsuccessful, as were all couples in the no-contact group. In fact, only one couple in the no-contact group actually completed treatment. The primary reason given for dropping out of the study was lack of time.

Mean latencies significantly increased in both the phone-contact and the standard treatment groups. Specifically, the standard treatment group means increased from approximately 1 minute to approximately 11 minutes; the phone-contact group means increased from approximately 2 minutes to 10 minutes when the treatment techniques were employed ($p < .005$). The increase in ejaculatory latency means of the 11 successful subjects was less when squeeze or pause techniques were not used, but still significantly greater than the pretreatment mean (posttreatment mean of four minutes versus the initial mean of two minutes). No significant differences were found at posttest on the Marital Adjustment Test. However, significant ($p < .001$) pre- and posttreatment differences were found on an index of sex quality assessed within the sexual background inventory for both males and females.

Of the 11 successfully treated couples, only eight returned three-month follow-up data, despite contingent remittance of $30.00. Of these eight, half were no longer considered successes, based on the above criteria (two each in the standard and phone-contact groups). Of the remaining four, three had been in the standard treatment group and one in the phone-contact group. The results of all eight couples indicated that, although mean latencies were still significantly higher than pretreatment, they had decreased significantly from posttreatment means [$t(7) = 3.81, p < .005$]. The sex quality ratings went through a similar (though nonsignificant) decline, as did the latencies.

Zeiss concluded that successful treatment of premature ejaculation is possible for couples who maintain minimal contact with a therapist who has had minimal training. However, given the dismal results from the no-contact group, it appears that some sort of contact is necessary to provide motivation for remaining in treatment (Zeiss, 1978). Regarding the maintenance of treatment gains, Zeiss hypothesized that specific sex therapy may not adequately address couples' needs for more general improvement in sexual relationships. Thus, improvements in target behaviors (e.g., ejaculatory latency) may be difficult to maintain if the general sexual relationship does not also improve. This hypothesis is based, in part, on Zeiss's finding that the males' ratings of sex quality at posttreatment were predictive of treatment maintenance (or lack thereof). Thus, therapists may need to address more general problems along with specific sexual dysfunctions in some cases, according to Zeiss.

Trudel and Proulx (1987) conducted a replication of Zeiss's (1978) study. The major differences in this study were (1) the inclusion of a control group in addition to the three experimental groups, (2) the use of "systematic positive reinforcement" for the experimental subjects' completion of each procedure (the reinforcer was money, taken from $70 initially deposited with the experimenters for this purpose), and (3) the translation from English into French of the treatment manual. Twenty-five subjects met inclusionary criteria similar to those described for Zeiss' 1978 study. Couples were randomly assigned to one of the four groups, and all subjects completed the Marital Adjustment Test (Locke & Wallace, 1959), the Sexual Interaction Inventory (LoPiccolo & Steger, 1974), a questionnaire about sexual problems, and a test of ejaculatory latency. Treatment procedures in the three experimental groups were similar to those of Zeiss (1978).

The results were also similar to those of Zeiss (1978). Significant increases in ejaculatory latencies were found in the three experimental groups at posttreatment, and the increases were greater when the treatment techniques were used. As in the Zeiss study, there was a higher dropout rate for couples in the no-contact group (45%) than in the standard and phone contact groups (14% and 33%, respectively). However, in contrast to the findings of Zeiss, there were no significant decreases in ejaculatory latency at follow-up, although length of follow-up and number of subjects who completed follow-up are not reported. The authors concluded that pairing a behavioral contract based on positive reinforcement with self-administered treatment may lead to significant treatment gains with subsequent maintenance. However, the small initial sample sizes, coupled with large dropout rates, leave Trudel and Proulx's conclusion open to questions. Furthermore, the lack of detail (e.g., on length of follow-up, number of subjects successfully followed) of this study make it difficult to adequately judge the merits of this study, although it does provide additional support for the use of self-administered treatment packages with minimal therapist contact.

The results of the studies reviewed thus far have provided some evidence in favor of Marks' (1986) argument that minimal direct contact with therapists who have minimal training may be all that is necessary for adequate treatment of cli-

ents with premature ejaculation, although complete lack of direct contact may negatively affect a client's motivation to stay in treatment (Zeiss, 1978). However, many therapists agree that some clients or couples may require more contact with specialized therapists (Lowe & Mikulas, 1975; Marks, 1986; Zeiss, 1978). Some evidence for this view is provided by Mathews et al. (1976), who concluded that the variability in response of their subjects to standard treatment and phone-contact treatment packages indicated that some couples responded well to self-administered treatment with minimal therapist input and contact, whereas the problems of other couples in this group may actually have been exacerbated by this aproach and may have warranted more therapeutic involvement.

Number of Therapists

Masters and Johnson (1970) have argued that several reasons necessitate the use of dual-sex cotherapist teams. For example, they believe that clients will respond more honestly to questioning from therapists of the opposite sex while in the presence of a therapist of the same sex. They also believe that the influence of personal biases on interpretations of clients' complaints is reduced when therapists of both sexes are involved. However, Mathews et al. (1976) failed to find significant differences between groups treated by one and by two therapists, and others have reported positive treatment effects when only one therapist was involved (Semans, 1956; Yulis, 1976; Zeiss, 1978).

In a comparison study, LoPiccolo et al. (1985) looked at the outcome of 65 sexually dysfunctional couples who were treated by either a male or female therapist or a cotherapist team. Of this sample, 21 of the males were diagnosed as premature ejaculators (defined as pretherapy intercourse duration of between one and three minutes). Treatment consisted of a cognitive-behavioral package involving 15 one-hour sessions (see LoPiccolo & Hogan, 1979). At two posttreatment assessment points, this duration had increased to between seven and ten minutes. There was no significant effect of a different number of therapists. However, the authors noted that the intense supervision and consultation all therapists received throughout this study may have caused their approaches to be more "teamlike" than individual—thus, more like that of a cotherapist team even when working alone.

Gender of Therapists

The case has been made that, because of biases potentially held by therapists, the gender of the therapist should be matched with that of the dysfunctional client (Broverman, Broverman, Clarkson, Rosenkrantz, & Vogel, 1970). In the study reviewed above, LoPiccolo et al. (1985) found no support for the view that male therapists have better results with male clients or female therapists with female clients. Similarly, Mathews and colleagues (1976) found no significant trends favoring treatment of sexually dysfunctional clients with therapists of the same sex.

Availability of a Partner

Nearly all of the treatment protocols reviewed here were designed in such a way that they necessitated involvement of a cooperative partner. Masters and Johnson (1970) argue against individual treatment of a sexually dysfunctional patient. Rather, they conceptualize sexual dysfunctions as problems of the marital unit. Similarly, Clement and Pfafflin (1980) concluded that "sexual dysfunction is a dysfunction of partnership" (p. 240). These authors based their claim on the finding that there were no significant differences between the personality scores of sexually dysfunctional subjects and their spouses. However, it seems feasible that men may gain ejaculatory control without the necessary involvement of a sexual partner (Hastings, 1966). Encouraging findings have been reported in one study involving only the dysfunctional clients (Zilbergeld, 1975), which reported on the initial results of group treatment of male-only

groups. These men either were not in a heterosexual relationship, were in a relatively new relationship, or were in a long-term relationship with a partner unwilling to participate in sexual therapy. For these reasons, the clients were unable to participate in traditional sex therapy.

Zilbergeld's group treatment focused on the correction of specific sexual dysfunctions and on the development of skills necessary to cope with sexual situations (Zilbergeld, 1975). Masturbatory exercises, self-disclosure, assertiveness training, relaxation training, and refutation of male "myths" were techniques employed in order to reach the two stated goals of this treatment. Groups were led either by two male cotherapists or (in one case) by a dual-sex cotherapist team.

Zilbergeld reported results based primarily on subjective assessment by group therapists and reports by the clients as to the effects of treatment. Accordingly, two-thirds of the clients reported achieving their goals by the end of treatment, and gains were generally reported to be maintained. Interestingly, men involved in long-term relationships appeared to be the most resistant to therapeutic change—indicating that, in these cases, the sexual dysfunction may be related to more broad relationship problems that interfere with the sex therapy (Zilbergeld, 1975). Another preliminary finding was that the one group composed of men with a single type of sexual dysfunction proceeded through treatment more quickly than the groups containing men with differing dysfunctions. Regarding the sex of the therapist, group members seen by a dual-sex co-therapist team indicated that they found the presence of the female therapist to be beneficial. Lastly, Zilbergeld presented the advantages of group versus individual treatment, such as cost-effectiveness, peer support, the opportunity for modeling, and a sense of camaraderie, which may improve or maintain treatment motivation.

The treatment programs of both Zilbergeld (1975) and Kaplan et al. (1974) were in preliminary stages when reported upon. It is hoped that more empirically rigorous designs will be executed with these programs, as they appear to offer benefits to men who are otherwise unable to receive sex therapy.

Group Treatment

The last treatment variable to be reviewed is optimal treatment group size (groups versus single couples). Kaplan et al. (1974) conducted a pilot study in which four couples were treated in group therapy for premature ejaculation. The program was designed to take six weeks, with one 45-minute session per week. Treatment was based on the theory that males who ejaculate reflexively (and therefore prematurely) are unaware of sexual sensations that signal impending ejaculation. Exercises based on Semans' stop-start techniques were presented verbally to the subjects, to be carried out at home. The group sessions were used primarily to discuss difficulties and obstacles with the exercises and to present new exercises to the couples. Exercises involved extravaginal or intravaginal stimulation. Specifically, couples were instructed how to employ the stop-start method during stimulation. For maintenance purposes, couples were told to employ the stop-start method occasionally, even after formal treatment had ended.

At the end of six weeks two couples reported that the male had learned voluntary ejaculatory control. The remaining two couples reported similar success at the end of an additional two months of treatment. At a four-month follow-up, three couples (the fourth could not be reached) reported maintenance of treatment gains. Noting that the small sample size precluded generalization, the authors concluded that the group format appeared to be an acceptable way to carry out sex therapy for premature ejaculation. The authors also note that therapist time was only 90 minutes per couple, a significant decrease from more traditional treatments. However, the authors did not comment on the fact that half of their sample required an extra two months before experiencing treatment effects. However, the group treatment format did result in an outcome similar to that of individual

treatment protocols; it warrants further investigation beyond the pilot phase.

Zeiss, Christensen, and Levine (1978) presented a study in which two male-only groups were treated for sexual dysfunctions ($N = 3$ in each group). Although only males attended therapy sessions, their female partners were included in the initial intake interviews, and it was emphasized that the subjects would be expected to share information learned in the treatment sessions with their female partners, who were in turn expected to participate in the exercises taught to their partners. Weekly phone contact between sessions allowed therapists to maintain contact with the female partners, as well as to monitor treatment progress.

The six-week treatment program developed by Zeiss et al. was modeled after Masters and Johnson's program and included the following components: (1) a ban on intercourse; (2) instruction on the squeeze and stop-start techniques of ejaculatory control; (3) instruction in sensate focus; and (4) a pairing of ejaculatory control techniques with masturbation, mutual manual stimulation, then with intercourse. In addition to these steps, the therapists gave assignments designed to increase sharing of intimate feelings. Subjective and objective (via stopwatch) estimates of ejaculation latencies were gathered three times during a baseline period, with averages computed for each couple. At posttreatment, all but one couple reported gains in objectively recorded and subjectively experienced ejaculatory latencies, with means for objectively recorded latencies increasing from one to approximately five minutes. Treatment maintenance was assessed at eight-month follow-up for the group in which all three subjects reported post-treatment gains. Two of these three couples had maintained treatment gains, and the third subject was experiencing premature ejaculation again. Follow-up for the other group was gathered at four months. In this second group, only one couple had experienced gains from the treatment sessions, and these were maintained at follow-up.

Based on the outcome for these two groups, the authors concluded that the group format may be a cost-effective and viable alternative to individual treatment, although more thorough testing needs to be carried out (Zeiss et al., 1978). The authors did not comment on the relatively minor gains in ejaculatory latency (as compared with other studies) or on their finding that the four couples who experienced treatment gains were still reporting premature ejaculation in 50% or more of their intercourse experiences posttreatment. As with the Kaplan et al. (1974) study, the small sample size and lack of a control or comparison group make it difficult to draw meaningful inferences. The relatively encouraging results from these two studies indicate that further, empirically sounder studies should be conducted with group formats.

CONCLUSIONS

There are real problems with the definition of premature ejaculation. The current definitions contain a level of subjectivity that can only lead to confusion and lowered diagnostic reliability. Also, premature ejaculation appears to be a very widespread phenomenon; from Kinsey's data, one would expect premature ejaculation to be the norm. If so, how can it be defined as a sexual dysfunction at all? Finally, by some definitions, the disorder can be seen as residing in the sexual partner. Masters and Johnson's (1970) classic definition of premature ejaculation—as occurring when, on more than half of the occasions of intercourse, the woman does not experience orgasm—defines the disorder in terms of the partner's reaction, thus relying on female orgasmic latency (a phenomenon even less well understood than ejaculatory control). Recognizing these definitional problems does not resolve them but will help the informed practitioner to grasp the complexities of premature ejaculation.

Our review of the literature does not reveal any solid conclusions concerning the causes of premature ejaculation. The data suggest simply that these individuals ejaculate at lower levels of stimulation than other individuals. That appears to be another way of defining the problem; it does not suggest any reasons for the differences in sensitivity levels. One suggestion, not always

borne out by the literature, is that premature ejaculation in some individuals may result from reduced levels of sexual activity. Although suggestions that premature ejaculation results from the individual being less in touch with his level of arousal are interesting, they have not garnered empirical support. The speculation that the problem reflects an evolutionarily selected behavioral pattern remains controversial and untested (and possibly untestable).

The assessment literature has also been found to have many gaps in the understanding of what constitutes appropriate assessment. There is agreement that the multiple response systems that characterize all behavior (verbal, motoric, and physiological) must be considered if assessment is to be adequate. However, this is much like being in favor of motherhood and apple pie. How can one disagree? The clinician will continue to rely on interview data for assessment of sexual dysfunctions; a wide variety of schedules are available. They range from assessment of the individual's arousal status to the assessment of relationships, heterosocial skills, and heterosexual skills. These instruments can prove useful in structuring data collection for clinicians.

Two difficult problems dog the assessment of premature ejaculation. The first is that assessment relies almost exclusively on self-report. We need not review the well-known problems with this sort of data, other than to note that information gathered in this way is of severely limited utility. This is particularly problematic when the self-report deals with material that is likely to be highly emotionally charged for the individual client or the couple. The second general problem with assessment is that assessment procedures themselves may influence the outcome (generally referred to as *reactivity*). We have very little information that allows us to evaluate and thus take into account the problems of reactivity and self-report. However, the conscientious clinician will be aware of these issues and perform careful evaluation in all cases of premature ejaculation.

Our final topic is treatment. It may be surprising to some that this topic has an extensive literature. The treatment regimen originally suggested by Semans (1956) has been widely used and was elaborated upon by Masters and Johnson (1970). Masters and Johnson reported successful treatment of essentially all men who complained of premature ejaculation. That would seem to be the end of it, but other investigators began reporting lower levels of success using what were felt to be quite similar procedures. Then questions were raised about the adequacy of the Masters and Johnson study. The bottom line is that the reports of almost complete success rates have not held up to further scrutiny. A series of investigations have examined alternative therapeutic strategies and examined variables within the original protocol to examine effectiveness. One of the more controversial findings is the suggestion (Marks, 1986) that premature ejaculation can be successfully treated by individuals with relatively low levels of training for psychological or behavioral treatment.

Despite the lower levels of successful outcome reported since 1970, it is still fair to say that the treatment of premature ejaculation remains a success story. With a variety of procedures available, the outlook for successful treatment is good. Considering the many problems in the definition and investigation of premature ejaculation, this is not only surprising but also satisfying.

REFERENCES

American Psychiatric Association. (1987). *Diagnostic and statistical manual of mental disorders* (3rd ed., rev.). Washington, DC: Author.

Bancroft, J., & Coles, L. (1976). Three years' experience in a sexual problems clinic. *British Medical Journal, 1,* 1575–1577.

Barlow, D. H., Sakheim, D. K., & Beck, J. G. (1983). Anxiety increases sexual arousal. *Journal of Abnormal Psychology, 92,* 49–54.

Beck, J. G., Barlow, D. H., Sakheim, D. K., & Abrahamson, D. J. (1987). Shock threat and sexual arousal: The role of selective attention, thought content and affective states. *Psychophysiology, 24,* 165–172.

Bell, A. P., & Weinberg, M. S. (1978). *Homosexualities.* New York: Simon & Schuster.

Bentler, P. (1968). Heterosexual behavior assessment. 1. Males. *Behavior Research and Therapy, 6,* 21–25.

Binik, Y. M., Servan-Schreiber, D. S., Freiwald, S., & Hall, K. S. (1988). Intelligent computer-based assessment and psychotherapy: An expert system for sexual dysfunction. *The Journal of Nervous and Mental Disease, 176,*(7), 387–400.

Bixler, R. H. (1986). Of apes and men (including females!). *Journal of Sex Research, 22,* 255–267.

Broverman, I. K., Broverman, D. M., Clarkson, F. E., Rosenkrantz, P. S., & Vogel, S. R. (1970). Sex role stereotypes and clinical judgments of mental health. *Journal of Consulting and Clinical Psychology, 34,* 1–7.

Casselman, D., & Durham, R. L. (1979). Demographic deferences for sexual knowledge and attitudes. *Journal of Sex Education and Therapy, 1,* 29–36.

Clement, U., & Pfafflin, F. (1980). Changes in personality scores among couples subsequent to sex therapy. *Archives of Sexual Behavior, 9*(3), 235–244.

Cooper, A. J., & Magnus, R. V. (1984). A clinical trial of the beta blocker Propranolol in premature ejaculation. *Psychosomatic Research, 28,* 331–336.

Damrav, F. (1963). Premature ejaculation: Use of ethyl amino benzoate to prolong coitus. *Journal of Urology, 89,* 936–939.

Dauw, D. C. (1988). Evaluating the effectiveness of the SECS surrogate-assisted sex therapy model. *Journal of Sex Research, 24,* 269–275.

Derogatis, L. R., & Melisaratos, N. (1979). The DSFI: A multidimensional measure of sexual functioning. *Journal of Sex and Marital Therapy, 5*(3), 244–281.

Earls, C. M., Morales, A., & Marshall, W. L. (1988). Penile sufficiency: An operational definition. *Journal of Urology, 139,* 536–538.

Frank, E., Andersen, C., & Rubenstein, D. (1978). Frequency of sexual dysfunction in "normal" couples. *New England Journal of Medicine, 299,* 111–115.

Freund, K., & Blanchard, R. (1981). Assessment of sexual dysfunction and deviation. In M. Hersen & A. S. Bellack (Eds.), *Behavioral assessment: A practical handbook* (2nd ed., pp. 427–455). New York: Pergamon.

Gebhard, P. H., & Johnson, A. B. (1979). *The Kinsey data: Marginal tabulations of the 1938–1963 inter-*

views conducted by the Institute for Sex Research. Philadelphia: Saunders.

Geer, H. H., & Fuhr, R. (1976). Cognitive factors in sexual arousal: The role of distraction. *Journal of Consulting and Clinical Psychology, 44,* 238–243.

Gentry, D. L. (1978). The treatment of premature ejaculation through brief therapy. *Psychotherapy Theory, Research, and Practice, 15*(1), 32–34.

Gough, H. G. (1974). A 24-item version of the Miller-Fisk Sexual Knowledge Questionnaire. *Journal of Psychology, 87,* 183–192.

Hartman, L. M., & Daly, E. M. (1983). Relationship factors in the treatment of sexual dysfunction. *Behaviour Research and Therapy, 21*(2), 153–160.

Hastings, D. W. (1966). *A doctor speaks on sexual expression in marriage.* Boston: Little, Brown.

Hatch, J. P. (1981). Psychophysiological aspects of sexual dysfunctions. *Archives of Sexual Behavior, 10,* 49–64.

Hawton, K. (1982). The behavioral treatment of sexual dysfunction. *British Journal of Psychiatry, 140,* 94–101.

Hawton, K. (1985). *Sex therapy: A practical guide.* Oxford, UK: Oxford University Press.

Hawton, K., & Catalan, J. (1986). Prognostic factors in sex therapy. *Behaviour Research and Therapy, 24*(4), 377–385.

Hong, L. K. (1984). Survival of the fastest: On the origin of premature ejaculation. *The Journal of Sex Research, 20,* 109–122.

Ince, L. P. (1973). Behavior modification of sexual disorders. *American Journal of Psychotherapy, 27*(3), 446–451.

Kaplan, H. (1974). *The new sex therapy.* London: Bailliere Tindall.

Kaplan, H. (1983). *The evaluation of sexual disorders.* New York: Brunner/Mazel.

Kaplan, H. S., Kohl, R. N., Pomeroy, W. B., Offit, A. K., & Hogan, B. (1974). Group treatment of premature ejaculation. *Archives of Sexual Behavior, 3*(5), 443–452.

Kilman, P. R., & Auerbach, R. (1979). Treatments of premature ejaculation and psychogenic impotence: A critical review of the literature. *Archives of Sexual Behavior, 8*(1), 81–100.

Kimmel, D., & Van der Veen, F. (1974). Factors of marital adjustment in Locke's Marital Adjustment Test. *Journal of Marriage and the Family, 36,* 57–63.

Kinsey, A. C., Pomeroy, W. B., & Martin, C. (1948).

Sexual behavior in the human male. Philadelphia: Saunders.

Kolodny, R. C., Masters, W. H., & Johnson, V. E. (1979). *Textbook of sexual medicine.* Boston: Little, Brown.

Lief, H., & Reed, D. (1972). *Sexual Knowledge and Attitude Test.* Philadelphia: University of Pennsylvania, Department of Psychiatry.

Locke, H. G., & Wallace, K. M. (1959). Short marital-adjustment and prediction tests: Their reliability and validity. *Marriage and Family Living, 21,* 251–255.

LoPiccolo, J. (1985). Diagnosis and treatment of male sexual dysfunction. *Journal of Sex & Marital Therapy, 11*(4), 215–232.

LoPiccolo, J., Heiman, J. R., Hogan, D. R., & Roberts, C. W. (1985). Effectiveness of single therapists versus cotherapy teams in sex therapy. *Journal of Consulting and Clinical Psychology, 53*(3), 287–294.

LoPiccolo, J., & Hogan, D. (1979). Multidimensional behavioral treatment of sexual dysfunction. In O. Pomerleau & J. Brady (Eds.), *Behavioral medicine.* Baltimore: Williams & Wilkins.

LoPiccolo, J., & Steger, J. (1974). The Sexual Interaction Inventory: A new instrument for the assessment of sexual dysfunction. *Archives of Sexual Behavior, 3,* 585–595.

LoPiccolo, J., & Stock, W. (1986). Treatment of sexual dysfunction. *Journal of Consulting and Clinical Psychology, 54*(2), 158–167.

Lowe, J. C., & Mikulas, W. L. (1975). Use of written material in learning self-control of premature ejaculation. *Psychological Reports, 37,* 295–298.

Malatesta, V. J., & Adams, H. E. (1986). Assessment of sexual behavior. In A. R. Ciminero, K. S. Calhoun, & H. E. Adams (Eds.), *Handbook of behavioral assessment* (2nd ed.). New York: Wiley.

Margolin, G., & Fernandez, V. (1983). Other marital and family questionnaires. In E. E. Filsinger (Ed.), *A sourcebook of marriage and family assessment.* Beverly Hills, CA: Sage.

Marks, I. (1986). Behavioural psychotherapy in general psychiatry: Helping patients help themselves. *British Journal of Psychiatry, 150,* 593–597.

Masters, W., & Johnson, V. (1970). *Human sexual inadequacy,* Boston: Little, Brown.

Mathews, A., Bancroft, J., Whitehead, A., Hackmann, A., Julier, D., Bancroft, J., Gath, D., & Shaw, P. (1976). The behavioural treatment of sexual inadequacy: A comparative study. *Behaviour Research and Therapy, 14*, 427–436.

Mathews, A., Whitehead, A., Kellett, J. M. (1983). Psychological and hormonal factors in the treatment of female sexual dysfunction. *Psychological Medicine, 13*(1), 83–92.

McCarthy, B. W. (1989). Cognitive-behavioral strategies and techniques in the treatment of early ejaculation. In S. Leiblum & R. Rosen (Eds.), *Principles and practice of sex therapy*. New York: Guilford.

Nathan, S. G. (1986). The epidemiology of the DSM-III psychosexual dysfunctions. *Journal of Sex and Marital Therapy, 12*, 267–281.

Nettelbladt, P., & Uddenberg, N. (1979). Sexual dysfunction and sexual satisfaction in 58 married Swedish men. *Journal of Psychosomatic Research, 23*, 141–147.

Nowinski, J., & LoPiccolo, J. (1979). Assessing sexual behavior in couples. *Journal of Sex and Marital Therapy, 5*(3), 225–243.

Renshaw, D. C. (1988). Profile of 2376 patients treated at Loyola Sex Clinic between 1972 and 1987. *Sexual and Marital Therapy, 3*, 111–117.

Rosen, R. C., & Beck, J. G. (1988). *Patterns of sexual arousal*. New York: Guilford.

Ruff, G. A., & St. Lawrence, J. S. (1985). Past research progress, future directions. *Clinical Psychology Review, 5*, 627–639.

Rust, R., & Golombok, S. (1985). The Golombok-Rust Inventory of Sexual Satisfaction (GRISS). *British Journal of Clinical Psychology, 24*, 63–64.

Shapiro, G. (1943). Premature ejaculation. *Journal of Urology, 50*, 374–379.

Semans, J. H. (1956). Premature ejaculation: A new approach. *Southern Medical Journal, 49*, 353–357.

Snyder, D. K., & Regts, J. M. (1982). Factor scales for assessing marital disharmony and disaffection. *Journal of Consulting and Clinical Psychology, 50*, 615–623.

Spanier, G. B. (1976). Measuring dyadic adjustment: New scales for assessing the quality of marriage and similar dyads. *Journal of Marriage and the Family, 38*(1), 15–28.

Spector, I. P., & Carey, M. P. (1990). Incidence and prevalence of the sexual dysfunctions: A critical review of the empirical literature. *Archives of Sexual Behavior, 19*, 389–408.

Spiess, W. F. J., Geer, J. H., & O'Donohue, W. T. (1984). Premature ejaculation: Investigation of factors in ejaculatory latency. *Journal of Abnormal Psychology, 93*, 242–245.

Strassberg, D. S., Kelly, M. P., Carroll, C., & Kircher, J. C. (1987). The psychophysiological nature of premature ejaculation. *Archives of Sexual Behavior, 16*, 327–336.

Strassberg, D. S., Mahoney, J. M., Schaugaard, M., & Hale, V. E. (1990). The role of anxiety in premature ejaculation: A psychophysiological model. *Archives of Sexual Behavior, 19*, 251–257.

Stravynski, A. (1986). Indirect behavioral treatment of erectile failure and premature ejaculation in a man without a partner. *Archives of Sexual Behavior, 15*(4), 355–361.

Symons, D. (1987). An evolutionary approach: Can Darwin's view of life shed light on human sexuality? In J. Geer & W. O'Donohue (Eds.), *Theories of human sexuality* (pp. 91–126). New York: Plenum.

Tollison, C. D., & Adams, H. E. (1979). *Sexual disorders: Treatment, theory, and research*. New York: Gardner.

Trudel, G., & Proulx, S. (1987). Treatment of premature ejaculation by bibliotherapy: An experimental study. *Sexual and Marital Therapy, 2*(2), 163–167.

Tuthill, J. F. (1955). Impotence. *Lancet, 111*, 124–128.

Twentyman, C. T., & McFall, R. M. (1975). Behavioral training of social skills in shy males. *Journal of Consulting and Clinical Psychology, 43*(3), 384–395.

Watson, D., & Friend, R. (1969). Measurement of social-evaluative anxiety. *Journal of Consulting and Clinical Psychology, 33*(4), 448–457.

Weiss, R. L., & Margolin, G. (1986). Assessment of marital conflict and accord. In A. Ciminero, K. Calhoun, & H. Adams (Eds.), *Handbook of behavioral assessment* (2nd ed.). New York: Wiley.

Wolpe, J. (1969). *The practice of behavior therapy*. London: Pergamon.

Yulis, S. (1976). Generalization of therapeutic gain in the treatment of premature ejaculation. *Behavior Therapy, 7*, 355–358.

Zeiss, R. A. (1978). Self-directed treatment for premature ejaculation. *Journal of Consulting and Clinical Psychology, 46*(6), 1243–1241.

Zeiss, R. A., Christensen, A., & Levine, A. G. (1978). Treatment for premature ejaculation through male-only groups. *Journal of Sex and Marital Therapy, 4*(2), 139–143.

Zeiss, R. A., & Zeiss, A. M. (1978). *Prolong your pleasure*. New York: Pocket Books.

Zilbergeld, B. (1975). Group treatment of sexual dysfunction in men without partners. *Journal of Sex and Marital Therapy, 1*(3), 204–214.

Zilbergeld, B., & Evans, M. (1980). The inadequacy of Masters and Johnson. *Psychology Today, 14,* 29–34.

CHAPTER 12

SEXUAL PAIN DISORDERS IN THE FEMALE

Richard Reid, Sinai Hospital, Detroit, Michigan;
   Wayne State University School of Medicine
Todd Lininger, Pontiac General Hospital, Pontiac, Michigan;
   Wayne State University School of Medicine

INTRODUCTION

Definition of Pain

Pain is a very common experience, yet one that both laymen and health care professionals have difficulty explaining. Historically, chronic pain has been subdivided according to whether symptoms are thought to be somatic (arising from a site of actual tissue injury) or psychogenic (discomfort caused or heavily influenced by emotional factors). Unfortunately, the connotations of "real pain" versus "histrionic overlay" force patients to seek multiple consultations, excessive testing, and potentially injurious therapies in order to legitimize their complaints. In reality, different medical disciplines advance contrasting definitions of pain. From a physiologic viewpoint, pain is a distressing sensation evoked by stimulation of a complex neuroanatomic and neurophysiologic system. Conversely, from a strictly psychological perspective, pain represents the outcome of multiple noxious psychological and social interactions. Bridging these two extremes, the Taxonomy Committee of the International Association for the Study of Pain defined pain in 1986 as "an unpleasant sensory and emotional experience associated with actual or potential tissue damage, or described in terms of such damage." The committee further stated that pain is always subjective, with each individual learning the application of the word through experience related to injury in early life. Since pain is always unpleasant, it is accepted as an emotional experience. The committee further recognized that people may report pain in the absence of any likely pathophysiologic cause—such symptoms being secondary to psychological reasons. However, since physical and psychological elements often coexist, attempts to determine the precipitating cause in chronic pain patients are not clinically helpful.

This chapter provides an overview of the principles underlying the assessment and management of gynecologic pain, with special emphasis on how chronic pain disrupts female sexuality. To aid the readers who are not physicians, a glossary of relevant medical terms is included at the end of the chapter, on pages 363–364.

Importance of Acute Pain Control

Afferent pain impulses are initiated within visceral or somatic structures by mechanical trauma, thermal injury, or ischemia. However, pain threshhold and tolerance are significantly influenced by cortical modulating factors. Pain sustained in sport or battle may not be perceived at the time, whereas the same injury inflicted in a surgical or experimental situation may evoke substantial discomfort. Thus, though more straightforward than chronic pain, acute pain still represents a complex activation of local, regional, and systemic reflexes, all of which significantly alter activity within the entire nervous system. In addition, the reaction to acute pain is significantly influenced by the same psychological factors that are usually discussed with regard to chronic pain: social class, cultural influences, personality, religious beliefs, and ethnic background (Peck & Cowan, 1986).

Traditionally, acute pain has been viewed as a warning system to identify threatening events, in hopes of limiting tissue damage. Once acute pain has served this goal, its beneficial role has been exhausted. Conversely, failure to control acute pain adequately may affect postoperative morbidity—and possibly mortality. For example, pain following an abdominal incision produces a "splinting" effect that reduces pulmonary function, potentially leading to atelectasis, hypoxemia, and pneumonitis. Elevated catecholamine levels induce tachycardia, hypertension, and increased systemic vascular resistance, all of which increase myocardial oxygen consumption and myocardial work. Decreased gastrointestinal motility may lead to gastric stasis and intestinal ileus, both of which will aggravate any pulmonary dysfunction. Prolonged hormonal stress will push the metabolism into a catabolic state, with consequent loss of muscle mass and impaired wound healing. Continued suffering will also sap the patient's mor-

ale, leading to anxiety, frustration, sleeplessness, and further decrease in functional performance (Bonica, 1953; Bonica, 1987; Kehlet, 1986).

Importance of Chronic Pain Control

The term *chronic pain* refers to the persistence of pain beyond normal healing time (e.g., 6–12 weeks), even if quality and severity are unchanged. When pain becomes chronic, all aspects of the patient's interaction with the environment are modified. Chronic pain makes patients irritable and withdrawn, with mood changes or even overt depression. Continued pain suppresses the appetite and disrupts sleeping patterns. Attention is increasingly focused on symptomatology. As patients become more and more fearful of their future, these complaints of prolonged pain are often interpreted as being secondary to an ongoing, life-threatening disease (Pilowski, 1986; Pilowski & Spence, 1976). Such dysfunctional behavior essentially destroys the quality of the patient's life.

The sick or injured role may allow the chronic pain patient to withdraw from social responsibility. However, this "privilege" is predicated on the patient's ability to demonstrate ongoing, intractable pain to the health care provider. As medical contact becomes more regular, both the patient and the health care provider may become increasingly frustrated with each other over how the pain should be managed. Patients often see a multitude of physicians, perhaps falling into the trap of polypharmacy and polysurgery. All of these characteristics make chronic pain patients extremely difficult to care for, thereby significantly worsening the prognosis.

Beyond the effect on the patient, chronic pain also has a tremendous impact on the family, the workplace, and society. After altering their activities to accommodate the patient's complaints, the family may also become disrupted and/or dysfunctional. Since the patient is frequently unable to return to work or to run the home, economic support becomes an expensive, long-term concern. Hence, chronic pain is currently one of society's costliest health care problems (Bonica, 1953: Bonica, 1983; Bonica, 1987).

GENERAL PAIN PATHWAYS

Recently, there has been tremendous growth in our knowledge of the neuroanatomy and neurophysiology of pain. These advances are best considered under the subheadings of peripheral mechanisms, spinal and brainstem modulating systems, and central pain mechanisms.

Peripheral Mechanisms

Mechanical, thermal, or ischemic stimuli trigger the release of peripheral mediators that excite the peripheral nerve terminal, thus initiating a series of neuroanatomical and neurophysiological events that may eventually lead to the cortical perception of pain. Such stimuli work through *nociceptors* (specialized peripheral receptors). Nociceptors are classified according to conduction velocity, the type of stimuli to which they respond, and the characteristics of such responses (Raja et al., 1988). Most important in pain perception are A-delta mechanical nociceptors and C polymodal nociceptors.

A-Delta Mechanical Nociceptors

The A-delta mechanical nociceptors are myelinated nerve fibers that conduct in the range of 15–25 meters per second. These sensory receptors are present in all skin, from which they transmit sharp, well-localized pain. As their name suggests, these nociceptors respond to high-threshold mechanical stimulation, but they are relatively resistent to thermal or chemical stimuli.

C Polymodal Nociceptors

The C polymodal nociceptors are unmyelinated fibers with a much slower conduction velocity (in the range of 2 meters per second). These nociceptors are also present in all skin, from which they transmit burning, aching, poorly lo-

calized pain. C polymodal nociceptors respond primarily to noxious chemical and thermal stimuli, with a variable but generally reduced response to mechanical stimuli. Principal chemical stimuli are hydrogen ions, potassium ions, histamine, acetylcholine, and bradykinin (Raja et al., 1988).

As a general rule, the nociceptors described above are activated by high-intensity physical stimuli. However, there are two abnormal conditions, primary and secondary hyperalgesia, wherein local trauma can produce long-lasting alterations in the transduction characteristics of the peripheral nociceptors. *Primary hyperalgesia* is an increased sensitivity to stimulation of the skin within the area of injury; *secondary hyperalgesia* refers to similar changes outside this area. During the initial local tissue damage, a variety of agents (including prostaglandins, leukotrienes, kinins, and substance P) are released (Raja, 1988). In hyperalgesia syndromes, these chemical agents may go on to sensitize the peripheral nociceptor, allowing excitation to be evoked by low-intensity, otherwise nonnoxious physical stimuli. In addition, there is local vasodilatation and increased capillary permeability, both of which can further contribute to hyperalgesia.

Spinal and Brain Stem Modulating Systems

Historically, it was believed that impulses from the pain receptors traveled rapidly to the cerebral cortex, much as a light bulb is illuminated by turning a switch. However, some 25 years ago, Melzack and Wall (1965) proposed the "gate control theory of pain" to account for the various factors influencing pain. This model best explains the diverse observations made about pain in both clinical and experimental settings. In essence, the gate control theory proposes that pain is not determined by tissue injury alone, but by a balance of influences competing at various levels of the nervous system. In other words, what the patient describes as pain is actually a summation of inhibitory and excitatory influences emanating both from the site of injury and from several higher modulating centers. Although modulation takes place at virtually every level, the two major sites that either amplify or dampen the nocioceptor pain impulses are the dorsal horn laminae of the spinal cord and certain brain stem nuclei.

Modulation within Adjacent Spinal Segments

Raw impulses from the A-delta and C nociceptors are transmitted along the afferent fibers of the primary neuron. The cell bodies of these primary neurons are located in the dorsal root ganglion, and the afferent fibers synapse within the dorsal horn of the spinal cord (LaMotte, 1986). See Figure 12.1. Recent research has shown that many of these afferent fibers synapse with interneurons—neurons whose fibers do not leave the immediate area of the first order synapse (Melzack & Wall, 1982). This means that afferent pain impulses must pass through a "gate" at the spinal cord level before they reach the brain. This gate can be closed through an increased input from touch-sensitive nociceptors—hence the efficacy of TENS units (see the Glossary at the end of this chapter). Descending (efferent) influences also modify the transmission of nociceptive input at the spinal cord and brain stem levels. Cognitive and affective factors can thus alter the severity of pain experienced, as well as the person's response to it.

Although the exact physiology is not yet known, this "prebrain" modulation by the interneurons does offer a potential therapeutic window. Neurochemicals involved in dorsal horn modulation include the following (Yaksh, 1988; Willis, 1985; Pearl, 1976):

1. Monoamines (serotonin, norepinephrine, and dopamine)
2. Amino acids (GABA, glycine, and glutamate)
3. Neuropeptides (substance P, cholecystokinin somatostatin, oxytocin, vasopressin, and enkephalins)

This knowledge has already provided new methods of managing certain pain syndromes, such as the intrathecal administration of very

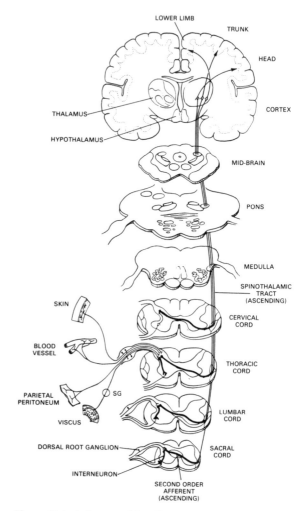

Figure 12.1. A diagram of the afferent pathways. First-order neurons link the nociceptors to each spinal segment. The second-order neuron links the dorsal horn to the higher centers, and the third-order neuron links the higher centers to the cerebral cortex.

low doses of opiods, clonidine, and norepinephrine. These agents then inhibit transmission at the dorsal horn level, thereby producing a segmental decrease in afferent pain impulses.

Modulation within Higher Centers

Ascending pathways (spinothalamic tract) and supraspinal modulating systems (thalamus, limbic system, reticular activating system, mesencephalon, and diencephalon) also exert important controls over the strength of the afferent pain impulse. The modulated impulse ascends through specific tracts in both the ventral and dorsal spinal cord, to terminate in the medulla, the mesencephalon, and the diencephalon (see Figure 12.1). These higher centers then influence whether the ascending impulses are perceived as pain—in one of two ways. First, the impulse itself may be modulated locally. Second, these higher centers are also the site of origin of descending pathways that, when stimulated, act to dampen pain perception at the first-order synapse in the dorsal horn (LaMotte, 1986; Yaksh, 1988; Willis, 1985). See Figure 12.2.

Central Pain Mechanisms

From these brain stem centers, a tertiary neuron runs to the cortex and limbic system, where these peripheral stimuli are now appreciated as "pain." Hence, such factors as anxiety, fear, motivation, and oppression may significantly amplify or dampen pain impulses arising at a more peripheral level. It appears that these central nervous system "states" exert their effects via fibers that descend from the cortex and subcortical structures, to decrease or increase pain significantly at a more peripheral level. These higher levels are adjusted to activate descending systems based on past experience, judgments, and current emotions. Further identifying these systems and the ways in which they can be controlled will advance pain management.

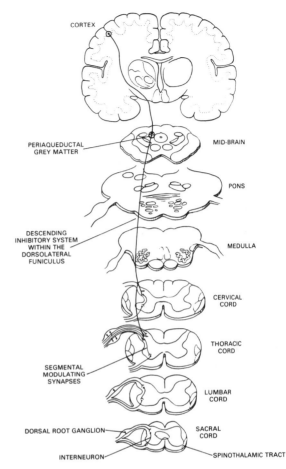

Figure 12.2. A schematic diagram of efferent pathways that modulate pain perception, traveling from cortex to basal nuclei (first order), and basal nuclei to dorsal horn (second order).

PATHWAYS SPECIFICALLY INVOLVED IN PELVIC PAIN

Somatic Innervation

The somatic nerve supply to the groin, vulva, and perineum arises predominately from the L1–L2 and S2–S4 spinal segments.

Fibers from the L1–L2 segments form the ilioinguinal and iliohypogastric nerves. After forming in the lumbar plexus, these peripheral nerves circle the abdominal wall to provide sensory innervation to the skin of the groin, mons pubis and anterior vulva.

Fibers from the S2–S4 segments fuse in the hollow of the sacrum to form the pudendal nerve. From there the pudendal nerve takes a complicated course along the back wall of the pelvis, exiting the pelvis via the greater sciatic foramen, crossing the ischial spine, then dividing into superficial and deep branches. The deep branch reenters Alcock's canal and runs to the top of the pubic arch, where it innervates the clitoris. The superficial branch splits into the inferior hemorrhoidal and posterior labial nerves, which innervate the perineum and posterior labia. Skin supplied by the posterior labial nerves (S2–S3) is overlapped laterally by the perineal branch of the posterior cutaneous nerve of the thigh (S1, S2, S3) and anteriorly by the ilioinguinal nerve.

Autonomic Innervation

In contrast to the somatic innervation of the skin and mucous membranes, the pelvic organs send sensory impulses via two groups of afferent fibers: sympathetic and parasympathetic. Although the peripheral anatomic distributions of these sympathetic and parasympathetic nerves overlap, impulses within these parallel pathways travel through different reflex arcs.

Sympathetic

The afferent sympathetic input from the vagina, uterus, and upper medial fallopian tube travel via the visceral afferent nerves to Frankenhauser's paracervical plexus, and then to the inferior, middle, and superior hypogastric plexus. In contrast, sympathetic nerves originating from the lateral fallopian tube, the ovary, the broad ligaments, and the adjacent peritoneum travel along the ovarian vessels to enter the aortic plexus directly. Finally, nerves from both sites join the lumbar and lower thoracic sympathetic chain and then enter the spinal cord at segmental levels T10–L1. Afferent sympathetic fibers also synapse in the dorsal horn before traversing the spinal cord en route to the cortex. Hence, visceral pain impulses are modulated both at the initial synapse and at multiple higher levels.

Parasympathetic

The parasympathetic fibers originate on the pelvic organs, travel along the pudendal nerve, and enter the spinal cord at segmental levels, S2–4. Noxious stimuli transmitted within the sympathetic and parasympathetic afferents are to the same segmental spinal modulatio scribed for afferent input arising within matic distribution. Hence, diseases of th organs commonly elicit the clinical synd "referred" pain. This phenomenon of convergence arises during the process modulation, because impulses conducte

the sympathetic and parasympathetic nerves stimulate somatic afferent fibers synapsing at the same spinal segment. Thus, ovarian pain may be referred to the anterior aspects of the leg. Likewise, pain arising from the uterus and cervix may be referred to the lower abdominal wall, the dorsum of the sacrum, or even the perianal skin.

A GENERAL APPROACH TO THE PATIENT WITH CHRONIC PAIN

In addition to the routine gynecological evaluation, the characteristics of the pain must be specifically defined. Since chronic pain is basically an unpleasant emotional experience, the ways in which long-standing pain have affected the patient's life must be evaluated, using a multidimensional approach (see Table 12.1).

Defining the Pain

Quality

The patient should be asked to describe carefully the nature of her pain (sharp or dull, diffuse or localized, burning or itchy, superficial or deep). Superficial pain tends to be sharp, burning, and well localized, whereas deep somatic or visceral pain is dull, diffuse, and often poorly localizable.

Table 12.1. The General Approach to a Patient with Chronic Pain

A. DEFINING THE PAIN
- Quality (superficial/deep)
- Severity (intensity/function)
- Location (dermatomic/peripheral nerve)
- Duration and periodicity
- Aggravating and relieving factors
- Previous therapy

B. EFFECT ON LIFESTYLE
- hange
- daily habits
- vithdrawal
- rsonal relationships

ING THE PSYCHOSOCIAL
ENT
- ve signs versus functional impairment
- "illness conviction"
- atric signs/symptoms
- nce abuse

Severity

This problem is best approached from two viewpoints: gauging intensity and quantifying functional impairment.

Intensity. This can be measured satisfactorily by any of three standard methods, applicable to pain at all anatomic sites:

1. A verbal severity scale, such as "none, mild, moderate, severe or excruciating" (Melzack, 1983).
2. A visual analog scale, which offers a more sensitive and more flexible alternative (Huskisson, 1983). This test is administered by drawing a 10 cm line and asking the patient to place her pain intensity somewhere on this visual scale. Zero is explained as being no pain and ten as the most intolerable pain imaginable. Severity is then gauged by measuring with a millimeter ruler. Differences of two centimeters or more indicate a clinically significant change.
3. Pain intensity can also be assessed by the McGill Pain Questionnaire (Melzack, 1983). This method was developed from a list of adjectives describing pain intensity and character. Each word was tested for its value in communicating pain experiences. Words were then arranged into weighted lists, such that a relatively reproductive numeric score could be generated to quantify pain intensity.

Functional Assessment. In contrast to the wide applicability of intensity measures, functional assessment requires the construction of a reasonably objective ordinal scale for each pain syndrome or physical activity. An example constructed to study chronic pain is shown in Table 12.2.

Location

An exact description of the location, plus any radiation patterns, is also important. At physical examination, points of maximum intensity and any associated tenderness should be carefully matched with the stated distribution of symptoms. Thought should be given to whether the location conforms to a dermatome, to the distribution of a specific peripheral nerve, or to the position of a specific anatomic structure.

Duration and Periodicity

The duration and periodicity of the pain should be described in detail. Is the pain always present? Are there short bouts of extreme pain? Is the pain ever gone completely? In addition, specific patterns can provide important diagnostic clues and may help determine therapeutic intervention when nonspecific therapies are under consideration. For example, pain syndromes that are paroxysmal in nature are more likely to respond to the anticonvulsant agents, whereas constant burning pain syndromes are more likely to respond to antidepressants. Unfortunately, mechanical pain syndromes (severe but shortlived pains, evoked by such mechanical manipulations as vaginal intercourse and reverting to little or no pain between episodes) respond poorly to nonspecific treatments.

Aggravating and Relieving Factors

The patient must also be asked what factors aggravate or improve the pain. Questions should not be directed only to the somatic aspect of the pain, but also to emotional situations that aggravate or alleviate it. Specific inquiries should be made as to whether episodes of increased pain are job-related or follow interpersonal problems.

Adequacy of Previous Therapy

Details of all therapeutic interventions should also be obtained. Were previous medical trials adequate? Were the classes or types of medications appropriate? Did previous surgical interventions change the intensity of the pain or the quality of pain? Did any of these interventions cause either temporary or permanent iatrogenic complications?

Table 12.2. The Functional Assessment Schema for Assessing the Impact of Chronic Gynecologic Pain on "Day-to-Day Activities" and "Ability to Have Intercourse"

A. DAY-TO-DAY ACTIVITIES

How do your day-to-day symptoms presently affect your life?

10) Incapacitating pain, destroying most facets of your life (e.g., unemployable, socially withdrawn, sense of personal desperation).

9) Severe burning or actual pain, dominating your daily thoughts and severe enough to cause regular absenteeism (e.g., 1 day/month), regular suspension of household tasks, and frequent restriction of social outings (e.g., 7 days/month).

8) Severe burning or actual pain, dominating your daily thoughts but not severe enough to cause more than occasional absenteeism, suspended housework, or social disruption.

7) Moderate vulvar discomfort (e.g., burning rather than pain). Severe enough to frequently break your concentration, but not severe enough to dominate your whole day's thoughts. Can be severe enough to restrict your personal activities (e.g., exercise, shopping, social outings).

6) Moderate vulvar discomfort, frequently breaking your concentration (but not dominating your thoughts). Severe enough to restrict your choice of clothing or sitting posture (but not enough to disrupt your personal activities).

5) Moderate vulvar discomfort, constant or almost constant. Severe enough to break your concentration, but not severe enough to limit your choice of clothing or sitting posture. Present at least 20 days/month (even if severity varies from week to week).

4) Moderate vulvar discomfort, intermittent but severe enough to break your concentration. Does not limit clothing/ sitting. Present less than 20 days/month.

3) Moderate vulvar discomfort (intermittent or constant), not severe enough to break your concentration when you are busy doing other things.

2) Nuisance-level vulvar symptoms (e.g., rawness, dryness, or stinging rather than distressing burning).

1) No vulvar discomfort.

B. SEXUAL DYSFUNCTION

How does your pain with intercourse affect your sex life?

10) Cannot have intercourse under any circumstances.

9) Intercourse extremely painful. Often have to discontinue and often have several days of subsequent pain. Frequency drastically reduced (less than once a month).

8) Intercourse always painful. Tolerable only at much reduced frequency (e.g., 1–2 times/month), and often have to discontinue. (Topical xylocaine: Yes/No?)

7) Intercourse almost always painful, tolerable only at much reduced frequency (e.g., 1–2 times/month), but do not usually have to discontinue. (Topical xylocaine: Yes/No?)

6) Intercourse always painful. Only tolerable at average frequency (1–2 times/week), if topical xylocaine and lubricants are used.

5) Intercourse almost always painful throughout. Tolerable at average frequency (1–2 times/week) without topical xylocaine and lubricants.

4) Intercourse partly painful (e.g., at entry), but often becomes partly pleasurable. May be followed by hours or days of postintercourse burning pain/burning.

3) Intercourse not painful during the act, but is followed by prolonged (2 or more days) flare-up of burning discomfort.

2) Intercourse not painful during the act, but is followed by short (less than 1 day) flare-up of burning discomfort.

1) No pain with intercourse/tampon use.

Effect on Lifestyle

In exploring the impact of the pain on the patient's current lifestyle, the patient should be asked to detail a typical day. Additional information may also be obtained through daily pain diaries and family interviews. Specific attention should be given to the following:

1. Mood changes. Chronic pain makes patients irritable and withdrawn and may even provoke overt depression. Has the pain interfered with self-image? Is there suicidal ideation?

2. Altered daily habits. Does the pain affect appetite and eating habits? Has weight changed? Has sexuality been affected? To what extent is attention focused continuously on the pain?

3. Social withdrawal. How has lifestyle changed since the onset of pain? What activities does the patient still enjoy? Has the sick or injured role allowed the patient to avoid social responsibilities (e.g., daily chores) or

to indulge herself in favored hobbies (e.g., reading, watching TV)?

4. Disrupted interpersonal relationships. Is the relationship with spouse and children strong, or is it now strained? What is the patient's employment status? Did the pain cause the patient to leave or be discharged from her job?

Some clinicians involved with chronic pain have developed questionnaires to cover these issues; others recommend that patients complete a Minnesota Multiphasic Personality Inventory (MMPI) during the initial evaluation process. When approaching the patient in this manner, one may meet a great deal of resistance. Patients may feel that the clinician is insinuating a psychological etiology to their pain—that their pain is viewed as "not real." It is important for the patient to realize that the clinician's evaluation in no way implies that the pain is psychogenic. The evaluator must develop ways of explaining how this information may be helpful. The devastating effects that chronic pain can have on other areas of the patient's life (such as disruption of familial, vocational, and social functioning) should be emphasized. After the multidimensional evaluation is completed, the results of the evaluation should be discussed with the patient and family. This will improve clinical outcome and also decrease the likelihood of fragmented health care delivery.

Warning Signs of an Undue Psychosocial Component

Warning signs of an unduly large psychological component include those discussed in the paragraphs that follow (Sullivan et al., 1991).

Great Disparity Between Objective Findings and Functional Disability

Although the inability of diagnostic testing to find a lesion does not prove psychogenesis, it might reasonably prompt the health care profes-

sional to look for psychosocial causes of "excess" disability. The degree to which the patient is able to avoid unpleasurable events or indulge herself in pleasurable activities should be carefully balanced against her pre-pain situation, as a means of assessing her potential for "secondary gain."

Strong "Illness Conviction"

Failure to accept her physician's assurance that no dangerous or progressive disease underlies her pain can be a sign that the patient's "illness conviction" is at variance with medical fact. Simply denying that there are unexplored medical or surgical options may alienate the patient, thereby initiating a search for other physicians who will offer answers that are easier to accept. An effective response to a strong "illness conviction" is to acknowledge that (1) the pain is objective (i.e., can be perceived in principle by a third party), (2) the pain is not of the patient's own making (i.e., illness, not behavior), and (3) the patient truly desires treatment. However, within this framework, the physician should try to minimize any sense of diagnostic ambiguity and (when appropriate) to change the focus of therapy from cure to rehabilitation.

Signs or Symptoms of Psychiatric Disorder

Concern, irritability, and sadness are appropriate responses to prolonged sexual disability. However, frustration at not getting better and fears of marital breakdown can excacerbate a treatable psychiatric disorder. The prevalence of major depressive and panic disorders (see the glossary at the end of this chapter) is greatly increased in chronic pain patients.

Opiate, Benzodiazepine or Alcohol Abuse

Substance abuse may arise in conjunction with the pain problem (e.g., opiates, benzodiazepines) or precede it (e.g., alcohol, marijuana, cocaine). In either form, substance abuse impedes rehabilitation and must be addressed aggressively. Abuse can manifest itself as signs of medication dependence (including escalating doses), maneuvering in the health care system to get drugs, and withdrawal symptoms. Physicians should avoid prescribing narcotics, since they are neither helpful nor safe in cases of chronic pain.

SPECIFIC APPROACH TO SEXUAL PAIN OR DISCOMFORT

Some women will spontaneously report difficulties to their gynecologist, but others are reluctant to discuss sexual complaints and will ask for help only if they are given a convenient opportunity. Hence, the extent of sexual dysfunction among patients is easily underestimated. Health care providers should routinely broach the subject of sexual health preferably in a situation of complete privacy.

Sexual difficulties in general, and dyspareunia in particular, may arise from solely physical causes, from solely emotional factors, or from a complex interaction of both. Sexual pain arising on an organic basis will create marital friction and can evoke feelings of guilt or despair, thereby leading to secondary pain behavior. Conversely, psychosomatic pain is readily accentuated by repeated tearing of the unlubricated vagina, producing chronic fissure formation and scarring. Hence, in making a diagnostic assessment, gynecologists must be very sensitive to the role of the behavioral problems or psychiatric disturbance, and psychologists must not overlook the operation of a physical disorder simply because of prominent psychological distress.

From the physical viewpoint, causes of dyspareunia (pain during intercourse) are best separated into those producing superficial discomfort versus those producing deep discomfort. Even so, arriving at a reasonably reliable provisional diagnosis, based upon history and physical examination, requires considerable gynecologic training. Even the most adroit clinician will often be unable to come to a firm clinical conclusion. Hence, in recent years, physicians have relied increasingly on laparoscopy and colposcopy to amplify physical findings and confirm clinical opinion.

Many patients who complain of chronic pelvic pain and deep dyspareunia have no demonstrable pelvic disorder, whereas others have quite remediable problems. In a series of 1194 consecutive pelvic pain patients, 839 (71%) had a plausible physical explanation detected at diagnostic laparoscopy (Cunanan et al., 1983), including 63% of the women whose initial clinical work-ups were normal. Hence, laparoscopy is indicated in all patients who complain of a consistent pattern of pain, present in the same location for six months or more.

Likewise, in a series of 100 women with chronic vulvar pain and introital dyspareunia, 74 had abnormalities that were either solely detectable or better visualized through the colposcope (Reid et al., 1988). Failure to examine such patients with the improved lighting and magnification of the colposcope repeatedly leads to an erroneous diagnosis of chronic candidiasis. For example, the Wayne State University Vaginitis Clinic (Sobel, 1990) was unable to demonstrate yeast forms in 85% of women referred for chronic candidiasis.

DIFFERENTIAL DIAGNOSIS AND SPECIFIC TREATMENT OF DEEP DYSPAREUNIA

Anatomic Distortion of the Upper Genital Tract

Dyspareunia on deep penetration may occur in the absence of any structural disorder, simply on the basis of a retroverted uterus that allows the ovaries to prolapse into the pouch of Douglas. Ovarian compression will produce a sharp, sickening discomfort, somewhat analogous to testicular trauma. Symptoms can generally be controlled by altering coital positions. However, in carefully considered cases, laparoscopic shortening of the round ligaments may be warranted.

Scarring or fixation of the vaginal vault is another significant but readily overlooked source of deep dyspareunia. Unless the physician specifically palpates for such a scar, the diagnosis will not be made. Causes of painful vaginal scarring include congenital septae, lateral extension of an obstetric cervical tear, and unskilled laser surgery (Reid & Dorsey, 1991) to vaginal and cervical lesions (generally because of such low power outputs and such low power densities as to produce thermal rather than optical tissue effects). Vaginal scars are readily correctible by the skilled surgeon, either by deep lateral incision with reverse direction suturing or by Z-plasty (Figure 12.3). The latter technique interrupts the lines of tension between the two attachments of the original scar, thus allowing these collagen fibers to relax and soften.

Chronic Vaginal Ulceration

Such chronic mucosal abnormalities as lichen planus or pemphigus can predominantly affect the vagina, producing copious purulent discharge and chronic painful ulcerations. Diagnosis will depend a biopsy, preferably one that incorporates both part of the ulcer crater and some viable vaginal epithelium at the crater edge. Treatment with potent topical corticosteroids and antibiotic vaginal suppositories can be helpful. However, in refractory cases, vaginectomy and myocutaneous flap construction may offer the only prospect of cure.

Organic Disease of the Uterus, Tubes, and Ovaries

Some diseases of the upper genital tract produce sufficient chronic interval pelvic pain to disrupt both the quality of daily life and any attempt at vaginal intercourse. However, other patients present only with dyspareunia, without intense pelvic pain. The latter group of diseases tend to manifest as a triad of related symptoms—

menorrhagia, secondary dysmenorrhea, and deep dyspareunia (Table 12.3). The most common causes are discussed in the subsections that follow.

Chronic Pelvic Inflammatory Disease

Pelvic inflammatory disease (PID) is infection of the upper genital tract (i.e., the uterus, fallopian tubes, and ovaries) by varying mixtures of facultative pathogens from the vaginal ecosystem. Common organisms include gram-negative aerobic rods (E. coli), gram-positive aerobes (streptocci and staphylococci), anaerobic rods or cocci (bacteroides, peptococci, and clostridia), and mycoplasma species. Events that can precipitate upper tract invasion by these facultative pathogens include:

1. Sexually transmitted infections (gonorrhoea and chylamydia)
2. Postpartum and postabortal infections
3. Atrogenic infection secondary to breaching the "cervical mucous barrier"
4. Infectious sequelae of an intrauterine device
5. Spread of intraperitoneal sepsis from appendicitis or diverticulosis

Most women recover from these acute episodes. However, a small proportion of acute PID patients progress to chronic pain syndromes. Some progress by repeated reinfection (e.g., from untreated male partners); others develop smoldering inflammation within avascular, scarred areas of the pelvic fascia. The clinical course consists of recurrent subacute episodes of salpingo-oophoritis, at increasingly frequent intervals, culminating in chronic pain and dyspareunia. Once extensive local damage has occurred, the progress of the disease is difficult to reverse, irrespective of how much antibiotic therapy is given. At least in Third World countries, tubercular salpingitis should also be considered a possibility in patients with "refractory PID."

Chronic pain arising as a sequel to recurrent or neglected PID is usually indicated by sug-

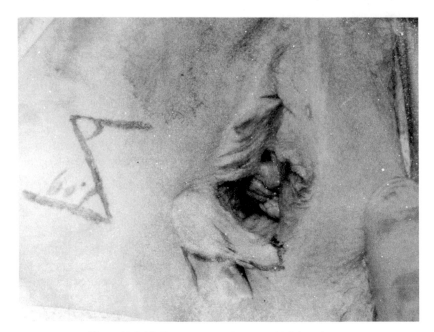

Figure 12.3 (a). Two symptomatic scars which have been marked for Z-plasty. The right-hand one is a perineal scar, which formed at the site of apposition of a previous pudendal flap. The left-hand one is an inguinal scar, which formed at the posterior edge of the pudendal flap donor site.

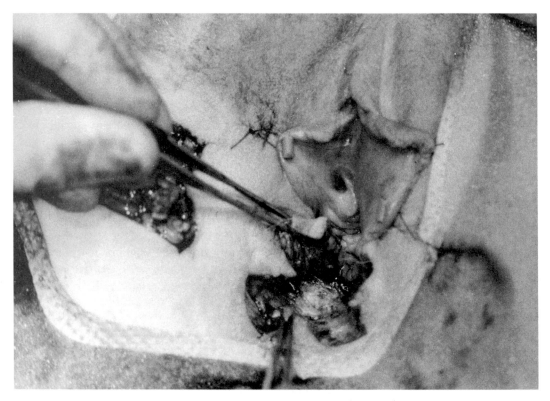

Figure 12.3 (b). Incision and transposition of the two sides of the perineal scar.

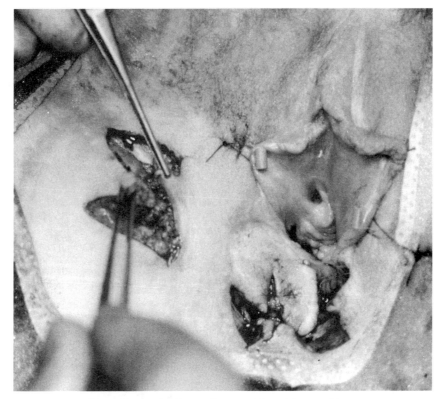

Figure 12.3 (c). Incision and transposition of the two sides of the inguinal scar.

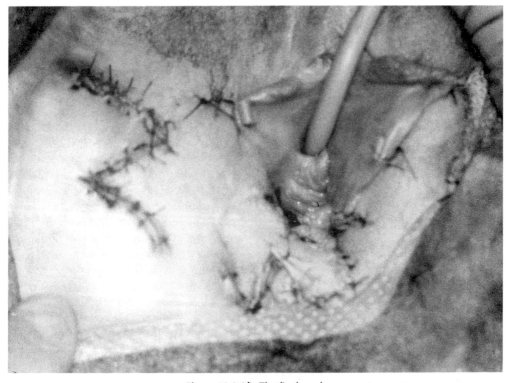

Figure 12.3 (d). The final result.

Table 12.3. Clinical Clues to Help Differentiate Between Organic Causes of Deep Dyspareunia

DIAGNOSTIC CLUE	PID	ENDOMETRIOSIS	ADENOMYOSIS
Patient profile	STD risks—young, poor, promiscuous	Nulliparous, late 20s/ early 30s	Multiparous, 35–50
Timing of flare-ups	Late menstrual or postmenstrual	Just before and throughout menses	Day 1 and 2 of period
Dyspareunia	Lateral more than central	Central, lateral, or both	Central
Characteristic symptoms	Recurrent febile episodes; chronic pain usually bilateral; uncommon after tubal ligation	Sacral backache; radiation to rectum; pain often unilateral; blood in stool/ urine	Burning, throbbing ache; pain central rather than lateral
Infertility	Very common	Common	Rare
Characteristic signs	Fixed retroversion; hydrosalpinges	Fixed retroversion; beading of uterosacral ligaments; adnexal scarring, with or without endometrioma	Globular, "woody," usually symmetric uterine enlargement; variations in tenderness

gestive events within the past medical history. In addition, at least 50% will give a previous history of recurrent abdominal pain, culminating in either outpatient or inpatient antibiotic therapy. About 15% will suffer involuntary infertility, and about 4% will have an ectopic pregnancy (Westrom, 1980).

Pain may be episodic or constant, and dyspareunia can be severe. At physical examination, diagnosis of chronic PID can be easy, especially if tubal obstruction results in chronic hydrosalpinges (Figure 12.4). Conversely, when the adnexae become small, fibrotic, and tethered to the posterior uterine surface, clinical or ultrasonic diagnosis can be virtually impossible.

Regretably, pain secondary to end-stage PID is essentially impossible to control medically. Nonetheless, until a definite diagnosis is established, gynecologists must be very cautious about advising surgery for chronic pelvic pain. Any decision to proceed to hysterectomy on the basis of chronic pelvic inflammatory disease requires prior laparoscopic documentation of organic disease (tubo-ovarian adhesions and/or hydrosalpinx formation).

Endometriosis

Endometriosis is an insidious, enigmatic disease, characterized by the presence of endometrial glands and stroma at various extrauterine locations. Especially common sites include the uterine ligaments, the pelvic peritoneum, the ovaries, and the sigmoid colon, appendix, or rectovaginal septum. This ectopic endometrium is hormone-responsive, resulting in endometrial proliferation during the follicular/luteal phases and bleeding during the menses. Although endometriosis is a benign condition, foci of ectopic endometrium can be locally invasive, and dissemination to pelvic lymph nodes, abdominal scars, or distant sites is seen in about one-third of severe cases. Repeated bleeding and local invasion create dense scarring, tender nodularity, and painful adhesions. The uterus is often fixed in retroversion, and the tubes and ovaries may be drawn into the midline, where they are vulnerable to compression during coitus. In severe cases, there may be obliteration of the pouch of Douglas or even the vaginal fornices. Dyspareunia results from a variety of mechanisms, including pressure on painful nodules, stretching of hyperesthetic scars, malplacement of even normally sensitive ovaries, and postaglandin release from areas of active endometriosis.

Events leading to the detection of endometriosis vary widely, depending on the site and the progression of disease. About one-third of patients are asymptomatic, and another third are diagnosed during an infertility workup (Figure 12.5). The remaining third present in a variety of ways, including cyclic pelvic pain, deep dyspareunia, a pelvic mass, bowel/bladder dysfunction, or an acute abdominal emergency. Beyond this diversity of clinical presentations, diagnosis is further complicated by incongruities between lesion size and symptom severity. Relatively small endometriotic deposits may produce substantial symptoms, whereas large endometriomas can be clinically silent until sudden rupture occurs.

Typically, endometriosis patients who present with the triad of cyclic pain, menorrhagia, and dyspareunia will be nulliparous women in their late 20s/early 30s. Secondary dysmenorrhea due to endometriosis tends to begin 24–48 hours before the onset of menstruation and to continue at high intensity for most of the duration of bleeding. Other clues include a tendence for pain to be worse on one side, an intense sacral/coccygeal backache, intense bloating, pain radiating down the recto-vaginal septum, and blood in the stool or urine. About 25% of these women will have undergone an infertility workup, and about 10% will have a history of unexplained acute abdominal pain.

Physical findings are as variable as the modes of presentation. Diagnosis is easy in patients who manifest an immoble retroverted uterus, adnexal enlargement, pelvic scarring, and diffuse tenderness (Figure 12.6). Conversely, vagi-

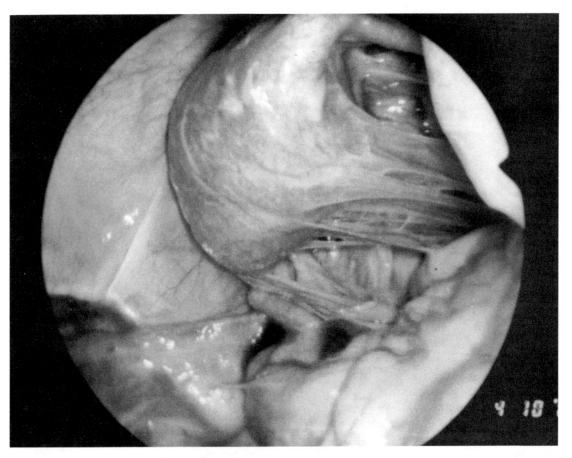

Figure 12.4. Appearances at laparoscopy, showing end-stage pelvic inflammatory disease, with distortion of the fallopian tubes and extensive adhesion formation (photograph courtesy of Dr. S. Osher, Cincinatti, Ohio).

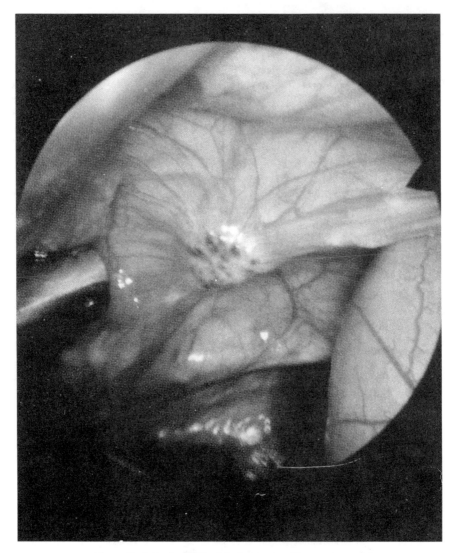

Figure 12.5. Puckered blue/black deposits of intraperitoneal endometriosis, typical of what is found in otherwise asymptomatic patients undergoing an infertility workup (photograph courtesy of Dr. D. Martin, Memphis, Tennessee).

nal exam can be entirely normal despite considerable occult pathology. Between these two extremes, abnormal findings (if present) can be completely nonspecific. Nonetheless, reasonable suspicion of occult endometriosis may come from one of three clues:

1. *Fixed retroversion.* In contrast to the mobile retroversion seen as a physiologic variation in 10% of normal women, fixed retroversion is an indication of chronic adhesion formation in the pouch of Douglas.

2. *Nodularity of the uterosacral ligaments.* Tenderness on rectovaginal exam can be highly diagnostic; findings range from small shot-like thickenings to discrete nodules 1 cm in diameter.

3. *Exacerbation during menstruation.* Reexam-

ination on the first day of bleeding, when organ swelling and peritoneal inflammation are maximal, will often resolve a previously ambiguous clinical picture.

Historically, endometriosis was managed through long-term, high-dose birth control pills (the ''pseudo-pregnancy regimen''), punctuated as necessary by conservative electrosurgical destruction of stubborn lesions (which was done through open abdominal incisions). When childbearing was complete or infertility was accepted as irreversible, patients with severe pelvic pain underwent total abdominal hysterectomy and bilateral salpingo-oophorectomy.

However, the advent of laser-adapted laporoscopy and the development of effective anti-estrogen and antigonadotrophin drugs have given both medical and surgical regimens a great deal more flexibility.

Today's physicians have several choices, depending on whether the objective is to forestall progression, to restore fertility, or to relieve chronic pain. Obviously, the equation reflects such factors as age, future reproductive plans, severity of symptomatology, and intrabdominal findings.

Pseudopregnancy regimens seldom (if ever) reversed the underlying pathology; the best that could be expected was that progression might be

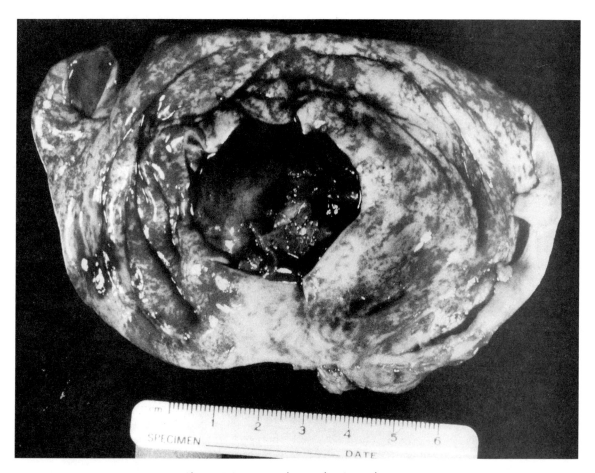

Figure 12.6. A resected ovary showing end-stage endometriosis, with large endometrioma formation (photograph courtesy of Dr. M. Husein, Southfield, Michigan).

delayed. However, the development of danazole (an attenuated androgen) in 1975 provided a medical regimen capable of inducing objective regression in about 90% of subjects. Unfortunately, there was a relapse rate of about 15–30% of patients within a year or so of discontinuing medication. Taken orally in doses of 200–800 mg per day, danazole will produce a "pseudomenopause." However, danazole is too expensive for long-term use (about $250 per month). Moreover, its side effects are substantial—mainly those attributable to estrogen deficiency (hot flashes, atrophic vaginitis, emotional lability, weight gain, and fluid retention) and those related to the underlying androgenicity of danazole (oily skin, acne, and sometimes facial hair or deepening of the voice).

Recently, gonadotrophin-releasing hormone antagonists, which completely block the hypothalamic-pituitary-ovarian axis, have enabled physicians to create a profound pseudomenopause without androgenic effects. Such regimens are an excellent alternative for short-term treatment, but they are too costly and induce too much osteporosis for long-term therapy.

Adaption of the argon and carbon dioxide lasers for laparascopic use has allowed sequential, noninvasive surgery for destruction of endometriotic deposits, lysis of adhesions, and removal of small endometriomas (endometriotic ovarian cysts). Particularly in combination with adjuvant medical regimens, serial laparoscopy should allow physicians to forestall the otherwise relentless progression of severe endometriosis. Nonetheless, open laparotomy is still indicated in some circumstances: acute rupture of an endometrioma, ovarian masses greater than 5 cm in diameter, retroperitoneal disease obstructing the ureters, and compromised bowel function.

Adenomyosis

Adenomyosis refers to the downward growth of the basalis layer of the endometrium, penetrating more than one low-power microscope field (2.5 mm) into the myometrium. Although basilar

endometrium is not fully hormone-responsive (perhaps because of low levels of hormone receptors), islands of entrapped bleeding can produce intense inflammation and hyperplasia of the adjacent uterine wall. Two distinct clinical patterns are seen, depending on whether the inflammatory response within the uterine wall is diffuse or focal. The diffuse pattern produces a "woody," globular, symmetrically enlarged (two or three times normal), deeply tender uterus (see Figure 12.7). Less commonly, focal adenoma formation can present as an asymmetric uterine deformity.

Confirming a suspicion of adenomyosis at physical examination is very difficult. Hysteroscopy may show characteristic crypt openings and distortion of the uterine cavity. However, final diagnosis generally relies on histologic examination of the extirpated uterus. Such a decision will be made if the patient and gynecologist have reached a consensus that symptoms are severe enough to warrant a surgical solution.

Residual Ovary Syndrome

Residual ovary syndrome is a very distressing but poorly recognized syndrome that can affect ovaries conserved after hysterectomy. Although adhesions from abdominal wall to bowel or from bowel to uterus are not painful, any such tethering of the ovarian cortex can be quite symptomatic. Principal complaints following postoperative fixation of the ovaries are chronic abdominal pain, bloating, intense dyspareunia, and even dyschezia.

Suppression of pituitary gonadotrophins with progestins, birth control pills, or even testosterone will control this syndrome in many women. More complete hypothalamic suppression with GnRH (Lupron or Synarel) or danocrine (danazole) is almost certain to relieve symptoms, but adverse side effects preclude long-term therapy. Hence, oophorectomy and hormone replacement are often the only realistic options.

Occasionally, a clinical picture suggestive of residual ovary syndrome is seen in a patient who has allegedly had a bilateral oophorectomy. Un-

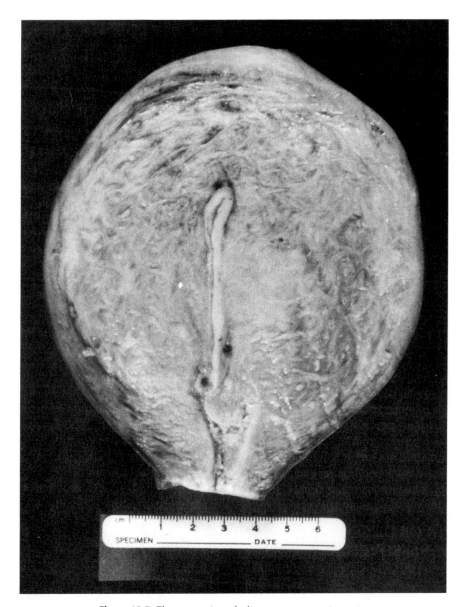

Figure 12.7. The cut section of a hysterectomy specimen, in which patchy areas of hemorrhage and fibrosis are visible within the deep myometrium; the uterus shows the globular, symmetric enlargement typical of adenomyosis (photograph courtesy of Dr. M. Husein, Southfield, Michigan).

der these circumstances, the physician should consider the possibility of a symptomatic ovarian remnant buried in the retroperitoneal space. Hence, ordering a hormone profile can help establish the diagnosis.

Pelvic Congestion Syndrome

Taylor (1949a, 1949b) defined the pelvic congestion syndrome as pain and heaviness in the pelvis, with the symptoms beginning after getting out of bed and worsening as the day progresses. Pelvic pain is classically described as having a burning or throbbing quality, and there may be deep dyspareunia secondary to low-grade uterine tenderness. On laparoscopic examination, the uterus appears dusky blue and mottled, and prominent varicosities are seen in the broad ligaments. When looking for these dilated vessels, it is important to watch as the intraabdominal pneumoperitoneum is being released, since a high level of intraperitoneal gas causes external vascular compression.

The role of these varicosities in causing chronic pelvic pain and dyspareunia is difficult to establish. Notably, not all women with such operative or laparoscopic findings complain of pelvic pain. Indeed, it is difficult to prove that these varicosities actually cause any symptoms whatsoever. Most experts believe this syndrome to be psychosomatic. The real cause of pelvic pain and dyspareunia is probably stress-related spasm of muscle fibers within the levatores ani (the broad, funnel-shaped muscular sheets that hold the abdominal contents within the pelvic cavity). Diagnosis depends on both the absence of a recognizable organic disorder and the positive identification of a predisposition toward other psychosomatic syndromes. Although a number of studies indicate that personality examinations do not differentiate between patients with psychogenic pain and those with organic pain, reassurance as to physical health plus general pain counseling is likely to be beneficial.

Treatment focuses on finding the means to reduce that patient's stress. Helpful strategies include education, teaching of relaxation techniques, psychologic counseling, and consideration of antidepressant or tranquilizing medications. Gynecologists must be extremely cautious about recommending surgery for any chronic pelvic pain that is not attributable to an organic disease. As a rule of thumb, good results from hysterectomy can be anticipated only in situations where secondary dysmenorrhea is a prominent part of the symptom complex (Stenchever, 1987).

"Universal Joint" Syndrome

Another complaint of pelvic pain/dyspareunia suspected to have a psychosomatic basis is the "universal joint" syndrome. In 1955, Allen and Masters (1955) theorized that pelvic pain could result from obstetric lacerations to the broad ligament, thereby allowing abnormal uterine mobility. Although operations have been designed to "repair these lacerations," it is difficult to establish any genuine surgical benefit for such intervention, beyond a simple placebo effect.

DIFFERENTIAL DIAGNOSIS AND SPECIFIC TREATMENT OF SUPERFICIAL DYSPAREUNIA

Anatomic Problems Affecting the Vestibule and Lower Vagina

Superficial dyspareunia is often due to narrowing or inelasticity of the vulvar vestibule or lower vagina. Specific causes include congenital bands or septae, rigid hymen, poorly repaired episiotomy scars, and burn contractures secondary to unskilled laser surgery (Figure 12.8). Skillful surgical correction, often by means of rotation flaps, will solve these problems (Reid & Dorsey, 1991).

Mucosal Atrophy and Chronic Ulceration

Unlike that of other mammalian species, human sexuality is not affected by fluctuations in ovarian sex hormone levels. Rather, female sexuality depends on a broad fabric of events, including socioeconomic status, cultural background, religious beliefs, general health, availability and function of partners, and the emotional quality of a woman's life at a particular time. However, during the perimenopausal and menopausal years, declining ovarian hormone function can emerge as a prominent factor. Mechanisms of genital atrophy include loss of cushioning due to

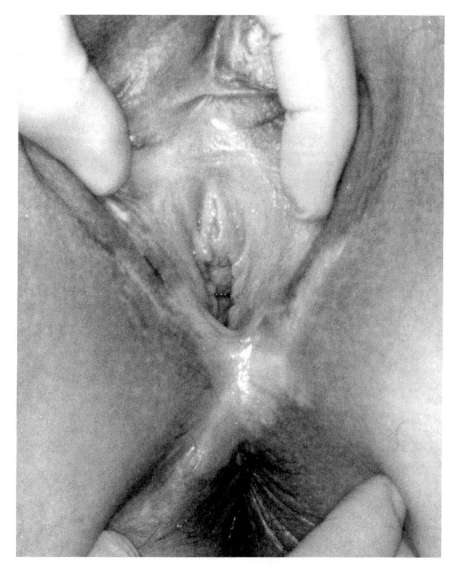

Figure 12.8. A classical burn contracture, following
unskilled CO_2 laser surgery to the vulva.

atrophy of the mons and labial fat pads, friability
of the mucosae due to combined epidermal and
dermal hypoplasia, chronic dryness due to declining vascularity, and a reduction in vaginal
lubrication capacity (Wallis, 1987). Even if the
patient does not actually complain of dyspareunia, the situation can be semiobjectively assessed by use of a subjective nominal scale (see

Table 12.4) (Leiblum et al., 1983). In a survey of
897 consecutive women seeking gynecologic
care, Bachmann (1989) reported that the likelihood of problems rose with advancing age. A
history of broad sexual dysfunction was obtained from 7.4% of teenagers, 18.1% of women
in their 20s and 30s, 22.5% of climacteric-age
women, and 28% of postmenopausal women.

Table 12.4. The Vaginal Atrophy Index*

CRITERIA	SCORE		
	0	1	2
Vulva	Pale, dry mucosa; loss of labial folds	Pale mucosa but normal contour	Moist, pink mucosae; full contour
Introitus	Less than 1 finger-breadth	1–2 finger-breadths	More than 2 finger-breadths
Speculum insertion	Minimal elasticity; difficulty with small speculum	Reducing elasticity; no difficulty with small speculum	Normal elasticity; accepts medium speculum
Vaginal mucosae	Pale, friable; numerous petechar	Pink mucosae; smooth vaginal walls	Pink, rugose vaginal walls

Scores: 0–2 Severe estrogen deficiency
3–5 Developing deficiency
6–8 Normal hormonal effect
*Modified with permission from Leiblum et al. (1983). Vaginal atrophy in the postmenopausal woman. The importance of sexual activity and hormones. *Journal of the American Medical Association, 249,* 2195. Copyright 1983, American Medical Association.

Nonetheless, most older women expressed an interest in sex, and the majority with a functional sexual partner continued to engage in coitus. Hence, although aging may cause difficulties, such difficulties must be viewed as obstacles to be overcome rather than as a signal that sexuality is ending.

Specifically, estrogen levels must not be allowed to fall to the point of vaginal mucosal atrophy and decreased capacity for lubrication. Estrogen replacement is efficacious, but it must include concomitant progestin administration if the uterus remains intact (Ettinger, 1990).

Urethral Diverticulum

Urethral diverticulae are small outpouchings that develop as a result of obstruction and infection in the periurethral glands. Presumably, spontaneous drainage of a small abscess into the urethral lumen can create a small but permanent cavity which will function as a nidus for chronic infection. Some patients are asymptomatic, others may present with only non-specific urinary symptoms, such as frequency and dysuria. However, many women with diverticulae will complain of introital or mid-vaginal dyspareunia. Some women may also be aware of a tender swelling beneath their anterior vaginal wall. Diagnosis can be easy, such as when the examining finger can palpate a mass, or can express pus by "milking" the urethra. Alternatively, a void-

ing cystometrogram (see Figure 12.9 on p. 357) or urethroscopy may be necessary.

Treatment is surgical. If the diverticulum is located in the distal third of the urethra (about 10% of cases), there is no risk of provoking urinary incontinence. Hence, the easiest and most successful approach is to marsupialize the cavity. However, the majority of cases require careful exploration of the vesicovaginal space, with accurate resection of the diverticulum and multilayered closure of the defect.

Idiopathic Vulvodynia

An illness characterized by itching or burning of the vulva, plus intense tenderness around the vaginal opening, was recognized by gynecologists during the last two decades of the nineteenth century (Skene, 1889). For mysterious reasons, this disease then disappeared from our society for the next 70 years. Unfortunately, since 1975, there has been a dramatic increase in the number of women who present with complaints of chronic vulvovaginal pain that are not explicable on other grounds (Freidrich, 1987).

Suspected Etiology

Suspected etiologic associations are similar in both variants of the vulvodynia syndrome. About 70% of affected women have a fair complexion and very sun-sensitive skin (R. Reid,

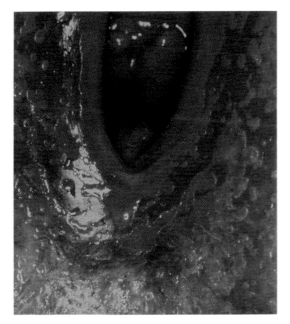

Figure 12.10. A color photograph showing chronically irritated vulvar skin, which would have appeared normal to examination by the naked eye but shows a dense acetowhite reaction after vinegar soaking.

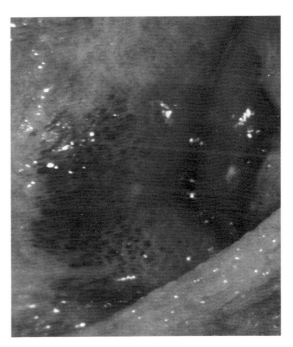

Figure 12.11. Painful hyperemic blood vessels adjacent to the right minor vestibular duct and Bartholin's ducts.

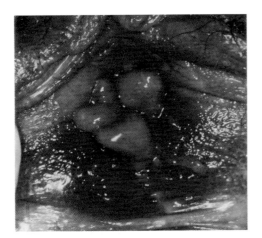

Figure 12.12(a). Painful hyperemic vessels radiating from a site of previous attempted destruction of erythematous minor vestibular gland. In addition to producing a dense carpet of reactive erythema, accompanying chronic inflammation within the Bartholin's gland has created substantial hymenal edema.

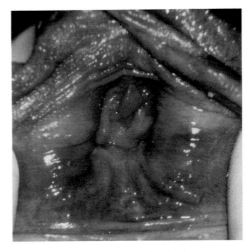

Figure 12.12(b). Appearance after dye laser surgery and removal of the Bartholin's gland.

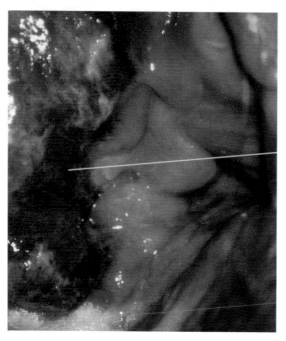

Figure 12.13(a). Intensely painful erythema surrounding the Bartholin's, minor vestibular, and Skene's glands.

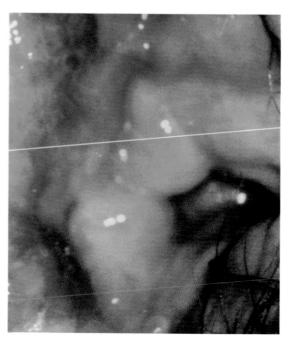

Figure 12.13(b). The same patient after argon laser photocoagulation of these painful vessels.

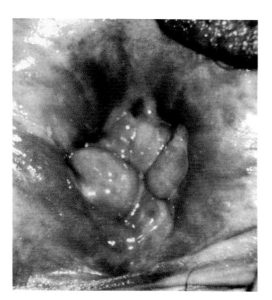

Figure 12.14(a). A view of the vulvar vestibule, showing intense, painful erythema surrounding the Bartholin's ducts. Note also the hymenal edema from underlying Bartholin's gland inflammation.

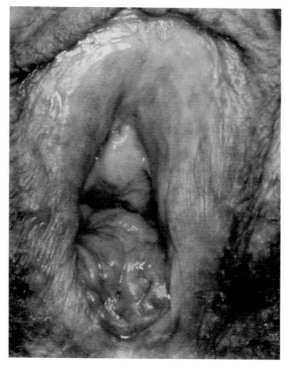

Figure 12.14(b). Appearance after treatment with bare-fiber argon laser energy.

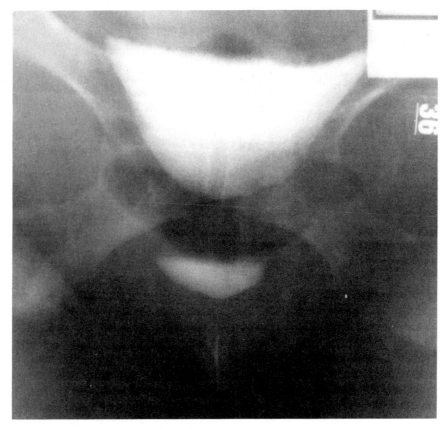

Figure 12.9. A voiding cystometrogram in a patient with a very painful urethral diverticulum. The upper white triangle is the bladder, filled with radio-opaque dye. The lower white triangle represents radio-opaque dye trapped in the diverticulum.

unpublished data). In addition, morphologic findings (through both the colposcope and the light microscope) are compatible with (but not diagnostic of) a low-grade human papillomavirus (HPV) infection. As evidenced by the prominent vascular changes accompanying condylomas and intraepithelial neoplasia, HPV infection has a well-defined capacity for producing both epithelial and vascular proliferation (Reid, 1989). Although attempts to detect HPV DNA (by Southern blot hybridization) have been unsuccessful (Reid et al., 1988), there remain many as yet unclassified HPV types that do not hybridize with the existing panel of probes. Analysis with polymerase chain reac-

tion techniques will be necessary to answer this question. Until these data are available, the exact role of HPV infection will remain uncertain. Nonetheless, the most plausible hypothesis available is that vulvodynia represents a hypersensitivity syndrome, seemingly triggered by some as yet uncharacterized papillomaviruses of low pathogenic potential in women of susceptible skin type.

Presenting Complaints

Presenting complaints center around two symptom complexes: interval vulvar burning or pain and introital dyspareunia. Although these symptoms have a demonstrable physical basis (eradication of which will cure the problem), the clinical picture is often clouded by a substantial overlay of anger (at not being believed by previous physicians), fear (of losing the partner), and depression.

Physical Findings

Physical examination will generally reveal several components, each of which contributes to symptomatology.

An irritative acetowhite reaction. Much of the vulvar epithelium shows an irritative whitening when soaked with vinegar during the colposcopic examination, as shown in Figure 12.10. (**Note:** Figures 12.10 through 12.14 are on the color insert page.) This irritative acetowhitening always involves the mucosa of the vestibule but also extends to the minimally keratinized, hairless skin of the interlabial grooves, clitoris, and perineum in about 50% of women.

A diffuse vascular ectasia. The blood vessels of the entire connective tissue of the vulvar vestibule generally show a hyperemic, ectatic effect. Although many of these foci of painful erythema will affect stroma immediately adjacent to vestibular gland epithelium (Figure 12.11), equally painful lesions can occur at other sites, as hyperemic telangiectatic vessels radiating to adjacent parts of the vestibule (Figure 12.12). These ectopic areas of painful erythema have proven to be more difficult to treat than initiating foci (those that surround the vestibular gland elements). In particular, such foci are aggravated (rather than relieved) by attempts at CO_2 laser photovaporization (Figure 12.13).

Painful inflammation of the minor vestibular glands. The minor vestibular glands are embryological remnants of the endothelial portion of the cloaca, which persists as shallow clefts located in the hymenal sulcus (Freidrich, 1982). In severe cases, this inflammation also involves the other structures derived from cloacal endothelium: Skene's complex (shallow glands adjacent to the external urethral meatus) and the ducts of Bartholin's gland (two small orifices

located just proximal to the mucocutaneous junction on the posteromedial surface of the labia minora). See Figure 12.14(a).

Deep pain upon palpation of the Bartholin's fossa. In the more severe 10–15%, this chronic inflammatory process descends into the Bartholin's ducts or glands, generally in association with squamous metaplasia. Under these circumstances, palpation at the junction of the bulbocavernosus and puborectalis muscles, just lateral to the anterior rectal wall, will evoke sharp discomfort.

Some authors distinguish vulvar papillomatosis from vestibular adenitis (McKay, 1989). However, in our view, these variations simply reflect differences of severity within the same clinicopathologic spectrum. Our experience has been that virtually everyone with "vestibular adenitis" will show features of "vulvar papillomatosis" if examined by a skilled colposcopist (Reid et al., 1988). As a general rule, the first two physical findings represent an earlier and milder manifestation, and the other two characterize a more severe form of the syndrome. An understanding of these facts is crucial, since accurate identification and careful eradication of the various physical components is the basis for successful therapy.

Treatment

A wide variety of antibacterial antibiotics, antifungal antibiotics, and antiinflammatory drugs have been used in an attempt to suppress the symptoms or cure the underlying disorder. None of these medications has proven successful. The only medical regimen of significant benefit in vulvodynia has been topical 5-fluorouracil cream (Efudex or Fluoroplex). Our group reported success in 16 of 24 women (75%) with mild to moderate degrees of vulvodynia, treated by a six-month course of 5-fluorouracil cream (Reid et al., 1988). Unfortunately, 5-fluorouracil cream was much less helpful in women with severe vulvodynia, being successful in only 1 of 13 cases (8%).

Recognition of the main sites of pain, and the fact that excision could cure some patients, represented a valuable initial step. The standard therapy has been an operation to excise the hymen and adjacent minor vestibular glands (Woodruff & Parmley, 1983). The wound is then closed by pulling down a 1½" to 2" sleeve of vaginal skin, to fill the defect left by excising the hymenal ring. However, in our experience, this surgery has several unsatisfactory aspects. (1) The operation has a 50% failure rate. (2) Some patients are made worse by this surgery. (3) Even if hymenal excision does control the symptoms of burning and pain, the cosmetic appearance can be distressing. Hence, various lasers have been tried, as a means of developing a more reliable, less mutilating first step.

In 1987, several patients with intractable vestibular vessel pain were successfully treated with an argon laser (Figure 12.14(b)) (Reid et al., 1988). However, because the long, slow pulses of blue-green argon light exhibit poor specifity for hemoglobin, this therapy produced extreme morbidity. Damage to adjacent stroma was almost as extensive as damage to the ectatic vessels. The following year, a protocol was initiated using a flash-pumped dye laser (a revolutionary instrument emitting ultrashort pulses of highly specific yellow light). The affinity of this laser beam for hemoglobin is such that extensive fields of subcutaneous vessels can be selectively coagulated, with negligible injury to the overlying epithelium. After an 18-month trial, 55% of patients were controlled by a single treatment, rising to 95% with additional treatment. Significantly, success rates of flash-pumped dye laser therapy paralleled physical findings, falling from 76% in those with just acetowhite epithelium or vascular ectasia, through 64% in those with painful red gland openings, down to just 5% in those with Bartholin's gland involvement (Table 12.5). Fortunately, 93% of the women with deep Bartholin's pain have responded to microsurgical resection of these glands.

NONSPECIFIC TREATMENT OF CHRONIC PAIN SYNDROMES

There are several nonspecific approaches to chronic pain syndromes, including selected medications, hormonal manipulation, surgery, individual psychotherapy, group therapy, biofeedback, and relaxation therapy. For the purpose of brevity, only drug therapy will be further discussed in this chapter.

When all specific therapies have failed, one may resort to several nonspecific medications. Each drug is given an adequate therapeutic trial, paying strict attention to risk-benefit analysis before each step. Although chronic pain patients will have tried multiple therapies previously, many are still searching for "an easy answer." Such patients are often inclined to give up too early in a pharmacologic trial. Hence, the con-

Table 12.5. Influence of Disease Pattern on Response Rates to Flashlamp-Excited Dye Laser Surgery

CLINICAL SEVERITY	INITIAL OUTCOME			
	SUCCESS	PARTIAL RESPONSE	FAILURE	TOTAL
Group A (colposcopic signs, limited to surface)	40 (74.1%)	9 (16.7%)	5 (9.3%)	54
Group B (macroscopic painful erythema, no deep pain)	32 (59.3%)	9 (16.7%)	13 (24.1%)	54
Group C (deep pain in Bartholin's glands)	3 (7.9%)	10 (26.3%)	25 (65.8%)	38
TOTAL	75	28	43	146

Overall comparison (Group A vs. Group B vs. Group C): $X^2 = 46.46$; $P < 0.0001$

Group A vs. Group B: $X^2 = 4.44$; not significant

Groups A & B vs. Group C: $X^2 = 43.30$; $P < 0.0001$

cept of an adequate trial of therapy (four to six weeks at full dose) and the importance of compliance must be explained to the patient and family.

Nonsteroidal Antiinflammatory Drugs

Nonsteroidal antiinflammatory drugs (NSAIDs) are a heterogenous group of drugs, all of which act by blocking biosynthetic enzymes involved in the formation of prostaglandins and eiocosanoids. Hence, by inhibiting the production of noxious chemicals, these drugs act as peripheral analgesics. NSAIDs are efficacious only for pain mediated by increased peripheral concentrations of prostaglandins, such as follows tissue injury or acute inflammation.

Although tolerance and physical dependence do not occur with NSAIDs, dosage shows a definite ceiling. Increasing dosage beyond that point cannot improve therapeutic efficacy but does significantly increase toxicity. Hence, each agent must be given an adequate trial, increasing the dosage to maximum levels while looking for either adequate pain control or unacceptable side effects. Once intolerable side effects are noted or the maximum dosage is reached, the patient should be switched to another chemical class of NSAIDs.

Available Agents

Principal pharmacologic classes of NSAIDs are as follows:

Carboxylic acids.

1. Acetylsalicylic acid (aspirin) is the most commonly used and least expensive NSAID. After aspirin, the next most commonly prescribed NSAIDs come from the other carboxilylic acids.
2. Propionic acids, including ibuprofin (Motrin), naproxen (Naprosyn), and ketoprofen (Orudis), are the best general first choice.
3. Acetic acids, including indomethacin (Indocin), sulindac (Clinoral), and tolmetin (Tolectin)

are also frequently effective. Most of these agents are often poorly tolerated and are best reserved as a second choice. However, ketorolac (Toradol), a new agent in this class, can be given parenterally. Toradol 60 mg Im is superior to 6 mg of morphine, but equipotent to 12 mg (O'Hara et al., 1987).

4. Anthranitic acids: Mefanamic acid (Ponstel) and meclofenamate (Meclomen) are a novel group of prostaglandin synthetase inhibitors that can be used in short courses, not to exceed one week. Although anthranitic acids are reasonably effective for primary dysmenorrhea, the frequency of such side effects as diarrhea, skin rash, elevation of blood urea nitrogen, and bone marrow depression nullify their potential clinical advantage (Halpern, 1989).

Oxicams. Piroxicam (Feldene) is a potent prostaglandin inhibitor, the main advantage of which is once-a-day dosing. Although chemically unrelated to carboxylic acids, piroxicam has similar side effects.

Pyrazoles. Penylbutazone is a derivative of phenacetin, which is used only for acute exacerbations of gout, tendinitis, or rheumatoid arthritis. Phenylbutazone (Butazolidine) should be given only for short periods of time (one week or less), because of the potential for significant side effects, including aplastic anemia, granulocytosis, nausea, vomiting, skin rashes, and sodium retention.

Side Effects

Gastrointestinal. All NSAIDs can cause GI distress, including nausea, dyspepsia, epigastric pain, superficial gastric erosions, bleeding, constipation, and diarrhea. Elderly patients seem to be at increased risk. In general, aspirin and indomethacin are less well tolerated than ibuprofen or naproxen.

Hematologic. All NSAIDs decrease thromboxane B2 biosynthesis, thereby inhibiting platelet aggregation and potentially prolonging bleeding time. Consequently, surgical hemostatasis is more difficult, and spontaneous gastrointestinal hemorrhage may occur. Aspirin inhibits platelet function in an irreversible, noncompetitive manner, lasting for the life span of that generation of platelets (approximately one week). Other NSAIDs inhibit platelet function in a competitive manner, such that platelet function will return to almost normal as serum concentrations decrease. Certainly, all patients taking NSAIDs should be instructed to contact their physician if significant gastrointestinal distress is noted or if blood is seen in the stool. In addition to this bleeding diathesis secondary to impaired platelet function, NSAIDs can also cause significant bone marrow depression (albeit rarely).

Renal. Chronic consumption of large doses of NSAIDs may lead to necrosis of the renal papilla or chronic interstitial nephritis. Such renal toxicity is thought to result from disruption of the normal prostaglandin control over renal circulation. Initially, these disorders may be detected by recognizing protein uria, renal casts, and a decreased ability to concentrate the urine. If damage continues unchecked, chronic renal failure will ensue.

Miscellaneous. NSAIDs can sometimes cause such nuisance side effects as skin rash, pruritus, headaches, tinnitus, and peripheral edema.

Antidepressants

Antidepressants are a second class of drugs commonly prescribed in chronic, nonspecific pain syndromes. Again, the risk-benefit ratio must be carefully assessed; the physician must be familiar with the chosen drug; and the dosage must be adjusted to ensure an adequate trial.

Mechanisms of Action

The mechanism by which antidepressants improve chronic pain is controversial. Correcting any affective component may produce an overall measure of pain relief. However, regimens used for chronic pain syndromes are typically just a fraction (often only 5–10%) of doses prescribed in depression. Hence, a more likely explanation is that antidepressants exert some kind of peripheral analgesic or local anaesthetic effect (Finemann et al., 1984; Finemann, 1985). Many investigators feel that chronic pain is secondary to biochemical abnormalities within the CNS, such as low brain serotonin or norepinephrine levels. Antidepressant drugs block the uptake of serotonin, norepinephrine, and dopamine from the central nervous system. It is thought that, by increasing brain concentrations of these chemicals, antidepressant drug therapy may enhance down-regulation at a number of pain-modulating sites. Moreover, increased brain serotonin levels may potentiate the action of endogenous systemic endorphins and enkephalins on the opioid receptors in the dorsal horn of the spinal cord (Finemann, 1985).

Though indications remain somewhat controversial, clinical experience has shown that many chronic pain patients will benefit from a trial of antidepressants. Favorable indicators are (1) a history that either pain or depression previously responded to antidepressants; (2) such associated endogenous symptoms as anorexia, early-morning wakening, psychomotor changes and anhedonia; and (3) pain syndromes of either musculoskeletal or neuralgic origin.

Most physicians should become familiar with and restrict themselves to the use of two or three antidepressants. Although there is little scientific evidence to recommend one drug over another, amitriptyline (Elavil) remains the most commonly prescribed formulation. There have been occasional reports of efficacy with the monoamine oxidase inhibitors (MAOIs). However, the potential for serious adverse side effects mandate that MAOIs be reserved for rare, complex patients and that they be prescribed only by physicians experienced in their use.

Dosage Schedules

Side effects can be significant, so dosage should start low and gradually increase until either intolerable side effects are noted or pain control is achieved. If an adequate dose (equivalent to 75–150 mg of amitriptyline per day) has been taken for four to six weeks without benefit, another agent from a different class should be tried (Finemann et al., 1984; Finemann, 1985; Sternbauch, 1976; Monks & Merskey, 1984). If the drug is found to be effective, our general plan is to continue treatment for at least six months. However, some patients may need very low doses of the antidepressant for even longer periods (i.e., 1–2 years) in order to control their chronic pain syndrome. Because mild withdrawal reactions (e.g., headache, diarrhea, unusual dreams) can occur, tricyclic antidepressants should be discontinued over a three-to-four-week period.

The main side effects of tricyclic antidepressants are sedation, orthostatic hypotension and anticholinergic effects (dry mouth, palpitations, blurred vision, constipation, and occasionally peripheral edema). More serious side effects include impotence, delirium, urinary retention, and exacerbation of narrow-angle glaucoma. Weight gain, hypersensitivity, and potentiation of other centrally acting drugs may also occur.

Anticonvulsants

A trial of anticonvulsants may be indicated for any pain thought to be neuralgic in origin. Classically, such syndromes are unilateral and often triggered by light touch over the affected area. Other neuralgic pains are atypical, presenting with a prominent continuous burning, aching, or throbbing component. However, even the atypical neuralgias tend to be distributed within an area innervated by a specific peripheral nerve. The most commonly used anticonvulsant is carbamazepine (Tegretol), but phenytoin (Dilantin) or baclofen (Lioresal) are sometimes tried.

Carbamazepine therapy must be started at a relatively low dose, such as 100 mg twice a day, and increased by 100 or 200 mg until either relief occurs or significant side effects are noted. Maintenance doses generally range around 400–800 mg per day, given in two to four doses. Once the pain has been adequately suppressed with this regimen for a number of weeks, the physician should attempt to decrease dosage gradually and then discontinue the agent (as described previously for tricyclic antidepressants).

Carbamazepine has a number of significant side effects, mainly involving the central nervous system and gastrointestinal tract. Patients commonly complain of drowsiness, dizziness, unsteadiness, nausea, and vomiting. These complaints may be seen at the initiation of drug therapy or as doses are escalated. There are case reports of serious bone marrow depression, as well as serious renal and hepatic dysfunction. Hence, prior to starting carbamazepine, the physician should obtain a complete blood count, together with liver and renal chemistries. These laboratory studies should be repeated after two weeks and thereafter at six- to eight-week intervals. If abnormalities are noted, medication must be discontinued.

Dilantin is less effective than carbamazepine but has less serious side effects. The usual starting dose with Dilantin is 100 mg three times per day.

Baclofen can be used alone or in combination with carbamazepine when side effects are noted. An initial dose of baclofen is on the order of 5 mg three times per day, dosage being gradually increased until the patient is receiving 40–80 mg per day. Principal side effects are drowsiness, dizziness, and fatigue.

Mexiletine

Mexiletine is an orally absorbed analogue of the local anaesthetic lidocaine. Mexiletine probably works by inhibiting the spontaneous nerve impulses that are thought to characterize many chronic pain states. The recommended protocol is to commence at 150 mg daily for three days, increase to 300 mg daily for the next three days, and thereafter plateau daily dosage at approximately 10 mg per kilogram of body weight. The commonest toxicity is nausea and tremor. Both side effects tend to be dose-related and can be generally avoided by raising the dosage gradually.

Topical Capsaicin

Capsaicin (Zostrix, Axsain), is a recently released topical agent, first used for postherpetic neuralgia. Subsequent reports have also claimed benefit in a number of other pain syndromes, including vulvar vestibulitis (Freidrich, 1988). Capsaicin is thought to work by selectively decreasing the functional capacity of the C-fiber afferent relaying pain impulses from somatic or visceral tissues. Secondarily, capsaicin also decreases tissue concentrations of substance P and other neurotransmitters. Capsaicin must be applied three to four times per day in order to achieve significant pain relief, and therapy must continue for not less than two to four weeks before the effects of an adequate trial can be determined. When attempting to treat patients with capsaicin, the most significant problem is significant burning on initial application. This response generally subsides over three to seven days. Thereafter, capsaicin applications are not painful (Lynn, 1990).

SUMMARY AND CONCLUSIONS

The dualistic approach to chronic pain (distinguishing somatic from psychogenic elements) is hazardous at any anatomic site. However, diagnosing sexual dysfunction as purely physical or purely psychosomatic is somewhat analogous to jogging blindfolded through a minefield. Difficulties arise from all sides. First, many causes of sexual pain or discomfort are not easily seen at physical examination. At the very least, ruling out a subtle physical malady requires consultation with an expert gynecologist; under most circumstances, colposcopic or laparoscopic examinations are also required to complete an adequate diagnostic workup. Second, manifestations of anxiety, irritability, or sadness, resulting from long-term disruption of the woman's sexuality, are perfectly appropriate! Moreover, stress provoked by friction within a close relationship can exacerbate preexisting neurotic or depressive traits. Because of this intricate interplay between emotional and physical factors, health care professionals must be especially cautious about labeling patients with prominent secondary pain behavior and a negative (but cursory) examination as sexual malingerers.

With acute pain, the physician's primary objectives are to identify and treat the causes of injury—pain relief being an important but subordinate goal. As pain becomes chronic, the goals of therapy change from curative to rehabilitative. Since afferent impulses from the original injury are substantially regulated by spinal and central modulating systems, the prospects of cure through retreatment of the original injury tend to diminish. Certainly, physicians must balance declining success rates against the risk of superimposed iatrogenic injury. Accepting the definition that pain is an "unpleasant sensory and emotional experience" helps to reduce the patient's need to "shop" from physician to physician in order to legitimize her complaints. Instead, the patient must be persuaded that her caregivers recognize the devastating effects of chronic pain on all aspects of her life, and that exploring the emotional elements of her problem is an essential component in effective rehabilitation. When specific therapies have failed, several nonspecific therapies offer an excellent prospect of improving the patient's quality of life, especially when applied through a multidisciplinary clinic.

GLOSSARY

Adnexae: the uterine appendages; the ovaries, uterine tubes, and ligaments of the uterus

Aplastic anemia: a severe form of anemia, in which the bone marrow fails to produce adequate numbers of peripheral blood cells (red cells, white cells, and platelets)

Atelectasis: collapse of some of the alveoli (air sacs) in a portion of a lung, often occurring as a result of shallow chest expansion after surgery

Candidiasis: infection with a fungus of the species *Candida;* usually a superficial infection of the moist cutaneous areas of the body, such as the vagina

Climacteric age: menopausal age (45–55 years)

Cloaca: termination of the hindgut, vagina, and urinary tract at a single orifice; during early intrauterine development, the human embryo goes through a cloacal stage, before having this common cavity subdivided into three distinctive compartments

Condylomas: fleshy papillomas (warts) affecting the mucous membranes or skin of the external genitals or in the perianal region; caused by a virus (HPV) that is infectious and linked to the causation of cervical and vulvar cancers

Depression: a psychobiological syndrome encompassing not only a sad mood or an inability to feel pleasure over a period of at least two weeks, but also a variety of vegetative symptoms involving disturbances in sleep, appetite, energy, concentration, and libido, and thoughts of death and suicide

Dermatome: the area of skin receiving sensory innervation from a single posterior spinal root

Diverticulum: A small pouch in the wall of the urethra or bowel

Dyschezia: difficult or painful evacuation of feces from the rectum

Dysmenorrhea: painful menstruation, generally subdivided as either primary or secondary

Ectasia: distension or prominence of small blood vessels

Epidural: the potential space between the inner and outer spinal membranes, that can be cannulated for repeated injections of analgesic medications over a period of days or weeks (see *Intrathecal*)

Erythema: redness of skin produced by congestion of the capillaries

Facultative pathogen: a microorganism normally present in the environment but capable of invading host tissues under specific conditions

Gastric stasis: a collection of gas and fluid in the stomach, due to interrupted bowel peristalsis

Granulocytosis: an abnormally large number of granulocytes (infection-fighting white corpuscles) in the bloodstream

Hydrosalpinx: A collection of watery fluid within a blocked dilated fallopian tube

Hyperemia: an excess of blood to a part, engorged

Hypoxemia: deficient oxygenation of the blood

Intestinal ileus: a collection of gas and fluid in the small intestines

Intraepithelial neoplasia: premalignant growth disorders within the epidermis of the cervix, vagina, vulva, or anus

Intrathecal: the fluid-filled space between the meninges and the spinal cord which can be used for direct injection of analgesic medications (e.g., as in a spinal anesthetic) (see *Epidural*)

Ischemia: insufficient blood flow, due to functional constriction or actual obstruction of a blood vessel

Menorrhagia: excessive uterine bleeding occuring at the regular intervals of menstruation

Myocutaneous flap: surgical creation of a flap (tube) of skin, fat, and muscle that can be used to repair a complicated defect

Oophorectomy: the removal of the ovary or ovaries

Pain attacks: episodic attacks of anxiety, generally unexpected and rapidly escalating, with such somatic symptoms as palpitations, shortness of breath, dizziness, nausea, and paresthesias

Papillomaviruses (HPVs): a group of species and site-specific DNA viruses that produce a variety of epithelial proliferations (warts), a small proportion of which can be premalignant

Pneumonitis: inflammation of the lungs

Prolapse: displacement of the uterus or vaginal walls, such that these structures may protrude outside the orifice

Pruritis: itching, an unpleasant cutaneous sensation that provokes the desire to rub or scratch the skin to obtain relief

Salpingo-oophoritis: inflammation of the tube and ovary

Septa: a dividing wall or partition

Stroma: the supporting tissue (matrix) of an organ, as distinguished from its functional element

TENS unit (transcutaneous electrical nerve stimulator): a low-voltage electrical device that can relieve surface pain by intense local stimulation of cutaneous touch receptors, thereby closing the spinal "gate"

Tinnitus: a noise in the ears, such as ringing, buzzing, roaring, clicking, etc.

Varicosities: varicose veins

REFERENCES

Allen, W. M., & Masters, W. H. (1955). Traumatic lacerations of uterine support. *American Journal of Obstetrics and Gynecology, 70,* 500.

Bachman, G. A., Leiblum, S. R., & Grill, J. (1989). Brief sexual inquiry in gynecologic practice. *Obstetrics and Gynecology, 73,* 425.

Bonica, J. J. (1953). *Management of pain.* Philadelphia: Lea & Febiger.

Bonica, J. J. (1983). IASP Presidential Address— Pain research and therapy: Achievements of the past and challenges of the future. In J. J. Bonica, U. Lindblom, & A. Iggo (Eds.), *Advances in pain research and therapy* (vol. 5, pp. 1–36). New York: Raven Press.

Bonica, J. J. (1987). Importance of effective pain control. *Acta Anaesthesiologica Scandinavia, 85,* S1–S16.

Cunanan, R. G., Courey, N. G., & Lippes, J. (1983). Laparoscopic findings in patients with pelvic pain. *American Journal of Obstetrics and Gynecology, 146,* 589.

Dejard, A., Peterson, P., & Kastrup, J. (1988). Mexiletine for treatment of chronic painful diabetic neuropathy. *Lancet, 1,* 9–11.

Ettinger, B. (1990). Hormonal replacement therapy and coronary heart disease. *Obstetric and Gynecologic Clinics of North America, 17,* 741–758.

Finemann, C. M. (1985). Pain relief by antidepressants: Possible modes of action. *Pain, 23,* 1–8.

Finemann, C. M., Harris, M., & Cawley, R. (1984). Psychogenic pain: Presentation and treatment. *British Medical Journal, 28,* 436–438.

Freidrich, E. G., Jr. (1983). The vulvar vestibule. *Journal of Reproductive Medicine, 28,* 773.

Freidrich, E. G., Jr. (1987). Vulvar vestibulitis syndrome. *Journal of Reproductive Medicine, 32,* 110.

Freidrich, E. G. (1988). Therapeutic studies on vulvar vestibulitis. *Journal of Reproductive Medicine, 33,* 514–518.

Halpern, L. M. (1989). Analgesic and anti-inflammatory medications. In C. D. Tollisond (Ed.), *Handbook of chronic pain management* (p. 58). Baltimore: Williams and Wilkins.

Huskisson, E. C. (1983). Visual analogue scales. In R. Melzack (Ed.), *Pain measurement and management* (pp. 33–37). New York: Raven Press.

Kehlet, H. (1986). Pain relief and modification of the stress response. In M. J. Cousins & G. D. Phillips (Eds.), *Acute pain management* (p. 49). New York: Churchill Livingstone.

LaMotte, C. C. (1986). Organization of dorsal horn neurotransmitter systems. In T. L. Yaksh (Ed.), *Spinal afferent processing* (p. 97). New York: Plenum.

Leiblum, S. R., Bachmann, G. A., Kemmann, E., et al. (1983). Vaginal atrophy in the postmenopausal woman. The importance of sexual activity and hormones. *Journal of the American Medical Association, 249,* 2195.

Lynn, B. (1990). Capsaicin: Actions on nociceptive C fibers and therapeutic potential. *Pain, 41,* 61–69.

McKay, M. (1989). Vulvodynia. A multifactorial clinical problem. *Archives of Dermatology, 125,* 256–262.

Melzack, R. (1983). The McGill Pain Questionnaire. In R. Melzack (Ed.), *Pain management and assessment* (pp. 41–47). New York: Raven Press.

Melzack, R., & Wall, P. D. (1965). Pain mechanisms: A new theory. *Science, 150,* 971–979.

Melzack, R., & Wall, P. D. (1982). *The challenge of pain.* New York: Basic Books.

Mims, B. C. (1989). Sociologic and cultural aspects of pain. In C. D. Tollison (Ed.), *Handbook of chronic pain management* (pp. 17–25). Baltimore: Williams and Wilkins.

Monks, R., & Merskey, H. (1984). Psychotropic drugs. In P. D. Wall & R. D. Melzack (Eds.), *Textbook of pain* (pp. 526–537). London: Churchill Livingstone.

O'Hara, D. A., Fragen, R. J., Kinzer, M., & Pemberton, D. (1987). Ketorolac tromethamine as compared with morphine sulfate for treatment of postoperative pain. *Clinical Pharmacological Therapy, 41*(5), 556–561.

Pearl, E. R. (1976). Sensitization of nociceptors in its relation to sensation. In J. J. Bonica & D. Aob-Fessard (Eds.), *Advances in pain research and therapy* (vol. 1, p. 17). New York: Raven Press.

Peck, C. L., & Cowan, P. (1986). Psychological factors in acute pain management. In M. J. Cousins & G. D. Phillips (Eds.), *Acute pain management* (p. 251). New York: Churchill Livingstone.

Pilowsky, I. (1986). Psychodynamic aspects of the pain experience. In R. A. Sternbauch (Ed.), *The psychology of pain* (2nd ed., pp. 181–195). New York: Raven Press.

Pilowsky, I., & Spence, M. D. (1976). Illness behaviour syndromes associated with intractable pain. *Pain, 2,* 61–71.

Prescott, L. F., Clements, J. A., & Pottage, A. (1977). Absorption, distribution and elimination of mexiletine. *Postgraduate Medicine Journal, 53,* 50–55.

Raja, S. N., Meyer, R. A., & Campbell, J. N. (1988). Peripheral mechanisms of somatic pain. *Anesthesiology, 68,* 571–590.

Reid, R. (1989). Human papillomavirus associated diseases of the lower genital tract: Implications for the laser surgeon. In W. Keye (Ed.), *Laser surgery in gynecology* (2nd ed., pp. 46–99). Chicago: Yearbook Publishers.

Reid, R., & Dorsey, J. (1991). Physical and surgical principles of carbon dioxide laser surgery in the lower genital tract. In M. Coppleson & J.

Monaghan (Eds.), *Gynecologic oncology* (2nd ed., pp. 1093–1137). New York: Churchill Livingstone.

Reid, R., Greenberg, M., Daoud, Y., et al. (1988). Colposcopic findings in women with vulvar pain syndromes. *Journal of Reproductive Medicine, 33,* 523.

Skene, A. J. C. (1889). *Treatise on the diseases of women.* New York: Appleton.

Sobel, J. (1990). Vaginitis in adult women. *Obstetric and Gynecologic Clinics of North America, 17,* 851–881.

Stenchever, M. A. (1987). Significant symptoms and signs in different age groups. In W. Droegemueller, A. L. Herbst, D. R. Mishell, & M. A. Stenchever (Eds.), *Comprehensive gynecology* (pp. 156–159). St. Louis: Mosby.

Sternbauch, R. (1976). The need for an animal model of chronic pain. *Pain, 2,* 2–4.

Sullivan, M., Turner, J. A., & Romano, J. (1991). Chronic pain in primary care. Identification and management of psychosocial factors. *Journal of Family Practice, 32,* 193–199.

Taylor, H. C. (1949a). Vascular congestion and hyperemia. I. Physiologic basis in history of the concept. *American Journal of Obstetrics and Gynecology, 57,* 211.

Taylor, H. C. (1949b). Vascular congestion and hyperemia. II. The clinical aspects of congestion-fibrosis syndrome. *American Journal of Obstetrics and Gynecology, 57,* 637.

Wallis, L. A. (1987). Management of dyspareunia in post-menopausal women. *Journal of the American Medical Association, 42,* 82.

Westrom, L. (1980). Incidence, prevalence and trends of acute pelvic inflammatory disease and its consequences in industrialized countries. *American Journal of Obstetrics and Gynecology, 138,* 888.

Willis, W. D., Jr. (1985). The pain system: The neural basis of nociceptive transmission in the mammalian nervous system. In P. L. Gildenberg (Ed.), *Pain and headache.*

Woodruff, J. D., & Parmley, T. H. (1983). Infection of the minor vestibular gland. *Obstetrics and Gynecology, 62,* 609.

Yaksh, T. L. (1988). Neurologic mechanisms of pain. In M. J. Cousins & P. O. Bridenbaugh (Eds.), *Clinical anesthesia and management of pain* (2nd ed., p. 791). Philadelphia: Lippincott.

CHAPTER 13

DYSPAREUNIA

Randal P. Quevillon, University of South Dakota

A recurrent pattern of genital pain before, during or immediately after coitus is the basis for the diagnosis of dyspareunia. This problem has an exceedingly long history; a detailed description of the symptoms can be found in an entry on the ancient Egyptian Raesseum Papyri IV scrolls (Fordney, 1978). The current edition of the *Diagnostic and Statistical Manual of Mental Disorders* (American Psychiatric Association, 1987) has included dyspareunia under the classification of sexual disorders—specifically, under the sexual pain disorders. This apparently will be maintained in the forthcoming edition of the DSM. Dyspareunia is defined as recurrent and persistent genital pain in either the male or female, associated with coitus. Additionally, the DSM-III-R criteria state that the problem cannot be caused exclusively by a lack of lubrication (a criterion for female sexual arousal disorder), or be due to vaginismus or another clinical syndrome. Dyspareunia is far more common in women than in men (Masters & Johnson, 1970; Wabrek & Wabrek, 1974), and female dyspareu-nia is more likely to involve psychological factors than is male dyspareunia (Abarbanel, 1978).

Dyspareunia and vaginismus are often linked, and repeated dyspareunia is likely to result in vaginismus (Lamont, 1978). Vaginismus may also be a causative factor in dyspareunia (Spano & Lamont, 1975). The difference between vaginismus and dyspareunia is that intromission is generally painful in the latter condition but virtually impossible in vaginismic women due to the involuntary contraction of the muscles controlling the vaginal opening (Leiblum, Pervin, & Campbell, 1988). If vaginismus is present, concurrent dyspareunia is not considered to be worthy of a dual diagnosis, as any persistence or success with forced penile entry is invariably painful (Fordney, 1978). If vaginismus is the cause of dyspareunia, the primary diagnosis is vaginismus (Levay & Sharpe, 1981). Many women with dyspareunia are also anorgasmic as well, and for a significant number, the anorgasmia precedes the dyspareunia (Fink, 1972; Fordney-Settlage, 1975).

DESCRIPTION AND CLASSIFICATION

Dyspareunic pain has been described and classified in a variety of ways. Fink (1972) separates pain experienced at the vaginal outlet from pain felt on deep penetration. Similarly, pain experienced during intercourse is described in terms of pressure, aching, tearing, or burning, and it may have a wide range of intensities and durations. Fordney (1978) states that for some individuals, coital pain is slight and very transient, and for others it is mild enough not to interfere with desire, receptivity, or orgasm. Therefore, Fordney reserves the syndrome diagnosis for those cases in which pain is usually persistent and severe. Her definition excludes occasional dyspareunia caused by a lack of arousal and resultant lack of lubrication, prolonged coital contact, or any transient condition caused by infections. Several authors hypothesize that women who experience dyspareunic pain without organic involvement are unable to localize or describe the character of their pain specifically, so they report it as diffuse and typically not persisting following termination of coitus (Fink, 1972; Masters & Johnson, 1970).

Sandberg and Quevillon (1987) comment on the confusing history of efforts to define, describe, and classify dyspareunia. They cite several examples of classification terms being used in differing ways. For example, according to Lamont (1978), a British practice was to use the term *dyspareunia* to label organically caused coital pain and *vaginismus* to denote all painful coitus that had no organic etiology (as opposed to the usages outlined above). This tradition of terminological confusion continues. Sarrel and Sarrel (1989) describe vaginismus as a subcategory of dyspareunia (in contrast to the DSM-III-R) and state that "dyspareunia not the result of vaginismus can almost always be traced to a specific physical cause or to total lack of sexual arousal" (p. 2291). They assert that two of the case examples cited by Lazarus (1980) in his chapter on dyspareunia might instead be cases of vaginismus (Sarrel & Sarrel, 1989).

Various systems have been used to delineate dyspareunia. Worchester (1955) used the terms *primary* and *secondary* to denote physical and psychological etiology, respectively. On the other hand, Hartnell (cited in Harlow, 1969) considered the terms quite differently: *primary* usually becoming manifest immediately after marriage and *secondary* appearing some years later (frequently after the birth of one or more children). Spano and Lamont (1975) used the term *primary* when penetration has always been painful and *secondary* when the onset of painful intercourse follows previously comfortable intromission.

Brant (1978) distinguishes superficial dyspareunia as stemming from a failure of vaginal relaxation and ballooning, which can occur intermittently. Currently, the general categorization of the term *superficial* denotes pain perceived at or near the introitus or vaginal barrel, and *deep* as located at the cervix or lower abdominal area (Fink, 1972; Fordney-Settlage, 1975).

Given this lack of consistency in term usage, the subclassification of sexual diagnoses utilized in the DSM-III-R provides a somewhat more comprehensive framework from which to assess and diagnose dyspareunia. The symptom can be described as primary or secondary and as complete or situational. *Primary* is defined as existing throughout the sexual lifetime of the individual, whereas a secondary symptom is one that develops after a significant symptom-free period. *Complete* means that the symptom is present under all circumstances rather than occurring selectively with specific situations (such as one particular partner, a type of stimulation, or other external variables). By definition, dyspareunia is restricted to coital activity (as a type of stimulation). Since more than one sexual dysfunction frequently occurs in the same individual (Kaplan, 1974; Masters & Johnson, 1970), the arrangement of these disorders by subclassification and relative time of onset can be extremely useful in providing clues to etiology and guiding the appropriate treatment (Fordney, 1978).

PREVALENCE AND ASSOCIATED FEATURES

Precise statistics regarding the incidence of dyspareunia are not available. Although some studies have recently become available (e.g., Glatt, Zinner, & McCormack, 1990), most statements are made from clinical experience. For example, Brant (1978) notes that the complaint of dyspareunia is an extremely common clinical presentation. Kaplan (1974) and Masters and Johnson (1970) report that next to anorgasmia, dyspareunia is the most frequently occurring sexual dysfunction among women. Lamont (1978) points out that probably every sexually active woman has had occasional dyspareunia, so the incidence of the isolated symptom might be said to be universal. Fordney-Settlage (1975) reports that in women of lower socioeconomic class, with a non-European white racial background, dyspareunia is a more disabling dysfunction than anorgasmia (cf. Davis, 1991). Fordney (1978) points out that women with fewer resources may live with the absence of orgasm without requesting treatment, but in the presence of pain that seriously alters their ability to engage in sexual behavior, they will seek assistance.

Despite being one of the most common sexual dysfunctions, dyspareunia has not been sufficiently studied to allow for a confident estimate of its prevalence. In their review of incidence and prevalence studies of sexual dysfunctions, Spector and Carey (1990) suggest that dyspareunia is a less common presenting problem at sex clinics than either arousal-phase disorders or orgasm-phase sexual dysfunctions. They go on to suggest, however, that the (albeit sparse) community prevalence data place the rates of dyspareunia noticeably higher in the general population, possibly because women may view pain as a medical symptom and are more likely to seek help from health professionals than sex therapists.

Certainly, a common complaint of women seeking gynecological services is coital pain. For example, 20 of the 98 sexually active women sampled by Plouffe (1985), from among women presenting to the gynecological wards of two university hospitals, had deep dyspareunia as a prominent complaint. Of these women, 35% defined their dyspareunia as a problem but sought no medical remedy, while the remaining 65% were asking for treatment. In another study, Bachman, Leiblum, and Grill (1989) found that out of 887 consecutive outpatient referrals for gynecologic evaluation, 83 women (9%) complained of dyspareunia—two-thirds insertional and one-third deep dyspareunia. Additionally, studies using patient tallies suggest that physicians across varied specialties frequently see individuals suffering from dyspareunia (Burnap & Golden, 1967; Frank, 1948).

Dyspareunia may be even more prevalent, however, owing to a high number of individuals who simply do not report their symptoms to any professional. In fact, the majority of women might fit a definition of dyspareunia broad enohug to include any instance of painful intercourse. A recent survey by Glatt et al. (1990) found a 61% overall rate of dyspareunia among 313 women responding to their survey. They sent questionnaires to a cohort of 428 women, mostly in their 30s, who had been part of a mid-1970s study on STDs (McCormack et al., 1981). This sample was composed of women presenting for any reason to a university student health service. Glatt et al. had kept in touch with most of the original sample and recontacted them for their 1990 survey. Of the 313 responders who had ever engaged in heterosexual intercourse, 105 (33.5%) reported current (persistent) dyspareunia. They categorized their persistent dyspareunia as follows: only on initial penetration (33 women), throughout intercourse (36 women), and only after intercourse (25 women). Eleven women either did not answer the question or were not able to be categorized (Glatt et al., 1990). For one-third of these women, the pain was diffuse or not localizable. About one-quarter each localized their pain either deep in the pelvis or in the vagina; 14 of the 105 reported introital pain; and three described a urethral or bladder location. Twenty-five women stated that they had pain only with certain partners; 29 reported discomfort across partners; and 46 reported having only one sexual partner since onset. Also noteworthy is the fact that only about 40% had sought professional medical assistance for their symptoms, and only a similar percent reported ever being asked about dyspareunia by their health care providers. One-half of these persistent dyspareunia sufferers did not know of any measures that could be used to alleviate their pain, and the half that did tended to get their relief by using natural or artificial lubrication (Glatt et al., 1990).

In addition to the 105 persistent sufferers, 86 other women reported primary or secondary dyspareunia that had resolved spontaneously or with treatment. The 39 instances of successful therapy were not described in the Glatt et al. (1990) report. Of the 105 persistent dyspareunia sufferers, only about one-third of those who sought medical/health care assistance received a specific diagnosis or any therapeutic benefit whatever.

RISK FACTORS

Several factors (sexual abuse history, drinking behavior, pregnancy and postpartum status, advanced age, and marital distress) have been hypothesized to increase the risk for sexual dysfunctions in general and dyspareunia in particular. Although the data are sparse, some relevant work has been reported.

Rape and incest victims have been shown to have an elevated rate of sexual dysfunctions generally, but the implications for dyspareunia are not as clear (Becker & Skinner, 1983). More studies are clearly needed, but sufficient anecdotal support exists to hypothesize that sexual abuse is one etiological factor.

Patterns of alcohol consumption, especially problem drinking and alcoholism, have been associated with high rates of sexual dysfunctions (Wilsnack, 1984). However, the best test, to date, of this association has come in the national survey reported by Klassen and Wilsnack (1986). Of the 917 respondents, 36% endorsed the item "Sexual relations have sometimes been

physically painful for me," and 177 endorsed "Sexual relations have sometimes been so painful I could not have intercourse" (p. 388). This does support a high overall incidence rate for dyspareunia, but the hypothesized relationship to drinking rates was not found. Thus, the jury is still out, but further study is warranted—especially in light of the effects of alcohol on arousal (Wilson & Lawson, 1978).

Older individuals appear to have a heightened risk of several sexual dysfunctions, including dyspareunia (Dagon, 1983). Several factors impinge on older persons including biological changes and health status as well as psychological and sociocultural factors. In particular, menopause has been associated with dyspareunia, due not only to the sequelae of changes in estrogen level but also to psychosocial problems (Sarrel & Whitehead, 1985). In the Bachman et al. (1989) survey, being over 50 years of age was associated with a significantly higher risk of dyspareunia.

Pregnancy, delivery events, postpartum factors, and abortion complications have been discussed as risk factors (Bachmann, 1986; Heisterberg, Hebjorn, Anderson & Petersen, 1986; Reamy and White, 1987). The episiotomy has received particular attention, since two-thirds of United States deliveries include this procedure, making it the second most common surgery after the cutting of the umbilical cord (Reamy & White, 1987).

Finally, factors such as marital strain, high individual levels of anxiety and/or depression, and personality problems can make dyspareunia more likely (Fordney, 1978; Lazarus, 1988; Wabrek & Wabrek, 1974). Case histories and anecdotes constitute most of the support for these variables in their influence on baseline rates of dyspareunia, and much more empirical work is needed.

In sum, the relatively low rates of dyspareunia in sex clinics (e.g., Renshaw, 1988) seem likely to be an artifact of referral patterns. More research is needed on incidence and prevalence, but the probable rates of this symptom make it among the most common sexual dysfunctions for women. The influence of several putative risk factors on dyspareunia rates, including those mentioned here, awaits further explication.

ETIOLOGY

The etiology of dyspareunia has traditionally been divided into two classes: organic and psychogenic (Spano & Lamont, 1975). The gynecologic literature on dyspareunia has tended to discuss conditions that could be treated medically or surgically; conversely, behavioral scientists and practitioners have expounded on the psychogenic causes of the syndrome (Lamont, 1980). Despite the fact that dyspareunia is a very common referral problem, and that gynecologists are frequently called upon by referring mental health professionals to rule out organic causes in dyspareunia, Grillo and Grillo (1980) state that most residency programs are woefully inadequate in this area of gynecology, and standard texts rarely devote even minimal attention to the disorder. Fink (1972) also comments on the existing gap between gynecologists and psychological science and stresses that it is essential to have an understanding of both organic and psychological causality in painful intercourse.

The literature presents dichotomous viewpoints. Organic pathology and psychological variables are alternatively proposed as the major factors in the causality of dyspareunia. As an illustration, two articles represent the poles. Huffman (1976) contends psychogenic dyspareunia is relatively uncommon; on the other hand, Spano and Lamont (1975) state that organic factors underlying dyspareunia are usually temporary, easily correctible, and rarely the cause of a continuing problem. Clearly, there is a need to integrate existing data and bring together the divergent viewpoints (Sandberg & Quevillon, 1987).

Dyspareunia is the only sexual dysfunction in which there is presumed to be a high incidence of physical disease etiology or association (Fordney, 1978). Among the physical factors commonly cited as causes of dyspareunia are a rigid hymen, painful hymenal tags, endometriosis, senile atrophy of the vagina, relaxation of the supporting uterine ligaments, pelvic tumors, pelvic inflammatory diseases, childbirth pathologies, stenosis of the vagina, and hemorrhoids (Kaplan, 1974). Imperforate and abnormally fibrous hymen and hymenal rings and remnants have been found to be a physical cause as well (Grillo & Grillo, 1980). Fink (1972) adds to the list episiotomy scars, Bartholin's gland inflammations, clitoral inflammation and adhesions, lesions of the vulva, a variety of vaginal infections, radiation vaginitis, iatrogenic causes, and allergic reactions to contraceptive and douching materials. Spano and Lamont (1975) report that many complaints of dyspareunia are caused by irritation from substances that the individual self-administers, such as feminine hygiene deodorants or restrictive clothing. They additionally contend that feminine hygiene products are unnecessary and may be damaging. Other possible organic causes of dyspareunia include trauma, irradiation of tumors, cystitis, constipation, proctitis, and ectopic pregnancy (Lamont, 1974).

Fordney (1978) points out that dyspareunia is not a constant symptom of any one pelvic disease, as there are well-recorded instances of extensive disease in which dyspareunia was conspicuously absent from the symptom complex. She reports that most women seeking treatment for dyspareunia have experienced chronic pain (two to six years in her sample), and that the presence of subtle or missed physical factors is common in women who have long-standing dyspareunia yet have been considered to be gynecologically normal. Wabrek and Wabrek (1975) stress that although it is difficult for gynecologists to determine whether the causality of a woman's dyspareunia is organic or functional, no woman should be labeled as having psychogenic dyspareunia without a thorough, extensive gynecological evaluation.

Many authors cite insufficient vaginal lubrication as a major causal factor in dyspareunia (Brant, 1978; Hastings, 1971; Masters & Johnson, 1970; Spano & Lamont, 1975). Insufficient lubrication may be a constant phenomenon or more situational in nature; it may be related to lack of interest, fear of pregnancy or loss of control, pain, minimal foreplay, or anger at the male partner (Wabrek & Wabrek, 1975). Anxiety has been implicated in the etiology of dyspareunia as a result of its interfering effect on lubrication, which can lead to pain, burning, itching, and aching during and following intercourse (Annon, 1976; Masters & Johnson, 1970). The female sexual response cycle includes vasocongestion and neuromuscular excitation, which produces lubrication of the vagina and erection of the clitoris, resulting in vaginal expansion and elevation of the uterus (Kaplan, 1974; Masters & Johnson, 1970). Spano and Lamont (1975) maintain that each of these steps is necessary if penetration is to be accomplished without pain being experienced. The DSM-III-R assigns lack of lubrication as a diagnostic criterion for female sexual arousal disorder and excludes it in the diagnosis of dyspareunia. Fordney (1978) states that in 60–70% of the cases of long-standing dyspareunia, organic factors cannot be identified. If no physical factors can be found after a thorough gynecological evaluation and the complaint of discomfort persists, dyspareunia is then often regarded solely as a symptom of underlying psychosexual dysfunction, and a diagnosis of psychogenic origin must be made (Lazarus, 1980).

Psychological theories about the causes of dyspareunia propose a number of factors, including fear-anxiety conflicts, phobic reactions, conversion reaction, and hostility toward sexual partners (Fink, 1972; Masters & Johnson, 1970; O'Connor, 1980). Psychoanalytic theory considers dyspareunia as constituting an hysterical or conversion symptom, conceptualized as the symbolic expression of a specific unconscious intrapsychic conflict (Kaplan, 1974). Learning theory, on the other hand, relates the development of the dyspareunic response to lack of learning or faulty learning; it is hypothesized that a dysfunctional pattern is reinforced with each succeeding sexual contact (Sotile & Kilman, 1977).

Lazarus (1988) contends that dyspareunia should not be viewed as a unitary disturbance, as it involves a broad spectrum of personalistic and idiosyncratic variables. Individual causes should be sought in specific cases, and treatments should be individualized as well. More generally, the DSM-III-R states that any negative attitude toward sexuality due to particular experiences, internal conflicts, or adherence to rigid subcultural values can predispose an individual to psychosexual dysfunction. Fear of pain or pregnancy and resulting aversion to coitus may have their origins in memories of distressing sexual experiences in childhood or adolescence or in the lessons of childhood (Huffman, 1976). Other significant contributing conditions include the presence of anxiety, depression, or self-esteem problems (Annon, 1976). Wabrek and Wabrek (1974) report that an anxiety response may be manifested in anticipation of pain during intercourse as a result of ignorance or misinformation. Kaplan (1974) reports on causes of psychogenic dyspareunia, including guilt about intercourse and erotic pleasure, fear of penetration, and anger at the partner. Masters and Johnson (1970) cite the residual aftereffects of associated psychological trauma resulting from rape as a cause of pain during intercourse.

A major variable in psychogenic dyspareunia involves the fundamental feelings and attitudes between sexual partners (Lazarus, 1988). Marital and communication problems are implicated in dyspareunia, as they are in many other forms of sexual dysfunction (Kaplan, 1974; Mira, 1988). Abarbanel (1978) reports that other psychological factors may be feelings of guilt, shame, or tension occasioned by new sexual situations, or inadequate foreplay contributing to a lack of arousal in the woman and ultimately resulting in insufficient lubrication and coital discomfort. Sexual issues, such as faulty information and intrapsychic problems, appear to be more prominent in primary dyspareunia, whereas relationship issues may be more important in secondary dyspareunia (Fordney-Settlage, 1975).

As long ago as 1931, Dickinson proposed an interesting conceptualization of dyspareunia that addressed both the organic and the psychogenic camps. He argued that physical dyspareunia is likely to be followed by psychic dyspareunia, as well as being often accompanied by it. This is due to the emotional trauma caused by the coital pain and by difficulties in intercourse. There is also reason to suspect that psychic dyspareunia may precede the physical in many cases. Psychic origins, such as anxiety or aversion, may take the form of physical pain, perhaps by a conversion process. In turn, these processes can lead to pain and avoidance, which can mask aversion; conversely, physical pain can be joined with psychological dissonance. Dickinson emphasized that although logical development is clearly difficult to establish in these cases, care should be taken to avoid one-way reasoning when the converse has an equal likelihood of proving to be true. Although some of the specifics of the model may be outdated, the attitude conveyed in Dickinson's argument still has validity. It clearly opposed to an either/or approach to the assessment and treatment of dyspareunia. Fink (1972) further strengthens this point of view by stressing that finding a physical cause for dyspareunic pain does not mean that all psychological matters can be set aside or considered solved.

Dickinson's discussion emphasizes careful evaluation of the emotional and psychological aspects of each case of dyspareunia, in addition to the physical. Although this conceptualization has been present in the literature for over 60 years, this balanced approach has been largely lacking in clinical and research reports. Authors have tended to align themselves with one side of the continuum, paying only lip service to alternative etiological factors. Everyone should give more genuine consideration to both organic and psychological factors in understanding cases of dyspareunia.

Implications

This review of organic and psychogenic causative factors in the development of dyspareunia suggests a general lack of agreement concerning the etiology of the disorder. Authors in both camps present factual and convincing arguments, but the singling out of organic or psychological causes is neither warranted nor essential; in fact, it could be counterproductive in many instances.

Practitioners from the medical and psychological communities should increase their level of awareness and expertise with regard to the complex factors involved in this syndrome. Heretofore rigid assumptions about the strict causality of this disorder appear to be erroneous and misinformed. I recommend approaching the problem in a stepwise fashion, emphasizing etiological factors as they are discovered. Viewing causality on a continuum from physical to psychogenic in nature, with the potential for both to be equal contributors to dyspareunic pain, more practical and efficacious than the either/or approach.

An integrated, rather than a dichotomous, view of dyspareunia, combined with better knowledge of all possible etiological factors (both organic and psychogenic) would enhance the chances for accurate assessment and appropriate treatment. Rather than medical and psychological professionals working at odds, there should be collaborative research efforts incorporating the knowledge and expertise of both disciplines. Additionally, reciprocal consultation and referral by physicians and mental health practitioners is essential in the approach I advocate.

ASSESSMENT

The assessment of dyspareunia is complicated by the complex and varied etiological picture and by the way in which individuals present for evaluation and treatment. First, women are likelier to seek help from their physicians or other medical health care workers than from sex therapists or psychologists (Spector & Carey, 1990). When they do seek help, many may not volunteer that dyspareunia is their concern. Only 3% of a sample of gynecology clinic outpatients spontaneously reported sexual concerns, whereas an additional 16% acknowledged sexual problems when specifically questioned (Bachman et al., 1989). The researchers simply asked two questions: "Are you sexually active?" and "Are you having sexual difficulties or problems at this time?" (p. 425), adding examples if needed. Of the 171 women with sexual problems, nearly half complained of vaginismus. Plouffe (1985) used essentially the same two questions to assess his sample of gynecology inpatients, but he added "Do you have any pain with intercourse?" (p. 167). Again, dyspareunia was by far the commonest sexual complaint. Unfortunately, though a few simple questions may fare quite well at eliciting information, the survey data of Glatt et al. (1990) suggest that these questions are asked less than half of the time. One obvious recommendation is that the relevant inquiries be made regarding sexual problems, and another is that both organic and psychogenic factors be thoroughly considered in each case (Sandberg & Quevillon, 1987).

A second limiting issue is the relative lack of measurement sophistication in this area. With the exception of several specific physical tests and biological assays, physical examination and psychological/behavioral assessment of dyspareunia leave much to be desired in specificity, generalizability, and cross-validation of validity (see Conte, 1983). What follows is a survey of current practices, recognizing the need for future refinement in this area.

Interviews

A staple of any assessment scheme for dyspareunia is a thorough interview, including a sexual history (Kaplan, 1974). Several outlines are available to guide the clinician (L. LoPiccolo & Heiman, 1978; Masters & Johnson, 1970). It is worth noting the caveat of Caird and Wincze (1977) that the intake interview may be quite intense for individuals unaccustomed to talking about intimate sexual behavior. They point out that compliance can be enhanced and anger diffused by carefully explaining the general purpose of the interview and the coverage areas as well as allowing the client (or clients) to express embarrassment or confusion.

Though interviews in this area have not been standardized and validated, they posses excellent bandwidth, flexibility, and opportunities for limited observation of nonverbal behavior. The interview can be tailored individually (see McConaghy, 1988), to detail dyspareunia symptoms but still allow for a range of other sexual and nonsexual data to be collected. Symptom chronology, impact, and prior attempts at solution should all be covered (see Steege, 1984). In addition, signs of anger, anxiety, or embarrassment can be observed— serving not only as another data source but also as a gauge of the client's willingness to proceed. Finally, the interview also presents opportunities to begin desensitizing the client to sexual content and to shape attitudes in a way consonant with therapeutic intent. Clinical sensitivity as well as cross-cultural sensitivity is at a premium (Davis, 1991; Wilkeson, Poussaint, Small, & Shapiro, 1983).

Paper-and-Pencil Measures

Available measures tend to have psychometric weaknesses (Conte, 1983), and many do not specifically address dyspareunia. One with the former but not the latter problem is the lengthy, multifaceted Sexual Adjustment Inventory by Stuart, Stuart, Maurice, and Szasz (1975). Similar in form to their better-known Marital Pre-Counseling Inventory (Stuart & Stuart, 1972), the SAI covers several areas and employs varied self-report styles, from Likert-type ratings to essays. Of direct relevance to dyspareunia assessment are an item requesting a percent rating for frequency of coital pain, as well as a health section that asks about present or past illnesses, medications, operations, genital infections, miscarriages or abortions, and drinking/drug use. Compliance may be a problem with the Sexual Adjustment Inventory; care must be taken so as not to embarrass or overwhelm the client while using it. It is recommended that the clinician at least begin the interview process first, to gain an impression as to whether or not the inventory would cause problems.

Another multiscale measure is the Derogatis Sexual Functioning Inventory (DSFI; Derogatis, 1980). This 261-item assessment tool yields a Global Sexual Satisfaction Index and 10 subtests: information, experience, drive, attitude, symptoms (general, not sexual), affects, role definition, fantasy, body image, and satisfaction. The DSFI produces much information, but none of the items bear directly on dyspareunia, and the clinical utility of the instrument has not yet been established with this population.

The Sexual Arousability Index (Hoon, Hoon, & Wincz, 1976) was designed to assess sexual arousal level in women by asking for projected arousal estimates in 28 erotic situations. The index is heuristically interesting, considering the findings of Caird and Wincze (1977) that anxiety reduction does not always lend to increases in arousal. Additionally, numerous clinical examples illustrate that high anxiety does not preclude sexual arousal (e.g., Resick & Quevillon, 1990). Despite its heuristic value, however, the fact that the SAI does not directly assess dyspareunia makes it a tenuous choice for clinical use.

The Sexual Interaction Inventory (SII; LoPiccolo & Steger, 1974) is a self-report scale of 17 heterosexual behaviors to which a couple responds separately on a series of six-point Likert-type scales. Of the resultant 11 scale scores, none directly assesses dyspareunia. As with the other scales, the SII does not fully meet the self-report assessment needs for comprehensive assessment of dyspareunia.

Physiological Assessment

Because of the interplay between psychological and physical features in dyspareunia, medical/gynecologic assessment is essential. The physical exam and gynecologic consultation should provide a thorough assessment of organic factors involved in the client's coital pain. Factors such as chronic pelvic infection, endometriosis, vulvovaginitis, estrogen deficiency, drug side effects, cancer, cystitis, and scarring must be carefully assessed (Abarbanel, 1978; Fordney, 1978; Huffman, 1983; Kaplan, 1979). Steege (1984) points out that, in addition to the obvious reason for conducting the physical exam, other

purposes can be served. These include illustrating for the dyspareunia sufferer that vaginal comfort is possible and that she might have a discernible success in lowering her own level of discomfort. Steege also employs a mirror in an effort to illustrate the conditioning basis for involuntary introital contractions. (This applies to vaginismus, though it might have application to general tensing or vaginismus-caused dyspareunia.) He also points out that the physical examination, if done with sensitivity, patience, and care, can be therapeutic as a source of reassurance (e.g., about the normality of genital size, etc.) and can serve as a first illustration of relaxation and/or Kegel exercises.

A thorough biological evaluation does, as LoPiccolo (1990) points out, go beyond a routine physical examination. The medical/gynecologic consultation outlined above would involve tests such as estrogen levels, thyroid function, or perhaps a glucose tolerance test. Additionally, research procedures such as vaginal plethysmography (Heiman, 1978) have promise, but to date they have not yielded as much clinically useful data as originally supposed (Schiavi, 1989). It is hoped that continued development in this area will produce measures with practical clinical utility.

Observations

Direct observation of sexual behavior and/or the use of videotaped segments for indirect observation might seem to have assessment advantages, in that these methods would seem to provide a direct, nondistorted sample of the behavior of interest. However, these methods have some overwhelming disadvantages (LoPiccolo, 1990). (1) The generalizability of taped or analogue observations is questionable. (2) The reactivity of a couple who are aware that observations are taking place limits their usefulness. (3) Lack of compliance with such procedures, since most couples would find them unacceptable, is a drawback. (4) Ethical problems are an obvious contraindication, particularly when the observation involves some direct contact between the therapist/assessor and the client, as is advocated by some authors (e.g., Hartman & Fithian, 1972).

Other Assessments

It is important to place an individual's sexual problems in the context of life circumstances, personal strengths and weaknesses, and co-existing psychopathology. Relationships, self-image, depression, anxiety level, and other adjustment variables should be assessed, possibly via self-reports and interview responses (see Kanfer & Saslow, 1969). Beyond general interviews and self-observations, an omnibus personality inventory such as the new revision of the Minnesota Multiphasic Personality Inventory (MMPI-2; Butcher, Dahlstrom, Graham, Tellegen, & Kaemmer, 1989) can prove very useful in providing a perspective on other problems or relevant personality features. Also, because of the importance of the marital relationship, the assessor should pay attention to marital adjustment (see, e.g., Stuart & Stuart, 1972). Some authors (e.g., Lazarus, 1988) suggest that clinicians must rule out individuals with pseudodyspareunia, a putative condition more related to malingering, conversion disorder, marital discord, or passive-aggressive or histrionic personality problems. However, this condition, if it exists, is essentially unstudied. In any case, personal context and factors that might interfere with successful treatment should be assessed.

TREATMENT

The general area of sexual dysfunctions is somewhat light on solid empirical evaluation of treatment outcomes. Dyspareunia is certainly no better off than other dysfunctions in its research base; in some ways, it is the worst of the lot. Of the relatively few outcome studies, some have not distinguished between dyspareunia and vaginismus (Haslam, 1965; Mira, 1988). Steger (1978) states that vaginismus and dyspareunia are "generally treated in the same manner behaviorally" (p. 81). Most reviews continue this blurring (Forney, 1978; Steege, 1984), or they omit dyspareunia altogether (LoPiccolo, 1990;

LoPiccolo & Stock, 1986). There is also the issue of dyspareunia that has its source in insufficient vaginal lubrication. The DSM-III-R criteria would suggest placing the former under vaginismus and the latter under female arousal disorder. If these diagnoses are eliminated from consideration, evaluation of outcome for dyspareunia treatment is often either missing (Lamont, 1978) or difficult to determine (Fordney-Settlage, 1975).

If one further eliminates the instances of dyspareunia that arise from primarily organic causes, the ground covered is essentially nil. Compare the research base on dyspareunia with that for vaginismus (Chapter 14), female arousal disorder (Chapter 6), and medical aspects of sexual pain disorders (Chapter 12). However, there follows a brief review of some techniques that might apply when the diagnosis is dyspareunia *or* when dyspareunia is the presenting problem. Some degree of overlap is unavoidable.

Medical Treatments

For the most part, medical procedures are designed to address the organic cause of an individual's dyspareunia (Abarbanel, 1978). For example, surgery for the removal of a troubling organic lesion (Huffman, 1983) or estrogen treatment for estrogen deprivation in the menopausal women (Dagon, 1983) can be effective. Noteworthy is the fact that various authors rate the importance of organic factors in different terms. Sarrel and Sarrel (1989) and Huffman (1983) have high estimates of the rate of organic causation, although in Huffman's report of his 220 private patients, the 17% psychogenic group should be supplemented by an unknown proportion of the 27% dysfunctional group, since they were made up of hormonal and psychically caused deficits in vaginal lubrication. Other authors (e.g., Fordney-Settlage, 1975) suggest a clear organic etiology in less than half of their cases, and Spano and Lamont (1975) indicate that physical causes are rare and usually temporary. Also noteworthy, however, is that subtle organic causes might easily be missed, so psychological factors might be mistakenly presumed to predominate.

Psychological factors still must be considered, even in cases where a clear organic cause is found. There can be psychological factors, such as negative attitudes, that reduce compliance with the treatment regimen (Steger, 1978). Furthermore, psychological variables exert a significant influence on the ability to profit from treatment and on subjective satisfaction. A good illustration of this is the second of three cases presented by Zuckerman, Goldberg, Neri, and Ovadia (1988). Despite declining the recommended surgery to correct the husband's congenital penile curvature, this couple was able to achieve pain relief and a satisfying sexual relationship with a combination of sex therapy, vaginal dilation practice, and a shift to rear entry position for intercourse.

Behavioral and Procedural Suggestions

Lazarus (1988) points out that couples can often be assisted with simple suggestions such as the use of artificial lubrication. In fact, in the survey by Glatt et al. (1990), natural and artificial lubrication was the most popular means for women to alleviate their coital pain. Sexual positions (specifically, changing to a female-superior position, which allows more control by the woman over timing and depth of penetration) can be useful (Abarbanel, 1978).

Depending on the location of pain and the etiology, suggestions such as cotton underwear, looser clothes, and the addition of a kleenex pinned in the woman's panties can provide benefits (Abarbanel, 1978). In an unusual case report, Greiss (1984) discusses two individuals who complained of dyspareunia that he attributed to muscle strain in the levator ani muscles. Greiss reported success after these individuals simply took a hiatus from their frequent horseback riding.

More commonly, anxiety plays a central role, and treatment recommendations are directed toward anxiety reduction. Relaxation training has been used (Kaplan, 1974), typically in association with other procedures. Several case studies have reported systematic desensitization used to treat dyspareunia (Haslam, 1965; Mira, 1988),

sometimes with hypnosis (Kroger & Fezler, 1976).

A typical package might involve (1) prohibition of intercourse; (2) initial finger exploration of the vagina, first by the woman, then by her partner (Mira, 1988); (3) sensate focus exercises (Masters & Johnson, 1970); (4) Kegel exercises building to 20 contractions four times per day (Fordney, 1978), followed in one week by (5) self-dilation using a finger and working up gradually to dilators of various sizes (see Kaplan, 1974; Masters & Johnson, 1970). Additional education and skill-building work might also be included to aid communication (Manara, 1991), as well as the partner's ability to provide stimulation (Kaplan, 1974).

Treatment of concurrent sexual dysfunctions is important as well. Fordney-Settlage (1975) found a high proportion of female orgasmic disorder problems in her dyspareunia sample, as well as premature ejaculation among their partners. In addition, work with problems such as depression or marital strife, if present, is part of responsible clinical practice.

Additional Cognitive Procedures

Beyond the imaginal and educational procedures outlined above, several specific cognitive foci might be profitable in treatment. For instance, Friedman and Czekala (1985) attempt to minimize compliance problems by communication to their clients that they consider dyspareunia to be genuine pain, whether or not an organic etiology is ever found, and that etiology does not determine whether or not psychological interventions are beneficial. Also useful for specific individuals might be the correction of misperceptions—such as about small genital capacity (Jarvis, 1984)—or ruminations that could interfere with therapy (Steger, 1978).

CONCLUSIONS

The present state of understanding of the etiology, assessment, and treatment of dyspareunia leaves much to be desired. Certainly, much has been gained at least in some areas since the days when dyspareunia might have been iatrogenically produced by the practice of having medical students gain experience by repairing episiotomies (Jarvis, 1984). Progress has also been made since the survey by Burnap and Golden (1967), where physicians clearly assumed that sex therapy had nothing to offer their patients. Instead, they offered support, reassurance, and reading material ("of these physicians three-fourths said they were not familiar with the material they recommended" p. 677). Today's practices need much refinement and validation, but the current climate of collaboration and interested inquiry is an improvement over the past.

REFERENCES

Abarbanel, A. (1978). Diagnosis and treatment of coital discomfort. In J. LoPiccolo & L. LoPiccolo (Eds.), *Handbook of sex therapy.* New York: Plenum.

American Psychiatric Association. (1987). *Diagnostic and statistical manual of mental disorders* (3rd ed., Rev.). Washington, DC: Author.

Annon, J. (1976). *Behavioral treatment of sexual problems: Brief therapy.* Hagerstown, MD: Harper & Row.

Araoz, D. L. (1982). *Hypnosis and sex therapy.* New York: Brunner/Mazel.

Bachmann, G. A. (1986). Dyspareunia, due to obstetrical trauma. *Medical Aspects of Human Sexuality, 20,* 21–25.

Bachmann, G. A., Leiblum, S. R., & Grill J. (1989). Brief sexual inquiry in gynecologic practice. *Obstetrics and Gynecology, 73,* 425–427.

Becker, J., & Skinner, L. J. (1983). Assessment and treatment of rape-related sexual dysfunctions. *Clinical Psychologist, 36,* 102–104.

Becker, J. V., Skinner, L. J., Abel, G. G., & Treacy, E. L. (1982). Incidence and types of sexual dysfunctions in rape and incest victims. *Journal of Sex and Marital Therapy, 8,* 65–74.

Brant, H. (1978). The psychosexual problems of women. Part 2: Female sexual dysfunctions. *Community Nurse, 14,* 73–76.

Burnap, D. W., & Golden, J. S. (1967). Sexual problems in medical practice. *Journal of Medical Education, 42,* 673–680.

Butcher, J. N., Dahlstrom, W. G., Graham, J. R., Tellegen, A., & Kaemmer, B. (1989). *Minnesota Multiphasic Personality Inventory (MMPI-2).*

Manual for administration and scoring. Minneapolis: University of Minnesota Press.

Caird, W. K., & Wincze, J. P. (1977). *Sex therapy: A behavioral approach.* Hagerstown, MD: Harper & Row.

Chapman, J. D. (1989). A longitudinal study of sexuality and gynecologic health in abused women. *Journal of the American Osteopathic Association, 89,* 619–624.

Conte, H. (1983). Development and use of self-report techniques for assessing sexual functioning: A review and critique. *Archives of Sexual Behavior, 12,* 555–576.

Dagon, E. M. (1983). Aging and sexuality. In C. C. Nadelson & D. B. Marcotte (Eds.), *Treatment interventions in human sexuality* (pp. 357–375). New York: Plenum.

David, D. L. (1991, April). *Cultural sensitivity and the sexual disorders of the DSM-IV: Review and Assessment.* Paper presented at the National Institute of Mental Health Conference on Culture and Diagnosis: Pittsburgh.

Derogatis, L. (1980). Psychological assessment of psychosexual functioning. *Psychiatric Clinics of North America, 3,* 113–131.

Dickinson, R. (1931). *A thousand marriages.* Baltimore: Williams & Wilkins.

Fink, P. (1972). Dyspareunia: Current concepts. *Medical Aspects of Human Sexuality, 6,* 28–33.

Fordney, D. (1978). Dyspareunia and vaginismus. *Clinical Obstetrics and Gynecology, 21,* 205–221.

Fordney-Settlage, D. (1975). Heterosexual dysfunction: Evaluation of treatment procedures. *Archives of Sexual Behavior, 4,* 367–387.

Frank, R. T. (1948). Dyspareunia: A problem for the general practitioner. *Journal of the American Medical Association, 136,* 361–365.

Friedman, J. M., & Czekala, J. (1985). Advances in sex therapy techniques. In P. A. Keller & L. G. Ritt (Eds.), *Innovations in clinical practice: A source book* (vol. 4, pp. 187–200). Sarasota, FL: Professional Resource Exchange.

Glatt, A. E., Zinner, S. H., & McCormack, W. M. (1990). The prevalence of dyspareunia. *Obstetrics and Gynecology, 75,* 433–436.

Greiss, F. C. (1984). Equestrian dyspareunia. *American Journal of Obstetrics and Gynecology, 150,* 168.

Grillo, I., & Grillo, D. (1980). Management of dyspareunia secondary to hymenal remnants. *Obstetrics and Gynecology, 56,* 510–514.

Harlow, R. (1969). Dyspareunia. *Practitioner, 202,* 393–397.

Hartman, W. E., & Fithian, M. A. (1972). *The treatment of sexual dysfunction.* Long Beach, CA: Center for Marital and Sexual Studies.

Haslam, M. T. (1965). The treatment of psychogenic dyspareunia by reciprocal inhibition. *British Journal of Psychiatry, 111,* 280–282.

Hastings, D. (1971). Impotence, premature ejaculation and lack of female response. *Psychiatric Annals. 1,* 25–31.

Heiman, J. (1978). Use of psychophysiology in the assessment and treatment of sexual dysfunction. In J. LoPiccolo & L. LoPiccolo (Eds.), *Handbook of sex therapy* (pp. 123–136). New York: Plenum.

Heisterberg, L., Hebjorn, S., Andersen, L. F., & Petersen H. (1986). Sequelae of induced first-trimester abortion. A prospective study assessing the role of postabortal pelvic inflammatory disease and prophylactic antibiotics. *American Journal of Obstetrics and Gynecology, 155,* 76–80.

Hoon, E. F., Hoon, P. W., and Wincze, J. (1976). The SAI: An inventory for measurement of female sexual arousal. *Archives of Sexual Behavior, 5,* 291–300.

Hoon, E. F., Hoon, P., & Wincze, J. (1976). An inventory for the measurement of female sexual arousability. *Archives of Sexual Behavior, 5,* 291–300.

Huffman, J. (1976). Office gynecology: Relieving dyspareunia. *Postgraduate Medicine, 59,* 223–226.

Huffman, J. W. (1983). Dyspareunia of vulvo-vaginal origin. Causes and management. *Postgraduate Medicine, 73,* 287–296.

Jarvis, G. J. (1984). Dyspareunia. *British Medical Journal, 228,* 1555–1556.

Kanfer, F., & Saslow, G. (1969). Behavioral diagnosis. In C. M. Franks (Ed.), *Behavior therapy: Appraisal and status* (pp. 417–444). New York: McGraw-Hill.

Kaplan, H. (1974). *The new sex therapy.* New York: Brunner/Mazel.

Kaplan, H. (1979). *Disorders of sexual desire.* New York: Brunner/Mazel.

Klassen, A. D., & Wilsnack, S. C. (1986). Sexual experience and drinking among women in a U. S. national survey. *Archives of Sexual Behavior, 15.* 363–392.

Kroger, W. S., & Fezler, W. D. (1976). *Hypnosis and behavior modification: Imagery conditioning.* Philadelphia: Lippincott.

Lamont, J. (1974). Female dyspareunia. *Canadian Family Physician, 20,* 53–57.

Lamont, J. (1978). Vaginismus. *American Journal of Obstetrics and Gynecology, 131,* 332–336.

Lamont, J. (1980). Female dyspareunia. *American Journal of Obstetrics, 136,* 282–285.

Lazarus, A. (1980). Psychological treatment of dyspareunia. In S. Leiblum, & L. Pervin (Eds.), *Principles and practice of sex therapy* (pp. 147–166). New York: Guilford.

Lazarus, A. (1988). Dyspareunia: A multimodal psychotherapeutic perspective. In S. Leiblum & R. C. Rosen (Eds.), *Principles and practice of sex therapy* (2nd ed.). New York: Guilford.

Leiblum, S., Pervin, L., & Campbell, E. (1988). The treatment of vaginismus: Success and failure. In S. Leiblum & R. C. Rosen (Eds.), *Principles and practice of sex therapy* (2nd ed., pp. 113–138). New York: Guilford.

Levay, A., & Sharpe, L. (1981). Sexual dysfunction: Diagnosis and treatment. In H. Lief (Ed.), *Sexual problems in medical practice.* Monroe, WI: American Medical Association.

Lobitz, W. C., & Lobitz, G. K. (1978). Clinical assessment in the treatment of sexual dysfunctions. In J. LoPiccolo & L. LoPiccolo (Eds.), *Handbook of sex therapy* (pp. 85–102). New York: Plenum.

LoPiccolo, J. (1990). Sexual dysfunction. In A. S. Bellack, M. Hersen, & A. E. Kazdin (Eds.), *International handbook of behavior modification and therapy* (2nd ed., pp. 547–564). New York: Plenum.

LoPiccolo, J., & Steger, J. (1974). The Sexual Interaction Inventory: A new instrument for assessment of sexual dysfunction. *Archives of Sexual behavior, 3,* 585–595.

LoPiccolo, J., & Stock, W. E. (1986). Treatment of sexual dysfunction. *Journal of Consulting and Clinical Psychology, 54,* 158–167.

LoPiccolo, L., & Heiman, J. R. (1978). Sexual assessment and history interview. In J. LoPiccolo & L. LoPiccolo (Eds.), *Handbook of sex therapy* (pp. 103–112). New York: Plenum.

Manara, F. (1991). Sex therapy for couples: An Italian perspective, *Journal of Sex Research, 28,* 157–162.

Masters, W., & Johnson, V. (1970). *Human sexual inadequacy.* Boston: Little, Brown.

McConaghy, N. (1988). Sexual dysfunction and deviation. In H. S. Bellack & M. Hersen (Eds.), *Behavioral assessment: A practical handbook* (3rd ed., pp. 490–541). New York: Pergamon.

McCormack, W. M., Evard, J. R., Laughlin, C. F., Rosner, B., Alpert, S., Crockett, V. A., McComb, D., & Zinner, S. H. (1981). Sexually transmitted conditions among women college students. *Ameri-*

can *Journal of Obstetrics and Gynecology, 139,* 130–133.

Mira, J. J. (1988). A therapeutic package for dyspareunia: A three case example. *Sexual and Marital Therapy, 3,* 77–82.

Newman, A. S., & Bertelson, A. D. (1986). Sexual dysfunction in diabetic women. *Journal of Behavioral Medicine, 9,* 261–270.

O'Connor, J. (1980). *Managing sexual dysfunction: A basic guide.* Oradell, NJ: Medical Economics Company.

Plouffe, L. (1985). Screening sexual problems through a simple questionnaire. *American Journal of Obstetrics and Gynecology, 151,* 166–169.

Quinn, J. T., Harbinson, J. J. M., Graham, J. P., & McAllister, H. (1974). A questionnaire measure of sexual interest. *Archives of Sexual Behavior, 3,* 357–366.

Reamy, K. J., & White, S. E. (1987). Sexuality in the puerperium: A review. *Archives of Sexual Behavior, 16,* 165–186.

Renshaw, D. C. (1988). Profile of 2376 patients treated at Loyola Sex Clinic between 1972 and 1987. *Sexual and Marital Therapy, 3,* 111–117.

Resick, P. A., & Quevillon, R. P. (1990, November). Working with victims of crime and disaster. Workshop presented at the annual meeting of the Association for Advancement of Behavior Therapy, San Francisco.

Sandberg, G., & Quevillon, R. P. (1987). Dyspareunia: An integrated approach to assessment and diagnosis. *Journal of Family Practice, 24,* 66–70.

Sarrel, P. M., & Sarrel, L. J. (1989). Dyspareunia and vaginismus. In American Psychiatric Association, *Treatments for psychiatric disorders: A task force report of the American Psychiatric Association* (vol. 3, pp. 2291–2299). Washington, DC: Author.

Sarrel, P. M., & Whitehead, M. I. (1985). Sex and menopause: Defining the issues. *Maturitas, 7*(3), 217–224.

Schiavi, R. C. (1989). Basic research relevant to treatment of psychosexual dysfunctions. In American Psychiatric Association, *Treatments of psychiatric disorders: A task force report of the American Psychiatric Association.* (pp. 2384–2394). Washington, DC: Author.

Schover, L. R., Fife, M., & Gershenson, D. M. (1989). Sexual dysfunction and treatment for early stage cervical cancer. *Cancer, 63,* 204–212.

Schover, L. R., Friedman, J., Weiler, S., Heiman, J. R., & LoPiccolo, J. (1982). A multi-axial diagnostic system for sexual dysfunctions: An alternative to DSM-III. *Archives of General Psychiatry, 39,* 614–619.

Sotile, W., & Kilman, P. (1977). Treatment of psychogenic female sexual dysfunctions. *Psychological Bulletin, 84,* 619–633.

Spano, L., & Lamont, J. (1975). Dyspareunia: A symptom of female sexual dysfunction. *Canadian Nurse, 71,* 22–25.

Spector, I. P., & Carey, M. P. (1990). Incidence and prevalence of sexual dysfunctions: A critical review of the empirical literature. *Archives of Sexual Behavior, 19,* 389–408.

Steege, J. F. (1984). Dyspareunia and vaginismus. *Clinical Obstetrics and Gynecology, 27,* 750–759.

Steger, J. C. (1978). Cognitive behavioral strategies in the treatment of sexual problems. In J. P. Foreyt & D. P. Rathjen (Eds.), *Cognitive behavior therapy: Research and application* (pp. 77–108). New York: Plenum.

Stuart, R. B., & Stuart, F. (1972). *Marital Pre-Counseling Inventory.* Champaign, IL: Research Press.

Stuart, R. B., Stuart, F., Maurice, W. L., & Szasz, G. (1975). *Sexual Adjustment Inventory.* Champaign, IL: Research Press.

Wabrek, A., & Wabrek, C. (1975). Dyspareunia. *Journal of Sex and Marital Therapy, 3,* 234–241.

Wabrek, C., & Wabrek, A. (1974). Sexual difficulties and the importance of the relationship. *Journal of Gynecological Nursing, 3,* 32–35.

Wilkeson, A. G., Poussaint, A. F., Small, E. C., & Shapiro, E. (1983). Human sexuality and the American minority experience. In C. C. Nadelson & D. B. Marcotte (Eds.), *Treatment interventions in human sexuality* (pp. 279–324). New York: Plenum.

Wilsnack, S. C. (1984). Drinking, sexuality and sexual dysfunction in women. In S. C. Wilsnack & L. J. Beckman (Eds.), *Alcohol problems in women: Antecedents, consequences, and intervention* (pp. 189–227). New York: Guilford.

Wilson, G. T., & Lawson, D. M. (1978). Expectancies, alcohol, and sexual arousal in women. *Journal of Abnormal Psychology, 87,* 358–367.

Worchester, R. (1955), cited in Harlow, R. (1969). Dyspareunia. *Practitioner, 202,* 393–397.

Zuckerman, Z., Goldberg, I., Neri, A., Ovadia, J. (1988). Couple sex therapy for dysfunctions associated with congenital penile curvature. *Journal of Urology, 139,* 1051–1052.

CHAPTER 14

VAGINISMUS

J. Gayle Beck, University of Houston

In certain respects, vaginismus has achieved a unique status among the sexual dysfunctions, because of the relative lack of available empirical knowledge and the large collection of clinical case material concerning this disorder. As a working definition, vaginismus is a sexual disorder that results from involuntary contraction of the vaginal muscles during attempted penetration. This involuntary response is the result of fear of painful penetration and has no organic basis. The phenomenon of vaginismus has been recognized for quite a long time, as illustrated in early Anglo-Saxon writings. These writings attributed the disorder to inadequate vaginal size; the recommended treatment involved the use of a "stretching" device for correction of the condition. Despite its long history, vaginismus has remained infrequently researched. As a result, it has been attributed to a wide array of factors: conditioned fear, castration fantasies, personality disturbance, sexual trauma, and various organic conditions (such as vaginal atrophy). Although the collec-

tion of writings about vaginismus makes for an interesting illustration of scientific neglect, this chapter will highlight the available knowledge concerning the disorder, focusing on relevant aspects of psychopathology, assessment, and treatment. It is the intent here to provide an overview that can guide further study of vaginismus.

DEFINITION AND DESCRIPTION

Vaginismus is defined as the involuntary spasm of the pelvic musculature surrounding the outer third of the vagina—specifically, the pubococcygeal, perineal, and the levator ani muscles (Masters & Johnson, 1970; Kaplan, 1974). (See Figure 14.1). Although women with vaginismus are capable of becoming sexually aroused, lubricating, and experiencing orgasm, penetration of the vagina is not possible. The specificity of vaginismus varies, ranging from spastic constriction that occurs only during attempts at penile insertion during sexual encounters to

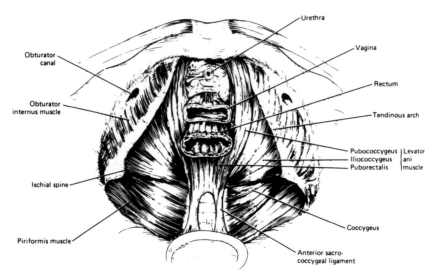

Figure 14.1. Female internal sexual anatomy. Reprinted
with permission from R. C. Benson (Ed.), *Current Obstetric
and Gynecologic Diagnosis and Treatment* (5th ed.). Los
Angeles: Lange Medical Publications, 1984.

constriction during any penetration attempt,
such as insertion of a tampon or a speculum
during a pelvic examination. Additionally, the
severity of the muscular spasm varies; severe
cases show generalized spasm that encom-
passes the adductor muscles of the thighs, the
rectus abdominis, and the gluteus muscles.

Although there is some disagreement among
authors in the differentiation of vaginismus
from dyspareunia, all agree that vaginismus is a
psychosomatic condition that results from contraction of the circumvaginal muscles and is
caused by a fear of penetration (J. LoPiccolo
& Stock, 1986). Pain is caused when penetration is forced, but there is no organic basis for
it. Despite the fact that a woman with vaginismus experiences pain during intercourse, dyspareunia is not diagnosed concurrently with
vaginismus, as the pain does not result from a
medical cause (Fordney, 1978). Although several authors have suggested that there indeed
may be an organic basis for vaginismus (e.g.,
Kaplan & Steege, 1983; Shortle & Jewelewicz,
1986), the traditional differentiation of these
two penetration disorders has centered on the
absence of a lesion, physical obstruction, in-

fection, or another organic cause in vaginismus.

Several authors have proposed different
classification schemes for vaginismus. Perhaps
the most time-honored is that of Masters and
Johnson (1970), which distinguishes between
absolute and *situational* vaginismus. According to this scheme, absolute vaginismus occurs
during any and all penetration attempts,
whereas situational vaginismus is limited to
specific situations such as penile insertion and
does not occur during forms of penetration
such as pelvic examinations. Another dimension of classification subsumes the woman's
prior sexual functioning. If she has had an interval of adequate sexual responding, including
successful penetration, the term *secondary*
vaginismus is applied, whereas if vaginismus
has been present since the first coital attempt,
the term *primary* is used (Masters & Johnson,
1970; Fordney, 1978). Lamont (1978) has proposed a five-part classification system based
on the woman's presenting symptoms and encompassing both vaginismus and dyspareunia. The following are included in Lamont's
system:

- *Primary apareunia:* complete inability to tolerate coitus
- *Secondary apareunia:* successful, comfortable coitus prior to the onset of the presenting symptoms, but no coitus since
- *Primary dyspareunia:* pain with each attempt since first coitus
- *Secondary dyspareunia:* comfortable coitus initially, followed by the onset of pain with each attempt
- *Primary vaginismus:* vasospasm during pelvic examination and self-examination in women who have never attempted coitus.

Historical Perspectives on Vaginismus

The first description of vaginismus appeared in the scientific literature in 1834, in a medical thesis presented by Huguier (Fuchs, 1980). A short time later, the term *vaginismus* was introduced by an American gynecologist, J. M. Sims, who described the treatment of the condition as easy, safe, and certain (Drenth, 1988). This treatment involved the complete excision of the hymen, a Y-shaped incision of the introitus to the perineum, transection of a portion of the sphincter muscle, and use of a glass bougie (or cylinder), which was worn four hours a day for several weeks. Although radical surgery such as this would be unheard of today for the treatment of vaginismus, the not-so-distant past contains echos of Sims' treatment, as surgical defloration was used commonly to treat vaginismus (Fuchs, 1980). In keeping with this approach, early psychoanalytic writings emphasized the woman's unconscious fear of her own castration, as exemplified in her fear of suffering pain and bleeding during intercourse (Drenth, 1988). Faure and Sireday (1909) noted that the 19th-century literature characterized vaginismus as the result of a specific excitability of the nervous system. Social factors such as arranged marriage were also implicated, particularly the consequences of traumatic defloration in the context of a woman's ignorance concerning sexuality and her spouse's lack of concern for her comfort and

satisfaction. Fortunately, the conceptualization of vaginismus has become more sophisticated since these early writings, with recognition that vaginal vasospasm is involuntary and based on the fear of penetration itself, rather than fears surrounding the loss of virginity or inadequate vaginal size.

THE PSYCHOPATHOLOGY OF VAGINISMUS: INCIDENCE, ASSOCIATED FEATURES, AND THEORIES OF ETIOLOGY

Incidence

Marked variability appears in the statistics concerning the number of women reporting vaginismus; indeed, we do not have an accurate estimate of the incidence of this disorder. In one of the earlier estimates of incidence, Masters and Johnson (1970) examined their clinic sample. Among the 510 "marital units" and 57 "single units" presenting to the Masters and Johnson clinic during an 11-year interval, only 29 cases of vaginismus were noted, a prevalence rate of 8.4% of 342 women total. Other American authors report similar statistics, as indicated by a recent survey of therapists who were members of the American Association of Sex Educators, Counselors, and Therapists (AASECT). Responses from 289 providers indicated that vaginismus was not a common presenting problem, with a 5% rate of presentation (Kilmann, Boland, Norton, Davidson, & Caid, 1986). However, this figure is biased by differences in the criteria providers used to diagnose vaginismus, as well as a low response rate to the mail survey.

Reports from other countries indicate a significantly higher rate of women presenting to clinics for help with vaginismus. For example, vaginismus appeared to be fairly common among patients at a sex clinic in Canada, as indicated by statistics from McMaster University. Eighty patients from a sample of 170 received a diagnosis of vaginismus, a rate of 47% of all patients seen from 1972 to 1976 (Lamont,

1978). Reports from Ireland indicate a high incidence, as well. One clinic reports that 55% of all referrals involved complaints of vaginismus, and the disorder accounted for 70% of the therapist work load (Barnes, Bowman, & Cullen, 1984). However, a survey of all patients presenting during a three-year interval to a sexual dysfunction clinic in England indicated that 12 of 188 female patients reported vaginismus, a rate of 6.3% (Bhugra, 1987). These incidence estimates are weakened by a lack of information on diagnostic reliability, as well as poor specification of assessment methods and diagnostic criteria.

Although it is tempting to speculate concerning the influence of cultural factors on the incidence of vaginismus, it is important to note that wide variations in the definition of vaginismus exist in these studies. It is likely that differences in the incidence estimates from these studies reflect method variance. Additionally, surveys of clinic samples do not offer true incidence or prevalence rates, although they do reflect patterns of help-seeking. For example, a woman may not initially report a sexual complaint—let alone vaginismus—as indicated by Ellison (1972). In 38% of 100 cases, Ellison noted that the presenting problem was identified by the patient as one or more nonsexual, physical symptoms, such as difficulty breathing, vomiting, and abdominal pain. After a thorough evaluation, these patients were identified correctly as suffering vaginismus. Additionally, vaginismus appears to occur to varying degrees as a sequela to stress and possibly to marital difficulties (Leiblum, Pervin, & Campbell, 1989). It is thus plausible that current estimates of incidence are influenced to a significant extent by patterns of symptom reporting, choice of care providers, and fluctuations in the severity of the disorder over time. In order to ascertain the true incidence of vaginismus, a representative community sample should be surveyed, using a clear operational definition of vaginismus and valid, reliable measures. Without this data, we have no sound estimate of the incidence of the disorder.

Additionally, it is possible that many women experience mild to moderate degrees of vaginismus, yet never seek help. For example, a probability sample of households in the United States (which was conducted to assess drinking patterns of women) indicated that 17% of the 917 respondents reported that sexual relations had sometimes been so painful that intercourse was not possible (Klassen & Wilsnack, 1986). Although it is impossible to discern the severity of vaginal vasospasm and the role of organic factors from such reports, these data indicate that vaginismus may occur in the general population at a rate much higher than that seen among sex clinic samples. Clearly, we need greater information concerning the incidence and prevalence of vaginismus, considering cross-cultural differences and the possibility that vaginismus may be underreported among sex clinic samples.

Associated Features

Probably more has been written about the psychological characteristics of women with vaginismus than about any other aspect of the diagnosis, assessment, or treatment of this disorder. The majority of this literature consists of case reports or clinical impressions—which may lull the reader into a perception that we know more about vaginismus than we actually do. All authors agree that vaginismus is characterized by a phobia-like quality and that the woman may avoid sexual contact of any form, for fear that it will lead to painful intercourse or another form of penetration. It is not unusual for a married woman to indicate that her marriage has not yet been consummated or to report that compliance with intercourse is accompanied by sensations described as "ripping," "tearing," "burning," "stinging," or "a sunburned vagina" (Crenshaw & Kessler, 1985). In some cases, these problems are long-standing and coexist with primary erectile dysfunction in the male partner (Masters & Johnson, 1970).

Despite experiencing painful vaginal spasms, women with vaginismus seem to experience adequate sexual responding in other respects.

Duddle (1977) assessed 32 women with vaginismus on measures of premarital sexual functioning. The length of marriage varied in this sample, ranging from three months to 15 years. In five cases, primary erectile dysfunction was present; in two other couples, the husband reported premature ejaculation. Relative to 50 sexually functional women, the dysfunctional sample reported greater experience in reaching orgasm during petting and during dreams prior to marriage. Of the dysfunctional women, 72% had reached orgasm prior to marriage, contrasted with 66% of the control sample. This suggests that the sexual arousal response is not significantly impaired in women with vaginismus, with the exception of the inability to tolerate penetration. It is not uncommon to hear reports of vaginismic women engaging in nonvaginal "intercourse," with the penis encompassed by the woman's adducted thighs. This position allows for sufficient friction for both partners to achieve orgasm, as women with vaginismus do not report difficulty in reaching orgasm with any greater frequency than sexually functional women (Stuntz, 1986).

Duddle's investigation also included an assessment of neuroticism, using the Eysenck Personality Inventory. The results indicated that the vaginismic sample was at the extreme end of the normal range for neuroticism and slightly below the norm for extraversion. These data agree with Cooper's report (1969) that women with sexual dysfunction scored within the normal range on the Neuroticism Scale Questionnaire of Scheier and Cattell. Cooper did note, however, that his sample showed elevated scores on measures of anxiety, intrapunitive hostility, and tough-mindedness, although this sample included women with the full range of sexual dysfunctions. Despite clinical lore that women with vaginismus choose passive men who will collude with them to avoid effective sexual functioning (e.g., Friedman, 1962; Ellison, 1968), Duddle noted that the husbands of her vaginismic sample showed no evidence of increased neuroticism or extraversion on the Eysenck scale.

The issue of marital functioning is an impor-

tant one in considering vaginismus. It is not unusual for complaints of vaginismus to remain untreated for prolonged intervals—up to 15 years in Duddle's sample. One wonders what the quality of marital functioning must be like for these couples, considering the long-standing sexual problems and the inability to have intercourse. Rust, Golombok, and Collier (1988) examined the correlation between marital distress and specific sexual dysfunctions in a sample of 28 couples presenting for sex therapy, using the Golombok Rust Inventory of Sexual Satisfaction (GRISS) and the Golombok Rust Inventory of Marital State (GRIMS). These data indicate nonsignificant correlations between reports of vaginismus on the GRISS and marital satisfaction (GRIMS) for both male and female partners. Although these findings may have been influenced by the small size of the vaginismic sample and the use of measures that have only recently been introduced, these data suggest that vaginismus does not necessarily disrupt marital harmony, contrary to expectation. (Discussion of the GRISS can be found below.) As noted by Leiblum et al. (1989), striking diversity in marital relationships appears among couples reporting vaginismus. Fertel (1977) and others had noted that the husbands of "virgin wives" are often overly considerate, weak, and dependent, but Leiblum et al., drawing on several case studies, have provided a clear illustration of the marked differences among husbands in their sexual attitudes and relationship with their vaginismic wives. Thus, it would appear that clinical observations may be biased toward viewing these marital relationships as pathological. Clearly, the conceptualization and treatment of vaginismus could benefit considerably from more adequate study of this important issue.

A related issue concerns the associated features and descriptive differences between women reporting primary, secondary, and situational vaginismus. Based purely on clinical observations, Shortle and Jewelewicz (1986) have indicated that women with primary vaginismus are likely to report the following characteristics: a history of long-term negative conditioning to sex; phobias about veneral disease, pregnancy, or illness; a prior traumatic pelvic examination; and misinformation regarding pain and bleeding at the time the hymen is ruptured. In contrast, women with secondary vaginismus are described as having been sexually traumatized in the past (e.g., rape, molestation in childhood), having a traumatic first coital attempt, having a history of psychologically painful sexual encounters, and experiencing marital discord. According to these authors, both forms of vaginismus are also allegedly associated with negative maternal attitudes regarding sexual hygiene, menstruation, and sexual maturation; a lesbian orientation; and a history of exposure to male sexual dysfunction, particularly erectile dysfunction or premature ejaculation. However, no data exist to confirm these observations, and this report serves as an example of the tendency within the field to speculate about the predisposing and etiological factors of vaginismus. Since treatment does not seem to be differentially effective for women with primary as against secondary vaginismus, this distinction may not be a critical one for understanding the disorder.

Of course, studies of the untreated course of vaginismus would be unethical to conduct, but it appears that the disorder does not spontaneously remit if left untreated. Given reports of long-standing difficulties with vaginal vasospasm among samples of vaginismic women, it would appear that the condition is fairly stable once it begins. In considering the reasons for this, Mowrer's (1939) two-factor theory appears applicable. Specifically, following a painful penetration attempt, in which the conditioned stimulus (CS) could be a speculum (as used in a pelvic examination) or a penis, conditioned pairing of the CS and the UCS (pain) is established. The reflexive response (UCR) to pain is withdrawl or escape from the UCS, exemplified in this instance by muscular spasm that prevents full penetration. Owing to the CS-UCS pairing, the UCR becomes the established conditioned response (CR) to penetration (CS). Depending on the severity of the

pain, this conditioned response could develop after only one CS-UCS pairing. Over time, escape generalizes into an avoidance response, which is reinforced via operant conditioning. Thus, the fact that vaginismuc women report an absence of any penetration attempts serves to maintain the CR of vaginal vasospasm. Two-factor theory has been questioned for its adequacy to account completely for the etiology of phobia (Rachman, 1976), but this model may explain the stability of the untreated course of vaginismus.

Thus, in considering the associated features of vaginismus, the issue of a prior history of painful penetration is relevant. Although the role of physical pathology is less obvious in vaginismus than it is in dyspareunia (see Sandberg & Quevillon, 1987), some authors contend that subtle organic pathology is involved in vaginismus. Kaplan and Steege (1983) have reported that many patients with vaginismus are found to suffer from "the urethral syndrome," a condition characterized by urinary frequency, urgency, and dysuria without significant urinary tract infection. Of 20 patients diagnosed with this syndrome, 14 reported vaginismus. These authors describe the typical patient profile as a woman with a lengthy medical history, which may have started with acute cystitis (an infection of the urinary bladder caused by bacterial growth). Although subsequent testing indicates no bacterial infection, the urinary symptoms persist and are accompanied by vaginal vasospasm. Other authors have identified organic causes of vaginismus such as atrophic vaginitis (atrophy of the vaginal lining caused by chronic inflammation), genital herpes, obstructing vaginal lesions, and other forms of pelvic pathology such as endometriosis (i.e., displacement of the endometrial tissue lining of the uterus into any abnormal place) (Shortle & Jewelewicz, 1986; Kaplan, 1974). In considering these reports, it is important to note that, according to all the authors, these various organic conditions have been medically resolved prior to the presentation of vaginismus. This suggests that vaginismus may develop following an interval of painful intercourse caused by physical pathology of some form. If the pathology exists concurrently with vaginal vasospasm, a diagnosis of dyspareunia is appropriate. However, if the physical condition has been treated successfully, a diagnosis of vaginismus is correct. This distinction most clearly reflects current diagnostic practices. Additionally, this perspective supports the observation that painful penetration, stemming (for example) from an organic cause, may be relevant in the etiology of vaginismus without serving a critical function in the maintenance of the disorder.

Another associated feature of vaginismus is a history of sexual trauma, including rape or childhood sexual abuse (e.g., J. LoPiccolo & Stock, 1986). Although the presence of this feature is consistent with a two-factor learning account of the etiology of vaginismus, it is important to note that sexual abuse may precipitate a variety of sexual dysfunctions in women and thus is not a specific cause of vaginismus. In reviews of this issue, Browne and Finkelhor (1986) and Jehu and Gazan (1983) have noted that abuse occurring in childhood is associated with a variety of problems in adult sexual adjustment, including sexual anxiety, avoidance or abstention from sex, diminished orgasmic ability, and a greater than average number of sexual partners. If abuse occurs in adulthood, the effects appear to be less generalized (Holmes & St. Lawrence, 1983). The majority of adult survivors of rape report sexual dysfunctions that were directly precipitated by the sexual assault, although the most frequently reported dysfunctions involve arousal or desire disorders (Becker, Skinner, Abel, & Treacy, 1982). In one study (Becker et al., 1982), vaginismus was reported by none of the 83 women surveyed after the assault, although multiple other sexual dysfunctions were present in 56% of these women. Thus, it would appear that vaginismus is rarely a direct consequence of sexual assault, based on available data. However, when a history of sexual abuse is associated with vaginismus, treatment can be more complicated, as the traumatic learning history warrants therapeutic attention separate from interventions designed to reduce involuntary vasospasm.

Theories of Etiology

In considering the various theories that have evolved to account for vaginismus, it is important to distinguish between accounts of initiating factors and processes involved in the maintenance of the disorder. Most existing theories have focused on the initiating etiological/causative factors, with surprising agreement concerning the processes that maintain the disorder. Interestingly, the most effective treatments available are those that address maintaining factors, often with little direct attention to etiology.

Psychoanalytic Accounts

Early psychoanalytic writers believed that vaginismus was caused by repressed fantasies of castrating the male (father figure), stemming from unresolved Oedipal conflicts (Fenichel, 1945). The disorder was viewed as a conversion reaction, and prolonged analysis was recommended to resolve the woman's unconscious wish to seek revenge for her own castration. Abraham (1956) was the first analyst to recommend a briefer form of treatment, noting that successful resolution of the problem could and did occur following short-term, insight-focused explorative therapy. Currently, psychoanalytic writers emphasize the causal role of unconscious fears and ambivalence, focusing on issues such as rejection of the female role and resistance against male sexual prerogatives (Leiblum et al., 1989). Other psychoanalytically oriented writers adopt a multicausal perspective. For example, despite inclusion of psychoanalytic concepts in her theory of the etiology of other sexual dysfunctions, Kaplan (1974) has questioned whether vaginismus represents a conversion symptom and conceptualizes the disorder as a conditioned response to aversive stimuli associated with vaginal penetration. In keeping with this formulation, Kaplan recommends treatment closely approximating that advocated by behavioral writers, based on the goal of extinction of conditioned vasospasm. To date, there is no empirical support for these various psychoanalytic models of vaginismus.

Personality Accounts

Several authors have theorized that key personality structures cause the development of vaginismus. Balint (1968) has described three types of vaginismic women. The first, termed the "Sleeping Beauty," is infantile woman who lives with her husband in a fraternal arrangement. The second, which Balint termed the "Brunhilde" type, is a woman who experiences sexuality as a battle of the sexes. For this woman, femininity is a sign of weakness and passivity, which must be avoided if the battle is to be won. The third personality structure is the "Queen Bee," type who desires to have a child but refuses sexuality, as she considers sex to be humiliating and unpleasant. Another personality-based theory has been proposed by Wolfromm (1954) who describes vaginismic women as either very masculine or infantile and their husbands as shy, timid, and compliant. According to this account, the relationship is maintained by a delicate interplay between these character structures, in which sex implicitly is avoided except to be used in the distribution of marital power. As discussed above, little information is available to validate these observations, although published reports suggest that considerable variation exists in the personalities and marital relationships of women presenting with vaginismus.

Psychosomatic Accounts

Although early writings about vaginismus emphasized that the disorder was caused by inadequate vaginal size, we now understand that the vagina functions as "potential space,"

which increases in length by approximately 50% during sexual arousal. The vagina itself is composed of smooth muscle, with the pubococcygeus (PC) muscle surrounding the outer one-third of the vagina (Rosen & Beck, 1988). This is the only vaginal muscle that is under voluntary control—an important factor for conceptualizing vaginismus as a psychosomatic condition. In this account, which is most clearly articulated by Masters and Johnson (1970), vaginismus results from "imagined, anticipated, or real attempts at vaginal penetration" (p. 243). The basis for vasospasm of the PC muscle is presumably a conditioned fear response, which may occur for various reasons. Masters and Johnson emphasize that the disorder may accompany erectile dysfunction in the male partner. Although these authors are careful to note the difficulty of establishing causality in this instance, they suggest that vaginismus may reflect the woman's high level of sexual frustration with a partner who has never been able to perform sexually. Additionally, vaginismus may result from excessive social and sexual control, such as might be learned during upbringing in a repressive, religiously orthodox home. Such a case involves fears based on the woman's ignorance of sexual mechanics and negative attitudes towards sex. Masters and Johnson also note that sexual trauma and attempted heterosexual functioning by a woman whose prior identification has been lesbian may result in vaginismus. A similar psychosomatic account has been presented by Ellison (1972).

It is noteworthy that the psychosomatic accounts of vaginismus emphasize the role of factors that maintain vasospasm—in particular, fear of penetration and the male partner's sexual skills. Thus, although multiple initiating factors are considered relevant, the theoretical focus is on those processes that are operative at the time when a women presents for sex therapy. The strongest support for this account consists of data examining the presence of sexual dysfunction in the partner and the general consensus regarding the important role of fear in maintaining vaginismus.

Conditioning Accounts

As outlined earlier, the conditioning model of vaginismus relies on a combination of classical and operant learning processes (two-factor theory) to explain the conditioned fear response to penetration (e.g., Wolpe, 1969). Additions to this model include a cognitive component—specifically, the belief that penetration will result in pain and considerable discomfort. Thus, vaginismus is likened to a sexual phobia, according to this account. A necessary factor in this model is the presence of at least one instance of painful penetration, which presumably could result from an organic cause, sexual trauma, or an unskilled pelvic examination (Taylor, 1975). As noted above, these factors can be associated with vaginismus, although they do not appear to occur frequently enough to account completely for its etiology. Unlike the psychosomatic model of etiology, the conditioning model emphasizes initiating factors, although the prescribed treatment approach relies on extinction of conditioned vasospasm via therapeutic attention to maintaining factors. To date, support for the conditioning model can be derived only from examination of the available literature concerning the effects of sexual trauma, although clinical reports support the utility of this account in formulating treatment.

Summary

With the possible exception of ''pure'' psychoanalytic and personality accounts, available theoretical models tend to arrive at the same conclusions regarding the relevant etiological/maintaining factors in vaginismus. Almost universally, these accounts emphasize the role of reflexive, involuntary vasospasm, which is accompanied by a fear of penetration. Although the possible originating causes for this response vary among theoretical schools, the implications for treatment are essentially the same: namely, that intervention must be focused on the elimination of vasospasm and fear. It is possible that, with greater empirical focus on this disorder, we will come to appreciate differences in the initiating causes, particularly as these differences impact a woman's response to treatment.

METHODS OF ASSESSMENT

Considerable consensus exists concerning the methods of assessment for a diagnosis of vaginismus. These include a careful sex history and a pelvic examination, although the latter may be greeted by the woman with vaginismus with considerable apprehension and possible refusal to participate. Most clinicians begin this process with a thorough sex history, including the sexual partner. Both Masters and Johnson (1970) and L. LoPiccolo and Heiman (1978) have provided outlines for interviewing a couple about their sex history. Although the content of this interview may vary for individual patients, areas of special importance include assessment of parental attitudes towards sexuality that were relevant in the individual's upbringing; early sexual experiences, including penetration experiences (if any); assessment of sexual trauma; how the couple met and their initial courtship experience; initial and current patterns of sexual contact; and the presence or absence of fantasies and sexual interest. Additionally, these interview formats include assessment of sexual arousal and orgasm for both partners; this is necessary for differential diagnosis and to determine if male sexual dysfunction is present in addition to vaginismus. No data concerning the diagnostic reliability or validity of these structured interviews are available, but these formats have been used widely and currently serve as the clinical standard for interviewing. Their continued use, despite the lack of psychometric support, reflects the lack of other, validated interview formats, as well as the relative underdevelopment of assessment strategies for vaginismus.

A pelvic examination is a necessity for diagnosing vaginismus, despite the fact that penetration in this context may not elicit vaginal vasospasm. However, owing to the fact that vaginismus may not be diagnosed simultaneously with organic conditions that produce pelvic pain or discomfort, this method of assessment is critical for determining the nature of the presenting complaint. The gynecological literature is replete with descriptions of special examination procedures designed to ease the process of examination for the patient and to help the physician determine if involuntary vasospasm is present (e.g., Shortle & Jewekewicz, 1986; Stuntz, 1986; Drenth, 1988). For instance, Stuntz (1986) suggests that the actual exam be preceded by a thorough explanation of the procedures involved, how these will be carried out, and the rationale for each. If the woman reacts to vaginal penetration with involuntary contraction and spasm of the levator ani and perineal muscles, which may be accompanied by fear or withdrawal from the examiner, further evidence of a conditioned response is provided. As in the case of structured interviews, the pelvic examination may vary for individual patients, and specific guidelines designed to ensure diagnostic reliability have yet to be established.

One of the more obvious gaps in the assessment of vaginismus is the relative absence of specialized questionnaire or self-report measures, which would aid in case formulation and the establishment of empirical information concerning this disorder. Many clinicians employ questionnaires such as the Sexual Interaction Inventory (SII; J. LoPiccolo & Steger, 1974), the Sexual Arousal Inventory (SAI; Hoon, Hoon, & Wincze, 1976), the Derogatis Sexual Functioning Inventory (DSFI; Derogatis, 1975), and the Self-Evaluation of Sexual Behavior and Gratification scale (SSBG; Lief, 1981), but none of these measures is aimed specifically at the assessment of vaginismus. Although psychometric data are available for the SAI and the DSFI, many of these questionnaires suffer from a lack of cross-validation, and several of them (such as the SII and the SSBG) can be used only with couples (Conte, 1986).

A notable exception is the GRISS (Rust & Golombok, 1985), a 28-item scale that is answered on a five-point category scale, ranging from "always" to "never." It is designed for heterosexual couples and administered to both parties, with separate sexual dysfunction scores produced for men and women. It also provides a profile for the couple on 12 subscales: erectile dysfunction, premature ejaculation, anorgasmia, vaginismus, sexual infrequency, noncommunication, nonsensuality, sexual avoidance, and dissatisfaction. (The last three subscales are derived separately for both the man and the woman.) The reliability of the overall scales has been found to be 0.94 for men and 0.87 for women (Rust & Golombok, 1986). The vaginismus subscale has been shown to have adequate test-retest reliability ($r = 0.82$) and internal consistency (0.73) when tested with a sample of 88 couples presenting for sex therapy in the United Kingdom. In this report, the clinical subscales differentiated patients with specific dysfunctions (e.g., vaginismus) from control subjects, and the overall dysfunction scale appeared sensitive to treatment effects. Although it is relatively new, this scale has shown promise and clearly warrants cross-validation in other settings.

Summary

There is a clear need for refinement of the available strategies for assessing vaginismus, particularly self-report measures. Seemingly, the field has focused on diagnostic concerns, as reflected in the emphasis on sexual history interviewing and physical examination. However, there appear to be various other dimensions that deserve attention with respect to psychometric assessment methods for vaginismus. The notable lack of behavioral assessment strategies is surprising, given the parallel between vaginismus and various anxiety disorders characterized by conditioned fear responses (e.g., simple phobia.) One could conceptualize the pelvic examination as an analogue behavioral test, but this would seem to be an overgeneralization, particularly since the pelvic examination shares few stimulus features with sexual intercourse. Additionally, some women with vaginismus are able to tolerate penetration in this context, so it seems a poor substitute for careful behavioral assessment. The development of strategies for standardized behavioral assessment would be a very useful addition; in particular, these strategies could be conducted in the patient's home environment, with both partners providing ratings or descriptive data of some form.

TREATMENT OF VAGINISMUS

Early approaches to the treatment of vaginismus emphasized interventions designed to affect the presumed physical causes of the disorder. Current treatment, however, involves psychosocial strategies aimed at reducing and eliminating vaginal vasospasm. Previously, surgical defloration under general anaesthesia was used, based on the belief that vaginismus was the result of fear of pain or injury during hymenial rupture (Fuchs, 1980). Although this approach was reported to be successful in some cases (Fuchs, Abramovici, Hoch, Timor-Tritsch, & Kleinhaus, 1975), it now is recognized that this procedure may be viewed by the woman as an iatrogenic "assault" (Shortle & Jewelwicz, 1986), so it is contraindicated by most authors. In its place, various approaches have been tried, including psychoanalytic psychotherapy, traditional sex therapy, behavior therapy (including biofeedback and systematic desensitization), and hypnosis.

Psychoanalytic Treatments

Based on the perspective that vaginismus is an unconscious expression of the woman's hostility toward men stemming from unresolved developmental conflicts, traditional psychoanalytic psychotherapy focuses on uncovering those inner processes that maintain vaginal vasospasm (Fenichel, 1945). To date, no systematic reports of the outcome of this approach have appeared, although various clinical reports have indicated success in 88% of 82 treated cases (e.g., Pasini, 1974). Considering the diversity of techniques among psychoanalytic therapists, combined with a general lack of criteria for determining treatment success and failure, it is

impossible to judge the efficacy of this treatment approach, relative to other intervention strategies.

Traditional Sex Therapy

What is currently referred to as "traditional" sex therapy was pioneered by Masters and Johnson in 1970 and rapidly revolutionized the field. Based on their account of vaginismus as multidetermined, this approach regards inclusion of both members of the couple as essential in treatment. Therapy is begun with a careful explanation of male and female sexual anatomy, followed by genital self-exploration and a temporary ban on coitus. Sensate focus exercises are introduced at the point when both parties are capable of touching their (external) genitals without discomfort. These exercises include instructions to attend to pleasurable sensations, without the performance demand of intercourse, and are combined with communication training. Hegar dilators of increasing sizes are used in conjunction with sensate focus exercises, designed to gradually expose the woman to vaginal penetration. Masters and Johnson recommend that once the larger-sized dilators can be accommodated without spasm, the woman should retain the dilator intravaginally for several hours per night for three to five days, in order to extinquish involuntary vaginal constriction completely. This treatment program was originally conducted with a dual-sex therapist team, and daily sessions were recommended.

The original success rates reported by Masters and Johnson were astounding: 100% of the 29 vaginismus cases. Although this study has been criticized on many features (e.g., Zilbergeld & Evans, 1980), it is difficult to dismiss a 100% "cure" rate. Masters and Johnson emphasize the importance of correcting sexual misconceptions and negative attitudes via direct sex education, as a critical ingredient of this treatment approach. Kaplan (1974) has advocated a very similar treatment strategy, with equally efficacious results. In her writings, Kaplan emphasizes the importance of instructing the woman to "stay with" her unpleasant feelings during the initial stages of vaginal dilation. This notion clearly is based on the proposition that avoidance of unpleasant affect and of the situations where these feelings arise is an important maintaining factor of vaginismus. In this respect, the "traditional" sex therapy approach resembles behavioral treatment methods, although Kaplan is careful to note that it seldom is necessary to address the phobic element of this disorder directly (presumably via systematic desensitization and/or relaxation training).

In considering the process and outcome of traditional sex therapy, all authors agree on the importance of partner cooperation and understanding of the disorder in reaching a successful outcome. A clear illustration of this point is provided by Leiblum et al. (1989), in a case presentation. There appear to be many ways in which an uncooperative partner can implicitly or explicitly undermine treatment, including refusal to comply with the ban on intercourse, with the dilation program, and with the sensate focus exercises. Overall, however, traditional sex therapy appears to be successful in the treatment of vaginismus, judging from measures taken at posttreatment or shortly thereafter (e.g., Hawton, 1982; Heiman & LoPiccolo, 1983).

Similarly, the long-term outcome of this approach is good. Although Masters and Johnson's figures are impossible to interpret, as the statistics from vaginismic women are combined with those from women with orgasmic dysfunction in the five-year follow-up data, other authors have examined the long-term results of sex therapy. Hawton, Catalan, Martin, and Fagg (1986) followed women who were treated with a modified Masters and Johnson approach. The primary modifications involved daily rather than weekly treatment sessions and the use of one therapist rather than two. There is considerable evidence that these modifications do not detract from the effectiveness of this approach (e.g., Heiman & LoPiccolo, 1983; Mathews, Whitehead, & Kellett, 1983). Of 24 cases originally presenting for treatment of vagi-

nismus, 20 women were followed successfully for an average of three years posttreatment. Posttreatment status was rated as complete problem resolution for ten women, partial resolution for seven women, and little or no improvement for three participants. At follow-up, eleven women were found to have complete resolution; seven had partial resolution; and two reported improvement but little change in vaginismus. These data indicate an excellent long-term outcome of sex therapy for this disorder. Among the factors that predicted follow-up status were a history of psychiatric disorder (poorer outcome), the couple's ability to communicate anger (better outcome), completion of treatment (better outcome), and satisfaction with the marital relationship (better outcome).

Over time, several revisions to the original Masters and Johnson approach have been proposed by other authors. In addition to changes in treatment format, several writers have suggested that self-dilation may be an improvement over mechanical dilators, using the woman's fingers or her partner's (e.g., Kaplan, 1974; Leiblum et al., 1989). There appears to be no difference in treatment outcome with these two strategies; the critical ingredient of the vaginal dilation program is that it is under the woman's control. Additionally, vaginal muscle exercises have been used in conjunction with other ingredients of the traditional sex therapy approach. Originally introduced by Kegel (1952), these exercises are designed to strengthen the PC muscle. They have been clinically reported to improve the awareness of vaginal sensations and the capacity for orgasm, although empirical tests are not supportive of this observation (Chambless, Stern, Sultan, Williams, Goldstein, Hazzard-Lineberger, Lifshitz, & Kelly, 1982; Chambless, Sultan, Stern, O'Neill, Garrison, & Jackson, 1984). However, Hall (1952) has suggested that Kegel exercises could be used to help the vaginismic woman learn to discriminate vaginal muscle contraction and to teach voluntary control over vasospasm. Other authors (e.g., Elliason, 1972; Colgan & Beautrais, 1977) have made similar suggestions, although controlled studies of the effect of Kegel exercises in the treatment of vaginismus have not appeared to date.

Behavior Therapy Approaches

Although many components of the traditional sex therapy approach have been interpreted within behavioral theory, a various behavior therapy strategies have been used in their own right to treat vaginismus. Among these interventions are biofeedback, systematic desensitization, rational restructuring, self-control, and fading. Many of these interventions have been reported in single-case studies, with a notable lack of controlled group studies. It is therefore difficult to determine their efficacy relative to the Masters and Johnson approach and its modifications.

In one of the more colorful applications of behavior therapy, Barnes et al. (1984) used biofeedback to treat five women with vaginismus. These authors developed a method of placing standard EMG electrodes on the lateral walls of the vagina, using graded dilators for this application. Following several sessions of sex education and instruction in pleasuring exercises, biofeedback was begun, beginning with a dilator 1.4 cm in diameter. Auditory feedback was used to provide an index of vaginal tension, with progression to dilators of increasing diameter in successive sessions. Each of the participants achieved therapeutic success with an average of 3.8 biofeedback sessions. This report was criticized by Perry (1985) on methodological and theoretical grounds, such as the placement of electrodes, the positioning of the subjects' body during feedback, and the absence of EMG criterion training. Nonetheless, the concept of gradual dilation, combined with feedback to help the woman learn to discriminate levels of vaginal tension, appears to reflect the general finding that these ingredients are necessary in the treatment of vaginismus.

Systematic desensitization has also been used to treat vaginismus. For example, Holroyd (1970) reports a successful case in which presentation of an individualized, graded hierarchy of scenes involving vaginal penetration was used

simultaneously with relaxation. Other authors, such as Caird and Wincze (1977), Husted (1975), and Haslam (1965), have advocated this type of approach. A modification of desensitization has been presented by Shahar and Jaffe (1978). These authors combined cognitive procedures, including rational restructuring to address self-defeating attitudes and beliefs, with self-control desensitization in the treatment of a 22-year-old woman. Following 20 treatment sessions, the woman and her husband reported that vaginismus was no longer a problem. These gains were maintained at eight-month follow-up. Overall, systematic desensitization has not been widely used recently, owing to the demonstrated efficacy of dilators, sex education, and sensate focus strategies.

Fading has also been used to treat vaginismus. Based on the concept of errorless discrimination training, fading was used by Alford (1979) in a successful single-case study. This approach involved gradual fading of clitoral self-stimulation, to digital stimulation by the partner, to penile insertion. It is difficult to distinguish this technique from the current practice of self- and partner dilation; it appears that, over time, a convergence of treatment approaches has occurred.

Hypnosis

Another treatment strategy that has been suggested for the alleviation of vaginismus is hypnosis. Drawn from a diverse background, including the original writings of Charcot (1882) and Janet (1925), current practice often involves self-hypnosis in combination with imagery and positive self-statements. Araoz (1986) has presented details of hypnotic imagery that are appropriate to use with vaginismic women. These involve the woman in images such as a fantasy trip inside her vagina, touching the vaginal walls, and admiring their beauty. Over time, the imagery proceeds to scenes in which the woman is engaging in sexual intercourse. There are striking similarities between hypnosis and systematic desensitization, suggesting a common mechanism of action in these treatments. To date, reports of the positive benefits of hypnosis have been made by several authors, including Delmonte (1988), Fuchs (1980), and Fuchs, Hoch, Paldi, Abramovici, Brandes, Timor-Tritsch, and Kleinhaus (1973). Controlled studies are lacking, however.

Summary

In reviewing the available treatment approaches for vaginismus, there is clear consensus concerning the essential ingredients for successful resolution of this disorder. In the intervention approaches, the elements that appear to have emerged as important and necessary components in treatment are progressive dilation, partner cooperation and support, provision of accurate information, and emphasis on sensual pleasuring and relaxation. Perhaps most striking is the convergence of treatment techniques, irrespective of theoretical derivation. Many of these approaches have placed emphasis on addressing relevant maintaining factors, and the current state of treatment reflects the consensus that vaginismus is the result of involuntary vasospasm and fear of penetration. Perhaps it is timely to call for greater focus on factors that predict individual treatment response, as illustrated by the Hawton et al. (1986) study. The treatment of vaginismus represents one of the success stories of sex therapy; overall rates of problem resolution have been high, as assessed both short- and long-term. However, we clearly have reached a point where more information about treatment failures is warranted.

CONCLUSIONS

As mentioned at the outset of this chapter, relatively little empirical information on vaginismus exists, when contrasted with the other sexual disorders. This may have resulted from the development of a successful treatment approach, since any field tends to focus on those disorders for which treatment is difficult or success rates less than acceptable. This relative neglect has left us with large gaps in our knowledge, particularly concerning the prevalence and incidence of vaginismus, associated features of the disorder, factors that predict treatment response, and the interface between vaginismus and male sexual dysfunction.

Overall, it appears that vaginismus may be considerably more common than our sex clinic statistics suggest and that the disorder, if untreated, may wax and wane over time, depending on the degree of life stress and (possibly) marital disharmony (Leiblum et al., 1989). From a theoretical standpoint, these nonclinical cases are quite important, as they offer the opportunity to understand factors that affect sexual functioning at the physiological and emotional levels. In particular, greater understanding of the role of anxiety in this process appears to be desirable. Also, the role of initiating influences (such as sexual trauma) could be explored in greated detail through the study of both clinical and nonclinical cases of vaginismus.

Despite the fact that vaginismus has remained a research orphan, a clinical lore has evolved about these women and their personalities, sexual attitudes, marriages, and willingness to change. Without an empirical base, this lore can potentially become dangerous in practice, since these assumptions tend to be negative. Clearly, it is time for greater understanding of the disorder of vaginismus, starting with controlled studies. In many respects, the account of vaginismus written by J. M. Sims in 1862 remains true today:

> I know of no disease [sic] capable of producing so much unhappiness to both parties of the marriage contract and I am happy to state that I know of no serious trouble that can be cured so easily, so safely, and so certainly (quoted in Drenth, 1988, p. 126).

Perhaps it is time for the field to advance in the understanding, assessment, and treatment of vaginismus.

REFERENCES

Abraham, H. C. (1956). A contribution to the problem of female sexuality. *International Journal of Psychoanalysis, 351,* 30.

Alford, G. (1979). Tactile stimulus fading in treating vaginismus. *Behavior Modification, 3,* 273–282.

Araoz, D. L. (1986). Uses of hypnosis in the treatment of psychogenic sexual dysfunctions. *Psychiatric Annals, 16,* 102–105.

Balint, M. (1968). *The basic fault.* London: Tavistock.

Barnes, J., Bowman, E. P., & Cullen, J. (1984). Biofeedback as an adjunct to psychotherapy in the treatment of vaginismus. *Biofeedback and Self-Regulation, 9,* 281–289.

Becker, J. V., Skinner, L. J., Abel, G. G., & Treacy, E. C. (1982). Incidence and types of sexual dysfunctions in rape and incest victims. *Journal of Sex and Marital Therapy, 8,* 65–74.

Bhugra, D. (1987). A retrospective view of a sexual dysfunction clinic, 1980–83. *Sexual and Marital Therapy, 2,* 73–82.

Browne, A., & Finkelhor, D. (1986). Impact of child sexual abuse: A review of the research. *Psychological Bulletin, 99,* 66–77.

Caird, W., & Wincze, J. P. (1977). *Sex therapy: A behavioral approach.* Hagerstown, MD: Harper & Row.

Chambless, D. L., Stern, T., Sultan, F. E., Williams, A. J., Goldstein, A. J., Hazzard-Lineberger, M., Lifshitz, J., & Kelly, L. (1982). The pubococcygeus and female orgasm: A correlational study with normal subjects. *Archives of Sexual Behavior, 11,* 479–490.

Chambless, D. L., Sultan, F. E., Stern, T. E., O'Neill, C., Garrison, S., & Jackson, A. (1984). Effects of pubococcygeal exercise on coital orgasm in women. *Journal of Consulting and Clinical Psychology, 52,* 114–118.

Charcot, J. M. (1882). Physiologie pathologique: L'hypnotization chez les hystériques. *CR Séances Academie Scientifique, 94,* 403–405.

Colgan, A. H., & Beautrais, P. G. (1977). Vaginal muscle control in vaginismus. *New Zealand Medical Journal, 36,* 300.

Conte, H. R. (1986). Multivariate assessment of sexual dysfunction. *Journal of Consulting and Clinical Psychology, 54,* 149–157.

Cooper, A. J. (1969). Some personality factors in frigidity. *Journal of Psychosomatic Research, 13,* 149–155.

Crenshaw, T. L., & Kessler, J. (1985). Vaginismus. *Medical Aspects of Human Sexuality, 19,* 21–32.

Delmonte, M. M. (1988). The use of relaxation and hypnotically-guided imagery in therapy as an intervention with a case of vaginismus. *Australian Journal of Clinical Hypnotherapy and Hypnosis, 9,* 1–7.

Derogatis, L. R. (1975). Derogatis Sexual Functioning Inventory. Baltimore: Clinical Psychometrics Research.

Drenth, J. J. (1988). Vaginismus and the desire for a child. *Journal of Psychosomatic Obstetrics and Gynecology, 9,* 125–138.

Duddle, M. (1977). Etiological factors in the unconsummated marriage. *Journal of Psychosomatic Research, 21,* 157–160.

Ellison, C. (1968). Psychosomatic factors in the unconsummated marriage. *Journal of Psychosomatic Research, 12,* 61–65.

Ellison, C. (1972). Vaginismus. *Medical Aspects of Human Sexuality, 6,* 34–54.

Faure, J. L., & Sireday, A. (1909). *Traité de gynecologie* (3rd ed.). Paris: Octave Doin.

Fenichel, L. (1945). *The psychoanalytic theory of neurosis.* New York: Norton.

Fertel, N. S. (1977). Vaginismus: A review. *Journal of Sex and Marital Therapy, 3,* 113–121.

Fordney, D. (1978). Dyspareunia and vaginimus. *Clinical Obstetrics and Gynecology, 21,* 205–221.

Friedman, L. J. (1962). *Virgin wives.* London: Tavistock.

Fuchs, K. (1980). Therapy of vaginismus by hypnotic desensitization. *American Journal of Obstetrics and Gynecology, 137,* 1–7.

Fuchs, K., Abramovici, H., Hoch, Z., Timor-Tritsch, I., & Kleinhaus, M. (1975). Vaginismus. The hypno-therapeutic approach. *Journal of Sex Research, 11,* 39–45.

Fuchs, K., Hoch, Z., Paldi, E., Abramovici, H., Brandes, J. M., Timor-Tritsch, I., & Kleinhaus, M. (1973). *International Journal of Clinical and Experimental Hypnosis, 21,* 144–156.

Hall, S. (1952). Vaginismus as cause of dyspareunia: Report of cases and method of treatment. *Western Journal of Clinical and Experimental Hypnosis, 60,* 117–120.

Haslam, M. T. (1965). The treatment of psychogenic dyspareunia by reciprocal inhibition. *British Journal of Psychiatry, 111,* 280–282.

Hawton, K. (1982). The behavioral treatment of sexual dysfunction. *British Journal of Psychiatry, 140,* 94–101.

Hawton, K., Catalan, J., Martin, P., & Fagg, J. (1986). Long-term outcome of sex therapy. *Behavior Research and Therapy, 24,* 665–675.

Heiman, J. R., & LoPiccolo, J. (1983). Clinical outcome of sex therapy. *Archives of General Psychiatry, 40,* 443–449.

Holmes, M. R., & St. Lawrence, J. S. (1983). Treatment of rape-induced trauma. *Clinical Psychology Review, 3,* 117–133.

Holroyd, J. (1970). Treatment of a married virgin by behavior therapy. *Obstetrics and Gynecology, 36,* 469–472.

Hoon, E. F., Hoon, P. W., & Wincze, J. (1976). An inventory for the measurement of female sexual arousability: The SAI. *Archives of Sexual Behavior, 5,* 291–300.

Husted, J. R. (1975). Desensitization procedures in dealing with female sexual dysfunction. *The Counseling Psychologist, 5,* 30–37.

Janet, J. (1925). *Psychological healing.* New York: Macmillan.

Jehu, D., & Gazan, M. (1983). Psychosocial adjustment of women who were sexually victimized in childhood or adolescence. *Canadian Journal of Community Mental Health, 2,* 71–82.

Kaplan, D. L., & Steege, J. F. (1983). The urethral syndrome: Sexual components. *Sexuality and Disability, 6,* 78–82.

Kaplan, H. S. (1974). *The new sex therapy.* New York: Brunner/Mazel.

Kegel, A. H. (1952). Sexual functions of the pubococcygeus muscle. *Western Journal of Surgery, Obstetrics, and Gynecology, 66,* 521–524.

Kilman, P. R., Boland, J. P., Norton, S. P., Davidson, E., & Caid, C. (1986). Perspectives of sex therapy outcome: A survey of AASECT providers. *Journal of Sex and Marital Therapy, 12,* 116–138.

Klassen, A. D., & Wilsnack, S. C. (1986). Sexual experience and drinking among women in a US national survey. *Archives of Sexual Behavior, 15,* 363–392.

Lamont, J. A. (1978). Vaginismus. *American Journal of Obstetrics and Gynecology, 131,* 632–636.

Leiblum, S. R., Pervin, L. A., & Campbell, E. H. (1989). The treatment of vaginismus: Success and failure. In S. R. Leiblum & R. C. Rosen (Eds.), *Principles and practice of sex therapy* (2nd ed., pp. 113–138). New York: Guilford.

Lief, H. I. (1981). Self-evaluation of sexual behavior and gratification. In H. I. Lief (Ed.), *Sexual problems in medical practice* (pp. 389–399). Monroe, WI: American Medical Association.

LoPiccolo, J., & Steger, J. (1974). The Sexual Interaction Inventory: A new instrument for as-

sessment of sexual dysfunction. *Archives of Sexual Behavior, 3,* 585–595.

LoPiccolo, J., & Stock, W. E. (1986). Treatment of sexual dysfunction. *Journal of Consulting and Clinical Psychology, 54,* 158–167.

LoPiccolo, L., & Heiman, J. R. (1978). Sexual assessment and history interview. In J. LoPiccolo & L. LoPiccolo (Eds.), *Handbook of sex therapy* (pp. 103–112). New York: Plenum.

Masters, W. H., & Johnson, V. E. (1970). *Human sexual inadequacy.* Boston: Little, Brown.

Mathews, A., Whitehead, A., & Kellett, J. (1983). Psychological and hormonal factors in the treatment of female sexual dysfunction. Psychological Medicine, 13, 83–92.

Mowrer, O. H. (1939). A stimulus-response analysis of anxiety and its role as a reinforcing agent. *Psychological Review, 46,* 553–565.

Perry, J. D. (1985). Letter to the editor. *Biofeedback and Self-Regulation, 10,* 199–200.

Rachman, S. (1976). The passing of the two stage theory of fear and avoidance: Fresh possibilities. *Behavior Research and Therapy, 14,* 125–131.

Rosen, R. C., & Beck, J. G. (1988). *Patterns of sexual arousal.* New York: Guilford.

Rust, J., & Golombok, S. (1985). The Golombok Rust Inventory of Sexual Satisfaction (GRISS). *British Journal of Psychology, 24,* 63–64.

Rust, J., & Golombok, S. (1986). The GRISS: A psychometric instrument for the assessment of sexual dysfunction. *Archives of Sexual Behavior, 15,* 157–165.

Rust, J., Golombok, S., & Collier, J. (1988). Marital problems and sexual dysfunction: How are they related? *British Journal of Psychiatry, 152,* 629–631.

Sandberg, G., & Quevillon, R. P. (1987). Dyspareunia: An integrated approach to assessment and diagnosis. *Journal of Family Practice, 24,* 66–69.

Shahar, A., & Jaffe, Y. (1978). Behavior and cognitive therapy in the treatment of vaginismus: A case study. *Cognitive Therapy and Research, 2,* 57–60.

Shortle, B., & Jewelewicz, R. (1986). Psychogenic vaginismus. *Medical Aspects of Human Sexuality, 20,* 82–87.

Stuntz, R. C. (1986). Physical obstructions to coitus in women. *Medical Aspects of Human Sexuality, 20,* 125–133.

Taylor, R. W. (1975). Some of the common sexual

disorders—problems mainly affecting the woman. *British Medical Journal, 3,* 32–34.

Wolfromm, M. H. (1954). Causes and treatment of vaginismus. *French Gynecology and Obstetrics, 30,* 49.

Wolpe, J. (1969). *The practice of behavior therapy.* New York: Pergamon.

Zilbergeld, B., & Evans, M. (1980). The inadequacy of Masters and Johnson. *Psychology Today, 14,* 29–43.

AUTHOR INDEX

SUBJECT INDEX

413